PROFESSIONAL NURSING

Concepts & Challenges

Sixth Edition

PROFESSIONAL NURSING
Concepts & Challenges

Kay Kittrell Chitty, RN, EdD
Adjunct Faculty
College of Nursing
Medical University of South Carolina
Charleston, South Carolina

Beth Perry Black, RN, PhD
Assistant Professor
School of Nursing
University of North Carolina at Chapel Hill
Chapel Hill, North Carolina

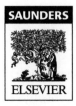

SAUNDERS

ELSEVIER

SAUNDERS
ELSEVIER

3251 Riverport Lane
Maryland Heights, Missouri 63043

PROFESSIONAL NURSING: CONCEPTS & CHALLENGES   ISBN: 978-1-4377-0719-9

Notices

Knowledge and best practice in this field are constantly changing. As new research and experience broaden our understanding, changes in research methods, professional practices, or medical treatment may become necessary.

Practitioners and researchers must always rely on their own experience and knowledge in evaluating and using any information, methods, compounds, or experiments described herein. In using such information or methods they should be mindful of their own safety and the safety of others, including parties for whom they have a professional responsibility.

With respect to any drug or pharmaceutical products identified, readers are advised to check the most current information provided (i) on procedures featured or (ii) by the manufacturer of each product to be administered, to verify the recommended dose or formula, the method and duration of administratiion, and contraindications. It is the responsibility of practitioners, relying on their own experience and knowledge of their patients, to make diagnoses, to determine dosages and the best treatment for each individual patient, and to take all appropriate safety precautions.

To the fullest extent of the law, neither the Publisher nor the authors, contributors, or editors, assume and liability for any injury and/or damage to persons or property as a matter of products liability, negligence or otherwise, or from any use or operation of any methods, products, instructions, or ideas contained in the material herein.

Library of Congress Control Number: 2009942417

Managing Editor: Maureen Iannuzzi
Associate Developmental Editor: Mary Ann Zimmerman
Publishing Services Manager: Anne Altepeter
Senior Project Manager: Beth Hayes
Design Direction: Margaret Reid

Printed in the United States of America

Last digit is the print number: 9   8   7   6   5   4   3

The sixth edition of this book is dedicated to Charlie, my husband of forty-two years,
with love and gratitude for his support and forbearance.
~~KKC

This edition is dedicated to my sister Laura Perry McLean, whom I love and admire,
and to my friend Greg Moore, who reminds me: "The language of Friendship is
not words but meanings." Thoreau was wise indeed.
~~BPB

Reviewers

Marie Ann Harris Ahrens, RN, BSN, MS
The University of Tulsa School of Nursing
Tulsa, Oklahoma

Barbara J. Braband, RN, MA, MSN, EdDc, CNE
Associate Professor
Mercy College of Health Sciences
Des Moines, Iowa

Mary E. Brune, RN, MS, CNE
Northwestern Oklahoma State University
Alva, Oklahoma

Denise R. Doliveira, RN, MSN
Community College of Allegheny County,
    Boyce Campus
Pittsburgh, Pennsylvania

Joellen W. Hawkins, RN, PhD, WHNP-BC, FAAN, FAANP
Professor Emeritus
William F. Connell School of Nursing,
    Boston College
Writer in Residence, Department of Nursing,
    Simmons College
Boston, Massachusetts

Jane Leach, RNC, PhD (c)
Midwestern State University
Wichita Falls, Texas

Grace Moodt, RN, MSN
Austin Peay State University
Clarksville, Tennessee

Janet P. Tracy, RN, PhD
William Paterson University
Wayne, New Jersey

Linda D. Wagner, RN, EdD, MSN
Central Connecticut State University
New Britain, Connecticut

Mary E. Weyer, EdD, APN, CNS
Professor
Elmhurst College
Elmurst, Illinois

Preface

Professions exist to serve society. When society changes, professions must also change. So it is with nursing. To maintain our relevance and dynamism today, professional nurses must possess skills that are more complex than previously have been required in the nursing profession.

To be effective, nurses must master more information than ever before available about human health and disease; they must be good leaders and good team members; they must think critically and creatively; they must communicate and collaborate with a diverse array of patients, families, and health care colleagues; they must be caring and businesslike; they must grapple with practical, ethical, and legal dilemmas not dreamed of even a decade ago; and they must practice their profession in both traditional and nontraditional settings. To be an effective professional nurse today poses a significant challenge.

The sixth edition of this text is designed to assist students to understand what it means to be a professional nurse; to appreciate the history of nursing; to understand and prize nursing's values, standards, and ethics; to recognize and deal effectively with the social and economic factors that influence how the profession is practiced; and to appreciate the need to be lifelong learners and contributing members of the nursing profession. This edition addresses concepts underlying the elements of the American Association of Colleges of Nursing's latest (2008) document, The Essentials of Baccalaureate Education for Professional Nursing Practice.

Feedback from users of earlier editions revealed that this text is used in RN-to-BSN "bridge" courses, in early courses in generic baccalaureate curricula, and as a resource for practicing nurses and graduate students. An increasing number of students in nursing programs are seeking second undergraduate degrees, such as mid-life adults seeking a career change and others who bring considerable experience to the learning situation. Accordingly, every effort has been made to present material that is comprehensive enough to challenge users at all levels without overwhelming the novice. The text has been designed to be "student friendly," and care has been taken to keep jargon to a minimum yet to provide a comprehensive glossary to assist in developing and refining a professional vocabulary. The visual features of the book have been carefully improved with today's visual learner in mind.

In addition to being revised and updated, the sixth edition has been streamlined. Users will notice this particularly in Chapters 5, 12, 14, and 15. Some of the material that was removed can now be found on the Evolve website.

As in previous editions, key terms are highlighted in the text itself. All terms in color print are in the Glossary. In addition, basic terms that may aid general student understanding have been added to the Glossary, even if they were not used in the book. We hope this will be valuable to students who are new to the profession.

Content in every chapter has been streamlined for greater focus. Photographs, illustrations, and other forms of visual interest have been added, as have real-life scenarios, personal viewpoints, and thought-provoking questions. The stand-alone feature that enables chapters to be read in any order remains a feature of the sixth edition. We realize that faculty may wish to teach the content in a different order and that the order that works best in one curriculum may not work in others.

Self-assessment exercises were retained and expanded in this revision. Evidence-Based Practice Notes have been expanded in keeping with the profession's progress. Critical Thinking Exercises have been expanded. Cultural Challenges have been added to several chapters, and the content on cultural care has been expanded and enhanced. Clinical examples have been increased.

The Evolve Resources, available at http://evolve.elsevier.com/Chitty/professional/, have been enhanced for both students and instructors. Students will find a collection of interesting and fun activities intended to further mastery of the chapter content. Instructors will now find a complete instructor suite including customizable PowerPoint Lectures, a comprehensive Test Bank, and Audience-Response Questions. Additionally, the Instructor's Manual has been revised based on user feedback to contain activities for both small and large groups. It contains in-class and out-of-class activities designed to enhance students' learning and to enrich classroom experiences. The Instructor's Manual also includes chapter outlines, chapter objectives, suggested readings, and critical thinking activities. Contact your sales representative or call our Sales Support Team at 1-800-222-9570 for further information.

As with earlier editions, it continues to be our heartfelt hope that the students and faculty who use this new edition will find it even more stimulating, enjoyable, and enlightening than the first five editions and that it will continue to contribute to the positive development of our profession.

Kay Kittrell Chitty
Beth Perry Black

Acknowledgments

The successful completion of any major project brings a sense both of accomplishment and relief. The completion of the sixth edition of *Professional Nursing: Concepts and Challenges* also brings overwhelming gratitude to the many individuals who participated in what has truly been a great team effort:

- To the faculty who used earlier editions and provided us their suggestions for revisions
- To students who sent e-mails, expressing their gratitude for an interesting and readable textbook while offering ideas for improvement
- To the reference librarians at the Medical University of South Carolina for their unselfish donation of time, talents, and energy
- To the many nurses who shared their experiences and perceptions in interviews and illustrative anecdotes
- To the staff at the American Nurses Association who took a personal interest in providing the latest available data.
- To all who assisted in gathering photographs

We are deeply indebted to them all.

Contents

16 NURSING'S FUTURE CHALLENGES, 380
Kay Kittrell Chitty

EPILOGUE, 403

GLOSSARY, 405

Nursing Today

Kay Kittrell Chitty

After studying this chapter, students will be able to:
- Describe the demographics of professional nursing today
- Identify the broad range of settings in which today's registered nurses practice
- Discuss emerging practice opportunities for nurses
- Cite similarities and differences among nursing roles in various practice settings
- Explain the roles of advanced practice nurses and the preparation required to assume these roles

What is the profile of the "typical" registered nurse (RN) today? Is there an average RN? Where do nurses work? What do they do? What type of preparation is required for various roles? How have new health care technologies and pressures to control health care costs affected nurses and nursing practice? As health care changes and nursing evolves to meet new challenges, the answers to these questions also change.

Far-reaching economic and social changes in the United States have profoundly affected the way health care is provided. Many of these changes have opened avenues to new and exciting employment opportunities for nurses. This chapter provides an overview of the RN population in the United States and briefly presents a selection of employment options available to nurses today in hospital and community settings. Integrated into this chapter are interviews with several nurses who describe their work and the rewards and challenges of their positions.

CURRENT STATUS OF NURSING IN THE UNITED STATES

To provide current information about practicing nurses, the federal government has conducted national surveys of actively licensed RNs in the United States regularly since the late 1970s. The most recent survey was conducted in March 2004. Data from this survey were published in 2006 by the U.S. Department of Health and Human Services, Division of Nursing, in a document titled *The Registered Nurse Population: Findings from the March 2004 National Sample Survey of Registered Nurses*. This document and information provided by the American Nurses Association (ANA), the National League for Nursing (NLN), and the American Association of Colleges of Nursing (AACN) provide a comprehensive look at the characteristics of RNs today.

Numbers

RNs represent the largest group of health care providers in the United States. More than 2.9 million individuals held licenses as RNs in 2004, but only 2.4 million (83.2%) of these individuals were actively working in nursing. The remainder of the RN population (16.8%) were either not working at all or working in fields other than nursing. Figures also indicated that fewer than two thirds (58.4%) of employed RNs worked full-time, whereas almost one fourth (24.8%) worked part-time. The total number of licensed RNs working full-time within nursing therefore is far lower than the 2.9 million figure indicates, as shown

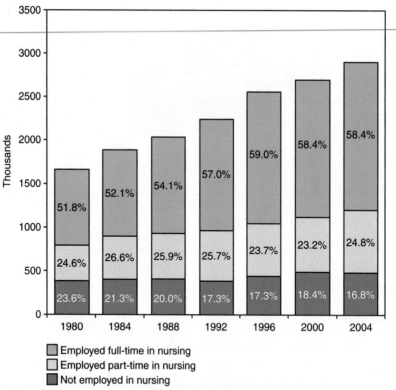

Figure 1-1 RN population by nursing employment status, 1980-2004. (Data from U.S. Department of Health and Human Services, Health Resources and Services Administration: *The registered nurse population: findings from the March 2004 National Sample Survey of Registered Nurses,* Washington, DC, 2006, Government Printing Office, p. 9 [website]: http://bhpr.hrsa.gov/healthworkforce/rnsurvey04/default.htm.)

in Figure 1-1. The number of nurses employed full-time is expected to increase as the economic recession continues.

Gender

Not surprisingly, the Division of Nursing's 2004 survey also showed that most RNs were women. Among employed RNs, only 5.7% were men. This figure seems to indicate a leveling off of the proportion of men in nursing, because the 2000 percentage was 5.4% and the 1996 percentage was also 5.4%. Even though the percentage of men in nursing has stabilized for the time being, the number of men is still growing at a rate faster than that for the total RN population. This is attributable to the fact that men accounted for 9.6% of all baccalaureate graduates in 2007 and 9.0% and

10.5%, respectively, of master's and doctoral program graduates (Fang et al, 2008).

In terms of absolute numbers, the 2004 survey revealed that there were 18,398 more male RNs in 2004 (when there were 161,300) than there were in 2000 (when there were 146,902). In addition, anecdotal reports from nursing faculty indicate that larger numbers of men are currently in the educational pipeline. The historic status of nursing as a female-dominated profession could eventually change as more male graduates of basic nursing programs enter the workforce.

Race and Ethnicity

As of 2004, the total RN population was overwhelmingly composed of white, non-Hispanic individuals (81.8%). The 2004 National Sample

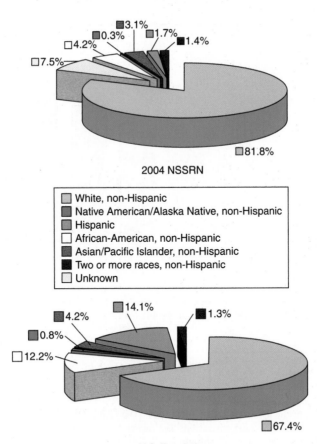

Figure 1-2 Distribution of RNs and the U.S. population by racial/ethnic background, March 2004. *NSSRN*, National Sample Survey of Registered Nurses. (Data from U.S. Department of Health and Human Services, Health Resources and Services Administration: *The registered nurse population: findings from the March 2004 National Sample Survey of Registered Nurses*, Washington, DC, 2006, Government Printing Office, p. 16 [website]: http://bhpr.hrsa.gov/healthworkforce/rnsurvey04/default.htm.)

Survey showed that distribution by ethnic/racial backgrounds of the 18.2% nonwhite RNs included African American, 4.2%; Asian/Pacific Islander, 3.1%; Hispanic, 1.7%; and Native American/Alaskan Native, 0.3%. The ethnic/racial backgrounds of the remainder (7.5%) were unknown, and 1.4% reported two or more categories.

Despite efforts to recruit and retain nonwhites in the nursing profession, the percentages in each nonwhite category decreased between 2000 and 2004. This indicates that nursing still has a long way to go before the racial/ethnic composition of the profession more accurately reflects that of American society as a whole. This disparity can easily be seen when nursing's percentages are compared with those of the country overall, reported by the U.S. Census Bureau in July 2004 to be 67.4% white and 32.6% nonwhite. Figure 1-2 compares the racial/ethnic distribution of RNs with that of the United States population.

There is better news on the horizon for minorities in nursing, however. The AACN's 2007 to 2008 data show that nearly 25.7% of undergraduate enrollees and 23.1% of graduate-level enrollees were from racial and ethnic minorities (Fang et al, 2008). The racial and ethnic composition of

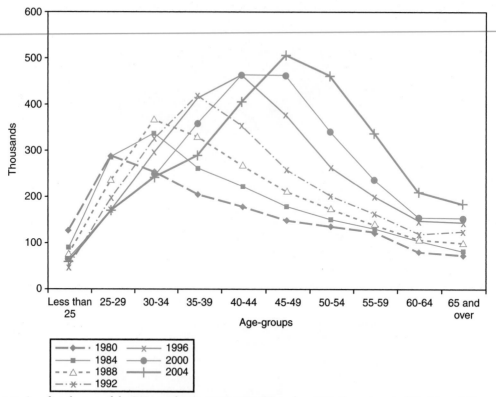

Figure 1-3 Age distribution of the RN population, 1980-2004. (Data from U.S. Department of Health and Human Services, Health Resources and Services Administration: *The registered nurse population: findings from the March 2004 National Sample Survey of Registered Nurses,* Washington, DC, 2006, Government Printing Office, p. 13 [website]: http://bhpr.hrsa.gov/healthworkforce/rnsurvey04/default.htm.)

the nursing profession will change to more accurately reflect the population as a whole as these students graduate and begin practice.

Age

With respect to age, the RN population is similar to the rest of American society: it is getting older. This "graying" of the workforce can be illustrated by comparing 1980 statistics with those from 2004. In 1980 the average age of all RNs was 40.3 years. This figure rose to 45.2 years by 2000 and increased to 46.8 years in 2004. The percentage of nurses more than 54 years of age rose to 25.5% in 2004, up from 24.3% in 2000 and 17.2% in 1980. With new nurses entering practice each year, the average age might be expected to remain the same or decline. Many new nurses are beginning second careers, however, and are significantly older than

the typical college graduate. Only 9.1% of newly licensed RNs in 2000 were younger than 30 years of age, and this number dropped to 8.1% in 2004 (Figure 1-3). Refer to this chapter's Cultural Considerations Challenge for insight into the adjustments required of an older second-degree student.

Are there second-degree students in your class? Are there students who are considerably older? After years of competence in another field, how must it feel to be back in the classroom as a beginner? How can you reach out to these students and assist in their transition to a second career in nursing?

Family Status

The family status of nurses has also been studied. In 2004, 70.5% of nurses were married, 18.1% were widowed/divorced/separated, and 9.2% had

Cultural Considerations Challenge*

Following a brush with death and quadruple bypass surgery, Randy Evans embarked on a second career as a nurse at the age of 55. After spending more than two decades in the editorial services business, Evans was a self-described "words person" who had never voluntarily taken a science course. What made him want to be a nurse? Following his surgery he watched as his nurses took care of both his and his family's needs. He was impressed with their dedication. "I just decided I'd like to be one of them."

Evans described his course work in microbiology and organic chemistry as "way out of my comfort zone," but his desire to become a nurse provided the necessary motivation for him to complete science prerequisites and enroll in the nursing program at Emory University. There, Evans says, "I felt like the aged mascot for a class of mostly women. I was older than most of my professors" (Mullen, 2008). Evans graduated with a BSN at 58, and today, at 59, works in the same coronary care unit where he was a patient.

*The original full-length version of this article first appeared in *Emory Health* (Mullen R: He was their patient. Now he's one of them, *Emory Health,* Fall 2008:12-15) and is excerpted here with permission. Online: http://whsc.emory.edu/_pubs/hsc/.

never been married. The marital status of 2.2% was unknown. Only 42.5% of all RNs had children at home, with 14.8% of those children reportedly younger than 6 years of age. RNs who were part of a two-parent family with children younger than 6 years were more likely to work part-time than any other group (USDHHS, 2006).

Education

Nursing has more levels of initial preparation than most professions because of the variety of educational pathways that one can take to become an RN. In 2004, of the 2,909,467 licensed RNs, 17.1% had diplomas as their highest nursing-related educational preparation; 33.7% held associate degrees; 34.2% had baccalaureate degrees; and 13% held master's or doctoral degrees (U.S. Department of Health and Human Services [USDHHS], 2006). These figures represent slight declines in the numbers of diploma-educated nurses and associate degree–prepared nurses and slight increases in the number of nurses with baccalaureate and higher degrees since 2000. Figure 1-4 illustrates trends in the initial educational preparation of RNs in the United States from 1980 to 2004. One must note, however, that initial preparation is only part of the educational picture for nurses because "increasing numbers of registered nurses receive baccalaureate and master's degrees, even if their initial preparation

for nursing was an associate degree or diploma" (USDHHS, 2006).

Foreign-educated nurses

Approximately 3.5% (100,791) of RNs practicing in the United States in 2004 completed their basic nursing education outside the United States and its territories. About half of these (50.2%) were from the Philippines, 20.2% from Canada, and 8.4% from the United Kingdom, followed by Nigeria, Ireland, India, Hong Kong, Jamaica, Israel, and South Korea. Foreign-educated nurses cited all 50 states and the District of Columbia as their principal nursing practice location. The largest number reported working in California (25.5%), followed by Florida (9.6%), New York (9.3%), Texas (6.7%), and New Jersey (6.1%). The educational levels achieved by foreign-educated nurses, exceed those of native-born American nurses with more than half (59.9%) having baccalaureate or higher degrees. Two percent reported being doctorally prepared, and more than 2% were advanced practice nurses (APNs). More than two thirds (68.5%) were multilingual (USDHHS, 2006).

The numbers reported in 2004 have increased rapidly. By 2007, an estimated 219,000 or 8% of practicing RNs were reported as being foreign-educated (Aiken, 2007). Nurse migration, the movement of nurses from one country to

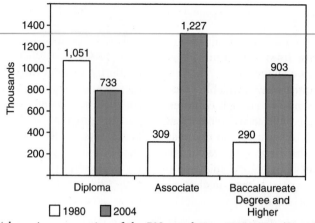

Figure 1-4 Trends in initial nursing preparation of the RN population, 1980-2004. (Data from U.S. Department of Health and Human Services, Health Resources and Services Administration: *The registered nurse population: findings from the March 2004 National Sample Survey of Registered Nurses,* Washington, DC, 2006, Government Printing Office, p. 10 [website]: http://bhpr.hrsa.gov/healthworkforce/rnsurvey04/default.htm.)

another in search of employment, is greater than at any time in history (Buchan, 2006; Huston, 2008) and is expected to continue. As a result of the influx of foreign-educated nurses, several nursing organizations have developed position statements about nurse migration. They include the International Council of Nurses (ICN) and Sigma Theta Tau International, honor society of nursing. You can read their position statements online at http://www.icn.ch/psrecruit01.htm and http://www.nursingsociety.org/aboutus/Position Papers/Pages/position_resource_papers.aspx.

Employment Opportunities for Nurses

As members of the largest health care profession in the United States, nurses practice in diverse settings such as hospitals, clinics, offices, homes, schools, workplaces, extended care facilities, the military, community centers, nursing homes, children's camps, and homeless shelters, among others. Increasingly, as state nurse practice acts are revised to cover independent advanced practice roles, RNs also work in private practice. Nurses in nurse-based practice must have advanced degrees or specialized education, training, and certification.

In 2004, hospitals remained the primary work site for RNs (reported by 56.2% of those employed, down from 59.1% in 2000). After

more than a decade of steady growth in numbers, employment in community health/public health settings, such as state or local health departments, home health services, community health centers, student health, occupational health, and faith community nursing, fell from an all-time high of 18.2% in 2000 to 14.9% of RNs in 2004. Ambulatory care settings, such as physician-based practices, nurse-based practices, free-standing emergency and surgical centers, or health maintenance organizations (HMOs), accounted for 11.5%. An additional 6.3% worked in nursing homes or extended care facilities. The remainder of employed RNs worked in settings such as schools of nursing; nursing associations; local, state, or federal governmental agencies; state boards of nursing; or insurance companies (USDHHS, 2006).

Not all nurses provide direct patient care as the primary part of their roles. A small but important group of nurses spend the majority of their time conducting research, teaching undergraduate and graduate students, managing companies as chief executives, and consulting with health care organizations. Nurses who have advanced levels of education, such as master's and doctoral degrees, are prepared to become researchers, educators, administrators, and APNs, including nurse practitioners (NPs), clinical nurse specialists (CNSs), certified nurse-midwives (CNMs), and certified registered nurse anesthetists (CRNAs). These advanced practice roles are discussed in greater detail later in this chapter.

In deciding which of the many available practice options to select, nurses should consider several salient points: educational preparation required; their special talents, likes, and dislikes; and whether their preparation, talents, and preferences are a good match with the employment opportunities under consideration. Although a majority of nurses are employed in hospitals, many others are pursuing challenges elsewhere. Numerous new opportunities and roles are being developed that use nurses' skills in different and exciting ways. What follows are descriptions of a sampling of the broad range of settings in which nurses now practice. In some instances, nurses are interviewed. It must be stressed that these areas represent only a sampling of the growing variety of opportunities available.

Hospital-based nursing

Nursing care originated and was practiced informally in home and community settings and moved into hospitals only within the last 150 years. Hospitals vary widely in size, comprehensiveness of services offered, and geographic location. In general, nurses in hospitals work with patients who have medical or surgical conditions, with sick children, with women and their newborns, with cancer patients, and with people who have had severe trauma or burns.

Within hospitals, nurses work in various units, such as in operating suites or emergency departments, in coronary and other special care units, on step-down or progressive care units, and in many other capacities. In addition to providing direct patient care, they serve as educators, managers, and administrators who teach or supervise others and establish the direction of nursing hospital-wide. Various generalist and specialist certification opportunities are appropriate for hospital-based nurses, including medical-surgical nurse, pediatric nurse, perinatal nurse, acute care nurse practitioner, gerontological

nurse, psychiatric and mental health nurse, nursing administration, nursing administration—advanced, nursing continuing education or staff development nurse, and informatics nurse. There is perhaps no other single work setting that offers so much employment variety to nurses as do hospitals.

The educational credentials required of RNs practicing in hospitals can range from associate degrees and diplomas to doctoral degrees. Generally, entry-level positions require only RN licensure. Many hospitals require nurses to hold baccalaureate degrees to advance on the clinical ladder or to assume management positions. A clinical coordinator, who is responsible for the management of more than one unit, is generally expected to have a master's degree.

Most new nurses choose to work in acute care hospitals initially to gain experience in organizing and delivering patient care to multiple patients. For many, staff nursing is extremely gratifying, and they continue in this role for their entire careers. Others pursue additional education, often provided by the hospital, to work in specialty units such as coronary care. Although specialty units usually require clinical experience and advanced training, some hospitals do allow exceptional new graduates to work in these units.

Some nurses find that management is their strength. **Nurse managers,** formerly called head nurses, are in charge of all activities on their units, including patient care, continuous quality improvement, personnel selection and evaluation, and resource management. Being a nurse manager in a hospital today is somewhat like running a business, and nurses need an entrepreneurial spirit and knowledge of business and financial principles to be most effective in this role.

Most nurses in hospitals provide direct patient care. In the past, it was necessary for nurses to assume administrative or management roles to be promoted or receive salary increases. Such positions removed them from bedside care. Today, in hospitals with clinical ladder programs, nurses no longer must make that choice; clinical ladder programs allow nurses to progress while staying in direct patient care roles.

A **clinical ladder** is a multiple-step program that begins with entry-level staff nurse positions. As nurses gain experience, participate in continuing education, demonstrate clinical competence, pursue formal education, and become certified, they are eligible to move up the rungs of the ladder.

At the top of most clinical ladders are **clinical nurse specialists** (CNSs), who are nurses with master's degrees in specialized areas of nursing, such as oncology. The role varies but generally includes responsibility for serving as a clinical mentor and role model for other nurses, as well as setting standards for nursing care on one or more particular units. The oncology clinical specialist, for example, works with the nurses on the oncology unit to help them stay informed of the latest research and skills useful in the care of patients with cancer. The clinical specialist is a resource person for the unit and may provide direct care to patients or families with particularly difficult or complex problems, establishes nursing protocols, and is responsible for ensuring that nurses adhere to high standards of care.

Salaries and responsibilities increase at the upper levels of clinical ladders. The clinical ladder concept benefits nurses by allowing them to advance while still working directly with patients. Hospitals also benefit by retaining experienced clinical nurses in direct patient care, thus improving the quality of nursing care throughout the hospital. Research has demonstrated that patient outcomes are more positive for patients cared for by baccalaureate (or higher)-prepared RNs. The Evidence-based Practice Note describes a landmark study reported in the *Journal of the American Medical Association* comparing surgical patient outcomes and educational levels of nurses.

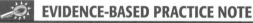

EVIDENCE-BASED PRACTICE NOTE

Several University of Pennsylvania researchers, led by distinguished nurse-researcher Dr. Linda Aiken, noted growing evidence suggesting "that nurse staffing affects the quality of care in hospitals, but little is known about whether the educational composition of registered nurses (RNs) in hospitals is related to patient outcomes." They wondered whether the proportion of a hospital's staff of baccalaureate or higher degree–prepared RNs contributed to improved patient outcomes. To answer this question, they undertook a large analysis of outcome data for 232,342 general, orthopedic, and vascular surgery patients discharged from 168 Pennsylvania hospitals over a 19-month period. They used statistical methods to control for risk factors such as age, sex, emergency or routine surgeries, type of surgery, preexisting conditions, surgeon qualifications, size of hospital, and other factors. Their findings were riveting:

To our knowledge, this study provides the first empirical evidence that hospitals' employment of nurses with BSN and higher degrees is associated with improved patient outcomes. Our findings indicate that surgical patients cared for in hospitals in which higher proportions of direct-care RNs held bachelor's degrees experienced a substantial survival advantage over those treated in hospitals in which fewer staff nurses had BSN or higher degrees. Similarly, surgical patients experiencing serious complications during hospitalization were significantly more likely to survive in hospitals with a higher proportion of nurses with baccalaureate education" (p. 1621).

Noting that fewer than half of all hospital staff nurses nationally are prepared at the baccalaureate level or higher, and citing the nursing shortage as a complicating factor, this group of researchers recommended "placing greater emphasis in national nurse workforce planning on policies to alter the educational composition of the future nurse workforce toward a greater proportion with baccalaureate or higher education as well as ensuring the adequacy of the overall supply" (p. 1623). They concluded that improved public financing of nursing education and increased employers' efforts to recruit and retain highly prepared bedside nurses could lead to substantial improvements in quality of care.

Modified from Aiken, et al: Educational levels of hospital nurses and surgical patient mortality, *JAMA* 290(12):1617-1623, 2003.

One of the greatest drawbacks to hospital nursing in the past was the necessity for nurses to work rigid schedules, which usually included evenings, nights, weekends, and holidays. Although hospital nurses still must work a fair share of undesirable times, **flexible staffing** is becoming the norm. Today, nurses on a particular unit often negotiate with one another and establish their own schedules to meet personal needs while still ensuring that appropriate patient care is provided. To facilitate self-scheduling, technology exists today that allows nurses to bid online for the days and shifts they prefer (Ellerbe, 2007).

Each hospital nursing role has its own unique characteristics. In the following profile, an RN discusses his role as a bedside nurse in a burn unit:

A burn nurse has to be gentle, strong, and patient enough to go slow. You must be confident enough to work alone; you must believe that what you're doing is in the patient's best interest because some of the procedures hurt far worse than anyone can imagine. Every burn is unique and a challenge. Fifteen years ago, the prognosis for surviving an extensive burn was not good, but with today's techniques for fluid replacement and the development of effective antibiotics, many patients are surviving the first few critical days. During the long hours of one-on-one care you really get to know your patient. There is nothing more rewarding.

When the "fit" between nurses and their role requirements is good, nursing is a gratifying profession, as an oncology nurse demonstrates in discussing her role:

Being an oncology nurse and working with people with potentially terminal illnesses brings you close to patients and their families. The family room for our patients and their families is very homelike. Families bring food in and have dinner with their loved one right here. Working with dying patients is a tall order. You must be able to support the family and the patient through many stages of the dying process, including anger and depression. Experiencing cancer is always traumatic, with the diagnosis, the treatment, and the struggle to cope. But today's statistics show that more people survive cancer. Because of research and early detection, being diagnosed with cancer is no longer the automatic death sentence it used to be. I love getting involved with patients and their families and feel that I can contribute to their positive mental attitude, which can have an impact on their disease process, or hold their hand and help them to die with dignity. They cry, I cry—it is part of my nursing, and I would have it no other way.

These are only two of the many possible roles nurses in hospital settings may choose. Although brief, these descriptions convey the flavor of the responsibility, complexity, and fulfillment to be found in hospital-based nursing (Figure 1-5).

Community health nursing

Lillian Wald (1867-1940) is credited with initiating community health nursing when she established the Henry Street Settlement in New York City in 1895. Community health nursing today is

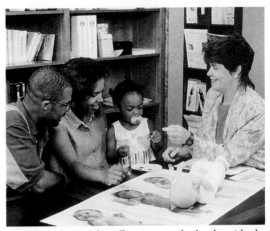

Figure 1-5 Hospital staff nurses work closely with the families of patients, as well as with the patients themselves. (Courtesy Memorial Health Care Systems, Chattanooga, Tenn.)

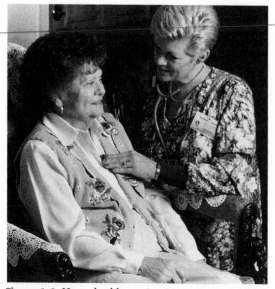

Figure 1-6 Home health nursing is a major component of the health care industry. (Courtesy Memorial Health Care Systems, Chattanooga, Tenn.)

a broad field encompassing areas formerly known as public health nursing and home health nursing. Community health nurses work in ambulatory clinics, health departments, hospices, and a variety of other community-based settings, including homes, where they provide nursing care to home-bound patients.

Community health nurses may work for either government or private agencies. Those working for public health departments provide care in clinics, schools, retirement communities, and other community settings. They focus on improving the overall health of communities by planning and implementing health programs, as well as delivering care for those with chronic health problems. These community health nurses provide educational programs in health maintenance, disease prevention, nutrition, and child care, among others. They conduct immunization clinics and health screenings and work with teachers, parents, physicians, and community leaders toward a healthier community.

Many health departments also have a home health component. Since 1980 there has been a tremendous increase in the number of public

and private agencies providing home health services, a form of community health nursing. In fact, home health care is a growing segment of the health care industry (Figure 1-6). Many home health nurses predict that most health care services in the future will be provided in the home.

Home health care has traditionally been, and will continue to be, nursing's "turf." Home health nurses across the United States provide quality care in the most cost-effective and, for patients, comfortable setting possible—the home. Patients cared for at home today tend to be more seriously ill than ever; this is largely because of early hospital discharges in efforts to control costs. As a result, more high-technology equipment is being used in the home. Equipment and procedures formerly unheard of outside of hospital settings, such as ventilators, intravenous pumps, and administration of chemotherapy and total parenteral nutrition, are routinely encountered in home care today.

Home health nurses must possess up-to-date nursing knowledge and be secure in their own nursing skills, because they do not have the immediate backup of more experienced nurses as they might in a hospital setting. These nurses must have strong assessment and communication skills. They must make independent judgments and be able to recognize patients' and families' teaching needs. Home health nurses must also know their limits and seek help when the patient's needs are beyond the scope of their abilities. An RN working in home health relates her experience:

I have always found a tremendous reward in working with the terminally ill and the elderly, and I get a great deal of contact with this particular population working in home health. One patient I cared for developed a pressure ulcer while at home. I was able to assess the patient's physiological needs as well as teach the family how to care for their loved one to prevent future skin breakdown. Within a few weeks the skin looked good, and the family felt important and involved. To me this is real nursing.

Community health nursing is growing as more and more nursing care is delivered outside the walls of hospitals. The American Nurses Credentialing Center offers certification in both community health and home health nursing at the generalist and clinical specialist levels. The increase in demand for nurses to work in a variety of community settings is expected to increase for the foreseeable future.

Nurse entrepreneurs

Some nurses are highly creative people who like finding new forms of expression and are challenged by the risks of starting a new enterprise. Such nurses may make good nurse entrepreneurs.

Similar to an entrepreneur in any field, a nurse entrepreneur identifies a need and creates a service to meet the identified need. Nurse entrepreneurs enjoy the autonomy (independent functioning) that is derived from owning and operating their own health-related businesses. Groups of nurses, some of whom are faculty members in schools of nursing, have opened nurse-managed centers to provide direct care to clients. Nurse entrepreneurs are self-employed as consultants to hospitals, nursing homes, and schools of nursing. Others have started nurse-based practices and carry their own caseloads of patients with physical or emotional needs. They are sometimes involved in presenting educational workshops and seminars. Some nurses establish their own apparel businesses, which provide articles of clothing for premature babies or physically challenged individuals. Others own and operate their own health equipment companies, health insurance agencies, and home health agencies. Still others invent products, such as stethoscope covers that can be changed between patients to prevent the spread of infection. In today's burgeoning health care environment, there is no limit to the opportunities available to nurses with the entrepreneurial spirit. Here are a few comments from one such entrepreneur, the chief executive officer of a privately owned home health agency:

I enjoy working for myself. I know that my success or failure in my business is up to me.

Having your own home health agency is a lot of work. You have to be very organized, manage other people effectively, and have excellent communication skills. You cannot be afraid to say no to the people. There is nothing better than the feeling I get when a family calls to say our nurses have made a difference in their loved one's life, but I also have to take the calls of complaint about my agency. Those are tough.

Increasingly, nurses are taking the business of health care into their own hands. They seem to agree that the opportunity to create their own companies has never been better. One such company offers nursing care for mothers, babies, and children. This company's emphasis is the care of women whose pregnancies may be complicated by diabetes, hypertension, or multiple births. The RN founder described the services offered by her company:

Our main specialty is managing high-risk pregnancies and high-risk newborns. Home care for these individuals is a boon not only to the patients themselves, but also to hospitals, insurance companies, and doctors. With the trend toward shorter hospital stays, risks are minimized if skilled maternity nurses are on hand to provide patients with specialty care in their homes.

As with almost any endeavor, disadvantages come with owning a small business. There is the risk for losing your investment if the business is unsuccessful. Fluctuations in income are common, especially in the early months, and regular paychecks may become a memory, at least in the beginning. A certain amount of pressure is created because of the total responsibility for meeting deadlines and paying bills, salaries, and taxes, but there is great opportunity as well.

In addition to financial incentives, there are also intangible rewards in entrepreneurship. For some people, the autonomy and freedom to control their own practice are more than enough to compensate for the increased pressure and initial uncertainty.

With rapid changes occurring daily in the health care system, new and exciting possibilities abound. Alert nurses who possess creativity, initiative, and business savvy have tremendous opportunities as entrepreneurs. The Evidence-based Practice Note describes the work of a pioneering nurse entrepreneur.

Office-based nursing

Nurses who are employed in medical office settings work in tandem with physicians or nurse practitioners and their patients. Office-based nursing activities include performing health assessments, drawing blood, giving immunizations, administering medications, and providing health teaching. Nurses in office settings also act as liaisons between patients and physicians or NPs. They amplify and clarify orders for patients, as well as provide emotional support to anxious patients. They may visit hospitalized patients, and some assist in surgery. Often, these nurses supervise other office workers, such as practical nurses, nurse aides, scheduling clerks, and record clerks. Educational requirements, hours of work, and

☀ EVIDENCE-BASED PRACTICE NOTE

Kathleen Vollman is a master's-prepared critical care nurse practicing in Detroit, Michigan. In the early 1980s she observed that about 60% to 70% of her patients with acute respiratory distress syndrome (ARDS) died of a lack of oxygen. Attempts to oxygenate them with ventilators often further injured their lungs. Inspired by an article on animal research left in the break room by a pulmonologist, Kathleen began to think about positioning patients for maximum oxygenation.

First, she tried turning her patients with ARDS from side to back to side every 30 minutes, as had been done in the animal study. She took blood gas readings in each position and developed a schedule for each patient based on that person's unique responses. Patients seemed to do better when she used this simple, noninvasive, independent nursing function of positioning.

Encouraged by her patients' responses, she read more research studies and found two articles dealing with the beneficial effect of prone (face down) positioning on gas exchange. She tried this with positive results but encountered problems turning very ill patients into the prone position. Solving this problem became the subject of her master's research.

Kathleen and a relative who is a mechanical engineer developed a turning frame and tested it in healthy people in a simulated critical care environment. After testing, the device was modified twice and then tested with patients with ARDS. Data were collected for more than 10 months and showed the usefulness of the frame in improving oxygenation of these critically ill patients. Kathleen has since won several research awards and has patented her device. She licensed the device to a major manufacturer of hospital beds, and now the Vollman Prone Positioner is marketed internationally. The device costs $2,000 and can be reused after disinfecting. Kathleen serves as a consultant to the company on the marketing of the device and the education of those who will use it. She is listed in *Who's Who of American Inventors*.

Kathleen Vollman's story is an example of how a practicing nurse, making an observation and thinking creatively through possible solutions, became a researcher, an inventor, and ultimately, an entrepreneur. This is not an overnight success story, however; it has been nearly 25 years since Kathleen made her initial observations. She continues her research in prone positioning science and prevention of complications in critical care unit patients today. You can read more about Kathleen Vollman's entrepreneurial activities online (http://www.vollman.com).

Modified from Vollman KM: My search to help patients breathe, *Reflections* 25(2):16-18, 1999; Vollman KM, Bander JL: Improved oxygenation utilizing a prone positioner in patients with acute respiratory distress syndrome, *Intensive Care Med* 22:1105-1111, 1996; Vollman KM: Nurse entrepreneurship: taking an invention from birth to the marketplace, *Clin Nurse Spec* 18(2):68-71, 2004; Vollman KM: Ventilator-associated pneumonia and pressure ulcer prevention as targets for quality improvement in the ICU, *Crit Care Nurs Clin North Am* 18:453-467, 2006.

specific responsibilities vary, depending on the preferences of the employer.

An RN who works for a group of three nephrologists describes a typical day:

I first make rounds independently on patients in the dialysis center, making sure that they are tolerating the dialysis procedure and answering questions regarding their treatments and diets. I then make rounds with one of the physicians in the hospital as he visits patients and orders new treatments. The afternoon is spent in the office assessing patients as they come for their physician's visit. I may draw blood for a diagnostic test on one patient and do patient teaching regarding diet to another. No two days are alike, and that is what I love about this position. I have a sense of independence but still have daily patient contact.

RNs considering employment in office settings need good communication skills, because a large part of their responsibilities includes communicating with patients, families, employers, pharmacists, and hospital admitting clerks. They should be careful to inquire about the specifics of the position because office practice nursing roles may range from routine task performance to the challenging, multifaceted functions described by the nurse interviewed above.

Occupational and environmental health nursing

Many large companies today employ **occupational and environmental health nurses** to provide basic health care services, health education, screenings, and emergency treatment to company employees at the workplace. Corporate executives have long known that good employee health reduces absenteeism, insurance costs, and worker errors, thereby improving company profitability. Occupational health nurses (OHNs) represent an important investment by companies. They are often asked to serve as consultants on health matters within the company. These nurses may participate in health-related policy development, such as policies governing employee smoking or family leaves (formerly limited to maternity leaves). Depending on the size of the company, the OHN may be the only health professional employed in a company and therefore may have a good deal of autonomy.

The minimum educational requirement for nurses in occupational health roles is licensure; however, the American Association of Occupational Health Nurses (AAOHN) recommends a baccalaureate degree. OHNs must possess knowledge and skills that enable them to perform routine physical assessments, including vision and hearing screenings, for all employees. Good interpersonal skills to provide counseling and referrals for lifestyle problems, such as stress or substance abuse, are a bonus for these nurses. They must also know first aid and cardiopulmonary resuscitation. If employed in a heavy industrial setting where burns or traumas are a risk, they must have special training in those medical emergencies.

OHNs also have responsibilities for identifying health risks in the entire work environment. They must be able to assess the environment for potential safety hazards and work with management to eliminate or reduce them. They need a working knowledge of governmental regulations, such as the requirements of the Occupational Safety and Health Administration, and must ensure that the company is complying with regulations. They may instruct new workers in the effective use of protective devices such as safety glasses and noise-canceling devices. These nurses also need to understand workers' compensation regulations and coordinate the care of injured workers with the treating physician.

Nurses in occupational settings have to be confident in their nursing skills, be effective communicators with both employees and managers, be able to motivate employees to adopt healthier habits, and be able to function independently in providing care. The AAOHN is the professional voice of OHNs. The AAOHN provides conferences, webcasts, a newsletter, a journal, and other resources to help OHNs stay up to date (online: http://www.aaohn.org). Certification for

OHNs is available through the American Board for Occupational Health Nurses (ABOHN).

Military nursing

Military nurses practice in peacetime and wartime settings in the army, navy, and air force. They may serve on active duty or in the reserves. They serve as staff nurses and supervisors in all major medical specialties. Both general and advanced practice opportunities are available in military nursing, and the settings in which these nurses practice have state-of-the-art technologies.

Military nurses often find themselves with broader responsibilities and scope of practice than do civilian nurses because of the demands of nursing "in the field," on aircraft, or onboard ship. Previous critical care, surgery, or trauma care experience is very desirable but not required. Military nurses are required to have a BSN degree for active duty. They enter active duty as officers and must be between the ages of 21 and 46½ years when they begin active duty.

A major benefit of military nursing is the opportunity for advanced education. Military nurses are encouraged to seek advanced degrees, and support is provided during schooling. The military pays for tuition, books, moving expenses, and even salary for nurses obtaining advanced degrees. This allows the student to focus on his or her studies. Nurses with advanced degrees are eligible for promotion in rank at an accelerated pace.

Travel and change are integral to military nursing, so these nurses must enjoy both. Military nurses in the reserves must be committed to readiness; they must be ready to go at a moment's notice. All military nurses may be called on for global wartime duty. These nurses take great pride in the fact that they are providing care to our fighting forces in every theater of operations.

A U.S. Army Reserve nurse wrote, "Events of 9/11 were the catalyst that made me realize that the right thing for me to do was to return to the military and merge that with my nursing career as an emergency nurse in the Army Nurse Corps"
(Hardin, 2006). Two years later he described his recent activities:

> My task is to teach combat lifesaver classes as part of a team of 16 other nurses. Our students are with us for four days, and we have between 180 and 200 students in a class. Our task is to teach the skills necessary to deal with chest wounds, amputations, and obstructed airways to National Guard soldiers and airmen. Our students are military police, truck drivers, truck refuelers, cooks, and similar individuals. Today I taught an 18-year-old soldier who normally works as a cashier in Iowa how to tourniquet her own leg should she fall victim to an IED (explosive device) in the next few months when she will be serving in Iraq (Hardin, 2008).

An Army major and nurse practitioner wrote:

> I have been working as the Officer in Charge of the Post-Deployment Health Reassessment program at Ft. Hood, the largest military post in the world. We care for over 65,000 soldiers and families and we see one in every ten soldiers in the US Army at some point in their careers. My team is in charge of seeing the post-deployed soldier within 90 to 180 days after returning from war. We evaluate them physically, emotionally, spiritually, and psychologically (Jandebeur, 2008).

Clearly, both these military nurses have vital responsibilities in support of U.S. troops at home and abroad. To learn more about military nursing, you can read an excellent article, "Esprit de Nurse Corps" by Barbara Barzoloski-O'Connor, in the online magazine *Nursing Spectrum*. This article can be found at http://include.nurse.com/apps/pbcs.dll/article?AID=20006260302.

School nursing

According to the National Association of School Nurses (2008), "School nursing is a specialized practice of professional nursing that advances the well-being, academic success, and life-long achievement of students." A **school nurse** should enjoy working with children, their families, teachers, school administrators, and parent-teacher organizations.

Although many states have well-developed school nurse programs, others do not. Very few states achieve the federally recommended ratio of 1:750 (a recommended minimum number of 1 school nurse for every 750 students). Reported ratios vary from a low of 1 RN to 305 students in Vermont to a high of 1 RN to 4952 students in Utah (Trossman, 2007). With higher than recommended ratios, it is difficult to imagine how children in these states can be deriving substantial health benefits from the school nurse program.

Health care futurists believe that school nursing is the wave of the future. In medically underserved areas and with the number of uninsured families increasing, the role of school nurse is sometimes expanded to include members of the schoolchild's immediate family. Obviously, this requires many more school nurses—along with willingness by state and local school boards to pay them. Without adequate qualified staffing, the nation's children cannot receive the full benefits of school nurse programs. The News Note on this page describes the impact of the school nurse shortage on school children.

Most school systems require nurses to have a minimum of a baccalaureate degree in nursing, whereas some school districts have higher educational requirements. Prior experience working

---

news note School Nurse Shortage Is Cause for Concern: How Bad Is It?

Thousands of children with asthma, attention deficit disorder, food allergies, injuries from accidents, and other health problems rely on teachers, school secretaries, or parent volunteers because there are not enough school nurses.

- More than 3.5 million school children take medications at school, including 200 types of prescription drugs.
- It is estimated that every 30 minutes of the school day a student suffers an injury significant enough to cause him or her to miss a half-day or more of school.
- Approximately two students per classroom suffer from asthma. During the 2002 school year, American students lost about 14.7 million school days to asthma.
- Allergies to peanuts doubled from 1997 to 2002.
- Students with diabetes, seizures, cerebral palsy, cystic fibrosis, and other serious disorders are in regular classroom situations with no one to monitor their medical conditions.
- A 1999 ruling by the U.S. Supreme Court requires public schools to provide care for students with disabilities. This means that someone must know how to use devices such as tracheostomy tubes, ventilators, feeding pumps, and catheters.

- In spite of the increasing demands for health care services in public schools, the number of school nurses is declining around the nation.
- In 3 years the Dearborn, Michigan, public schools cut school nurses at 32 schools from nine nurses to only five. They now depend on school secretaries to take care of minor health problems.
- Three of the seven school nurses in Baldwin County, Georgia, were laid off in 2005 because of lack of money.
- The number of California schools with full-time nurses fell from 7% in 1998 to 5% in 2003.
- In Florida schools during 2003-2004, 6007 calls were made to 9-1-1 for injuries or illness because no school nurse was available.

Children's advocates underscore the urgency of the situation. "Schools without nurses are putting children in harm's way," says William Sears, a pediatrician and author of more than 30 books on child care. "If we can't afford school nurses, we've got our priorities skewed." U.S. Representative Lois Capps, a Democrat from California and former school nurse, agrees. She worries "that staff members at schools without nurses might fail to spot illnesses among students" or be unable to respond during emergencies. "It's a ticking time bomb," she says.

Modified from Horovitz B, McCoy K: Nurse shortage puts school kids at risk, *USA Today,* Dec 14, 2005, p. A-1, and other sources.

with children is also usually required. School health has become a specialty in its own right, and in states where school health is a priority, graduate programs in school health nursing have been established. The National Board for Certification of School Nurses (NBCSN) is the official certifying body for school nurses.

School nurses need a working knowledge of human growth and development to detect developmental problems early and refer children to appropriate therapists. Counseling skills are important because many children turn to the school nurse as counselor. School nurses keep records of children's required immunizations and are responsible for ensuring that immunizations are current. When an outbreak of a childhood communicable disease occurs, school nurses educate parents, teachers, and students about treatment and prevention of disease transmission.

Although the essentially well child is the focus of the school nurse's work, the practice of mainstreaming has brought many chronically ill, injured, developmentally delayed, and physically challenged students into regular school classrooms. School nurses must work closely with families, teachers, and the community to provide these children with the special care they need while at school—and these needs can be significant.

School nurses work closely with teachers to incorporate health concepts into the curriculum. They endorse the teaching of basic hygiene, such as hand washing after bathroom use and dental hygiene. School nurses encourage the inclusion of age-appropriate nutritional information in school curricula and healthful foods in cafeteria and vending machine choices. They conduct vision and hearing screenings and make referrals to qualified physicians or other health care providers when routine screenings identify problems outside the nurses' scope of practice.

School nurses must be prepared to handle both routine illnesses of children and adolescents and emergencies. One of their major concerns is safety. Accidents are the leading cause of death in children of all ages, yet accidents are preventable. Prevention includes both protection from obvious hazards and education of teachers, parents, and students about how to avoid accidents. School nurses work with teachers, school bus drivers, cafeteria workers, and other school employees to provide the safest possible environment. When accidents occur, first aid for minor injuries and emergency care for more severe ones are additional skills school nurses use. Detection of evidence of child neglect and abuse is a sensitive but essential aspect of school nursing. School violence or bullying can also result in injury, absenteeism, and anxiety.

School nursing is a complex and multifaceted field that is constantly expanding. It represents a challenge for those nurses who choose it as a career.

You can learn more about school nursing by reading the ANA position statement, "Assuring Safe, High Quality Health Care in Pre-K through 12 Educational Settings" online at http://www.nursingworld.org under "health care policy" and then "position statements."

Hospice and palliative care nursing

Hospice and palliative care nursing is a rapidly developing specialty in nursing dedicated to improving the experience of seriously ill and dying patients and their families. It was initiated as a result of a $28 million study by the Robert Wood Johnson Foundation in the mid-1990s. This study found that there were significant problems associated with the care of seriously ill and dying patients. The problems reported included poor communication, continued aggressive treatment after treatment was no longer effective, and high levels of pain. The study pointed out the "overriding need to change the kind of care dying Americans receive" (Last Acts Task Force, 1998, p. 109). In the years since that report was issued, a number of nursing schools and organizations have increased attention to this important realm of care.

According to the ANA document *Hospice and Palliative Care Nursing: Scope and Standards of Practice*, "Hospice and palliative care nursing reflects a holistic philosophy of care implemented across the life span and across diverse health settings. . . . The goal of hospice and palliative nursing is to promote and improve the patient's quality of life through the relief of suffering along the course of the illness, through the death of the patient, and into the bereavement period of the family" (ANA, 2007, p. 1). The ANA (2007) identified three major precepts underlying hospice and end-of-life care:

- Persons are living until the moment of death.
- Coordinated care should be offered by a variety of professionals, with attention to the physical, psychological, social, and spiritual needs of patients and their families.
- Care should be sensitive to patient/family diversity (or cultural beliefs).

Nursing curricula traditionally have not included extensive content to prepare nurses to deal effectively with dying patients and their families. The AACN used the three precepts identified above to develop a document titled "Peaceful Death." This document identifies the competencies needed by baccalaureate nurses for palliative/hospice care and outlines where these competencies can fit into nursing curricula. You can review this document and other resources online (http://www.aacn.nche.edu/Publications/deathfin.htm).

End-of-life care is largely the responsibility of nurses. In recognition of this fact, the ANA formulated a position statement regarding the promotion of comfort and relief of pain of dying patients, reinforcing the nurse's obligation to promote comfort and ensure aggressive efforts to relieve pain and suffering (ANA, 2003). This position statement can be found online (http://www.nursingworld.org/readroom/position/ethics/etpain.htm).

Hospice and palliative care nurses work in a variety of settings, including inpatient palliative/hospice units, free-standing residential hospices, community-based or home hospice programs, ambulatory palliative care programs, teams of consultants in palliative care, and skilled nursing facilities. Both generalist and advanced practice nurses work in palliative care. The certifying agency is the National Board for the Certification

of Hospice and Palliative Nurses (NBCHPN). By 2007 more than 10,000 RNs had become certified hospice and palliative nurses (ANA, 2007).

With the aging population, end-of-life needs are expected to increase. Every nurse, not just specialists in hospice and palliative care, should be familiar with the precepts of palliative and end-of-life nursing care. You can learn more about end-of-life care online at http://www.nursingcenter.com/prodev/ce_article.asp?tid=411607.

Case management nursing

Case management is a dynamic, challenging, and growing field in nursing that evolved in the mid-1980s as a way of managing health care costs and patient length of stay (LOS). It involves systematic collaboration with patients, their significant others, and their health care providers to coordinate high-quality health care services in a cost-effective manner with positive patient outcomes. Another aspect of nursing case management includes decreasing fragmentation and duplication of care (Tahan, Huber, and Downey, 2006). The case manager is the person responsible for this process, and although RNs are not the only professionals who act as case managers, they are uniquely prepared for this role. Because of their broad educational backgrounds, skill in arranging and providing patient education and referrals, orientation toward holistic care and health promotion, and communication and interpersonal skills, nurses are particularly well suited for case management.

Depending on the case management model being used—and there are many—the nursing case manager may follow the patient from the diagnostic phase through hospitalization, rehabilitation, and back to home care. When necessary he or she helps the patient get assistance with transportation, home care, and housekeeping. Through careful planning, every step of the patient's care can be coordinated in a timely manner. "Case managers help patients with everything from avoiding duplicated tests to finding the best-priced prescriptions and other services" (Mincer, 2008).

Although there are challenges for nurses who make the transition from direct caregiver to case manager, both patient satisfaction and nurse satisfaction are high with the one-on-one relationship fostered with case management. Patients like the security of having one familiar person managing their care, and a nursing case manager has the satisfaction of coordinating a patient's care from beginning to end. Certification in nursing case management is offered by the American Nurses Credentialing Center. You may also hear case management nursing referred to as "care management nursing," a name more consistent with nursing's values.

Telehealth nursing

Telehealth is defined as the delivery of health care services and related health care activities through telecommunication technologies. Telehealth nursing may or may not be a separate nursing role because few nurses use telehealth exclusively in their practices. Rather, it is most often found as a part of other nursing roles. At the most basic level, nurses have always used the telephone to communicate with physicians, patients, and other health care providers. Today's technologies have evolved far beyond the telephone to include bedside computers, interactive audio and video linkages, teleconferencing, real-time transmission of patients' diagnostic and clinical data, electronic mail, and more.

The use of telehealth expands access to health care for underserved populations and individuals in both urban and rural areas. It also serves to reduce the sense of professional isolation experienced by those who work in such areas and may assist in attracting and retaining health care professionals in remote areas.

Practical uses of telehealth technology include faxing a change in a patient's drug order; consulting by telephone with other care providers; accessing a laboratory report from a remote site with a wireless, handheld computer; counseling patients on medications, diet, activity, or other therapy over the telephone or computer; or participating in interactive video sessions such as an interdisciplinary team consultation about a complex patient issue. Although the fundamentals of basic nursing practice do not change because nurses use telehealth technologies, their use may require adaptation or modification of usual procedures. In addition, telenurses must develop competence in the use of each new type of telehealth technology, and these may change rapidly.

Numerous legal and regulatory issues surround nursing care delivered through telehealth technologies. The *Online Journal of Issues in Nursing* has posted a comprehensive article enumerating these (http://www.nursingworld.org/MainMenu Categories/ANAMarketplace/ANAPeriodicals/ OJIN/TableofContents/Volume62001/No3Sept01/ TelehealthOverview.aspx). The American Academy of Ambulatory Care Nursing (2007) has developed practice standards for this emerging specialty to define and describe telehealth nursing practice and outline expectations for the telehealth nurse.

You can learn more about telehealth, an area of growing interest in nursing and other health professions, as well as some controversy, from the Association of Telehealth Service Providers (http://www.atsp.org), from the American Telemedicine Association (http://www.americantelemed. org), and from the American Academy of Ambulatory Care Nursing (http://www.aaacn.org).

Faith community nursing

Interest in spirituality and its relation to wellness and healing in recent years prompted the development of a practice area known as faith community nursing. This area of nursing, formerly termed parish nursing, takes a holistic approach to healing that involves partnerships between congregations, their pastoral staffs, and health care providers. Since its development in the Chicago area in the 1980s by a hospital chaplain, Dr. Granger E. Westberg, faith community nursing has spread rapidly and now includes more than 10,000 nurses in paid and volunteer positions across the country. According to the ANA definition: "Faith community nursing is the specialized practice of professional nursing that focuses on the intentional care of the spirit as part of the process of promoting holistic health and preventing or minimizing illness in a faith community" (ANA, 2005, p. 1).

The spiritual dimension is central to faith community nursing practice. The nurse's own spiritual journey is an essential aspect of this nursing role. Faith community nursing is based on the belief that spiritual health is central to well-being and influences a person's entire being.

Faith community nurses serve as members of the ministry staff or clergy of a church or other faith community. They practice independently, within the legal scope of the individual state's nurse practice act. Roles of the faith community nurse include health educator and counselor, advocate for health services, referral agent, coordinator of volunteer health ministers, developer of support groups, and integrator of spiritual practices and health. The Interview provides a discussion with a faith community nurse who describes her calling and her practice.

As faith community nursing has evolved, so have the standards for minimum preparation for nurses entering the specialty. Present preferred preparation includes a baccalaureate or higher degree in nursing, including preparation in community nursing, experience as an RN using the nursing process, knowledge of the health care assets of the community, specialized knowledge of the spiritual beliefs and practices of the faith community, and knowledge and skills to implement Faith Community Nursing: Scope and Standards of Practice (ANA, 2005, p. 5). This document, which sets forth the responsibilities for which faith community nurses are accountable and reflects the values and priorities of the specialty, can be obtained from the ANA. Certification is not yet available for faith community nurses.

INTERVIEW   Amy Corder, RN, MSN, CRRN *Faith Community Nurse*

Interviewer: Describe a typical day in your practice.

Corder: There is no "typical" day. Every day is different, which is what I love about faith community nursing. There are many aspects of my work, a number of which are not usually thought of as nursing. I help the congregation understand the interaction and connection between body, mind, and spirit. This is important because unhealthy behaviors or emotions often affect us physically in harmful ways.

Interviewer: What is the focus of your practice?

Corder: One aspect is health maintenance, such as teaching nutrition and diet, dental health, medication management, blood pressure screenings, and the like. I also visit parishioners in their homes, mostly older adults. Recently I visited a lady with a stasis ulcer on her leg. After my assessment and much discussion, she agreed to let me make a referral to a wound specialist. I don't do invasive procedures like a home health nurse might do. My focus is in the role of teaching, counseling, supporting, and often just encouraging people about how to improve their lives physically, mentally, and spiritually both within the congregation and the community.

Interviewer: What has surprised you about faith community nursing?

Corder: It surprised me how much writing I do. I am frequently asked to write an article for a newsletter or a small local paper about my current programs or about what I do as a faith community nurse. I also make a lot of presentations, which takes some research. I sure didn't appreciate writing all of those papers in school, but now I'm glad because it gave me confidence in my writing and research skills.

Interviewer: How did you prepare yourself to be a faith community nurse?

Corder: By searching and establishing my own spiritual foundation and having an open mind and heart, in order to hear God's calling. Faith community nursing is a calling by God. I do not believe you can be totally effective in assisting others in discovering and improving their spirituality for better health unless you have achieved a certain amount of spiritual awareness within your own life. Education-wise, I have a BSN and a master's degree in gerontological nursing. I have primarily worked in the areas of rehabilitation nursing and long-term care, which has prepared me well for what I do.

Interviewer: What is the most challenging part of your work?

Corder: The most challenging part of my work is learning about the philosophy of health ministry and faith community nursing and applying it to my practice. Although faith community nursing has been around for 15 to 20 years, it is still a relatively new field. I am the first faith community nurse for my congregation, and there are fewer than two dozen other faith community nurses in our community, although that number is growing. This is an exciting time for our congregation as we explore the role of health ministry and faith community nursing together.

Nursing informatics

Another exciting specialty area evolving in nursing is nursing informatics (NI). If you have an aptitude for information technology (IT) and would like to help bridge the gap between IT and nursing practice, NI may be a field for you. The **informatics nurse** combines nursing science with information management science and computer science to manage information nurses need and to make that information accessible. This field encompasses the full range of activities that focus on information handling in nursing (ANA, 2008) and assists nurses to carry out the work of nursing efficiently and effectively. Because it "has been estimated that nurses spend as much as 50 percent of their time gathering, coordinating, and documenting information" (Meadows, 2002), it is easy to understand the potential benefits of streamlining this process. Benefits of clinical information systems include improved patient safety, reduction in variability of care, improved communication, improved clinical decision making, and increased efficiency of staff.

In contrast to computer science systems analysts, informatics nurses must clearly understand the information they handle and how other nurses will use it. Nursing knowledge is specialized and must be accessible by nurse users; otherwise, it is useless in improving patient care. Complex information systems are more likely to fail when end users are not consulted during the planning and design process (ANA, 2008). Because they are nurses themselves, informatics nurses are best able to understand the needs of nurses who use the systems and can design them with the needs, skills, and time constraints of those nurses in mind.

Informatics nurses may work in clinical areas, ensuring that the direct caregiver nurse is provided with complete and accurate information about patients' health needs and nursing care requirements. They may also practice in nonclinical areas such as nursing education or administration, where they design ways to make information needed by teachers, students, and managers easily accessible. In addition to practicing in hospitals and universities, informatics nurses also work in the military, health maintenance organizations, and research settings.

All nurses must be prepared to use informatics to communicate, manage knowledge, mitigate error, and support decision making. This is considered so important that it is one of the five core competencies identified in the Institute of Medicine's 2003 report, *Health Professions Education: A Bridge to Quality*. IT can help nurses deliver more effective care in a number of ways. Some examples include computerizing a nursing document or system; writing a program to support nursing care of patients; developing an interactive video disk system for educational purposes; helping nurse managers develop systems to use nursing resources effectively (such as people, money, supplies); or designing systems to collect and aggregate clinical data so they can be analyzed to assess the cost and outcomes of nursing care.

As a minimum, nurses specializing in informatics should have a bachelor's degree in nursing and additional knowledge and experience in the field of informatics. Advanced practice in nursing informatics requires preparation at the graduate level in nursing (ANA, 2008). Certification as an informatics nurse is available through the American Nurses Credentialing Center.

Travel nursing

If you love adventure and flexibility, travel nursing may be for you. Travel nurses choose where they work and when they will begin working, depending on the availability of a position in their chosen facility. "Travellers are fixed-term, temporary nurses who usually work at the same hospital for 13 weeks and are scheduled at least 2 months in advance. Hospitals are likely to depend on travellers for specific or strategic staffing needs, such as to provide continuity of care when covering for maternity leaves, vacations, or sick leaves" (Shaffer, 2007). Travel nurses work in their clinical specialty and often have bachelor's or higher degrees. In most instances they are as well qualified as permanent staff nurses. The field of travel nursing has evolved to the point that staffing firms, the companies that assist travel nurses in placements, now may offer benefits such as insurance, retirement plans, and other benefits. The staffing firm also may pay for licensure and housing costs. Hospitals hire travel nurses for a variety of reasons: to augment their own staff and reduce nurse-patient ratios, to relieve regular staff so they can attend training sessions or participate in other projects, or to serve as interim nurse-managers and recruiters (Shaffer, 2007). If you are interested in travel nursing, be sure to use a certified staffing firm. You can find a list of certified staffing firms at The Joint Commission's website: http://www.jointcommission.org/Certification-Programs/HealthCareStaffingServices.

NURSING OPPORTUNITIES REQUIRING HIGHER DEGREES

Many RNs choose to pursue roles that require a master's degree, doctoral degree, or specialized education in a specific area. These roles include CNSs, nurse managers, nurse executives in hospital settings, nurse educators (whether in clinical or academic settings), nurse anesthetists, nurse-midwives, and other APNs including the newly designated clinical nurse leader.

Nurse Educators

In 2004, 48,666 RNs worked in nursing education (USDHHS, 2006). These nurses teach in licensed practical nurse/licensed vocational nurse programs, diploma programs, associate degree programs, baccalaureate and higher degree programs, and programs preparing nursing assistants. Nurse educators in accredited schools of nursing offering a baccalaureate or higher degree must hold a minimum of a master's degree in nursing; in 2006 43.2% had doctoral degrees in nursing or other fields (National League for Nursing, 2006).

Most nursing faculty (95.9%) are women, and 10.7% are members of minority groups (National League for Nursing, 2006). In 2007 to 2008 16.8% of master's students chose nursing education to prepare for a teaching role, compared with 10.7% in 2005 to 2006 (Fang et al, 2008). This represents an increase, which, if continued, may mitigate somewhat the downward trend of

the past decade. Concerns about a critical shortage of nursing faculty in the future, however, continue. A discussion of the nursing faculty shortage can be found in Chapter 7, The Education of Nurses.

Advanced Practice Nursing

APN is an umbrella term applied to an RN who has met advanced educational and clinical practice requirements beyond the 2 to 4 years of basic nursing education demanded of all RNs. Advanced practice nursing has grown since APN practice evolved more than 40 years ago. In 2004, approximately 240,461 of RNs (8.3%) held the required credentials to work as APNs, up from 196,279 in 2000. This growth was spurred by several factors, including increased demand for primary care coupled with increased specialization of physicians and heightened demand for efficient and cost-effective treatment. The push for health care reform by the Obama administration is expected to stimulate even greater interest and growth in the numbers of APNs.

Patient acceptance of APNs is high. A growing body of evidence is accumulating that confirms that APNs deliver high-quality care, exceeding that delivered by physicians on several measures. It is estimated that 60% to 80% of primary and preventive care measures traditionally performed by physicians can be safely accomplished by APNs.

There are four categories of APNs: nurse practitioner, clinical nurse specialist, certified nurse-midwife, and certified registered nurse anesthetist. Figure 1-7 shows the breakdown of APNs by area of specialty in 2004.

Nurse practitioner

Opportunities for nurses in expanded roles in health care have created a boom in nurse practitioner (NP) education. There were 150 NP education programs in 1992. By 2005 this number had risen to 334 (AACN, 2006). These programs grant master's degrees or post-master's certificates and prepare nurses to sit for national certification examinations as NPs. The length of the programs varies, depending on prior education of

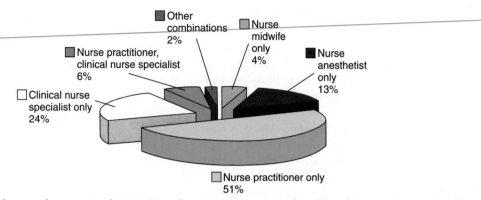

Figure 1-7 APNs by specialty area, March 2004. (Data from U.S. Department of Health and Human Services, Health Resources and Services Administration: *The registered nurse population: findings from the March 2004 National Sample Survey of Registered Nurses,* Washington, DC, 2006, Government Printing Office, p. 33 [website]: http://bhpr.hrsa.gov/ healthworkforce/rnsurvey04/default.htm.)

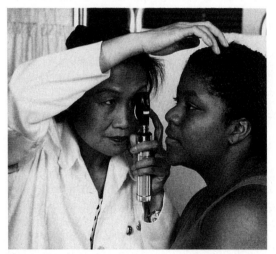

Figure 1-8 A nurse practitioner assesses her patient. (Photo by Fielding Freed.)

the students. In 2004 there were 141,209 NPs in the United States. This figure includes the 14,699 who are also CNSs (USDHHS, 2006).

States vary in the amount of practice autonomy accorded to NPs. According to the annual survey conducted by *The Nurse Practitioner: The American Journal of Primary Health Care* (Phillips, 2008), in 24 states and the District of Columbia the board of nursing has sole authority in NP scope of practice. In those states there

are no statutory or regulatory requirements for physician collaboration, direction, or supervision. An additional 16 states require some physician collaboration. Physician supervision of NP practice is required in 5 states. In 5 states, the scope of NP practice is determined jointly by the board of nursing and the board of medicine (Phillips, 2008). NPs beginning practice in a new state should check the status of the advanced practice laws in that state before making firm commitments because some states still place limitations on NP independence, termed "barriers to practice."

NPs work in clinics, nursing homes, their own offices, or physicians' offices. Others work for hospitals, HMOs, or private industry. Most NPs choose a specialty area such as adult, family, or pediatric health care. They are qualified to handle a wide range of basic health problems. These nurses can perform physical examinations, take medical histories, diagnose and treat common acute and chronic illnesses and injuries, order and interpret laboratory tests and x-ray films, and counsel and educate clients (Figure 1-8).

In 2008 NPs could legally write prescriptions in 37 states with some physician supervision, whereas in 13 states and the District of Columbia, NPs could prescribe independently of physician involvement (Phillips, 2008). Some NPs are independent practitioners and can be directly reimbursed by Medicare, Medicaid, and military and private insurers for their work.

Clinical nurse specialist

CNSs work in a variety of settings, including hospitals, clinics, nursing homes, their own offices, industry, home care, and HMOs. These nurses hold advanced nursing degrees—master's or doctoral—and are qualified to handle a wide range of physical and mental health problems. They are experts in a particular field of clinical practice, such as mental health, gerontology, cardiac care, cancer care, community health, or neonatal health, and they perform health assessments, make diagnoses, deliver treatment, and develop quality control methods. Additionally, CNSs work in consultation, research, education, and administration. Direct reimbursement to some CNSs is possible through Medicare, Medicaid, and military and private insurers. In 2004 there were 72,521 CNSs in the United States, including 14,689 who were both NPs and CNSs (USDHHS, 2006).

Certified nurse-midwife

In 2004 there were an estimated 13,684 nurse-midwives in the United States (USDHHS, 2006), 93.7% of whom are nationally certified. Certified nurse-midwives (CNMs) provide well-woman care and attend to or assist in childbirth in various settings, including hospitals, birthing centers, private practice, and home birthing services. They are prepared in formal nurse-midwife courses of at least 9 months in length. Of the 43 nurse-midwife programs accredited by the American College of Nurse-Midwives, 39 offer a master's degree, accounting for an average of 1.5 years of specialized education beyond basic nursing education (American College of Nurse-Midwives, 2009). As of 2010, all programs are required to award a MS or MSN degree.

Births attended by nurse-midwives are among the safest. According to the National Center for Health Statistics, CNMs attended 317,168 births in 2006. This represented 10.8% of all spontaneous vaginal births in the United States in 2006

(Martin, Hamilton, Sutton, et al, 2009). Historically, births attended by nurse-midwives have had half the national average rates for cesarean sections and higher rates of successful vaginal births after a previous cesarean, both considered measures of high-quality obstetric care. A study published in the June 2003 edition of the *American Journal of Public Health* documents that "low-risk patients receiving collaborative midwifery care had birth success rates comparable to those who saw only physicians, with fewer interventions, more options, and lower cost to the health care system" (Jackson, Lang, Swartz, et al, 2003, p. 1003).

CNMs have the widest prescriptive rights of all APNs. As of 2009, CNMs were able to prescribe medication in all 50 states and 3 jurisdictions, including the District of Columbia (American College of Nurse-Midwives, 2009).

Because of patient acceptance and a good safety record, deliveries attended by nurse-midwives have increased every year since 1975 (Martin, Hamilton, Sutton, et al, 2007) and are expected to increase in the future.

Certified registered nurse anesthetist

There were approximately 39,000 certified registered nurse anesthetists (CRNAs) and CRNA students in the United States in 2007 (American Association of Nurse Anesthetists, 2008). Nurse anesthetists administer approximately 30 million anesthetics each year and are the only anesthesia providers in nearly one third of U.S. hospitals (American Association of Nurse Anesthetists, 2008). Collaborating with physician anesthesiologists or working independently, they are found in a variety of settings, including operating suites; obstetric delivery rooms; the offices of dentists, podiatrists, ophthalmologists, and plastic surgeons; ambulatory surgical facilities; and in military and governmental health services (American Association of Nurse Anesthetists, 2008).

To become a CRNA, nurses must complete 2 to 3 years of specialized education in a master's program beyond the required bachelor's degree. There are 109 accredited nurse anesthesia programs in the United States, ranging from 24 to 36 months in length. Nurse anesthetists must also meet national certification and recertification requirements. According to the American Association of Nurse Anesthetists, 44% of the nation's CRNAs are men, as compared with under 10% in all nursing fields (American Association of Nurse Anesthetists, 2008).

The safety of care delivered by CRNAs is well established. Anesthesia care today is safer than in the past, and numerous outcome studies have demonstrated that there is "no difference in the quality of care provided by CRNAs and their physician counterparts" (American Association of Nurse Anesthetists, 2008).

Clinical nurse leader

In January 2008, after comprehensive review of nursing roles and several years of study and discussion with many health care leaders and experts, the AACN proposed a new credential, the **clinical nurse leader** (CNL). This designation was intended as a means of allowing master's-prepared nurses to oversee and manage care delivery in various settings. CNLs are not intended to be administrators or managers but are clinical experts who are involved in the care of a distinct group of patients and who may, on occasion, actively provide direct patient care themselves. They "coordinate the direct care activities of other nursing staff and healthcare professionals, gather and evaluate patient outcomes, and have the authority to change plans of care when necessary" (Brown, 2008, p. 40). According to the AACN, the CNL role is intended "to assure the highest quality nursing workforce for our nation's health care needs" (AACN, 2004).

This proposal was not without controversy and objections from CNSs who saw the proposed role as duplicating and potentially disenfranchising CNSs. By January 2009, however, nearly 90 clinical agencies in 35 states and Puerto Rico were involved in a pilot program designed to study the education needed by CNLs and to evaluate their effectiveness. You will be hearing more about this emerging role in the future. More information can be found on the AACN's website: http://www.aacn.nche.edu/CNL/about.htm.

Issues in advanced practice nursing

Each year in January, *The Nurse Practitioner: The American Journal of Primary Health Care* publishes an update on legislation affecting advanced practice nursing. Over the years, advances have been made toward removing the barriers to autonomous practice for APNs in many, but not all, states.

In the past, substantial barriers to APN autonomy existed because of the overlap between traditional medical and nursing functions. A decade ago, the picture was considerably less optimistic than it is now. The issue of APNs practicing autonomously was a politically charged arena, with organized medicine positioned firmly against all efforts of nurses to be recognized as independent health care providers receiving direct reimbursement for their services. Organized nursing, however, persevered. Nurses, through their professional associations, continued their efforts to change laws that limit the scope of nursing practice. Their efforts were aided by the fact that numerous published studies validated the safety, cost-efficiency, and high patient acceptance of APN care.

According to the 2008 *Nurse Practitioner* update (Phillips, 2008), both the public and legislators at state and national levels have begun to appreciate the role that APNs have played in increasing the efficiency and availability of primary health care delivery while reducing costs. However, opposition to APN autonomy persists. Roadblocks to full practice autonomy continue, primarily because of the resistance of organized physicians in spite of positive patient outcome data. Although progress has been made, there remains the need for all APNs to continue to work with their professional organizations to promote legislation mandating full autonomy. Until the U.S. Congress approves legislation to provide primary health care for all citizens and makes provisions for APNs to share fully in the provision of that care, the practice parameters of APNs are at the mercy of the various state legislatures.

EMPLOYMENT OUTLOOK IN NURSING

The Bureau of Labor Statistics, a division of the U.S. Department of Labor, is confident about nursing's overall employment prospects in the near and distant future. According to the Bureau (U.S. Department of Labor, 2008), nurses can expect their employment opportunities to grow "much faster than the average" (meaning a 23% increase) through the year 2016. The Bureau estimates that, during this time, 587,000 new RN jobs will be created to meet growing patient needs and to replace retiring nurses. RNs were first on the Bureau's list of the 30 occupations with the largest projected job growth in the years 2006-2016 (U.S. Department of Labor, 2008). Several factors are fueling this growth, including technologic advances and the increasing emphasis on primary care. The aging of the nation's population also has a significant impact, because older people are more likely to require medical care. As aging nurses retire, many additional job openings will result.

Opportunities in hospitals, traditionally the largest employers of nurses, will grow more slowly than those in community-based sectors. The most rapid hospital-based growth is projected to occur in outpatient facilities, such as same-day surgery centers, rehabilitation programs, and outpatient cancer centers.

Home health care positions are expected to increase the fastest of all. This is in response to the expanding elderly population's needs and the preference for and cost-effectiveness of home care. Furthermore, technologic advances are making it possible to bring increasingly complex treatments into the home.

Another expected area of high growth will occur in assisted living and nursing home care; this is primarily in response to the larger number of frail elderly in their 80s and 90s requiring long-term care. As hospitals come under greater pressure to decrease the average patient LOS, nursing home admissions will increase, as will growth in long-term rehabilitation units (U.S. Department of Labor, 2008).

An additional factor influencing employment patterns for RNs is the tendency for sophisticated medical procedures to be performed in physicians' offices, clinics, ambulatory surgical centers, and other outpatient settings. RNs' expertise will be needed to care for patients undergoing procedures formerly performed only in hospital settings.

APNs can also expect to find themselves in higher demand for the foreseeable future. The evolution of integrated health care networks focusing on primary care and health maintenance and pressure for cost-effective care are ideal conditions for advanced nursing practice.

Nursing Salaries

Salaries in the nursing profession vary widely according to practice setting, level of preparation and credentials, experience, and region of the country. The latest survey report, *The Registered Nurse Population: Findings from the March 2004 National Sample Survey of Registered Nurses* (USDHHS, 2006), reported that the average full-time earnings of RNs in 2004 were $57,785. *Nursing2007*'s salary survey reported that the average annual full-time income was $54,900 for RNs nationwide in 2006, and the Bureau of Labor Statistics' *Occupational Handbook* (2008) reported a median annual salary of RNs as $57,280 for 2006. In addition, *RN* magazine's earnings survey reported base pay as $58,383 for full- and part-time RNs working in acute care hospitals for the year 2007 (Eriksen, 2007). Needless to say, it is difficult to pin down exactly what nursing salaries are at any given point in time.

Although salaries have generally increased nationwide, discussing salary trends from a national perspective is often misleading. For instance, salaries in urban areas are much higher than those in rural communities, and so is the cost of living. Readers should bear this in mind when reviewing these figures. Regional salaries tend to be more realistic measures. Figure 1-9 shows the average annual salaries of staff nurses in each geographic area of the United States in 2006. Regional variations are apparent. It should be noted that these figures do not include salaries of APNs, whose

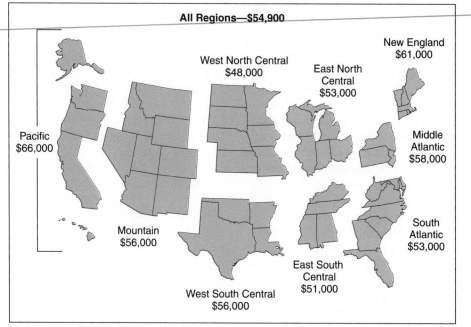

Figure 1-9 Average annual salaries of full-time staff RNs by region. (Data from Mee CL: A closer look at nurses' salaries, *Nursing 2007*, 37 [Career Directory]:8-10, 2007.)

earnings are higher than the averages shown for staff nurses.

Nationwide in 2007, the average salary of NPs was $81,397 (Rollet and Lebo, 2008). For CNMs, the average in 2007 was more than $79,000 (American College of Nurse-Midwives, 2007). CRNAs in 2007 averaged $152,819, the highest average salary of any advanced practice specialty group (Horton, 2008). Clearly, in nursing as in most other professions, additional preparation and responsibility increase earning potential.

Most of the wage growth for nurses occurs early in their careers and tapers off in time as nurses "top out" on the salary scale. This leads to a flattening of salaries for more experienced nurses (O'Brien, 2008). This decreased potential for salary improvements may account for nurses leaving patient care for additional education and/ or other careers in nursing or outside the profession, an issue that must be addressed to improve retention of the seasoned nurses that are badly needed in the profession.

Summary of Key Points

- There are more than 2.9 million RNs in the United States, and more than 2.4 million are actively practicing. Fewer than 60% work full-time.
- Approximately 56.2% of working nurses are employed in hospitals, a traditional setting for nursing practice, but one that will see dramatic changes as health care in the United States continues to become more community based.
- A continuing trend is the growth of opportunities for nurses in practice settings outside the traditional hospital.
- Increased use of APNs as providers of primary care may be part of the solution to the U.S. health care crisis that is caused by the aging of the baby boom generation, the fast-growing group of frail elderly, technologic advances, and the critical need for cost-containment measures in the health care sector.
- APNs are capable of delivering high-quality care to many segments of the population not

currently receiving health care or receiving substandard care. It is anticipated that APNs will be a key to delivering primary care under any health care reform package endorsed by the Obama administration.

- If the nation is to benefit from the services of APNs, legal barriers to their practice must be removed through the political action of organized nursing and politically active nurses.
- Government projections are for the demand for nurses, including APNs, to increase through the year 2016 and beyond.

Critical Thinking Questions

1. What characteristics do today's nurses have in common, and in what ways do they differ?
2. Think of the areas of nursing that interest you most. How do your personal and professional qualifications compare with the characteristics needed in the roles discussed in this chapter?
3. Interview nurses in various practice settings, especially those not covered in this chapter. Find out how they prepared for their positions, what their daily activities are, and what they find most challenging and rewarding about their work.
4. Call the nurse recruiter or personnel office of a nearby hospital and inquire about salaries and other benefits for entry-level and APN positions. How do they compare with those listed in this chapter? Is there a clinical ladder program? How does it work?
5. Interview an APN working in your community. What does he or she see as the major barriers to practice?
6. Contact your state nurses' association to find out what legislative initiatives are being undertaken to remove barriers to full APN practice in your state.

ⓔvolve *To enhance your understanding of this chapter, try the Student Exercises on the Evolve site at http://evolve.elsevier.com/Chitty/professional.*

REFERENCES

Aiken LH: U.S. nurse labor market dynamics are key to global nurse sufficiency, *Health Serv Res* 42 (32):1299-1320, 2007.

Aiken LH, Clarke SP, Cheung RB, et al: Educational levels of hospital nurses and surgical patient mortality, *JAMA* 290(12):1617-1623, 2003.

American Academy of Ambulatory Care Nursing: *Telehealth nursing practice administration and practice standards,* ed 4, Pitman, NJ, 2007, American Academy of Ambulatory Care Nursing.

American Association of Colleges of Nursing: *AACN board decisions regarding the clinical nurse leader initiative,* 2004 (website): http://www.aacn.nche.edu/CNL/TalkingPoints.htm.

American Association of Colleges of Nursing: *Enrollment and graduations in baccalaureate and graduate programs in nursing, 2005-2006,* Washington, DC, 2006, American Association of Colleges of Nursing.

American Association of Nurse Anesthetists: *Certified Registered Nurse Anesthetists at a glance,* 2008 (website): http://www.aana.com/aboutaana.aspx?ucNavMenu_TSMenuTargetID=179&ucNavMenu_TSMenuTargetType=4&ucNavMenu_TSMenuID=6&id=265.

American College of Nurse-Midwives: *ACNM compensation and benefits survey, 2007: Results* (website): http://www.midwife.org/siteFiles/education/ACNM_salary_survey_2007.pdf.

American College of Nurse-Midwives: *Essential facts about certified nurse-midwives,* 2009 (website):http://www.midwife.org/Essential_Facts.pdf.

American Nurses Association: *Position statement on pain management and control of distressing symptoms in dying patients,* Washington, DC, 2003, American Nurses Association.

American Nurses Association [in collaboration with the Health Ministries Association]: *Faith community nursing: scope and standards of practice,* Washington, DC, 2005, American Nurses Association.

American Nurses Association: *Hospice and palliative care nursing: scope and standards of practice,* Silver Spring, MD, 2007, American Nurses Association.

American Nurses Association: *Nursing informatics: scope and standards of practice,* Silver Spring, MD, 2008, American Nurses Association.

Brown AB: Understanding the role of the clinical nurse leader, *Am Nurse Today* 3(6):40-41, 2008.

Buchan J: The impact of global nursing migration on health services delivery, *Policy Polit Nurs Pract* 7(3 Suppl):16S-25S, 2006.

Ellerbe S: Staffing through web-based open shift bidding, *American Nurse Today* 2(4):32-35, 2007.

Ericksen AB: 2007 earnings survey: how does it add up? *RN* 70(10):42-48, 2007.

Fang D, Htut A, Bednash GD: *2007-2008 enrollment and graduations in baccalaureate and graduate programs in nursing*, Washington, DC, 2008, American Association of Colleges of Nursing.

Hardin C: Captain, United States Army Reserve, *Personal communication*, 2006.

Hardin C, Captain: United States Army Reserve, *Personal communication*, 2008.

Horovitz B, McCoy K: Nurse shortage puts school kids at risk, *USA Today*, Dec 14, 2005, p A-1.

Horton S: Manager of Offices and Fulfillment Services, American Association of Nurse Anesthetists, *Personal communication*, 2008.

Huston C: Letter from the president, *Create the Future* 5(12):1-2, 2008.

Institute of Medicine: *Health professions education: a bridge to quality*, Washington, DC, 2003, National Academy of Sciences.

Jackson DJ, Lang JM, Swartz WH, et al: Outcomes, safety, and resource utilization in a collaborative care birth center program, *Am J Public Health* 93(6):999-1006, 2003.

Jandebeur R: Major, United States Army, Personal communication, 2008.

Last Acts Task Force: National policy statements on end of life care: precepts of palliative care, *J Palliative Med* 1(2):109-112, 1998.

Martin JA, Hamilton BE, Sutton PD, et al: *Births: final data for 2006, National Vital Statistics Reports, 57:7,* Hyattsville, Md, 2009, National Center for Health Statistics.

Meadows G: Nursing informatics: an evolving specialty, *Nurs Econ* 20(6):300-301, 2002.

Mee CL: A closer look at nurses' salaries, *Nursing2007* 37(Career Directory):8-10, 2007.

Mincer J: Aid from unlikely sources, *Wall Street Journal Online*, Aug 24, 2008 (website): http://finance.yahoo.com/insurance/article/105619/Aid-From-Unlikely-Sources.

Mullen R: He was their patient. Now he's one of them, *Emory Health*, Fall 2008:12-15. Online: http://www.whsc.emory.edu/_pubs/hsc.

National Association of School Nurses: *Definition of school nursing*, 2008 (website): http://www.nasn.org/Default.aspx?tabid=57.

National League for Nursing: *Nurse educators 2006: a report of the faculty census survey of RN and graduate programs*, New York, 2006, National League for Nursing.

O'Brien A: Advance salary survey 2008, *Advance for Nurses* (website): http://nursing.advanceweb.com/Editorial/Content/Editorial.aspx?CC=108359.

Phillips SJ: Twentieth annual legislative update: after 20 years, APNs are still standing together, *Nurse Practitioner: Am J Prim Health Care* 33(1):10-34, 2008.

Rollet J, Lebo S: 2007 National salary and workplace survey of NPs, 2008, *Advance for Nurse Practitioners* (website): http://nurse-practitioners.advanceweb.com/Editorial/Content/Editorial.aspx?CC=105234.

Shaffer F: Travel nursing: is it right for you? *American Nurse Today* 2(2), 2007.

Tahan HA, Huber DL, Downey WT: Case managers' roles and functions, *Lippincott's Case Manage* 11(1):4-22, 2006.

Trossman S: Issues up close: is the school nurse in? ANA promotes strategies to help meet students' health and safety needs, *AJN* 2(8):38-40, 2007.

U.S. Census Bureau: *Statistical Abstract of the United States: Resident population by sex, race, and Hispanic origin status*: 15, 2000 to 2004, Table 13.

U.S. Department of Health and Human Services: *Health Resources and Services Administration: The registered nurse population: findings from the March 2004 National Sample Survey of Registered Nurses*, Washington, DC, 2006, Government Printing Office.

U.S. Department of Labor, Bureau of Labor Statistics: *Occupational outlook handbook: 2008-09*, Washington, DC, 2008, Government Printing Office (website): http://www.bls.gov/oco/ocos083.htm.

Vollman KM: My search to help patients breathe, *Reflections* 25(2):16-18, 1999.

Vollman KM: Nurse entrepreneurship: taking an invention from birth to the marketplace, *Clin Nurse Specialist* 18(2):68-71, 2004.

Vollman KM: Ventilator-associated pneumonia and pressure ulcer prevention as targets for quality improvement in the ICU, *Crit Care Nurs Clin North Am* 18:453-467, 2006.

Vollman KM, Bander JL: Improved oxygenation utilizing a prone positioner in patients with acute respiratory distress syndrome, *Intensive Care Med* 22:1105-1111, 1996.

The History and Social Context of Nursing

Beth Perry Black

After studying this chapter, students will be able to:
- Identify the social, political, and economic factors and trends that influenced the development of professional nursing in the United States
- Describe the influence of Florence Nightingale on the development of the nursing profession
- Identify early nursing leaders and identify their significance to nursing
- Describe the development of early schools of nursing
- Explain the role that the military and wars have had on the development of the nursing profession
- Describe the struggles and contributions of minorities and men in nursing
- Discuss the development of advanced practice nursing in nursing's history in the United States
- Describe how common stereotypes of women have affected the development of the nursing profession
- Explain the impact of the media on the image of nursing
- Evaluate the implications for nursing as technology continues to be developed
- Describe the impact of societal violence on nursing
- Describe the causes and effects of imbalances in supply of and demand for nurses in the United States
- Explain how nursing shortages affect patient outcomes

HISTORICAL CONTEXT OF NURSING

From the work of Florence Nightingale in the Crimea in the mid-1800s to the present, the profession has been influenced by the social, political, and economic climate of the times, as well as by technologic advances and theoretical shifts in medicine and science. This chapter presents an overview of some of the highlights of nursing's history and several of its leaders, as well as a discussion of current and past social forces that have shaped the discipline's course of development.

Mid–Nineteenth-Century Nursing in England: The Influence of Florence Nightingale

Nursing's most notable early figure, Florence Nightingale, was born into the aristocratic social sphere of Victorian England in 1820. As a young woman, Nightingale (Figure 2-1) often felt stifled by her privileged and protected social position. As was customary at the time, aristocratic women visited and brought comfort to the sick and poor. The young Florence often accompanied her mother on these visits. At the age of 30 years, against her parents' wishes, Nightingale entered the nurses' training program in Kaiserswerth, Germany, where she spent 3 years learning the basics of nursing under the guidance of the Protestant deaconesses. She also studied under the Sisters of Charity in Paris. Care of the sick was often in the purview of women and men in religious orders.

On hearing of the horrible conditions suffered by the sick and wounded British soldiers in Turkey during the Crimean War, Nightingale took a small band of untrained women to the British hospital in Scutari. With great compassion, and despite the opposition of military officers,

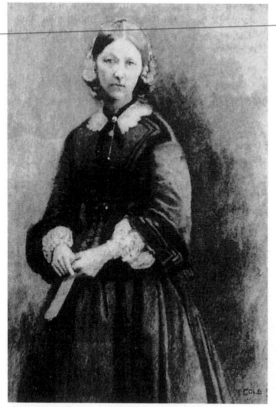

Figure 2-1 Florence Nightingale (1820-1910), founder of modern nursing. (T. Cole, wood engraving, National Library of Medicine, Bethesda, Md.)

of those wishing to practice professional nursing (Nightingale, 1859).

Her publications, dedication to hospital reform, commitment to upgrading conditions for the sick and wounded in the military, and establishment of training schools for nurses all greatly affected the development of nursing in the United States, as well as in her native England.

1861-1873: The American Civil War—An Impetus for Training for Nursing

At the onset of the American Civil War, there were no professional nurses available to tend the wounded and no organized system of medical care in either the Union or the Confederacy. Conditions on the battlefield and in military hospitals were horrible, with wounded and dying men lying in agony in filthy conditions. Appeals for nurses were made, and women on both sides responded. Most significant perhaps was the response by the Catholic orders, particularly the Sisters of Charity, the Sisters of Mercy, and the Sisters of the Holy Cross, who had a long history of providing care for the sick (Wall, 1995). Doubtless the most skillful and devoted of the women who nursed in the Civil War, these religious sisters were highly disciplined, organized, and efficient.

On both the Union and the Confederate sides of the war, as well as on the war's Western Front, women arose to meet the needs of the sick and wounded. A number of leaders emerged, including Dorothea L. Dix, a long-time advocate for the mentally ill in prewar years. She was appointed Superintendent of Women Nurses of the (Union) Army. In that position she was instrumental in creating a month-long training program at two New York hospitals for women who wished to serve. Thousands of women volunteered. Among the women who served the Union forces were several African-American women, including Sojourner Truth, a famous abolitionist, and Harriet Tubman, a former field slave who established the "underground railroad" and herself led numerous slaves to freedom. Another former slave, Susie King Taylor, first worked as a laundress but was called on to assist as a nurse. She is noted for teaching soldiers, African-American and white, how to read and write.

Nightingale set about the task of organizing and cleaning the hospital and providing care to the wounded soldiers. Armed with an excellent education in statistics, Nightingale collected very detailed data on morbidity and mortality of the soldiers in Scutari. Using this supportive evidence, she effectively argued the case for reform of the entire British Army medical system.

Following the Crimean War, Nightingale founded the first training school for nurses at St. Thomas's Hospital in London (1860), which would become the model for nursing education in the United States. Perhaps her most famous publication is the 1859 *Notes on Nursing: What It Is and What It Is Not.* In this document Nightingale stated clearly for the first time that mastering a unique body of knowledge was required

Mary Ann ("Mother") Bickerdyke, an uneducated, widowed housekeeper known locally for her nursing ability, was sent to the Western Front to investigate the situation in the hospital camp at Cairo, Illinois, where she found appalling conditions. Bickerdyke had no official authority and was opposed by the camp surgeons, but this did not deter her efforts to bring order out of chaos and create clean, if not sanitary, conditions. Even though she was not a formally trained nurse she provided much needed nursing services and deserves her place in history.

Clara Barton is another well-known nursing pioneer. Barton, a Massachusetts woman who worked as a copyist in the U.S. Patent Office, began an independent campaign to provide relief for the soldiers. Appealing to the nation for supplies of woolen shirts, blankets, towels, lanterns, camp kettles, and other necessities (Barton, 1862), she established her own system of distribution, refusing to enlist in the military nurse corps headed by Dorothea Dix (Oates, 1994). Barton took a leave of absence from her patent job, and traveled to Culpeper, Virginia. At the scene of the battle, she set up a makeshift field hospital and cared for the wounded and dying. During this battle, Barton gained her famous title, "Angel of the Battlefield." Her efforts did not end with the war. Barton went on to found an organization whose name is synonymous with compassionate service: the American Red Cross.

The women of the South also responded by demonstrating a vast outpouring of support for their soldiers. Until the last months of 1861 and early 1862, Confederate hospitals were staffed by female volunteers or wounded soldiers. When the Confederate government assumed control, several women were appointed as superintendents of hospitals. Superintendent Sallie Thompkins, who had earlier established a private hospital in Richmond, Virginia, was commissioned a "captain of Cavalry, unassigned" by Confederate President Jefferson Davis, and was the only woman in the Confederacy to hold military rank.

Although thousands of women supported the war effort, only a few were appointed as matrons of hospitals. One of the earliest to be placed in charge was Phoebe Pember. Before her September 1862 assignment to Chimborazo Hospital, a sprawling government-run institution on the western boundary of Richmond, Virginia, the care was provided by "sick or wounded men, convalescing and placed in that position, however ignorant they might be—until strong enough for field duty" (Pember, 1959, p. 18).

The Civil War, for all of its destruction and horror, helped to advance the cause of professional nursing as these leaders, even though largely untrained, demonstrated dramatic improvements in care. The success in the reform of military hospitals would open the doors for reform of civilian hospital facilities throughout the country (Rosenberg, 1987).

After the Civil War: Moving Toward Education and Licensure Under the Challenges of Segregation

The move toward formal education and training for nurses grew after the Civil War. Support was garnered from physicians, as well as the United States Sanitary Commission. At the American Medical Association meeting of 1869, Dr. Samuel Gross, chair of the Committee on the Training of Nurses, put forth three proposals regarding nursing training. The most important of these was the recommendation that large hospitals begin the process of developing training schools for nurses. Simultaneously, members of the United States Sanitary Commission, who had served during the war and learned its lessons, began to lobby for the creation of nursing schools (Donahue, 1996). Support for their efforts gained momentum as advocates of social reform reported the shockingly inadequate conditions that existed in many hospitals.

The first training schools for nurses and the feminization of nursing

The first three American training schools for nurses, modeled after Nightingale's famous school at St. Thomas's Hospital in London, opened in 1873. They were the Bellevue Training School for Nurses in New York City, Connecticut Training School for Nurses in New Haven, and

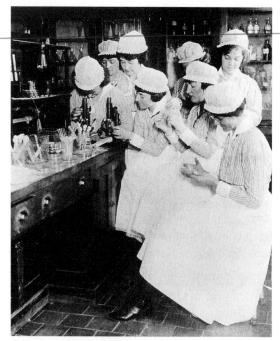

Figure 2-2 Nurses training in the bacteriologic laboratory at Bellevue Hospital, New York City, circa 1900. (The Bettman Archive, New York.)

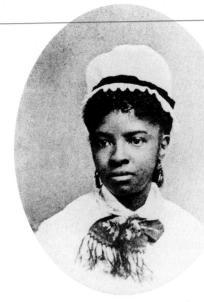

Figure 2-3 Mary Eliza Mahoney (1845-1926), the first trained African-American nurse in the United States.

the Boston Training School for Nurses at Massachusetts General Hospital in Boston (Donahue, 1996). The first trained nurse in the United States, Linda Richards, graduated in 1874.

The Victorian belief in women's innate sensitivity and high morals led to the early requirement that applicants to these programs be women, for it was thought that these feminine qualities were useful qualities of in a nurse. Thus sensitivity, "good breeding," intelligence, and characteristics of "ladylike" behavior, including submission to authority, were highly desired personal characteristics for applicants. There was a concomitant discrimination against men entering the profession. The number of training schools increased steadily during the last decades of the nineteenth century, and by 1900 they played a critical role in providing hospitals with a stable, subservient, female workforce, as hospitals came to be staffed primarily by students (Figure 2-2).

Some schools in the North admitted a small number of African-American students to their programs. The training school at the New England Hospital for Women and Children agreed to admit one African-American and one Jewish student in each of their classes if they met all entrance qualifications. Mary Eliza Mahoney (Figure 2-3), the first African-American professionally educated nurse, received her training there. Historical Note 2-1 gives some details about Mahoney.

The development of separate nursing schools for African Americans reflected the segregated American society. African Americans received care at separate hospitals from whites and were cared for by black nurses. The first program established exclusively for training of African-American women in nursing was established at the Atlanta Baptist Female Seminary (later Spelman Seminary, now Spelman College) in Atlanta, Georgia, in 1886. This program was 2 years long and led to a diploma in nursing. Spelman closed its program in 1928 after graduating 117 nurses (Carnegie, 1995).

Male students were not allowed in the early nursing schools that enrolled women. The earliest school established exclusively for the training of men in nursing was the School for Male Nurses

HISTORICAL NOTE 2-1

Mary Eliza Mahoney (1845-1926) is known as the first educated, professionally trained African-American nurse (Miller, 1986). She began her nursing training at the New England Hospital for Women and Children at age 33 years. An inscription in records from the New England Hospital reads "Mary E. Mahoney, first coloured girl admitted" (Miller, p 19). The course of study was rigorous and admission highly competitive. When Ms. Mahoney applied, there were 40 applicants; 18 were accepted for a probationary period, only half of those (9) were kept after probation, and only 3 received the diploma. Mahoney was one of the three. As was common in her day, her practice mainly consisted of private duty nursing with families in the Boston area. To celebrate her accomplishments and her status as the first African-American professional nurse, the Mary Mahoney Award was established by the National Association of Colored Graduate Nurses in 1935, with the first award given in 1936. This organization was later blended with the American Nurses Association.

at the New York City Training School, established in 1886. The Mills College of Nursing at Bellevue Hospital was the second male school, founded in 1888. In 1898 the Alexian Brothers Hospital in Chicago established a nursing school to train males. They opened a second school in 1928 in St. Louis. Nursing was stratified into black/white/male/female in the late nineteenth century.

Professionalization through organization

The 1893 Chicago World's Fair was an unlikely setting for a turning point in nursing's history. Several influential nursing leaders of the century, including Isabel Hampton (Robb), Lavinia Lloyd Dock, and Bedford Fenwick of Great Britain, gathered to share ideas and discuss issues pertaining to nursing education. Isabel Hampton (Robb) presented a paper in which she protested the lack of uniformity across nursing schools, which led to inadequate curriculum development and nursing education. A paper by Florence Nightingale on the need for scientific training of nurses was presented at this same meeting. Also at this event the precursor to the National League for Nursing, the American Society of Superintendents of Training Schools for Nurses, was formed to address issues in nursing education. The society changed its name in 1912 to the National League of Nursing Education (NLNE) and in 1952 became the National League for Nursing (NLN). This event held during the Chicago World's Fair became a pivotal point in nursing history.

Three years later, in 1896, Isabel Hampton Robb founded the group that eventually became the American Nurses Association (ANA) in 1911. Originally known as the Nurses' Associated Alumnae of the United States and Canada, the initial mission of this group was to enhance collaboration among practicing nurses and educators.

At the close of the century, in 1899, this same group of energetic American nursing leaders, along with nursing leaders from abroad, collaborated with Bedford Fenwick of Britain to found the International Council of Nurses (ICN). The ICN was dedicated to uniting nursing organizations of all nations, and, fittingly, the first meeting was held at the World Exposition in Buffalo, New York, in 1901. At that meeting, a major topic of discussion was one that would dramatically change the practice of nursing: state registration of nurses.

Early nursing professional organizations reflected the segregation that characterized post–Civil War America. Initially, minority group nurses were excluded from the ANA. After 1916, African-American nurses were admitted to membership through their constituent (state) associations in parts of the country, but states in the South and the District of Columbia barred their membership. African-American nurses recognized the need for their own professional organization to manage their specific challenges. Martha Franklin sent 1500 letters to African-American nurses and nursing schools across the country to gather support for this idea (Carnegie, 1995). In response, the National Association of Colored Graduate Nurses (NACGN) was formed in 1908 in New York with the objectives of achieving

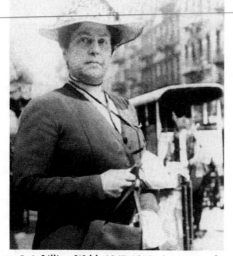

Figure 2-4 Lillian Wald, 1867-1940. A nurse and social activist, Wald founded the Henry Street Settlement, which is still in operation today, and was one of the founders of the NAACP.

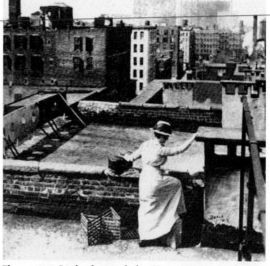

Figure 2-5 Little deterred the Henry Street Settlement nurses from making their daily rounds on their patients in New York's Lower East Side.

higher professional standards, breaking down discriminatory practices faced by "Negro" nurses in schools of nursing and nursing organizations, and developing leadership among African-American nurses. The group dissolved in 1951 after deciding it had met these objectives. The ANA had by that time committed full support to minority groups, as well as abolishment of discrimination in all aspects of the profession.

Nursing's focus on social justice: The Henry Street Settlement

Early in the twentieth century, the young profession of nursing was called on to address the serious health conditions related to the influx of immigrants who came seeking work in the factories of the Northeast. Poverty-stricken and overcrowded, primitive living conditions in inner city tenements became a target for infectious diseases. It was in response to these conditions that the Henry Street Settlement was established on New York's Lower East Side. Its founder, Lillian Wald (Figure 2-4), obtained financial assistance from private sources and began the first formalized

public health nursing practice. Her colleague Lavinia Dock, a social activist and reformer, assisted Wald in providing services through visiting nurses and clinics that cared for well babies, treated minor illnesses, prevented disease transmission, and provided health education to the neighborhood (Cherry and Jacob, 2005). The nurses were relentless in their goal to improve the health of the immigrants who were seeking better lives in America (Figure 2-5). Historical Note 2-2 describes another pioneering nurse, Margaret Sanger, whose work was inspired by the plight of immigrant women on the Lower East Side. Sanger became the face of the battle for safe contraception and family planning for women. Her work was sometimes dangerous and always controversial, yet she persisted in her work to preserve reproductive and contraceptive rights for women. The Henry Street Settlement still functions today to fight urban poverty in New York's Lower East Side (http://www.henrystreet.org).

A common cause but still segregated

Tuberculosis was a major health problem in the teeming slums of the newly developing cities. Dr. Edward T. Devine, president of the Charity

HISTORICAL NOTE 2-2

Margaret Sanger, a nurse who worked on the Lower East Side of New York City in 1912, was struck by the lack of knowledge of immigrant women about pregnancy and contraception. After witnessing the death of Sadie Sachs from a self-attempted abortion, Sanger was inspired to action by the tragedy and became determined to teach women about birth control. A radical activist in her early years, Sanger devoted the remainder of her life to the birth control movement and became a national figure in that cause (Kennedy, 1970).

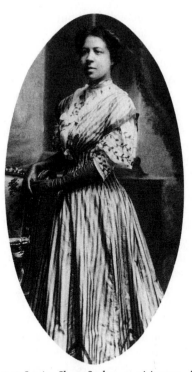

Figure 2-6 Jessie Sleet Scales, a visionary African-American nurse, was among the first to bring community health nursing principles to the slums of New York City around 1900. (Reproduced with permission of the E. M. Carnegie Collection, Archives of Hampton University.)

Organization Society, noted the high incidence of tuberculosis among New York City's African-American population. Aware of racial barriers and cultural resistance to seeking medical care, Dr. Devine determined that a "Negro" district nurse should be hired to work in the African-American community to persuade people to accept treatment. Jessie Sleet Scales (Figure 2-6), an African-American nurse who had been trained at Providence Hospital in Chicago, a hospital exclusively for "colored people," was hired as a district nurse on a trial basis. Her report to the Charity Organization Society was published in the *American Journal of Nursing* in 1901, titled "A Successful Experiment":

> *I beg to render to you a report of the work done by me as a district nurse among the colored people of New York City during the months of October and November. . . . I have visited forty-one families and made 156 calls in connection with these families, caring for nine cases of consumption, four cases of peritonitis, two cases of chickenpox, two cases of cancer, one case of diphtheria, two cases of heart disease, two cases of tumor, one case of gastric catarrh, two cases of pneumonia, four cases of rheumatism, and two cases of scalp wound. I have given baths, applied poultices, dressed wounds, washed and dressed newborn babies, cared for mothers. . . . (Sleet, 1901, p. 729).*

Jessie Sleet Scales later recommended to Lillian Wald that Elizabeth Tyler, a graduate of Freedmen's Hospital Training School for Nurses, work with African-American patients at the Henry Street Settlement. Working within the confines of segregation, Scales and Tyler established the Stillman House, a branch of the Henry Street Settlement serving "colored people" in a small store on West 61st Street. For community health nursing, the addition of these pioneer African-American nurses to the ranks of the Henry Street Settlement signified activism, expansion, and growth. Despite the ever-present racial barriers and deplorable living and health conditions, these courageous young women succeeded in providing excellent nursing care to underserved families with burgeoning but manageable health problems. The common focus on prevention of illness and management of illness bound these visionary nurses across racial lines.

War again creates the need for nurses: Spanish-American War

In 1898, the United States Congress declared war on Spain, and once again, nursing had a major role in the care of the sick and injured in war. Anita M. McGee, MD, was appointed head of the Hospital Corps, a group formed to recruit nurses. Encouraged by Isabel Hampton Robb and the fledgling Nurses' Associated Alumnae of the United States and Canada, McGee initially wanted only graduates of nurse training schools in the Hospital Corps (Wall, 1995). It soon became apparent that this requirement could not be met. A widespread epidemic of typhoid fever created a greater need than anticipated, and as a result others, including the Sisters of the Holy Cross and untrained African-American nurses who had had typhoid fever in the past, were accepted for service (Wall, 1995). Namahyoke Curtis was employed as a contract nurse by the War Department during the Spanish-American War, making her the first trained African-American nurse in this capacity. Although McGee and Robb had to enlist untrained persons to care for the sick and wounded during the Spanish-American War, their efforts set the stage for the development of a permanent Army Nurse Corps (1901) and Navy Nurse Corps (1908) (Figure 2-7).

Professionalization and Standardization of Nursing Through Licensure

The institution of state licensure for nurses was a huge milestone for nursing in the early twentieth century. Early efforts at licensure were not well received. After an educational campaign, the ICN passed a resolution asking each country and state to provide for licensure of the nurses working there. As a result, state legislatures in North Carolina, New Jersey, New York, and Virginia passed what were termed permissive licensure laws for nursing in 1903. Nurses did not have to be registered to practice but could not use the title of registered nurse (RN) unless they were registered.

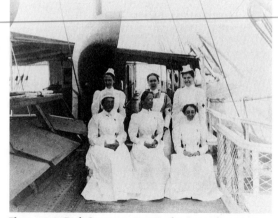

Figure 2-7 Red Cross nursing in the Spanish-American War, circa 1898. Nurses on deck of the hospital ship *Relief* near Cuba. (National Library of Medicine, Bethesda, Md.)

By 1923 all states required examinations for permissive licensure, but these examination were not standardized (Cherry and Jacob, 2005). It was not until the 1930s that New York became the first state to have mandatory licensure; however, this was not fully mandated until 1947. In 1950 the NLN assumed responsibility for administering the first nationwide State Board Test Pool Examination.

A key event during this decade was the publication of the first edition of the *American Journal of Nursing* in October 1900. Those working to bring this project to fruition included nurse leaders Isabel Hampton Robb, Mary Adelaide Nutting, Lavinia L. Dock, Sophia Palmer, and Mary E. Davis. Sophia Palmer, director of nursing at Rochester City Hospital, New York, was appointed as the first editor, with "the aim of the editors to present month by month the most useful facts, the most progressive thought and the latest news that the profession has to offer in the most attractive form that can be secured" (Palmer, 1900, p. 64).

1917-1930: The Challenges of the Flu Epidemic, World War I, and the Early Depression Era

Two significant events coincided in 1917 to challenge nursing: the United States entered World War I, and an influenza epidemic swept the

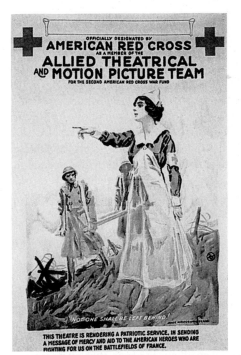

Figure 2-8 A World War I Red Cross nursing poster, 1918. "Not one shall be left behind!" by James Montgomery Flagg is typical of World War I recruitment posters. Nurses answered the call in record numbers. (Collection of the Library of Congress.)

country. The concept of using trained female nurses to care for soldiers had been proved in earlier wars; therefore when the United States entered the war in Europe, the National Committee on Nursing was formed (Dock and Stewart, 1920). This committee was chaired by Mary Adelaide Nutting, professor of Nursing and Health at Columbia University, and included Jane A. Delano, director of Nursing in the American Red Cross, among others. Charged with supplying an adequate number of trained nurses to U.S. Army hospitals abroad, the committee initiated a national publicity campaign to recruit young women to enter nurses training (Figure 2-8), established the Army School of Nursing with Annie Goodrich as dean, introduced college women to nursing in the Vassar Training Camp for Nurses, and began widespread public education in home nursing and hygiene through Red

HISTORICAL NOTE 2-3

On the home front, the flu epidemic of 1917 to 1919 increased the public's awareness of the necessity of public health nursing. Across the nation, the public health service, American Red Cross, and Visiting Nursing Associations mobilized to provide care for the thousands of citizens struck with influenza. In spring 1919, the second wave of the flu epidemic struck the East Coast and swept across the country. Although not as lethal as the first, the flu epidemic closed businesses, schools, and churches and increased demands for nursing services.

Cross nursing. Historical Note 2-3 describes the impact of the influenza epidemic on the nation and the profession.

By the time World War I ended, nursing had demonstrated its ability both to provide care to the war wounded and to respond effectively to the influenza epidemic at home. In 1920 Congress passed a bill that provided nurses with military rank (Dock and Stewart, 1920). The 1920s also saw increased use of hospitals and an acceptance of the scientific basis of medicine.

Two other noteworthy events of the decade included the publication of the Goldmark Report, a study of nursing education (discussed in Chapter 7) that advocated the establishment of collegiate schools of nursing rather than hospital-based diploma programs, and establishment of programs in rural midwifery.

An important development in the pre-Depression eras was the establishment of the Frontier Nursing Service (FNS) in 1925. Mary Breckinridge, a nurse and midwife, established the Kentucky Committee for Mothers and Babies, later known as the FNS. This service provided the first organized midwifery program in the United States. Nurses of the FNS worked in isolated rural areas in the Appalachian Mountains, traveling by horseback to serve the health needs of the poverty-stricken mountain people (Figure 2-9). FNS nurses delivered babies, provided prenatal and postnatal care, educated mothers and

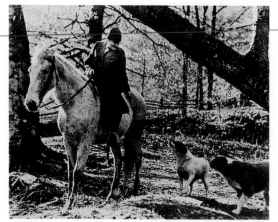

Figure 2-9 Mary Breckinridge, founder of the FNS, on her way to visit patients in rural Kentucky. (Used with permission of the Frontier Nursing Service, Wendover, Ky.)

their families about nutrition and hygiene, and cared for the sick. Through this rural midwifery service, Breckinridge demonstrated that nurses could play a significant role in providing primary rural health care.

1931-1945: Challenges of the Great Depression and World War II

With hospitals largely staffed by nursing students, most graduate nurses worked as private duty nurses in patients' homes. The Great Depression meant that many families could no longer afford nursing services, forcing many nurses into unemployment. In 1933 President Franklin D. Roosevelt established the Civil Works Administration (CWA) in which nurses participated by providing rural and school health services. They also took part in specific projects, such as conducting health surveys on communicable disease and nutrition of children (Fitzpatrick, 1975). Hospitals, also affected by economic turmoil, were forced to close their schools of nursing. As a result, they no longer had a reliable, inexpensive student workforce at the time there was a dramatic increase in the number of patients needing charity care. The solution soon became apparent: unemployed graduate nurses, willing to work for minimum pay, were recruited to work in the hospitals rather than doing private duty for wealthy

families. This had a lasting impact on the staffing of hospitals.

The Social Security Act (SSA) of 1935, a significant part of President Roosevelt's plans to bring the nation out of the Depression, enhanced the practice of public health nursing. One of its purposes was to strengthen public health services and to provide medical care for crippled children and the blind. With funds from the SSA, public health nursing became the major avenue for the provision of care to dependent mothers and children, the blind, and crippled children (Cherry and Jacob, 2005).

World War II: Challenges and opportunities for nursing

During World War II, the nation's military once again found itself without an adequate supply of nurses. In response Congress enacted legislation to provide $1 million for nursing education. The military and collegiate programs of nursing formed an alliance to train student nurses in what was known as the Cadet Nurse Corps. Students received tuition, books, a stipend, and a uniform in return for a promise to serve as nurses for the duration of the war in either civilian or military hospitals, the Indian Health Service, or public health facilities (Robinson and Perry, 2001). Approximately 124,000 nurses volunteered, graduated, and were certified for military services in the Army and Navy Nurse Corps during the years 1943-1948. Despite ongoing racial segregation, African-American collegiate programs, as well as the NACGN, were active participants in the Cadet Nurse Corps.

Historical Note 2-4 describes the courage of nurses in the Philippines at Corregidor and the Bataan during the World War II, who were held in captivity for 3 years in an internment camp.

1945-1960: The Rise of Hospitals— Bureaucracy, Science, and Shortages

The professionalization of nursing continued after the end of World War II. In 1947 military nurses were awarded full commissioned officer status in both the Army and the Navy Nurse Corps, and segregation of African-American nurses was

HISTORICAL NOTE 2-4

Hours after Pearl Harbor was attacked on December 7, 1941, a successful surprise attack on U.S. installations in the Philippines crippled the air force in the South Pacific. Over 100 nurses were enlisted with the U.S. Army and Navy units in the Philippines at that time. Some of the most dramatic stories in nursing's history played out over the next weeks and months during the Japanese take-over of the Bataan peninsula, a large land mass at the northern tip of the Philippines, and then Corregidor, a small island (about 6 square miles) in a strategically advantageous location at the opening on the Manila Bay. Nurses proved their ingenuity, commitment, and intelligence during the first months of 1942 as they were forced to provide care under the most extreme conditions. By the end of March, 1942, the 2 field hospitals that were built to handle 1,000 patients each had 11,000 patients. One month later, there were 24,000 sick and wounded. The field hospitals themselves were bombed twice. With the fall of the Bataan to Japanese control imminent, the nurses were evacuated to Corregidor.

Corregidor contained a huge bomb-proof tunnel system, a complex of a main tunnel (the Malinta Tunnel 1,400 feet long and 30 feet wide) and numerous lateral tunnels, with electricity and ventilation, and a hospital (see figure). The conditions deep in the tunnel were a stark contrast to the horrors of the Bataan. Over the next few weeks, conditions deteriorated in the tunnel. Corregidor was under relentless air attack by the Japanese; the numbers of wounded soldiers increased, until finally 1000 young men were being cared for by the nurses in a space where power outages, poor ventilation, oppressive heat, and vermin were common

Although many nurses were evacuated from Corregidor before the final takeover of the island fortress

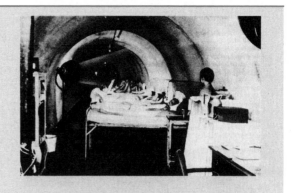

by Japan, about 85 American and Filipino nurses remained in the tunnel hospital, attending to the wounded. On May 4, 1942, the American forces on Corregidor surrendered. The nurses remaining on Corregidor were confined to the tunnel hospital, not allowed to go outside for fresh air, were given two small meals a day, and continued to provide care for 1000 sick and injured soldiers. This continued for 6 weeks, until they were moved to the old hospital site outside the tunnel. One week later, they were bound for Manila, not knowing that they were soon to be providing care at an internment camp, where they would spend the next 33 months in captivity. On February 3, 1945, U.S. troops liberated the internment camp.

For more details of the nurses ordeal at Bataan, Corregidor and the internment camp, these are excellent resources:

Kalisch PA, Kalisch, BJ: Nurses under fire: the World War II experiences of nurses on Bataan and Corregidor, *Nurs Res* 44(5): 260-271.

Norman E: *We band of angels: the untold story of American nurses trapped on Bataan by the Japanese*, New York, 1999, Random House.

---

ended. Julie O. Flikke was the first nurse to be promoted to the rank of colonel in the U.S. Army. In 1954 men were allowed to enter the military nursing corps.

In 1946 the Hill-Burton Act was enacted, providing funds to construct hospitals and leading to a surge in the growth of new facilities. This rapid expansion in the number of hospital beds resulted

in an acute shortage of nurses and increasingly difficult working conditions. Long hours, inadequate salaries, and increasing patient loads made many nurses unhappy with their jobs, and threats of strikes and collective bargaining ensued.

In response to the shortages, "team nursing" was introduced. Team nursing involved the provision of care to a group of patients by a group of care providers. Although efficient, the method fragmented patient care and removed the RN from the bedside. Another response to the shortage was the institution of the associate degree in nursing, discussed in more detail in Chapter 7. As nursing continued to search for its identity, it focused on the scientific bases for nursing practice. Clinical nursing research began in earnest, and the *Journal of Nursing Research* was first published.

1961-1985: The Great Society, Vietnam, and the Change in Roles for Women

Two 1965 amendments to the SSA, designed to ensure access to health care for elderly, poor, and disabled Americans, resulted in the establishment of Medicare and Medicaid. Soon after, hospitals began to rely heavily on reimbursements from Medicare and Medicaid. Because the majority of the care for the sick was taking place in hospitals rather than homes, the hospital setting became the preferred place of employment for nurses. This gave rise to new opportunities and roles for nurses.

The 1960s were the era of specialty care and clinical specialization for nurses. The successful development of the clinical specialist role in psychiatric nursing—combined with the proliferation of intensive care units and technologic advances of the period—fostered the growth of clinical specialization in many areas of nursing, including cardiac-thoracic surgery and coronary care. The increase in medical specialization, along with the concurrent shortage of primary care physicians and the public demand for improved access to health care that grew out of President Lyndon B. Johnson's "Great Society" reforms, fostered the emergence of the nurse practitioner (NP) in primary care. In 1971 Idaho became the first state to recognize diagnosis and treatment as part of the legal scope of practice for NPs.

Again, war—this time in Vietnam—provided nurses with opportunities to stretch the boundaries of the discipline. The Vietnam War occurred in jungles not easily accessed by rescue workers or medics and without clearly drawn lines of combat. Mobile hospital units were set up in the jungles, where nurses often worked without the direct supervision of physicians as they fought to save lives of the wounded. They performed emergency procedures such as tracheotomies and chest tube insertions, never before executed by nurses. They also had to deal with the lack of support on home soil, where the Vietnam War was controversial and often the cause for widespread protests. The trauma of the battlefield would be intensified by this lack of support at home, and many nurses suffered posttraumatic stress disorder (PTSD), as did the returning soldiers.

1986-2010: Challenges for Nursing: Managed Care, Technology, Diversity, Terrorism

With the advent of managed care in the late 1980s and the resulting emphasis on health care reform as a way to continue to cut the costs of medical care, nursing was caught up in the whirlwind of change. Determined to take a proactive stance in the reform effort, the nursing profession wrote its Agenda for Health Care Reform in 1992. The plan for reform was comprehensive and focused on restructuring the health care system in the United States to reduce costs and improve access to care. Although health care reform did not pass in Congress in the early days of the Clinton administration, insurance companies nevertheless demanded accountability for costs. The system of diagnostic-related groups (DRGs) and managed care were instituted in efforts to improve quality of care within the context of reducing costs. This era is marked by attempts to obtain third-party reimbursement for advanced practice nurses in both primary and acute care.

Another major development in the last years of the twentieth century was the incredibly rapid influx of medical and informational technology. Electronic medical records became common, with a goal for the U.S. health care system to go paperless completely. Digitized medical records allow for access across disciplines and across distance, with the goal to improve continuity of health care no matter where a person requires medical treatment. In many institutions, nurses enter patient data into computers at the bedside. Life-sustaining medical technologies have created new ethical challenges for nurses, who continue to be the first line of defense on behalf of their vulnerable patients. This role has never changed for nurses.

Many of the issues that confronted nurses of the past still confront nurses today. War, epidemic, poverty, and immigration are still threats to the public welfare. With an increasing interest in global health, nurses are finding that, although many infectious diseases have been managed, HIV/AIDS and malaria still threaten the health of a generation of people in Africa and other underdeveloped parts of the world. Nurses are increasingly aware of the need for cultural humility in providing care to others with whom nurses share little in common demographically. Significant language barriers exist as nurses manage the care of large numbers of Latinos who have immigrated into the United States in recent years. And with ongoing conflicts in Iraq and Afghanistan, many soldiers are returning to the United States with significant injuries that will need management for a very long time. Understanding the past helps us meet the challenges of the present and plan for the future.

SOCIAL CONTEXT OF NURSING

No endeavor functions separately from its social and historical context. Nursing is no exception. The influences on nursing in several contexts are identified and discussed in the remaining pages of this chapter. The social context also influences who chooses nursing as a career.

As you read this section, think about what drew you into the profession of nursing. What is the story of your individual journey into nursing? One nurse's story is found in the Critical Thinking Challenge 2-1. As you read her story, identify factors that influenced her choice of career. Then think of your own story and identify social forces that have influenced your career choice. Spend a few minutes now to reflect on your own individual journey toward nursing.

Several social factors that have influenced the development of professional nursing will be explored in this section, including:

- Gender
- The image of nursing
- National population trends
- Technology
- The shortage of nursing

Gender

Gender is a social construction of behaviors, roles, beliefs, and values that are specific to females or males. Gender is not the same as sex, which is a biologic entity. A fundamental example has to do with asking a pregnant woman whether she is having a girl or a boy. This is a question of

---

CRITICAL THINKING *Challenge 2-1*

One Nurse's Journey Into Nursing

Instructions: Analyze the story below and determine some of the factors that influenced this nurse's choice of a career. What assumptions did she make about the profession before entering it? Were her assumptions accurate or inaccurate? How would her assumptions hold up today?

"During childhood I had taken care of wounded dogs and played nurse to numerous dolls. I watched as my grandmother made cough syrup with tree bark, applied snuff to wasp bites, and practiced a variety of other healing treatments for our extended family. But maybe my real fascination for nursing can be attributed to my neighbor who was a nurse.

During the summers or other times when school was out I watched her leave for work in her crisp white uniform, white hose, and white shoes. When I was in fourth grade she came and talked to our class about health. Throughout my years in school I was an excellent student but never considered any other career. My algebra and trigonometry teacher tried relentlessly to steer me to major in math since that was my favorite subject in school, but for the life of me I could not fathom how a career in math could be exciting or challenging. And so it was that I entered a baccalaureate program in nursing following high school graduation."

☼ EVIDENCE-BASED PRACTICE NOTE

Kimberly Powell and Lori Abels are researchers who examined children's television programs to assess the manner in which gender roles were presented. They defined sex-role as "a set of activities deemed appropriate for one sex but not the other" and sex-role stereotypes as existing when "actions are thought of as simply masculine or feminine and tend to be resistant to change" (p. 14). Powell and Abels decided to focus on two popular television programs aimed at preschool (aged 2 to 5 years) children—*Barney & Friends* and *Teletubbies*—for gendered themes, characteristics, and messages within the programs. For a theme to be identified, both researchers must have spotted it and it had to appear in at least half the episodes, which they viewed separately to avoid influencing each other.

After studying 10 episodes of each program, these researchers found that gendered messages and behaviors were presented in a number of ways. For example, female characters were usually followers; they looked feminine, that is, small or petite; they were underrepresented in the occupations portrayed; they played feminine roles such as

caretaker or peacemaker; and they were shown in activities such as braiding hair, cooking, and washing dishes. Male characters were usually leaders; appeared in a variety of masculine occupations and roles, such as playing basketball, driving a bulldozer, or building a wall; were larger physically; and were stereotypically male in appearance. Socially, males were active and females passive.

The researchers concluded that both programs did well at opening up acceptable behavior choices for boys, such as being cooperative and social, yet they maintained sex-role stereotypes such as caretaker and follower for girls. They made three suggestions for improving gender representation in preschool television programs:

1. Depict women as construction workers or men as child care providers to present children with more options in learning what men and women can do.
2. Alternate males and females as leaders.
3. Design some programs that show females in action with males observing, or better yet, all working together and equally active.

Powell KA, Abels L: Sex-role stereotypes in TV programs aimed at the preschool audience: an analysis of *Teletubbies* and *Barney & Friends*, *Women Language* 25(2):14-22, 2002.

biology—is she pregnant with an XX or an XY? If the woman responds, "It's a boy—he's big and strong, and he moves so much that I can tell he's going to be a professional football player someday!", she has assigned a gender to the biologic entity of a male fetus. Because the fetus is large and active, she has interpreted this behavior in light of the fetal sex—he is going to be a huge, professional athlete.

Assignment of gender roles starts early (even before birth in some cases!), as part of socialization, the process through which values and expectations are transmitted from generation to generation. See the Evidence-Based Practice Note. Parents and others in a child's sphere of influence teach lessons about gender roles and behavior, both intentionally and unintentionally.

A consequence of this is that gender role stereotyping occurs. Stereotypes are also social constructions that portray how men and women "ought" to behave in society or within their cultural group. Some common gender role stereotypes of women identified by Cummings (1995) are found in Box 2-1.

Gender role stereotyping can be subtle. For instance, the pregnant woman described above is probably very unlikely to paint the nursery pink—a color associated with "girls," although it may be the mother's favorite color and she would love to have a pink room.

Gender-specific stereotypes have affected nursing for 160 years. When nursing as a modern profession began in the mid-1800s, the most common roles assumed by women were within

Box 2-1   Common Gender Role Stereotypes of Women

MOTHER
- Subrogates own needs
- Freely gives advice
- Becomes the peacemaker
- Fosters dependence
- Is passive, wants recognition

IRON MAIDEN
- Is competitive versus collaborative
- Possesses the ability to "be in charge"
- Gives critical feedback
- Sets rigid interpersonal boundaries
- Can be unapproachable

SUPERWOMAN
- Demands perfection
- Will not delegate
- Overcommits her time
- Assumes multiple roles
- Feels isolated, not supported

Based on Cummings SH: Attila the Hun versus Attila the hen: gender socialization of the American nurse, *Nurs Adm Q* 19(2):25, 1995.

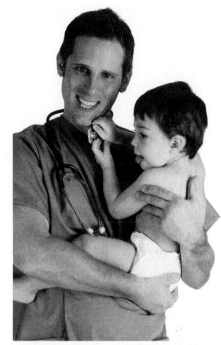

Figure 2-10 Nurses who are men are found in every setting in U.S. hospitals today. This RN enjoys his work with children. (iStockphoto.com.)

their families and involved caring for others, maintaining a household, and pleasing their husbands. "Respectable" women did not work outside the home for money but rather relied on their husbands or families for support. The first formal schools of nursing in the United States were developed to attract these "respectable women" into nursing, which was designed to increase the value society put on nursing. Stereotyping of women also included the notion that women were intellectually inferior to men, and hence women were not called on to make decisions or think. This type of stereotyping shaped the type of training that nurses received, basically task oriented, and this form of instruction persisted for many years.

Men are not new to the profession of nursing. During the eleventh, twelfth, and thirteenth centuries in Europe they supplied much of the nursing care, often within the authority of military or religious orders. Florence Nightingale worked hard to establish nursing as a worthy career for respectable women, largely ignoring the historical contributions of men. The male role as she saw it was confined to supplying physical strength, such as lifting, moving, or controlling patients, when needed. Early schools of nursing in the United States did not admit men, establishing an early tradition of discrimination in the profession. An exception was psychiatric nursing, which often required physical stamina and strength and was therefore considered an appropriate setting for men in nursing (Figure 2-10).

Today, about 8% of students enrolled in undergraduate programs are men. Men in nursing, as compared to women in nursing, are likely to be younger, to be employed full-time in nursing, to have more nonnursing education, and to have chosen nursing as a second career. Their motivations for entering nursing, however, are similar to those of their female counterparts. The top three reasons identified by men for becoming nurses

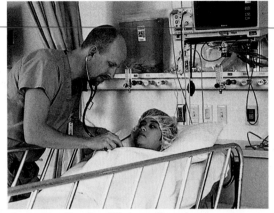

Figure 2-11 In spite of their small numbers, men in nursing play an important role in the profession.

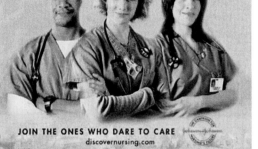

Figure 2-12 An example of an advertisement that depicts men in nursing in a favorable way. (Reprinted with permission from Johnson & Johnson, Campaign for Nursing's Future.)

are (1) a desire to help people, (2) the perception that nursing is a growth profession with many career paths, and (3) the desire to have a stable career (Hart, 2005) (Figures 2-11 and 2-12).

In 1974, the American Assembly for Men in Nursing (AAMN) was organized to address, discuss, and influence factors that affect men in nursing. Open to men and women, this national organization has local chapters, most of which are clustered in the mid-Atlantic states. The goals for this organization are as follows:

- Encourage men of all ages to become nurses and join together with all nurses in strengthening and humanizing health care
- Support men who are nurses to grow professionally and demonstrate to one another and to society the increasing contributions being made by men within the nursing profession
- Advocate for continued research, education, and dissemination of information about men's health issues, men in nursing, and nursing knowledge at the local and national levels
- Support members' full participation in the nursing profession and its organizations and use this assembly for the limited objectives stated above (AAMN, 2003).

Traditionally, men interested in health care became physicians and, later, dentists or physical therapists; women became nurses. Men who

elect to become nurses report feeling role strain, an emotional reaction that may be felt by a person in a profession that has a social structure dominated by members of the opposite sex. Role strain can create anxiety and discontent. The public lacks awareness that men can be well suited for nursing. Patients commonly assume that a man delivering health care is either a physician or a medical student. A popular movie referred to a man in nursing as a "murse," and a great many disparaging comments were made about his chosen profession.

Social change in the 1960s had a profound effect on society and has both hurt and helped the nursing profession. Women began to recognize that they had career opportunities beyond the traditional "female" ones such as teaching and nursing. Gifted women who might have otherwise become nurses pursued careers in a variety of other fields. This meant that nursing faced more competition for students than it once did because of the heightened interest in other careers by young women. Women sought opportunities that offered more competitive salaries, better working conditions, and schedules more accommodating to family life.

An interesting recent phenomenon has occurred, however. Across the United States nursing programs are seeing an increasing number of applicants who have degrees in other areas or who have had careers in other disciplines such as schoolteachers, attorneys, engineers, computer programmers, accountants, businesspeople, and other health-related occupations. The current appeal of nursing to both men and women in this category seems to be related to the fact that a career in nursing can provide economic and job security. A more significant reason for this trend is that in spite of the wide array of career choices available to men and women, nursing's appeal is strong to people of both genders who want to make a difference in the lives of others.

The women's movement helped nursing by bringing economic issues such as low salaries and poor working conditions into the open. The movement provoked a conscious awareness that equality and autonomy for women were inherent rights, not privileges, and stimulated the passage of legislation to ensure those rights.

Nursing also benefited from the women's movement in more subtle ways. As nursing students were increasingly educated in colleges and universities, they were exposed to campus activism, protests, and organizations that were trying to change the status of women. Learning informal lessons about power and how to bring about change had a positive effect on students, who later used this knowledge to improve the status of nursing. With the firm commitment of all of its practitioners, the profession of nursing can give voice to all its members, male and female, and ultimately contribute to the advancement of society at large.

Image of Nursing

A quick "moderate safe" search of images available on a popular search engine using the word "nurse" recently resulted in 12.5 million results. Of the first 10 images, three were cartoons in which the nurse is holding an oversized syringe. Three others were of pleasant-looking young white women, all holding clipboards, two wearing scrubs, the third in a traditional white cap and dress. One was of a white man wearing scrubs,

leaning forward while sitting on a bench, looking soulfully into the camera. Only the caption gave any indication that he was a nurse. Two others were highly sexualized images of white women—one with a red cross on a cap, wearing a tight white top with a plunging neckline (and holding an oversized capsule); the other was a nurse wearing a garter, white stockings, and a very short skirt, and she too was holding an oversized syringe. (This image was in a print ad for a popular shoe in the not-too-distant past that was widely denounced by nurses.) The tenth image—the only one that represented nursing and the work of nursing well—was of a young black nurse, professionally dressed in a white top with a name badge in place, leaning over a patient with her hand over his. She appeared to be making eye contact with him. If this was a representative sample of nursing, it is no wonder that we have a shortage. If this is a representative sample of the public's image of nursing, we have an image problem.

Images are powerful. They surround us, and we become saturated by images. The images of nurses seen in advertisements and on television shows may be the first impression that people have of nursing. First impressions based on media images affect public attitudes toward the profession. Although the public's view of nursing has changed over time, most people do not appreciate the complexity and range of today's professional nursing role.

Nurses are not so identifiable in health care settings as they once were. Once worn by nurses everywhere, caps were for decades a symbol of the profession (Figure 2-13). In the United States each school had a unique cap that was instantly recognizable. Nursing schools held capping ceremonies during which they presented caps to students as a symbol of their progress toward graduation. The cap saw its demise by the late 1970s; many, if not most, nurses were glad to forgo wearing a cap, believing it was part of the stereotypical image of nursing. Some speculate, however, that a part of nursing's identity problem is attributable to the disappearance of the traditional mode of dress. With many different

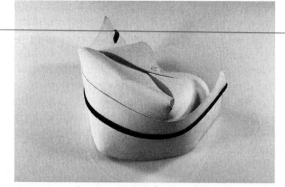

Figure 2-13 Caps were strongly identified with nursing. Each school of nursing's cap had its own shape and design. (iStockphoto.com.)

health care providers involved in the care of patients, there is no distinct way of determining who is an RN. Identification badges carry titles but are difficult to see. Interestingly, in the interest of safety, some personnel on certain units, such as urban emergency departments, are no longer putting their last names on their badges or have them in a font so small as to be unreadable in usual emergency department lighting. Some medical centers and hospitals have recently made some movement toward reestablishing identifiable dress norms across health care disciplines.

The manner in which health professionals address one another is a matter of image. Nurses in most agencies refer to themselves by first name, for example: "Good morning, my name is Dennis and I'm going to be your nurse for this shift." Physicians usually introduce themselves by title and last name, for example: "I am Dr. Roberts." It is rare to hear nurses refer to each other as "Ms. White" or "Mr. Johnson," and even rarer to hear them refer to each other as "Nurse White" or "Nurse Johnson." Nurses have reported being uncomfortable with this practice, thinking that it establishes a formality that could interfere with the nurse-patient relationship. Gordon (2005) in an informal survey of approximately 30 lay people found that the respondents did not think it would be odd for nurses to refer to themselves more

formally. Nursing educators could take the lead in restoring more professional modes of address as a norm during educational experiences. One of the most damaging images of nursing was the portrayal of a cold, sadistic, and controlling psychiatric nurse in the 1975 movie *One Flew Over the Cuckoo's Nest* by Louise Fletcher, who won an Academy Award for her role as "Nurse Ratched," a name that has become synonymous for a cold, uncaring nurse.

In spite of challenges facing the nursing profession, nurses are well respected by the public and enjoy a generally positive image (Ulmer, 2000). Results of a Harris poll in July 2000, which surveyed more than 1000 people about their attitudes toward nursing, showed the following results: 92% trusted information given by nurses, and 85% would be "pleased" if their child became a nurse (Ulrich, 2003). The accuracy of this high public regard was reinforced by annual Gallup polls from 1999 to 2005. Nurses came out on top of these polls on honesty and ethics in the professions surveyed. In 6 of the last 7 years since the nursing profession was added to the poll, nursing has rated number 1. The only exception was in 2001, when nursing ranked second to firefighters in the wake of the September 11 attacks, at a time when a great deal of positive media coverage focused on firefighters.

Foundations and corporations, as well as nursing groups, have undertaken initiatives to analyze and/or improve nursing's image. Three major initiatives are discussed here.

The Woodhull Study on Nursing and the Media

The Woodhull Study on Nursing and the Media was a comprehensive study of nursing in the print media conducted in September 1997 by 17 students and three faculty coordinators from the University of Rochester (New York) School of Nursing (URSN). In this study, sponsored by Sigma Theta Tau International (STTI) and URSN, students examined approximately 20,000 articles from 16 newspapers, magazines, and trade publications. The study was named in memory of Nancy Woodhull, a founding editor of *USA*

Box 2-2   The Woodhull Study at a Glance: Purpose, Findings, and Recommendations

---

PURPOSE OF THE STUDY

The Woodhull Study was designed to survey and analyze the portrayal of health care and nursing in U.S. newspapers, news magazines, and health care industry trade publications.

KEY STUDY FINDINGS

Nurses and the nursing profession are essentially invisible in media coverage of health care and, consequently, to the American public.

1. Nurses were cited only 4% of the time in the more than 2000 health-related articles gathered from 16 major news publications.
2. The few references to nurses or nursing that did occur were simply mentioned in passing.
3. In many of the stories, nurses and nursing would have been sources more germane to the story subject matter than the references selected.
4. Health care industry publications were no more likely to take advantage of nursing expertise, focusing more attention on bottom-line issues such as business or policy.

KEY STUDY RECOMMENDATIONS

1. Both media and nursing should take more proactive roles in establishing an ongoing dialogue.
2. The often-repeated advice in media articles and advertisements to "consult your doctor" ignores the role of nurses in health care and needs to be changed to "consult your primary health care provider."
3. Journalists should distinguish researchers with doctoral degrees from medical doctors to add clarity to health care coverage.
4. To provide comprehensive coverage of health care, the media should include information by and about nurses.
5. It is essential to distinguish health care from medicine as subject matter in the media.

Modified from Sigma Theta Tau International: *The Woodhull Study on Nursing and the Media: health care's invisible partner,* Indianapolis, Ind, 1998, Sigma Theta Tau International-Center Nursing Press.

Today. Woodhull became an advocate of nursing after her diagnosis of lung cancer, when she was impressed with the comprehensive nursing care she received. She suggested the study and assisted in the design of the survey after she became concerned about the absence of media attention to nurses and nursing.

In December 1997 the students presented their findings and recommendations to a mixed audience of nurses and national media representatives at the STTI Biennial Convention. The key finding was "Nurses and the nursing profession are essentially invisible to the media and, consequently, to the American public" (STTI, 1998, p. 8). The purpose of the Woodhull Study, its major findings, and strategies to guide the nursing profession's collective response are found in Box 2-2.

The Johnson & Johnson campaign

Johnson & Johnson, the giant health care corporation, began a multimillion dollar campaign, the Campaign for Nursing's Future, in 2002 "to enhance the image of the nursing profession, recruit new nurses and educators, and to retain nurses currently in the system" (Donelan, Buerhaus, Ulrich et al, 2005). This campaign included initiatives in print media, television advertising, student scholarships, fund raising, and research. Half of the money allotted to the campaign through 2006 was spent on publications such as posters, videos, and pamphlets, as well as television advertisement. Part of the company's efforts is also focused on increasing the number of individuals choosing nursing careers through recruitment and retention of nursing students. The campaign's website, http://www.discovernursing.com, is popular among nursing students and prospective students. The site has an easy menu of "who," "what," "why," and "how" with drop-down menus that give thorough information about nursing. Johnson & Johnson offers free materials to help promote nursing and has approximately 11 videos promoting nursing in various setting available on http://www.youtube.com through links on the Johnson & Johnson home page.

Johnson & Johnson has granted more than 500 student scholarships and more than 100 renewable faculty fellowships, and more than 100 grants to nursing schools were established and/or awarded (Smith, 2005). A survey of nursing students, chief nursing officers, and RNs (Donelan et al, 2005) found that the campaign had positive effects for nursing. Participants in this study reported significant awareness of the advertisements and the website. Even though the campaign is ongoing and the total impact has not been evaluated, early reports indicate that the positive impact will be far-reaching. This landmark effort by a major American corporation provides a stimulus to the nursing profession to partner with other entities to continue the quest for an accurate image of professional nursing, thereby addressing the nursing shortage.

Ultimately it is the professional responsibility of all nurses to reinforce positive images of nursing and, equally important, to speak out against negative ones. Nurses cannot and should not attribute their image problems to any other group, including physicians or the media. The nursing profession has the major responsibility for improving its own image. The major avenue for changing the image of nursing occurs one nurse-patient encounter at a time, where nurses demonstrate what it is nurses do and look and behave professionally. Additionally, organizations such as the ANA can enhance nursing's image by offering services as consultants to media and setting professional standards.

Box 2-3 presents a checklist for monitoring media images of nurses and nursing. Use this checklist as you view television, watch movies, read books and newspapers, and look at advertisements. Then take action:

- Write letters to those responsible for negative nursing images on television and in films.
- Write to the companies that sponsor television programs with negative images of nurses.
- Write letters to the editors of publications that present nursing in a less than favorable light.
- Boycott programs, films, and products that promote negative images of nurses and nursing.

National Population Trends

Over the course of American nursing history, nurses have responded as individuals and as a profession to wars, poverty, epidemics, and various social movements. Contemporary nursing also seeks to respond as a profession to social changes that shape our nation and the world. Two in particular will be examined here: the aging population and increasing diversity.

Aging of America

Persons in America are living longer because of more sophisticated health care and better health in general. In 2006, 37.3 million residents of the United States were aged 65 years and over (Centers for Disease Control and Prevention [CDC], 2006). Currently, the life expectancy for men at 65 years of age is 17.2 years, and for women at age 65 years the life expectancy is 20.0 years (CDC, 2006). This means that the people who have lived to 65 years of age are expected to live into their early to mid-80s. The number of people 75 years of age or older in 2020—well within the working lives of most of today's nursing students—is projected to reach 21.8 million. The very old (>85 years) represent the fastest-growing segment of the total population (see Figure 2-14). In contrast, the number of 35- to 44-year-old Americans is expected to decline from 44.7 million in 2000 to 39.6 million by 2020. This phenomenon is often referred to as "the graying of America."

People older than age 75 years are more likely than younger people to be poor, widowed, female, living alone, and suffering from chronic conditions such as arthritis, hypertension, and heart disease. As a consequence of these and other factors, this age-group uses a disproportionately higher share of health services than other

Box 2-3   Checklist for Monitoring Media Images of Nurses and Nursing

PROMINENCE IN THE PLOT

1. Are nurse characters seen in leading or supportive roles?
2. Are nurse characters shown taking an active part in the proceedings, or are they shown primarily in the background (e.g., handing instruments, carrying trays, pushing wheelchairs)?
3. To what extent are nurse characters shown in professional roles, engaged in nursing practice?
4. Do nurse characters or other characters provide the actual nursing care?
5. In scenes with nonnursing professionals (e.g., physicians, hospital administrators), who does most of the talking?

DEMOGRAPHICS

6. Does the portrayal show that men, as well as women, may aspire to a career in nursing?
7. Are nurse characters shown to be of varying ages?
8. Are some nurse characters single and others married?

PERSONALITY TRAITS

9. Are nurse characters portrayed as:

    a. Intelligent
    b. Rational
    c. Confident
    d. Ambitious

    e. Sophisticated
    f. Problem solvers
    g. Assertive
    h. Powerful

    i. Nurturant
    j. Empathic
    k. Sincere
    l. Kind

10. If other health care providers are included in the program, what differences are seen in their personality traits as compared with nurse characters?
11. When nurse characters exhibit personality traits 9a through 9h listed above, do such portrayals show them to be abnormal in some way?

PRIMARY VALUES

12. Do nurse characters exhibit values for:

    a. Service to others, humanism   b. Scholarship, achievement

13. If other health care providers are included in the program, what differences are seen in their primary values as compared with nurse characters?
14. When nurse characters exhibit the primary values of scholarship and achievement, do such portrayals show them to be abnormal in some way?

SEX OBJECTS

15. Are nurse characters portrayed as sex objects?
16. Are nurse characters referred to in sexually demeaning terms?
17. Are nurse characters presented as appealing because of their physical attractiveness or "cuteness" as opposed to their intellectual capacity, professional commitment, or skill?

ROLE OF THE NURSE

18. Is the profession of nursing shown to be an attractive and fulfilling long-term career?
19. Is the work of the nurse characters shown to be creative and exciting?

(Continued)

Box 2-3   Checklist for Monitoring Media Images of Nurses and Nursing—cont'd

CAREER ORIENTATION

20. How important is the career of nursing to the nurse character portrayed?
21. How does this compare with other professionals depicted in the program?

PROFESSIONAL COMPETENCE

22. Are nurse characters praised for their professional capabilities by other characters?
23. Do nurse characters praise other professionals?
24. Do nurse characters exhibit autonomous judgment in professional matters?
25. Is there a gratuitous message that a nurse's role in health care is a supportive rather than central one?
26. Do nurse characters positively influence patient/family welfare?
27. Are nurse characters shown harming or acting to the detriment of patients?
28. How does the professional competence of nurse characters compare with the professional competence of other health care providers?
29. When nurse characters exhibit professional competence, are they shown to be abnormal in some way?

EDUCATION

30. Who actually teaches the nursing students?
31. Who appears to be in charge of nursing education?
32. Is there evidence that the practice of nursing requires special knowledge and skills?
33. What is actually taught to nursing students?

ADMINISTRATION

34. Are any roles filled by nurse administrators or managers, or are all nurse characters shown as staff nurses or students?
35. Is there evidence of an administrative hierarchy in nursing, or are nurses shown answering to physicians or hospital administrators?
36. Are nurse characters shown turning to other nurses for assistance, or are they depicted as relying on a physician or other character (generally male) for guidance, strength, or rescuing?

OVERALL ASSESSMENT AND COMMENTS

37. Overall, is this a positive or negative portrayal of nursing? Why or why not?

age-groups. In 2006, persons 65 years of age and over recorded 229.8 million visits to physician offices. The leading causes of death in persons 65 of age and over are heart disease, cancer, and stroke (CDC, 2006). The oldest baby boomers, those Americans born between 1946 and 1964, will create a bulge in the aging population between the years 2010 and 2030. As these postwar babies age, their large numbers are expected to create an additional strain on the health care system. For the first time in U.S. history, the portion of elders is increasing as the numbers of early midlife adults are decreasing. This new disproportion that is projected to occur in the next 20 years will create stress on the economic and social systems of our nation. The graying of America will have a profound impact on the health care system and the nursing profession, stretching an already-challenged capacity to provide adequate medical and nursing care.

The nursing profession has responded to the aging population by increasing courses offered in gerontological nursing to prepare nurses to care for elders more effectively. Most nursing programs

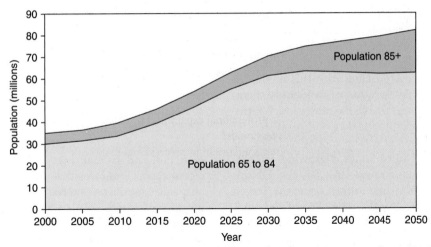

Figure 2-14 Population projections, ages 65 to 84 years and ages 85 years and over: 2000-2050. (From U.S. Department of Health and Human Services, Health Resources and Services Administration: Projected supply, demand, and shortages of registered nurses: 2000-2020, Washington, DC, 2002, Government Printing Office.)

have basic content on nursing care of the elderly integrated into the curriculum, and many baccalaureate programs have separate gerontology courses for their undergraduates. Gerontological nursing is now a specialty in which a nurse can get certification as a generalist, specialist, and NP from the American Nurses Credentialing Center (ANCC). Colleges of nursing offer master's-level preparation for gerontological clinical specialists and NPs. In spite of these responses, much remains to be done to prepare nurses for the dramatic increase in the number of aging patients they will encounter in the next few decades.

Cultural diversity

America has always been called a "melting pot" of cultures, ethnicities, and races. The means and circumstances under which persons of varying nationalities have come to the United States range considerably; however, the health care system has always been affected by the change in demographic characteristics of its population. In eras past, immigrants were most often from European and Asian countries and frequently found themselves in cultural enclaves within major cities. The residents of the tenements of the New York City Lower East Side were often immigrants; Lillian

Wald and her colleagues responded to their needs by starting what was to become the first visiting nurse association in the United States. Although descendants of Africans are part of the diverse culture of America, early Africans did not enter the country as immigrants but rather as merchandise. Modern-day African Americans' perceptions of the health care system are rooted in this unique and troublesome history and pose challenges to health care providers.

The first decade of the twenty-first century in the United States was characterized by significant immigration of Latinos from Mexico and other Central and South American countries. People from other lands often have different values, health beliefs, and practices and find that assimilation into the dominant culture is difficult. Instead of blending, as in a melting pot, individuals from other countries are increasingly appreciated for the uniqueness and flavor they bring to life in the United States. Many prefer to preserve their own cultural heritage rather than becoming "Americanized."

The exact number of persons in the various racial/ethnic groups is difficult to pinpoint. Identifying by race does not necessarily capture all the different cultures that may have migrated from a country. The concept of race as used by the U.S. Census Bureau depends on "self-identification by respondents; that is, the individual's perception of his/her racial identity" (U.S. Bureau of the Census, 2002, p. 5). A problem with this method is that biracial people are forced to identify themselves as either one race or the other, which introduces inaccuracy into the data.

The population of most minority racial/ethnic groups in the United States is growing. In 2002 the total population was 284,797,000. Of this number, non-Hispanic whites were the largest group with 196,219,000, or 68.9% of the total. The second largest and fastest growing minority group were persons of Hispanic origin, with 36,972,000, or 13%. Next in size was the African-American population, numbering 36,247,000, or 12.7%. Asians numbered 10,983,000 (3.9%) followed by Native Americans at 2,726,000 (<1%). The group identified as "other," which includes anyone who does not mark one of the five major categories on the census form, was reported at 4,552,000, or 1.6% of the total population (U.S. Census Bureau, 2002).

Projections indicate that the historically dominant Anglo-American (white) culture will become a minority by the middle of the twenty-first century. This represents a radical change in the historical demographics and attitudes of the nation. Nursing must also change to meet the requirements of the ethnic groups it serves. Propensities toward certain illnesses vary across race, ethnicity, and sex. The changing demographics of America represent a significant challenge to nursing.

Diversity in the profession

To meet the challenge of an increasingly diverse population entering the health care system, nurses need to be educated to be aware of and respectful of culture differences among their patients. The language of cultural education changes, from "cultural competence" to "cultural sensitivity" to a more recent phrase "cultural humility." This is the view that one understands that he or she cannot be competent in another's culture, but one can take a posture of willingness

to learn and gain experience about other cultures from those who inhabit the culture. Nurses from minority groups are an even smaller minority in nursing, never reaching the same proportions in the profession as they hold in the population in large. In 2000, minorities represented only 12% of all RNs, up from 10% in 1996 but still far less than the percentage of minorities in the overall population, which was 30% in 2000 (U.S. Department of Health and Human Services, 2001). A more recent report indicates that African Americans, Hispanic Americans, and Native Americans make up approximately 25% of the U.S. population but only 9% of its nurses (Maxwell, 2005). Preliminary findings from the 2004 National Sample Survey of Registered Nurses (U.S. Department of Health and Human Services, 2005) show that ethnic minority group nurses comprise 10.6% of the total number of RNs. Managers, educators, and other nursing leaders will require training so they can be culturally competent leaders for nurses and students who may have backgrounds different from their own.

Attention to the development of nurses who are attuned to culture and cultural differences has become an integral part of progressive nursing education programs so that "nurses know what health and illness mean to patients in the context of their cultural heritage" (Johnson, 2005, p. 53). You will learn more about cultural competence in Chapter 10.

Technologic Developments

The word "technology" seems to be everywhere today and has a place in many domains in health care. For purposes of this basic introduction, four types of technologic developments will be discussed: genetic, biomedical, information, and knowledge (Yoder-Wise, 2003).

Genetics, genomics, and epigenetics are three important words that have shaped and will continue to shape health care for the foreseeable future. Genetics is the science of heredity, and genomics is the study of genomes—DNA sequences. Epigenetics is a new and important field of study—the examination of the causes of changes in phenotypes or gene expressions that are not explained by the underlying DNA sequence. The Human Genome Project was a study funded by the National Institutes of Health in which the 20,000 to 25,000 genes on the human genome were mapped out. This took 13 years. The data are still being analyzed but will likely have significant impact on our understanding of health and illness.

The new fields of pharmacogenetics will have significant impact on nursing practice eventually, in which the mechanisms and actions of medications can be determined by their genetic structures. This will mean that medications can be prescribed that will be more effective than those that are given generically. Advances are being made in chemotherapy for certain cancers, such as leukemias and lymphomas, where methylation that occurs at the gene level causes the expression of the genes to be aberrant, that is, to go wrong, leading to the development of malignant cell growth. Certain drugs used in these cancers are "hypomethylating" agents that reverse the increased or "hyper" methylation that is occurring. Dr. Theresa Swift-Scanlan, a nurse researcher whom you will read about in Chapter 11, examines the epigenetics of breast cancer, that is, looking for those agents that cause certain genetic changes that are not explained by normal gene expression.

Biomedical technology involves complex machines or implantable devices used in patient care settings for a variety of reasons—for example, pacemakers, internal automated defibrillators, insulin pumps, artificial organs, and various invasive monitoring systems such as those used to measure intracranial pressure. This form of technology affects nursing practice because nurses assume responsibility for monitoring the data generated from these machines and for assessing the safety and effectiveness of implantable equipment in relation to patient well-being. In many instances the nurse is called on to react to the data and revise the plan of care on the basis of the data received. An important consideration in nursing when working in a high-tech environment: do not forget that there is a "human in there" under all of the lines and monitors. The human

touch and a word of reassurance to your patient are comforting to patients, and no technology can replace you. Family members usually need help in distinguishing monitoring equipment from those technologies that are used to support the patient's basic functions, such as a ventilator. Showing them what you are reading and seeing can be reassuring to them at a time when families are in a great deal of distress.

Information technology refers to a variety of computer-based applications used to communicate, store, manage, retrieve, and process information. Nurses assumed much of the responsibility for data entry and retrieval with the development of this technology. Computers are common on nursing units and at the bedside, and most hospitals have at least some degree of computerization of the medical records. The Obama administration's goals for health care reform include going "paperless," that is, that all medical orders, patient records, and other documents will be digitally stored and available for convenient transmittal across various record systems and health care facilities. Any other care provider can access data at any time, as opposed to the single "hard copy" chart that only one person can view or use at a time.

In some health care organizations, nursing information systems are handheld, allowing nurses to enter and access data about the patient directly from the patient's side, whether in an inpatient, outpatient, or home setting. This type of technology allows for more timely documentation of care, and because documentation is done at the time of care, the information is likely to be more accurate. This convenience can come at the expense of patient privacy, and the privacy and confidentiality of patient information is both an ethical and a legal issue. The Health Insurance Portability and Accountability Act (HIPAA) of 1996 is legislation designed to protect patients' health care information from misuse. A more complete discussion of HIPAA's provisions is found in Chapter 4.

Knowledge technology is described as "technology of the mind." It involves the use of computer systems to transform information into knowledge and to generate new knowledge. Through the creation of "expert systems," this form of technology assists nurses with clinical judgments about patient management problems. An example of knowledge technology includes medication administration carts that prompt the nurse for data needed before giving a particular medication. Nurse clinicians and nurse leaders should play a role in programming these devices to maximize their effectiveness in improving nursing care and patient outcomes. Human simulation mannequins are gaining popularity in schools of nursing (Figure 2-15). They make it possible to simulate a clinical event such as a cardiac arrest or pneumothorax, allowing the student to practice clinical assessment and intervention skills. One of the benefits of computerized expert systems is that they can provide practice in decision making for novice nurses and nurses who may be working outside their area of expertise without increased risk to a patient.

As technology becomes more pervasive, nurses must be very intentional in providing compassionate, personalized care for the patient. Technologic advances now allow nurses to monitor their patients' conditions on computer screens at remote sites. Without even seeing the patient, nurses can gather large amounts of information and make nursing decisions based on that information. As nurses rely more on technology, they may actually spend less time with the patient, creating dissatisfaction on the part of patients and families. Although being able to monitor one's patient on a telemetry unit from the nurses' station is very convenient and practical, monitoring of a contraction pattern and fetal heart rate from the nurses' station diminished the nurse's role to one of labor surveillance rather than labor support. The use of technology must be applied carefully and never take the place of human-to-human contact and interaction (Figure 2-16).

Successfully combining technology and caring requires sensitivity to patients' physical, emotional, and spiritual needs. This has always been a part of nursing's skill set. This type of emotional connectivity has been termed emotional intelligence (Simpson and Keegan, 2003).

Periodic imbalances are not uncommon between the numbers of nurses working and the number of available nursing positions. Over many decades there have been rare, brief periods of oversupply of nurses and more frequent and longer-lasting nursing shortages. By far the more common concern is an inadequate supply of RNs to meet the health care needs of the nation.

The term "nursing shortage" is misleading because actual shortages are usually confined to institutional settings such as hospitals and nursing homes. Causes of shortages may be seen as

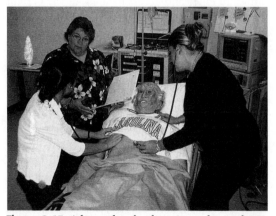

Figure 2-15 Advanced technology is used to enhance clinical decision making in novices. Here students use a human simulator in a lab setting to refine their skills. (Photo courtesy of the University of North Carolina at Chapel Hill School of Nursing.)

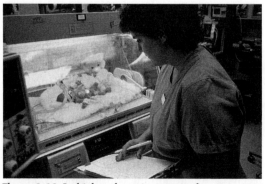

Figure 2-16 In high-tech environments the nurse must remember the significance of human touch in healing and in demonstrating care and compassion. (Courtesy Emory University.)

either external or internal. Internal causes include salary issues, long hours, increased responsibility for unlicensed workers, and significant responsibility with little authority. External causes include changes in demand for nursing services, the increasing age of the American population, greater acuity (degree of illness) of hospitalized individuals, public perceptions of nursing as a profession, and ever-widening career options for women.

One of the key aspects of the current nursing shortage is the shortage of nursing faculty. In 2008, 50,000 otherwise qualified applicants were denied admission to U.S. schools of nursing because of insufficient numbers of faculty, clinical sites, and classroom space. Faculty shortages are attributed to several factors. First, doctorally prepared and master's degree–prepared faculty now average over 50 years of age, foreshadowing a large number of retirements in the next decade. Second, nurses with advanced degrees who are otherwise eligible for faculty appointments are being hired into more lucrative private-sector positions. Third, not enough doctoral and master's-level graduates are being produced to meet the demands of nursing education. The American Association of Colleges of Nursing (AACN) is looking at several remedies for this situation (AACN, 2009).

In the past, each time a shortage of RNs became serious, two solutions were attempted: (1) increase the supply of nurses, and (2) create a less-trained worker to supplement the number of nurses. Practical nursing programs, which produce graduates in only 1 year, were created to meet civilian and military needs of the United States during World War II. The nursing shortage of the 1950s stimulated a desire to shorten basic RN programs, and 2-year associate degree programs were the result. In the 1960s shortages led to the creation of the position of unit manager; this manager was expected to take over certain tasks to relieve nurses, who could then concentrate on providing patient care. The 1970s produced other new positions, such as emergency medical technicians (EMTs), physician's assistants, respiratory therapists, and others who took on various aspects of patient care formerly performed by nurses. The shortage of nurses in the late 1980s resulted in a proposal by the American Medical Association to create yet another "nurse extender" called the registered care technician. However, this initiative was short-lived as nurses responded quickly and negatively, with nurse leaders stating that nurses could not be responsible for direct caregivers that nurses had not trained.

Another method of increasing the supply of nurses is to import them from other English-speaking countries. Nurses from the United Kingdom, Australia, New Zealand, certain Caribbean islands, South Africa, and the Philippines are targeted for recruitment. Companies have been established to prepare them to take the National Council Licensure Examination for Registered Nurses (NCLEX-RN®) successfully to practice in this country. The ethics of this solution are addressed in Chapter 5.

Shortages are often limited to certain geographic areas or specialties. In those cases, redistributing already-licensed RNs can be seen as a solution. Many agencies specialize in providing nurses for short-term assignments, often called "traveling nurses." The American Hospital Association reported in 2003 that 56% of hospitals surveyed were using traveling or agency nurses—at great expense—to fill vacancies (Joint Commission on Accreditation of Healthcare Organizations, 2003). Travel nursing can provide individual nurses with good opportunities to live in and experience different parts of the country and world, but there is little incentive for traveling nurses to work toward long-term goals on the units where they are, for all practical purposes, filling in until a permanent nurse can be hired.

The current nursing shortage, which began in 2000, is deepening and will continue to do so for the foreseeable future (Figure 2-17). Explaining why there is a shortage is complex. Like many issues in nursing there is no simple explanation, and the issue is multifaceted. What is known is that the shortage exists and is more crucial in traditional settings such as hospitals and long-term care facilities. One reason for the shortage

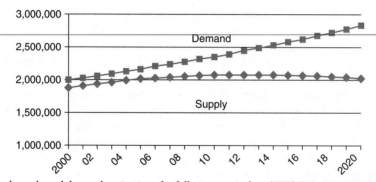

Figure 2-17 National supply and demand projections for full-time equivalent (FTE) RNs, 2000-2020. In 2000 the national supply of FTE RNs was estimated at 1.89 million, whereas the demand was estimated at 2 million, a shortage of 110,000, or 6%. On the basis of what is known about trends in the supply of RNs and the anticipated demand, the shortage is expected to grow relatively slowly until 2010, by which time it will have reached 12%. At that point, demand will begin to exceed supply at an accelerated rate, and by 2015 the shortage will have almost quadrupled to 20%. If not addressed, and if current trends continue, the shortage is projected to grow to 29% by 2020. Factors driving the growth in demand include an 18% increase in population, a larger proportion of elderly persons, and medical advances that heighten the need for nurses. (From U.S. Department of Health and Human Services, Health Resources and Services Administration: Projected supply, demand, and shortages of registered nurses: 2000-2020, Washington, DC, 2002, Government Printing Office, pp. 2-3.)

is an increased demand for nurses because of the growth in total population, especially an aging population that has extensive health care needs. The shortage is also compounded by the fact that the nursing workforce is aging and the number of new entrants to the profession is not keeping pace with the numbers who are exiting. The 2004 National Sample Survey of Registered Nurses identified three factors that seem to be contributing to the aging of the RN workforce:

- A decline in the total number of nursing school graduates
- The higher average age of recent graduates
- The aging of the entire existing pool of licensed nurses

Shortages are sometimes blamed on the phenomenon of nurses leaving hospital work for nonhospital nursing positions, such as in the insurance industry or in pharmaceutical sales. In spite of the fact that in 2004 8.5% of licensed nurses were estimated to be employed in fields other than hospitals, long-term care, nursing education, public health, or ambulatory care, hospitals employ nearly the same proportion of the total pool of RNs, 56%, as they did in 2000, when they employed 59%. The total number of RNs working

in hospitals was greater than in 2000 even though the overall percentage was constant. This is attributable to several factors:

- More nursing care hours per capita are being provided to hospitalized patients today because of a higher acuity of their illnesses and needs that demand more time.
- Technologic advances in medical care have created the need for special care units, staffed with specialized nurses. In these units, because patients are critically ill, one nurse can safely care for only one or two patients.
- Advances in technology prolong lives of chronically ill patients, which in turn creates more need for long-term nursing care.
- Cost-containment measures have caused hospital consolidations, downsizing, and reengineering. The result is more patients in fewer hospitals staffed with reduced numbers of personnel.

Initiatives to provide a stable supply of registered nurses

Recognizing that dramatic swings in the supply of and demand for RNs harm the profession, jeopardize patient care, and are costly to nurses and their employers, organizations inside and outside of nursing have called for mechanisms to ensure more even distribution of the workforce. Here are four major initiatives making an impact:

- The American Recovery and Reinvestment Act of 2009, the goal of which is to stimulate the U.S. economy, has a provision for $500 million to strengthen the U.S. health care work force. This includes the training and education of the next generation of nurses and physicians.
- The Robert Wood Johnson Foundation (RWJF), a private foundation that funds innovative health care initiatives, committed tens of millions of dollars to pursuing programs that help nursing schools, hospitals, and other health care agencies create regional workforce development systems. This initiative was named Colleagues in Caring.
- Johnson & Johnson's Campaign for Nursing's Future was mentioned earlier. Johnson & Johnson is working in partnership with the National Student Nurses Association (NSNA), the NLN, the ANA, the Association of Nurse Executives (AONE), and STTI Honor Society of Nursing.
- The ANCC Magnet Recognition Program is a model for employers to earn the designation "employer of choice" by implementing a model program designed to attract and retain nurses in acute hospital settings.

Numerous other initiatives by nursing associations, colleges of nursing, and states are also underway.

Two national surveys conducted in 2002 and 2004 examined the impact of the nursing shortage on patient outcomes and quality of care (Buerhaus et al, 2005a). Findings from these surveys indicate that hospital nurses and nursing officers believe that a shortage of RNs presents a major problem for the quality of patient care (Buerhaus et al, 2005b). In 2002, 62% of nurses and, in 2004, 67% of nurses believed that the nursing shortage created problems in early detection of patient complications; 68% of 2002 participants and 71% of 2004 participants identified that the ability of nurses to maintain patient safety was a problem (Buerhaus et al, 2005b). Overwhelmingly, both groups thought that the shortage had affected

the amount of time the nurse could spend with patients (93% and 92%, respectively). The gap between a desirable level of care and the care these nurses were able to provide created both stress and moral distress.

The author acknowledges the contributions of Shielda Rodgers in the preparation of this chapter.

Summary of Key Points

- In 1860 Florence Nightingale founded a school for nurses at St. Thomas's Hospital, London, that became the model for nursing education in the United States.
- Formal educational programs for U.S. nurses were established in 1873.
- The period between the 1893 World's Fair and 1908 marked a time of organizing for nurses. During that time the forerunners of the NLN, the ANA, the ICN, and the NACGN were formed.
- The initiation of state licensure in 1903 heralded standardization of nursing education programs that, until this time, had varied widely.
- The establishment of the Henry Street Settlement and the rise of community health nursing played a major role in the widespread public acceptance of nurses, particularly African-American nurses.
- World War I and the influenza epidemic of 1917-1919 created a strong demand for nursing services. Many nursing schools were opened in response, mostly in hospitals.
- The Great Depression and World War II created new opportunities for nurses, including the Cadet Nurse Corps, which added 124,000 new RNs to the profession by the end of the war, but denied membership to men.
- Since World War II, hospital expansion, technologic advances, and social changes have created new and progressively autonomous roles for nurses, especially advanced practice nurses.
- Social trends that have affected nursing include the "graying of America," cultural diversity, men in nursing, and technologic advances in genetics, health care, and information management.

- Numerous nurses from ethnically diverse groups and men have made major contributions to the development of the profession of nursing.
- Individual nurses must take direct action when nursing is presented in an unfavorable light in the media.
- The number of men in nursing has stabilized.
- Nurses are expected to be culturally aware to meet the needs of an increasingly diverse population of both patients and colleagues.
- Nurses must not forget the art of nursing that involves compassionate care despite the presence of an array of technology.
- Imbalances in the supply of and demand for nurses arise periodically because of changes in society and in health care itself. A number of ongoing initiatives have been designed to ensure an adequate supply of RNs, yet shortages continue.

Critical Thinking Questions

1. Florence Nightingale is often credited with being the first nurse researcher. Why do you think this is so?
2. Discuss the significance of the events that occurred during the Chicago World's Fair, 1893, to the advancement of the nursing profession.
3. Do you agree with the view that nursing is inevitably tied to the greater issues of the women's movement throughout the world? Why or why not? How has this attitude affected the entry of men into nursing?
4. Wars have often been the driving force in creating social change. How have wars influenced the profession of nursing?
5. What role did the military have in integrating the profession of nursing for African Americans and other minorities?
6. Discuss the role the military played in perpetuating discriminatory practices against men in nursing.
7. Explain how being a female-dominated profession has affected the development of the nursing profession.

8. Describe your ideal nurse. What social stereotypes does your description reveal? Does your "ideal nurse" belong to a particular gender, race, ethnic group, or generation?
9. What positive and negative impact has the consumer movement had on health care in the United States? How do you reflect consumerism when using the health care system?
10. Why is a bill of rights necessary in health care? Examine the document found at the following website and give a rationale for each "right" listed: http://www.hospitalconnect.com:80/aha/ptcommunication/index.html.
11. List three social factors that have the potential to stimulate or squelch interest in nursing as a profession and explain their impact. Recommend ways the profession can capitalize on or combat each factor you listed.
12. If everyone in a health care setting dresses alike, how does this affect nursing's image? In addition to attire, what would you recommend as an appropriate or acceptable look for nurses? Be sure to address hair, makeup, facial hair for men, jewelry, piercings, and tattoos.
13. The nursing shortage is projected to worsen in the next few years. Discuss the reasons for the deepening of this shortage and strategies to address it.

⊝volve *To enhance your understanding of this chapter, try the Student Exercises on the Evolve site at http://evolve.elsevier.com/Chitty/professional.*

REFERENCES

American Assembly for Men in Nursing: Purpose and objectives, 2003 (website): http://www.aamn.org.

American Association of Colleges of Nursing: Media paper on the nursing and nursing faculty shortage, March 2009, http://www.aacn.nche.edu/Media/NewsReleases/2009/workforcedata.html.

Barton C: *Diary: the papers of Clara Barton (1812-1912)*, Washington, DC, 1862, Library of Congress, Manuscript Division.

Buerhaus PI, Donelan K, Ulrich BT et al: Is the shortage of hospital registered nurses getting better or worse? Findings from two recent national surveys of RNs, *Nurs Econ* 23(2):61-71, 96, 2005a.

Buerhaus PI, Donelan K, Ulrich BT et al: Hospital RNs' and CNOs' perceptions of the impact of the nursing shortage on the quality of care, *Nurs Econ* 23(5): 214-221, 2005b.

Carnegie ME: *The path we tread: blacks in nursing, 1854-1994*, Philadelphia, 1995, JB Lippincott.

Centers for Disease Control and Prevention: Older person's health, 2006 (website): http://www.cdc.gov/nchs/fastats/older_americans.htm.

Cherry B, Jacob S: *Contemporary nursing: issues, trends and management*, St Louis, 2005, Mosby.

Cummings SH: Attila the Hun versus Attila the hen: gender socialization of the American nurse, *Nurs Adm Q* 19(2):19-29, 1995.

Dock LL, Stewart IM: *A short history of nursing*, New York, 1920, Putnam.

Donahue MP: *Nursing: the finest art: an illustrated history*, ed 2, Philadelphia, 1996, Mosby.

Donelan K, Buerhaus PI, Ulrich BT, et al: Awareness and perceptions of the Johnson & Johnson Campaign for Nursing's Future: views from nursing students, RNs, and CNOs, *Nursing Economic$* 23(4):150-156, 2005:180.

Fitzpatrick ML: Nursing and the Great Depression, *Am J Nurs* 75(12):2188-2190, 1975.

Gordon S: *Nursing against the odds: how health care cost cutting, media stereotypes and medical hubris undermine nurses and patient care*, Ithaca, NY, 2005, Cornell University Press.

Hart KA: What do men in nursing really want? *Nursing2005* 35(11):46-48, 2005.

Johnson LD: The role of cultural competency in eliminating health disparities, *Minority Nurse Winter* 52-55, 2005.

Joint Commission on Accreditation of Healthcare Organizations: Quick statistics on the nursing shortage, 2003 (website): http://www.jcaho.org/News?Room/Press?Kits/quick?statistics?on?the?nursing?shortage.htm.

Kalisch PA, Kalisch, BJ: Nurses under fire: the World War II experiences of nurses on Bataan and Corregidor, Nurs Res 44(5): 260-271.

Kennedy D: *Birth control in America: the career of Margaret Sanger*, New Haven, Conn, 1970, Yale University Press.

Maxwell M: It's not just black and white: how diverse is your workforce? *Nurs Econ* 23(3):139-140, 2005.

Miller HS: *America's first black professional nurse*, Atlanta, 1986, Wright Publishing.

Nightingale F: *Notes on nursing: what it is and what it is not [Reprint]*, Philadelphia, 1946, JB Lippincott (originally published in 1859).

Norman E: *We band of angels: the untold story of American nurses trapped on Bataan by the Japanese*, New York, 1999, Random House.

Oates SB: *A woman of valor*, New York, 1994, The Free Press.

Palmer S: The editor, *Am J Nurs* 1(1):64, 1900.

Pember PY: *A Southern woman's story*, Atlanta, 1959, Bill Wiley.

Powell KA, Abels L: Sex-role stereotypes in TV programs aimed at the preschool audience: an analysis of *Teletubbies* and *Barney & Friends, Women Language* 25(2):14-22, 2002.

Rosenberg CE: *The care of strangers*, New York, 1987, Basic Books.

Robinson TM, Perry PM: *Cadet nurse stories: the call for and response of women during World War II*, Indianapolis, 2001, Sigma Theta Tau International-Center for Nursing Press.

Sigma Theta Tau International: *The Woodhull Study on Nursing and the Media: health care's invisible partner*, Indianapolis, 1998, Sigma Theta Tau International-Center Nursing Press.

Simpson RL, Keegan AJ: How connected are you? Emotional intelligence in a high-tech world, *Nurs Adm Q* 26(2):80-86, 2003.

Sleet J: A successful experiment, *Am J Nurs* 2:729, 1901.

Smith A: J & J's campaign for nursing's future: the gift that keeps on giving, *Nurs Econ* 23(4):199-200, 2005.

Ulmer BC: The image of nursing, *AORN J* 71(6):26-27, 2000.

Ulrich B: A matter of trust, NurseWeek, 2003 (website): http://www.nurseweek.com/ednote/03/121803_ca_sc_print.html.

U.S. Bureau of the Census: *Statistical abstract of the United States: 2002*, ed 122, Washington, DC, 2002, Government Printing Office.

U.S. Department of Health and Human Services: *Division of Nursing: The registered nurse population, March 2000: findings from national sample survey of registered nurses*, Washington, DC, 2001, Government Printing Office.

U.S. Department of Health and Human Services: *Division of Nursing: The registered nurse population, March 2004: national sample survey of registered nurses, preliminary findings*, Washington, DC, 2005, Government Printing Office.

Wall BM: Courage to care: the Sisters of the Holy Cross in the Spanish-American War, *Nurs Hist Rev* 3:55-77, 1995.

Yoder-Wise P: *Leading and managing in nursing*, St Louis, 2003, Mosby.

Nursing's Pathway to Professionalism

Kay Kittrell Chitty

LEARNING OUTCOMES

After studying this chapter, students will be able to:
- Identify the characteristics of a profession
- Distinguish between the characteristics of professions and occupations
- Describe how professions evolve
- Evaluate nursing's position on the professionalism continuum
- Explain the elements of nursing's contract with society
- Recognize characteristic behaviors that exemplify professional nurses
- Describe outcomes of professional nursing practice
- Assess themselves in the development of professional conduct

What is a profession, and who can be called a professional? These terms are used loosely in everyday conversation. Historically, only medicine, law, and the ministry were considered professions. Today, however, professional is a term commonly used to identify many types of people, ranging from wrestlers to pharmacists. Are all these individuals professionals? Is the value of the term professional diminished when it is used indiscriminately to describe any work done by any group? Does possession of a license to practice as a registered nurse make a person a professional nurse? Knowledge, skills, and expertise are part of being a professional. As you will see in this chapter, there are many other criteria to be examined in a discussion of what contributes to professionalism in general and in nursing specifically.

HISTORICAL REVIEW: CHARACTERISTICS OF A PROFESSION

For nearly a century scholars have grappled with the meaning of profession. They have generally agreed that a profession is an occupational group with a set of attitudes or behaviors, or both. In this section we will briefly review several definitions by scholars through the years and identify major similarities.

Abraham Flexner

Every serious study of professions must begin with a review of Abraham Flexner's seminal work on professions and the education of professionals. In the early 1900s, the Carnegie Foundation issued a series of papers about professional schools. The first of these reports was based on sociologist Abraham Flexner's 1910 study of medical education (Flexner, 1910). The Flexner Report, as it became known, is a classic piece of educational literature that provided the impetus for the much-needed reform of medical education and is still highly regarded today.

Flexner went on to study other disciplines and later, in a paper about social work, published a list of criteria that he believed were characteristic of all true professions (Flexner, 1915). Flexner's work has stood the test of time. Since his original criteria were published, they have been widely used as a benchmark for determining the status of various occupations in terms of professionalism and have had a profound influence on professional education in several disciplines, including nursing.

Flexner's criteria stipulate that a profession:

1. Is basically intellectual (as opposed to physical) and is accompanied by a high degree of individual responsibility
2. Is based on a body of knowledge that can be learned and is refreshed and refined through research (today, this is known as evidence-based practice)
3. Is practical, in addition to being theoretical
4. Can be taught through a process of highly specialized professional education
5. Has a strong internal organization of members and a well-developed group consciousness
6. Has practitioners who are motivated by altruism (the desire to help others) and who are responsive to public interests (Figure 3-1)

Since this early work, other authorities have identified criteria for professions, building on but varying slightly from Flexner's.

Richard H. Hall

Another sociologist, Richard H. Hall, published his work on professionalism in 1968. Hall described a professional model that classified attributes such as educational qualifications, professional organizations, and sense of calling. He identified five indicators of an individual's attitude toward professionalism (1968):

1. Use of a professional organization as a primary point of reference
2. Belief in the value of public service
3. Belief in self-regulation
4. Commitment to a profession that goes beyond economic incentives
5. A sense of autonomy in practice

Hall recommended that each profession needed to develop its own methods of measuring professionalism that recognize the uniqueness of that discipline.

Contemporary Conceptualizations of Profession

In recent years, individuals and groups have continued to identify what professionals believe, think, and do. Muller (1998) wrote that "professionalism involves the application of knowledge and skills, a high standard of practice, leadership,

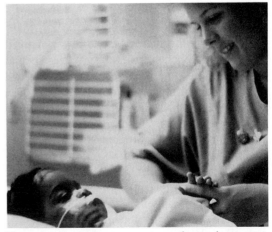

Figure 3-1 According to experts, professionals are motivated by altruism, a desire to help others. (Courtesy Medical University of South Carolina.)

self-regulation, professional commitment, social values, and service-directed activity."

More recently, a pharmacy profession task force spent 5 years studying and promoting pharmacy student professionalism (Task Force on Professionalism, 2000). They reached back into the history of professional development in the broad sense, reviewing the work of numerous scholars. From this review they distilled a list of 10 common characteristics of the members of a profession:

1. Prolonged specialized training in a body of abstract knowledge
2. A service orientation
3. An ideology based on the original faith professed by members
4. An ethic that is binding on the practitioners
5. A body of knowledge unique to the members
6. A set of skills that forms the technique of the profession
7. A guild of those entitled to practice the profession
8. Authority granted by society in the form of licensure or certification
9. A recognized setting in which the profession is practiced
10. A theory of societal benefits derived from the ideology

Major Similarities

As you see, authorities have not always agreed about the number of criteria and the types of behaviors and characteristics of professions. A review of a variety of publications on this topic, however, reveals that there are three criteria that consistently appear: service/altruism, specialized knowledge, and autonomy/ethics (Flexner, 1915; Hall, 1968, 1982; Carr-Saunders and Wilson, 1933; Adams, Miller, and Beck, 1996; Huber, 2000).

1. Service implies a sense of calling to the discipline, a sense of mission, and a responsibility to the public.
2. Knowledge implies specialized education, including both theoretical knowledge and techniques or skills.
3. Practice autonomy implies having control over one's own practice. It also implies having a code of ethics governing standards of conduct within the profession (Huber, 2000).

After nearly a century of study, contemplation, and deliberation, there is still no clear-cut consensus about what constitutes a profession, nor is there likely to be. Occupational groups are constantly pushing to become more professional and to receive public acknowledgment of their professional status. As they do so, conceptions of profession change.

FROM OCCUPATION TO PROFESSION

Professions usually evolved from occupations that originally consisted of tasks but developed more specialized educational pathways and publicly legitimized status. The established professions, such as law, medicine, and the ministry, generally followed a typical developmental pattern of stages that occurred sequentially. First, practitioners performed full-time work in the discipline. They then determined work standards, identified a body of knowledge, and established educational programs in institutions of higher learning. Next, they promoted organization into effective occupational associations. Then they worked toward legal protection that limited practice of their unique skills by outsiders. Finally, they established codes of ethics (Carr-Saunders and Wilson, 1933). This process can be termed *professionalization*.

Another analysis of the evolution from occupation to profession was done by Houle (1980). He identified a number of characteristics that indicate that an occupational group is moving along the continuum toward professional status. First is the definition of the group's mission and foundations of practice. Then comes mastery of theoretical knowledge, development of the capacity to solve problems, the use of practical knowledge, and self-enhancement (continued learning and development). Finally, Houle identified nine characteristics that indicate that an occupation is developing a **collective identity** or group identification, which is necessary for professions. These include formal training, credentialing, creation of a subculture, legal right to practice, public acceptance, ethical practice, discipline of incompetent/unethical practitioners, relationship to other practitioners, and relationship to users of services.

The term *occupation* is often used interchangeably with profession, but their definitions differ. *Webster's New World Dictionary* (1996) defines occupation as "what occupies, or engages, one's time; business; employment." In this discussion we define *profession* as "a calling, vocation, or form of employment that provides a needed service to society and possesses characteristics of expertise, autonomy, long academic preparation, commitment, and responsibility" (Huber, 2000, p. 34).

There is widespread, overall agreement that a profession is different from an occupation in at least two major ways—preparation and commitment.

Professional Preparation

Professional preparation usually takes place in a college or university setting. Preparation is prolonged to include instruction in the specialized body of knowledge and techniques of the profession. Professional preparation includes more than knowledge and skills, however. It also includes orientation to the beliefs, values, and attitudes expected of the members of the profession. Standards of practice and ethical considerations are also included. These components of professional education are part of the process of socialization into a profession and are discussed in more detail in Chapter 6. According to Miller (1985), preparation enables professional practitioners to act in a logical, rational manner rather than relying on custom, intuition, or trial and error. An ever-expanding base of knowledge in all disciplines complicates the challenges of professional preparation.

The belief that there are "core competencies" that should be included in all health professional education was suggested by the Institute of Medicine in 2003 after study by a task force of more than 150 health professionals of all disciplines in a Health Professions Education Summit. The report issued after this summit identified five core competencies that all students of health professions should acquire (Greiner and Knebel, 2003).

1. Provide patient-centered care.
2. Work in interdisciplinary teams.
3. Employ evidence-based practice.
4. Apply quality improvement principles.
5. Utilize informatics.

In the past decade an emphasis on evidence-based practice has evolved, particularly in medicine and nursing. Basing one's practice and decisions about patient care on research findings rather than tradition has come to be recognized as a characteristic of professional nursing practice. The Evidence-Based Practice Note below describes a study that examined nursing students' beliefs about what it means to be a professional.

Professional Commitment

Professionals' commitment to their profession is strong. They derive much of their personal identification from their work and consider it an integral part of their lives. People engaging in a profession often consider it their "calling." Historically, professionals' commitment to their profession has transcended their expectation of material reward. Although people may readily change occupations, it is less common for people to change professions. Several critical differences between occupations and professions are summarized in Table 3-1.

☀ EVIDENCE-BASED PRACTICE NOTE

Three professors at a Tennessee university sought to understand how students develop professional identity. They conducted a qualitative, existential-phenomenological study of baccalaureate students to determine their ideas of what it means to be a professional. Sixty-nine nursing students at various levels of education were asked to describe specific experiences in which they "felt professional." The researchers analyzed these figural (outstanding) experiences for common patterns or themes. Three interrelated themes were identified: belonging, knowing, and affirmation.

- An example of belonging: "I knew...that I had acted as a professional and knowledgeable nurse and even though that man died, the team did everything they could to keep him alive and I was a team member. It was a satisfying moment."

- An example of knowing: "For myself, my nursing knowledge and actions make me a professional. However, when this nursing knowledge is applied and the client and family express their appreciation of my nursing efforts, then I feel professional."

- An example of affirmation: "I had one family who just couldn't believe I was in nursing school. They stated that I was so 'professional and caring' and that I was a 'great nurse.' Then I said, 'Well, I'm not a nurse yet; I'll be graduating in one year.' That made me feel like I was actually a nurse."

The researchers suggested that courses encouraging students to reflect on the meaning of the profession and being a professional should be offered early in the curriculum. They stated their belief that "developing a sense of professionalism is equally important as knowledge and skills."

Modified from Secrest J, Norwood BR, Keatley VM: "I was actually a nurse": the meaning of professionalism for baccalaureate nursing students, *J Nurs Educ* 42(2):77-82, 2003.

Table 3-1   Comparison of Characteristics of Occupations and Professions

Occupation	Profession
Training may occur on the job.	Education takes place in a college or university.
Length of training varies.	Education is prolonged.
Work is largely manual.	Work involves mental creativity.
Decision making is guided largely by experience or by trial and error.	Decision making is based largely on science or theoretical constructs (evidence-based practice).
Values, beliefs, and ethics are not prominent features of preparation.	Values, beliefs, and ethics are an integral part of preparation.
Commitment and personal identification vary.	Commitment and personal identification are strong.
Workers are supervised.	Workers are autonomous.
People often change jobs.	People are unlikely to change professions.
Material reward is main motivation.	Commitment transcends material reward.
Accountability rests primarily with employer.	Accountability rests with individual.

BARRIERS TO PROFESSIONALISM IN NURSING

As a group, nurses must strive to reduce the barriers to professionalization. The first step in that process is developing an awareness of those barriers. Several major barriers will be discussed here.

Variability in Educational Preparation

The most obvious barrier to nursing's achievement of professional status is the variability of educational backgrounds of its practitioners. There is no other profession that allows entry into practice at less than the baccalaureate level. To the contrary, many professions, such as law, medicine, and physical therapy, require postgraduate preparation for professional practice. Because professional status and power increase with education, a legitimate question is, "How can nursing take its place as a peer among the professions when most nurses currently in practice do not hold the baccalaureate degree?" The differentiation between professional nursing and technical nursing is a challenging issue that has not yet been resolved. Educational diversity within nursing has slowed the progress toward acceptance of the baccalaureate or higher degree as the prerequisite for professional practice. Nurses prepared in three different types of basic educational programs—diploma, associate degree, and baccalaureate—have thus far failed to develop a unified identity that would

allow them to move the profession forward together. Lack of resolution of these differences threatens to undermine nursing's continued steady development as a profession (Christman, 1998; Kidder and Cornelius, 2006). This is a painful issue for nurses, creating division, defensiveness, and anger whenever it is discussed in groups large and small. For the profession as a whole to progress, we must move beyond personal feelings to look objectively at how nursing stacks up when compared with other groups—groups with whom we wish to be compared and by whom we wish to be treated as equals—and adjust our educational and credentialing requirements accordingly.

Gender Issues

Although gender was not identified as a criterion by any of the scholars of professionalism, it plays a major role in the perceived value of female-dominated professions such as teaching, social work, and nursing. Although the number of men in nursing is gradually increasing, a gender balance may never be achieved. This will continue to be a hindrance, because of the persistent prevalence of outmoded thinking and the resultant devaluing of "women's work" in our society.

Historical Influences

Nursing's historical connections with religious orders and the military continue to have influence, both positive and negative, today. Aspects that have become liabilities with the passage of time include unquestioning obedience, which runs counter to the professional values of autonomy and self-determination, and altruism, which mitigates against the fair economic valuation of the work of nursing. Nurses should be aware that unquestioning obedience stifles the creative thinking and problem solving required for professional practice. Similar to other helping professionals, nurses must resist pressures to feel guilty or greedy for expecting to be paid well for their complex and demanding work.

External Conflicts

As nurses have become more highly educated and able to provide services that were formerly part of medical practice, conflicts with medicine have inevitably arisen. Much of the power, influence, and resources of organized nursing has gone toward lobbying efforts in state legislatures to ensure that the legal scope of nursing practice is protected and appropriately enhanced. These efforts should and will continue on the professional association level. On the personal level, however, nurses must strive for collaboration, not competition, with physicians and other health personnel with whom they work. Nurses must demonstrate their unique knowledge, expertise, and skills so that professional autonomy can be exercised within the various bureaucratic organizations in which they work.

Internal Conflicts

Professional nursing's power is fragmented by subgroups and dissension. Rivalry among diploma-educated, associate degree–educated, and baccalaureate-educated nurses saps the vitality of the profession. The proliferation of nursing organizations (see a list of nursing organizations at http://www.nurse.org/orgs.shtml) and competition among them for members also diminish nursing's potential. Fewer than 10 percent of the 2.9 million registered nurses in the United States are members of the American Nurses Association (ANA), the largest professional nursing organization. The fact that most nurses are not members of any professional organization hampers nursing's ability to govern itself, set standards, and use its

collective power to lobby effectively for positive changes in health care. These are major challenges for nursing if it is to realize its potential collective professional power and autonomy.

NURSING'S PATHWAY TO PROFESSIONALISM

As can be seen, nursing's pathway to professionalism has not been smooth. For decades an ongoing subject for discussion in nursing circles has been the following question: "Is nursing a profession?" Much has been spoken and written on both sides of this issue. Nursing sociologists do not all agree that nursing is a profession. Some believe that it is, at best, an emerging profession. Others cite the progress nursing has made toward meeting the commonly accepted criteria for full-fledged professional status. Still others believe that nursing leaders, by embracing the masculine orientation to professionalism embodied in the work of Flexner and others, have supported the existing patriarchal order, thereby prolonging the subordination of nursing to male-dominated professions such as medicine. Setting our personal biases aside, let us now look objectively at various criteria for professions and nursing's status in relation to them.

Bixler and Bixler's Criteria

Roy and Genevieve Bixler, a husband and wife team of nonnurses who were advocates and supporters of nursing, first wrote about the status of nursing as a profession in 1945. In 1959 they again appraised nursing according to their original seven criteria, noting the progress made (Bixler and Bixler, 1959). Their criteria included the following:

1. "A profession utilizes in its practice a well-defined and well-organized body of specialized knowledge which is on the intellectual level of higher learning" (p. 1142).
2. "A profession constantly enlarges the body of knowledge it uses and improves its techniques of education and service by the use of the scientific method" (p. 1143).
3. "A profession entrusts the education of its practitioners to institutions of higher education" (p. 1144).

4. "A profession applies its body of knowledge in practical services which are vital to human and social welfare" (p. 1145).
5. "A profession functions autonomously in the formulation of professional policy and in the control of professional activity thereby" (p. 1145).
6. "A profession attracts individuals of intellectual and personal qualities who exalt service above personal gain and who recognize their chosen occupation as a life work" (p. 1146).
7. "A profession strives to compensate its practitioners by providing freedom of action, opportunity for continuous professional growth, and economic security" (p. 1146).

Kelly's Criteria

Lucie Kelly, RN, PhD, FAAN, is an outstanding nurse writer, teacher, and influential leader. She was editor of the journal *Nursing Outlook* and president of Sigma Theta Tau International Honor Society of Nursing, among many career highlights. Dr. Kelly has spent much of her nursing career exploring the dimensions of professional nursing. She compiled the following set of eight characteristics of a profession many years ago (Kelly, 1981, p. 157), but they remain relevant today:

1. The services provided are vital to humanity and the welfare of society.
2. There is a special body of knowledge that is continually enlarged through research.
3. The services involve intellectual activities; individual responsibility (accountability) is a strong feature.
4. Practitioners are educated in institutions of higher learning.
5. Practitioners are relatively independent and control their own policies and activities (autonomy).
6. Practitioners are motivated by service (altruism) and consider their work an important component of their lives.
7. There is a code of ethics to guide the decisions and conduct of practitioners.
8. There is an organization (association) that encourages and supports high standards of practice.

Let us examine how well contemporary nursing fulfills these eight characteristics.

"The services provided are vital to humanity and the welfare of society."

If random students were asked why they chose nursing, most would reply, "To help people." Certainly nursing is a service that is essential to the well-being of people and to society as a whole. Nursing promotes the maintenance and restoration of health of individuals, groups, and communities. The goal of nursing is to assist others to attain the highest level of wellness of which they are capable. Caring—meaning nurturing and helping others— is a basic component of professional nursing.

"There is a special body of knowledge that is continually enlarged through research."

In the past, nursing was based on principles borrowed from the physical and social sciences and other disciplines. Today, however, there is a body of knowledge that is uniquely nursing's own. Although this was not always so, the amount of investigation and analysis of nursing care has expanded rapidly in the past 30 years. Nursing theory development is also proceeding swiftly. Nursing is no longer based on trial and error but increasingly relies on theory development and research as a basis for practice. We call the reliance on research as a basis for nursing practice *evidence-based practice.* You will learn more about theory, research, and evidence-based practice later in this book.

"The services involve intellectual activities; individual responsibility (accountability) is a strong feature."

Nursing developed and refined its own unique approach to practice, called the nursing process. The nursing process is essentially a cognitive (mental) activity that requires both critical and creative thinking and serves as the basis for providing nursing care. The profession is now engaged in an ongoing effort to identify and standardize nursing diagnoses, interventions, and outcomes, all of which are parts of the nursing process.

Individual accountability in nursing has become the hallmark of practice. Accountability, according to the ANA's *Code of Ethics for Nurses* (2001), is being answerable to someone for something one has done. Provision 4 of the Code states, "The nurse is responsible and accountable for individual nursing practice and determines the appropriate delegation of tasks consistent with the nurse's obligation to provide optimum patient care" (p. 5). Through legal opinions and court cases, society has demonstrated that it, too, holds nurses individually responsible for their actions, as well as for those of unlicensed personnel under their supervision.

"Practitioners are educated in institutions of higher learning."

As presented in Chapter 7, the first university-based nursing program began in 1909 at the University of Minnesota. Several studies, including Esther Lucille Brown's 1948 report, *Nursing for the Future,* called for nursing education to be based in universities and colleges (Brown, 1948). Another milestone was the 1965 position paper of the ANA, which called for all nursing education to take place in institutions of higher education (ANA, 1965).

The majority of programs offering basic nursing education are now associate degree and baccalaureate programs located in colleges and universities. There are growing numbers of master's and doctoral programs in nursing, although the number of graduates is small compared with other health professions.

"Practitioners are relatively independent and control their own policies and activities (autonomy)."

Autonomy, or control over one's practice, is another controversial area for nursing. Although many nursing actions are independent, most nurses are employed in hospitals, where authority resides in one's position. One's place in the hierarchy, rather than expertise, often confers or denies power and status. Physicians are widely regarded as gatekeepers, and their authorization or supervision is required before many activities can occur. Nurse practice acts in many states reinforce nursing's tenuous self-determination by requiring that nurses perform certain actions only when authorized by supervising physicians or hospital protocols.

There are at least three groups that have historically attempted to control nursing practice: organized medicine, health service administration, and organized nursing. Both the medical profession and health service administration have attempted to maintain control of nursing because they believe it is in their best interest to keep nurses dependent on them. Both are well organized and well funded and have powerful lobbies at state and national levels. This is a major challenge to full autonomy for nurses.

The **magnet hospital** program, sponsored by the ANA, recognizes hospitals that attract and retain nurses and achieve better patient outcomes. In 1983, the first published study of what would come to be called magnet hospitals identified nurse staffing, nursing autonomy, and control over nursing practice as crucial to a "magnetic" environment. Now, a quarter-century later, these are still hot-button issues (McClure and Hinshaw, 2007). Clearly, the issue of nursing autonomy represents a challenge to nursing's professionalism.

"Practitioners are motivated by service (altruism) and consider their work an important component of their lives."

As a group, nurses are dedicated to the ideal of service to others, also known as altruism. This ideal has sometimes become intertwined with economic issues and historically has been exploited by employers of nurses. No one questions the right of other professionals to charge reasonable fees for the services they render; when nurses want higher salaries, however, others sometimes call their altruism into question. Nurses must take responsibility for their own financial well-being and for the economic health of the profession. This will, in turn, ensure its continued attractiveness to those who might choose nursing as a career. If there are to be adequate numbers of nurses to meet society's needs, salaries must be comparable with those in competing disciplines. Being motivated by salary does nothing to diminish a nurse's altruism or professionalism.

Another issue, consideration of work as a primary component of life, has been a thornier problem for nurses. Commitment to a career is not a value equally shared by all nurses. Some still regard nursing as a job and drop in and out of practice depending on economic and family needs. This flexible approach, although appealing to many nurses and conducive to traditional family management, has retarded the development of professional attitudes and behaviors for the profession as a whole.

"There is a code of ethics to guide the decisions and conduct of practitioners."

An ethical code does not stipulate how an individual should act in a specific situation; rather, it provides professional standards and a framework for decision making. The trust placed in the nursing profession by the public requires that nurses act with integrity. To aid them in doing so, both the International Council of Nurses (ICN) and the ANA, among others, have established codes of nursing ethics through which profession-wide standards of practice are established, promoted, and refined. The *Code of Ethics for Nurses,* which will be discussed later in the chapter, can be found on the inside back cover of this text.

In 1893 long before these codes were written, "The Florence Nightingale Pledge" (Box 3-1) was created by a committee headed by Lystra Eggert Gretter and presented to the Farrand Training School for Nurses located at Harper Hospital in Detroit, Michigan (Dock and Stewart, 1920). Its similarities to the medical profession's Hippocratic Oath are apparent. The Nightingale Pledge can be considered nursing's first code of ethics. It is presented here not only for its historic value but also because it established the roots for our current code.

"There is an organization (association) that encourages and supports high standards of practice."

As will be discussed in Chapter 15, a number of professional associations have been formed to promote the improvement of the nursing profession. Among these is the ANA, which all

---

Box 3-1   The Florence Nightingale Pledge

I solemnly pledge myself before God and in the presence of this assembly to pass my life in purity and to practice my profession faithfully.

I will abstain from whatever is deleterious and mischievous, and will not take or knowingly administer any harmful drug. I will do all in my power to maintain and elevate the standard of my profession, and will hold in confidence all personal matters committed to my keeping and all family affairs coming to my knowledge in the practice of my calling.

With loyalty will I endeavor to aid the physician in his work and devote myself to the welfare of those committed to my care.

From Dock LL, Stewart IM: *A short history of nursing,* New York, 1920, Putnam.

---

registered nurses are eligible to join. According to its bylaws, the purposes of the ANA are to work for the improvement of health standards and the availability of health care services for all people, to foster high standards of nursing, and to stimulate and promote the professional development of nurses and advance their economic and general welfare (ANA, 2008). The ANA is also the official voice of nursing and therefore is the primary advocate for nursing interests in general. As mentioned earlier, fewer than 1 of 10 nurses belongs to this official professional organization. The political power that could be derived from the unified efforts of 2.9 million registered nurses nationwide would be impressive; sadly, that goal has not yet been realized. Figure 3-2 shows the house of delegates in session at a state nurses association convention.

Miller's Wheel of Professionalism in Nursing

Using commonalities she detected in the work of sociologists and nursing leaders, as well as statements from *Nursing's Social Policy Statement* and *Code of Ethics for Nurses,* Miller (1985; Adams and Miller, 2001) created a model (or visual expression) to conceptualize nursing professionalism. She titled this model the Wheel of Professionalism (Figure 3-3).

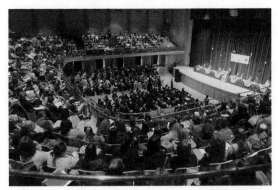

Figure 3-2 Professionals belong to associations that work for the improvement and availability of health care for all people, set practice standards, encourage and support ethical standards of practice, promote the professional development of nurses, and advance their economic and general welfare. (Courtesy Tennessee Nurses Association.)

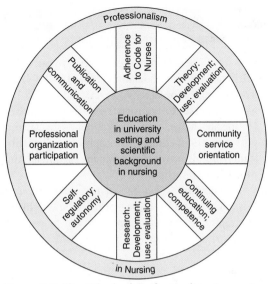

Figure 3-3 The Wheel of Professionalism in nursing. (Copyright 1984 Barbara Kemp Miller.)

In Miller's wheel, the center represents the essential foundation of nursing education in an institution of higher learning. According to Adams, et al (1996),

> *Each of the eight spokes represents other behaviors deemed necessary in maintaining or increasing nurses' professionalism. They are competence and continuing education; adherence to the code of ethics; participation in the primary and referent professional organization, i.e., ANA and state constituent member association; publication and communication; orientation toward community services; theory and research development and utilization; and self-regulation and autonomy (p. 79).*

To assist you in evaluating your own professional growth, complete Critical Thinking Challenge 3-1.

Standards Established by the Profession Itself

Any exploration of nursing's development as a profession would be incomplete without a discussion of three major documents that guide all nurses in their professional commitments. These are *Nursing's Social Policy Statement*, second edition (ANA, 2010b), *Nursing: Scope and Standards of Practice*, second edition (2004), and the *Code of Ethics for Nurses With Interpretive Statements* (ANA, 2010a).

Nursing's Social Policy Statement: A Contract With Society

Although criteria for professions vary, all professions have one criterion in common: an obligation to the recipients of their services. Nursing, therefore, has an obligation to those who receive nursing care. The nature of the social contract between the members of the nursing profession and society is summarized in *Nursing's Social Policy Statement*, second edition. This edition is the result of several years of work by literally hundreds of nurses. It serves as a framework for understanding professional nursing's relationship with society and nursing's obligation to those who receive professional nursing care. It also includes the ANA's contemporary definition of nursing and pertinent discussions related to the knowledge base of nursing, specialty and advanced practice, and professional regulation. A careful reading of this brief document will provide the reader with the essence of nursing's professionalism. (It is available from American Nurses Publishing; see References.)

Nursing: Scope and Standards of Practice

Nursing: Scope and Standards of Practice, second edition, outlines the expectations of the professional role within which all registered nurses must practice and delineates the standards of care and associated competencies for professional nursing. The goal of establishing standards is to improve the health and well-being of all recipients of nursing care and to establish the responsibilities for which nurses are accountable. There have been several editions of *Standards* issued by the ANA since the first one was written in 1973. Each edition has been painstakingly revised by large numbers of nurse volunteers under the leadership of the ANA.

The current document (2010a) itemizes the Standards of Practice and Standards of Professional Performance. For each standard there are numerous competencies by which practice for that standard can be assessed. Although all the standards are important to the practice of nursing, the Standards of Professional Performance are particularly germane to this chapter's emphasis on professionalism. One cannot fail to be impressed with the depth and scope of this document, and it is worthy of your time.

The Code of Ethics for Nurses

As you will recall, most of the early scholars attempting to define profession mentioned ethical behavior as a hallmark of a profession. In fact, a code of ethics is generally considered a tool that guides a group toward professional self-definition and provides evidence of professional legitimacy.

A code of ethics is a written, public document that reminds practitioners and the public they serve of the specific responsibilities and obligations accepted by the profession's practitioners. Since the inception of formalized education for nurses, the practice of nursing has been guided by ethical standards promoted first by Florence Nightingale and thereafter by nursing groups. The *Code of Ethics for Nurses* has been modified over the years as nursing and its social context have evolved. It is intended to guide the practice of registered nurses in all practice settings with all types of clients. The most recent version, *Code of Ethics for Nurses With Interpretive Statements*, was approved in 2001.

There are nine provisions in the 2001 Code, each of which is accompanied by interpretive statements intended to clarify the provision. The first three provisions describe "the fundamental values and commitments of the nurse;

Box 3-2   Self-Assessment: Am I a Patient-Centered Nurse?

1. Do I refrain from talking about myself and my problems to patients and their families?
2. Do I always introduce myself to patients and families when I first meet them?
3. When a patient or family member approaches me, do I immediately acknowledge them and turn my attention to them as soon as possible?
4. Do I really listen when patients and family members attempt to express a problem or concern? Do I try to understand what they are feeling?
5. Do I clarify patients' reasons for refusing medications or treatments without becoming defensive or taking the refusal personally?
6. Do I give prompt attention to all my patients, even those who are "difficult"?
7. Do I make every effort to be pleasant and polite to patients, family members, co-workers, and students, even when I am pressed for time or am having a bad day?
8. Do I explain procedures to patients and take every opportunity to educate them about their medications and conditions?
9. Am I alert to patient anxiety and attempt to "talk them through" anxiety-laden procedures?
10. Do I project high self-regard through my professional image, which includes tidy hair style, clean and polished shoes, neat uniform, short nails, and conservative makeup/grooming?
11. Do I recognize that I am accountable for both my actions and my omissions?
12. Do I take every opportunity to learn, grow, and enhance my competence as a nurse?

Modified from Cooper PG: A call for a return to patient-centered care, *Nurs Forum* 40(3):73-74, 2005.

the next three address boundaries of duty and loyalty; and the last three address aspects of duties beyond individual patient encounters" (p. 2). Read the provisions of the *Code of Ethics for Nurses* on the inside back cover of this text. The entire document, including interpretive statements, is available for review online (http://nursingworld.org/ethics/code/protected_nwcoe 303.htm).

Today's health care environment often presents challenges to nurses' ethics. Cost-conscious hospitals, managed care plans, and staffing insufficiencies created by both economic factors and nursing shortages are just a few of the many strains on nursing practice (Hook, 2001). The Code exists to strengthen and guide nurses' decision making as they navigate the troubled waters that now exist in many practice settings. The Code empowers nurses to maintain their focus on the patient as the center of health care.

Current concerns about professionalism in nursing have arisen in the last few years as some nurses seem to have become more nurse centered than patient centered. Is nursing losing its

patient-centered focus? Patients and their families have reported that "nursing has changed" and identified conduct by nurses that is at odds with their perceptions of "what nurses do." This has caused concerned nurses to think deeply about the profession and where it is going (Roberts, 2005). Regardless of the responsibility and workloads of today's nurses, the fact remains that nurses are paid to take care of patients and their loved ones (Cooper, 2005). Nursing has long prided itself as being the health care profession that cares. Certainly the behaviors exhibited by an individual nurse reflect the character and values of that individual and can enhance patient well-being and patient outcomes. You can assess your patient-centered focus using the self-assessment exercise found in Box 3-2.

COLLEGIALITY AS AN ATTRIBUTE OF THE PROFESSIONAL NURSE

A sometimes overlooked but increasingly important aspect of professionalism in nursing is collegiality. The promotion of a supportive and healthy work environment, cooperation, and recognition of interdependence among members of the nursing profession is the essence of collegiality. Professional nurses demonstrate collegiality by sharing with, supporting, assisting, and counseling other nurses and nursing students. These behaviors can be seen when nurses, for example, share knowledge with colleagues and students, take part in professional organizations, mentor less-experienced nurses, willingly serve as role models for nursing students, welcome learners and their instructors in the practice setting, assist researchers with data gathering, publish in professional literature, and support peer-assistance programs for impaired nurses.

The value placed on collegiality as a professional attribute can be seen in the ANA's 2004 *Nursing: Scope and Standards of Practice*, which includes collegiality as one of nine standards of professional performance. The practice of nursing would be enhanced if the commitment nurses feel toward their patients were equaled by their commitment to one another, to assistive personnel for whom they are legally responsible, and to nurturing the next generation of professional nurses.

An article titled "Being Good and Doing Good" by Bruhn (2001) outlines 12 points on professionalism, a number of which serve as reminders of the value of collegiality (Box 3-3).

NEED FOR A NEW PARADIGM

As society and health care have become more complex, perhaps the time has come to shift away from a rigid conceptualization of profession toward viewing the achievement of professional status as a dynamic, ongoing process. Huber (2000) recommends that we view professionalization as a continuum from nonprofessional to semiprofessional to professional, related to the degree to which an occupational group is characterized by the achievement of identified professional criteria. Instead of asking, "Is nursing a profession?" it may be more fruitful to ask,

---

Box 3-3   Points on Professionalism

- Be civil—Treat people with respect. You do not have to like or agree with a person to treat him or her as you would want to be treated.
- Be ethical—Stand up for personal and professional standards. Do what is right, not what is expected.
- Be honest—Be forthright; do not participate in gossip and rumor.
- Be the best—Strive to be better than good.
- Be consistent—Behavior should coincide with values and beliefs.
- Be a communicator—Invite ideas, opinions, and feedback from patients and colleagues.
- Be accountable—Do what you say you will do. Take responsibility for your own actions.
- Be collaborative—Work in partnership with others for the benefit of patients.
- Be forgiving—Everyone makes mistakes; give people a fair chance.
- Be current—Keep knowledge and skills up to date.
- Be involved—Be active at local, state, and national levels.
- Be a model—What a person says and does reflects on his or her profession.
- Be responsible for self—Take responsibility for your own learning needs and be assertive in making them known to teachers and mentors.
- Be prepared—Do assignments for classes and prepare for labs and clinicals in advance, brushing up on skills if needed.

Modified from Bruhn JG: Being good and doing good: the culture of professionalism in the health professions, *Health Care Manag* 19(4):47-58, 2001; and Cheyne D: Take responsibility for your learning needs, *Nurs Standard* 20(7):88, 2005.

"How is nursing progressing in the dynamic process of professionalization?" or "Where on the professional continuum is nursing right now?" Although barriers remain, some of which were identified earlier in this chapter, nursing has made a great deal of progress in the past few decades and is poised to continue that progress in the future.

To summarize this discussion of professionalism in nursing, read Critical Thinking Challenge 3-2 and identify the professional behaviors exhibited in the case study presented.

CRITICAL THINKING *Challenge 3-2*

Identifying Professional Nursing Behaviors

Instructions: *If being a professional nurse is different from practicing the occupation of nursing, there must be certain behaviors that differentiate the two. Read the case study below; then, using various criteria for professions presented in this chapter and the* Code of Ethics for Nurses, *identify professional behaviors exhibited by Joan. For each behavior you identify, state which source or document, such as the Code or Social Policy Statement, promotes that behavior.*

Joan is a 32-year-old married mother of two. She graduated from River City College of Nursing at the age of 26 years and has been practicing since her graduation. Her first position was as a staff nurse at Providence Hospital, a 300-bed private hospital. Nursing administration at Providence encourages nurses to provide individualized nursing care while protecting the dignity and autonomy of each patient and family. She chose Providence because the hospital's philosophy of nursing paralleled her own. Another reason Joan selected this hospital was that she wanted to practice oncology (cancer) nursing, and there is an oncology unit at Providence.

Each day Joan arrives promptly on her nursing unit. Her neat grooming and positive attitude convey pride in herself and her profession. She uses the nursing process in caring for her patients and in dealing with their families. That means she assesses their condition, plans and implements their care, and evaluates the care she has given. Then she documents what she has done in each patient's database in the accepted format. She communicates clearly to the other members of the nursing staff and collaborates with other health care professionals involved in the care of the patients on her unit but is careful not to discuss her patients with others not involved in their direct care.

After 2 years as a staff nurse, Joan accepted a position as a team leader. This means that now she takes responsibility not only for her own practice but also for that of licensed practical nurses and nursing assistants on her team. To do this effectively, she stays abreast of changes in her state's nurse practice act and Providence Hospital's policies and procedures. In addition, she updates her knowledge by reading current journals and research periodicals to base her practice on evidence rather than intuition. She makes it a policy to attend at least two nursing conferences each year to stay on top of trends. She belongs to her professional organization and participates as an active member. She finds that this is another source of the latest information on professional issues.

Joan looks forward to working with the nursing students at Providence Hospital. She remembers when she was a student and how a word from a practicing nurse could make or break her day. Of course, students do mean extra work, but she sees this as a part of her role and patiently provides the guidance they need, even when she is busy.

In the course of her daily work, Joan sometimes has questions. She is not embarrassed to seek help from more experienced nurses, from textbooks, or from other health professionals. Sometimes she offers suggestions to the head nurse and the

(Continued)

Identifying Professional Nursing Behaviors

oncology clinical nurse specialist about possible research questions and participates in gathering data when the unit takes on a research study.

Providence Hospital uses a shared governance model, which means nurses serve on committees that develop and interpret nursing policies and procedures. Joan serves on two committees and chairs another. Right now the hospital is preparing a self-study for an upcoming accreditation, so the meetings are frequent. Instead of complaining about the meetings, Joan prepares and organizes her portion of the meeting so that everyone's time is used most effectively. She has to delegate some of her patient care responsibilities to others while she is attending meetings. Because she has taken the time to know the other workers' skills and abilities, she does not worry about what happens while she is gone and asks for a full report when she returns to her unit.

At the end of the day when Joan goes home, she occasionally gets a call from a friend with a health-related question or a request to give a neighbor's child an allergy injection. Although she is tired, she recognizes that, in the eyes of others, she represents the nursing profession. She is proud to be trusted and respected for her knowledge, skills, and dedication. Helping others through nursing care is something Joan has wanted to do since she was small, and she finds it very fulfilling.

Lately, Joan has recognized in herself some troubling signs: She has been irritable and impatient with family and coworkers and generally out of sorts. She has gained weight and is exercising less than usual. She wonders whether working with terminally ill patients and their families is the source of her stress and recognizes that her work/life balance is out of kilter. Joan's husband has suggested that she take "a break" from nursing and stay home with the children, but, after talking it over with her nurse manager, she has decided to ask for assignment to different nursing responsibilities for a while. She knows that she needs to be her own advocate and take care of herself. Next week she will begin a 3-month stint in outpatient surgery, where she believes the emotional intensity will be a bit lower. She hopes to return to her first love, oncology nursing, at the end of that time.

Summary of Key Points

- Commitment to a profession is different from having a job or an occupation.
- A review of scholarly writing about professions reveals that there are several characteristics that all professions have in common.
- A body of knowledge, specialized education, service to society, accountability, autonomy, and ethical standards are a few of the hallmarks of professions.
- Although nursing has a briefer history than some traditional professions and is still dealing with autonomy, preparation, and commitment issues, great progress has been made in moving nursing along the professionalization continuum.
- An awareness of the characteristics of professions and professional behavior helps nurses assume leadership in continuing progress toward professionalism.
- *Nursing's Social Policy Statement* is considered nursing's contract with society.
- Being a professional is a dynamic process, not a condition or state of being.
- Professional growth begins during professional education and evolves throughout the different stages of nurses' careers.

Critical Thinking Questions

1. What is the relationship between training and education?
2. On a scale of 1 to 10, rate nursing on each of the criteria for professions identified by two of the following: Flexner, Hall, Bixler and Bixler, and Kelly.
3. Describe at least five characteristic behaviors of professional nurses.
4. Discuss the Nightingale Pledge (see Box 3-1) as a historical document, as an ethical statement, and as a reflection of Florence Nightingale's social and cultural environment. What value does this document have for today's nurse?
5. Using Miller's Wheel of Professionalism, identify specific activities that fit under each of the "spokes." How might a novice nurse's behaviors in relation to each spoke differ from those of a seasoned practitioner? Where does evidence-based practice fit into this model?
6. How might nursing be different today if all its practitioners viewed it as their profession rather than a job?

⊖volve *To enhance your understanding of this chapter, try the Student Exercises on the Evolve site at http://evolve.elsevier.com/Chitty/professional.*

REFERENCES

Adams D, Miller BK: Professionalism in nursing behaviors of nurse practitioners, *J Prof Nurs* 17(4): 203–210, 2001.

Adams D, Miller BK, Beck L: Professionalism behaviors of hospital nurse executives and middle managers in 10 western states, *West J Nurs Res* 18(1):77–89, 1996.

American Nurses Association: *Educational preparation for nurse practitioners and assistants to nurses: a position paper*, Kansas City, Mo, 1965, American Nurses Association.

American Nurses Association: *Code of ethics for nurses with interpretive statements*, Washington, DC, 2001, American Nurses Association.

American Nurses Association: *Association bylaws*, Silver Spring, MD, 2008, American Nurses Association.

American Nurses Association: *Nursing: scope and standards of practice*, ed 2, Washington, DC, 2010a, American Nurses Association.

American Nurses Association: *Nursing's social policy statement*, ed 2, Washington, DC, 2010b, American Nurses Association.

Bixler GK, Bixler RW: The professional status of nursing, *Am J Nurs* 59(8):1142–1147, 1959.

Brown EL: *Nursing for the future*, New York, 1948, Russell Sage Foundation.

Bruhn JG: Being good and doing good: the culture of professionalism in the health professions, *Health Care Manag* 19(4):47–58, 2001.

Carr-Saunders AM, Wilson PA: *The professions*, Oxford, 1933, Clarendon Press.

Cheyne D: Take responsibility for your learning needs, *Nurs Standard* 20(7):88, 2005.

Christman L: Who is a nurse? *Image J Nurs Sch* 30(3):211–214, 1998.

Cooper PG: A call for a return to patient-centered care, *Nurs Forum* 40(3):73–74, 2005.

Dock LL, Stewart IM: *A short history of nursing*, New York, 1920, Putnam.

Ervin N: 101 ways to improve nursing culture, *Mich Nurse* 79(1):15, 2006.

Flexner A: *Medical education in the United States and Canada: a report to the Carnegie Foundation for the advancement of teaching*, Bethesda, Md, 1910, Science & Health Publications.

Flexner A: Is social work a profession? *School Soc* 1(26):901, 1915.

Greiner AC, Knebel E, editors: *Health professions education: a bridge to quality*, Washington, DC, 2003, Institute of Medicine, National Academies Press.

Hall RH: Professionalization and bureaucratization, *Am Sociol Rev* 33:92–104, 1968.

Hall RH: The professionals, employed professionals, and the professional association. In *Professionalism and the empowerment of nursing*, Kansas City, Mo, 1982, American Nurses Association.

Hook K: Empowered caring and the code of ethics, *ANA Ethics & Human Rights Issues Update* 1(2), 2001 (website): http://www.nursingworld.org/MainMenu Categories/EthicsStandards/IssuesUpdate/Update Archive/IssuesUpdateFall2001/CodeofEthics.aspx.

Houle C: *Continuing learning in the professions*, San Francisco, Calif, 1980, Jossey-Bass.

Huber D: *Leadership and nursing care management*, Philadelphia, 2000, WB Saunders.

Kelly L: *Dimensions of professional nursing*, ed 4, New York, 1981, Macmillan.

Kidder MM, Cornelius PB: Licensure is not synonymous with professionalism: it's time to stop the hypocrisy, *Nurse Educ* 31(1):15–19, 2006.

LaSala KB, Nelson J: What contributes to professionalism? *MedSurg Nurs* 14(1):63–67, 2005.

McClure ML, Hinshaw AS: Spotlight on nurse staffing, autonomy, and control over practice, *American Nurse Today* 2(4):15–17, 2007.

Miller BK: Just what is a professional? *Nurs Success Today* 2(4):21–27, 1985.

Muller M: *Nursing dynamics*, ed 2, Sandton, South Africa, 1998, Heinemann.

Roberts D: Competence and professionalism, *MedSurg Nurs* 14(4):211, 2005.

Secrest J, Norwood BR, Keatley VM: "I was actually a nurse": the meaning of professionalism for baccalaureate nursing students, *J Nurs Educ* 42(2):77–82, 2003.

Task Force on Professionalism: White paper on pharmacy student professionalism, *J Am Pharm Assoc* 40(1):96–100, 2000.

Webster's new world dictionary, New York, 1996, Simon & Schuster.

Legal Aspects of Nursing

Beth Perry Black

LEARNING OUTCOMES

After studying this chapter, students will be able to:
- Describe the components of a model nurse practice act
- Discuss the authority of state boards of nursing
- Explain the conditions that must be present for malpractice to occur
- Identify nursing concerns related to delegation, assault and battery, informed consent, and confidentiality
- Describe strategies nurses can use to protect their patients, thereby protecting themselves from legal actions

Professional nursing has many complex and intertwined relationships in the legal arena that are important to identify and understand. The legal aspects of nursing are an area that is both extremely important and constantly changing. Schools of nursing and continuing education providers offer "Nursing and the Law" courses that are very popular among nurses. This chapter highlights key legal issues that affect professional nurses. Maintaining a working knowledge of the law as it relates to professional nursing practice is even more critical now in a time of great change in health care, as roles and practice settings change and expand. Nurses who do not understand and stay current with the changes in laws and regulations that govern nursing practice may find themselves with an increased exposure to liability, disciplinary measures, fines, or litigation (Aiken, 2004). This chapter will give you a beginning perspective on the various ways that nursing practice is affected by the legal system. It is common for nurses, especially early in their careers, to be very concerned about "breaking the law" regarding nursing practice or to misinterpret the meaning and purposes of laws. Laws are actually protective of both nurses and the patients for whom they are providing care.

AMERICAN LEGAL SYSTEM

The U.S. Constitution is the framework on which governance in this country is built. The purpose of the law in the United States is found in the Preamble to the U.S. Constitution: to ensure order, protect the individual person, resolve disputes, and promote the general welfare. To achieve these broad objectives, the law concerns itself with the legal relationships between persons and the government. All law in the United States flows from the U.S. Constitution and must conform to its principles. This means that although states themselves have the power to set laws for their citizens, no state or municipality can make laws that are not in accordance with the intentions of the framers of the Constitution. These intentions are subject to interpretation; hence the constitutionality of a particular law or ruling is argued in the court system.

The Constitution established a government in which the balance of power was divided among three separate but equal branches: (1) the executive branch, charged to implement law, and which includes the Office of the President at its highest level; (2) the legislative branch, charged to create law, and which includes the U.S. Congress

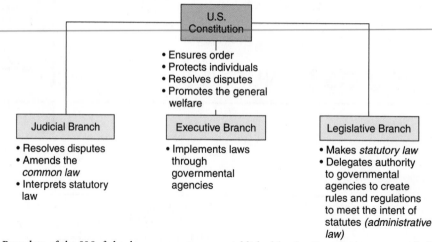

Figure 4-1 Branches of the U.S. federal government were established by the Constitution to provide for a balance of power.

and other regulatory agencies that set law; and (3) the judicial branch, charged to interpret law, and which includes the Supreme Court and federal court system (Figure 4-1).

Laws are rules of conduct that are authored and enforced by formal authorities and hold people accountable for compliance (Helm, 2003). Three major types of laws govern American society: common law, statutory law, and administrative law. Common law is decisional, meaning that judges' rulings become law. U.S. law has its foundation in centuries-old English common law. Every time a judge makes a legal decision, the body of common law expands.

Statutory laws—statutes—are those established through formal legislative processes. Every time the U.S. Congress or a state legislature passes legislation, the body of statutory law expands.

Administrative laws result when the legislative branch of a government delegates authority to governmental agencies to create laws that meet the intent of a statute. Both federal and state administrative laws have the force and effect of statutory law.

Laws are further categorized as either civil or criminal. Civil law recognizes and enforces the rights of individuals in disputes over legal rights or duties of individuals in relation to one another.

In civil cases, the party judged responsible for the harm may be required to pay compensation to the injured party. In contrast, criminal law involves public concerns regarding an individual's unlawful behavior that threatens society, such as murder, robbery, or fraud. The criminal court system both defines what constitutes a crime and also may mandate specific punishments (Aiken, 2004). Individuals convicted of criminal charges are punished, usually through the loss of some degree of their freedom, ranging from probation to imprisonment. They may also be required to pay fines. Administrative cases result when a person violates the regulations and rules established by administrative law, such as when a nurse or physician practices without a valid license. Punishment may involve having a license revoked or suspended or being placed on probation. In egregious cases, imprisonment may be required, especially if malicious intent or gross negligence is demonstrated.

For nurses, the statutory authority governing practice is of particular importance, including the executive authority of state boards of nursing (SBNs), the civil law areas of torts, privacy rights, and the evolving common law related to health care. The remainder of this chapter focuses on these key areas.

NURSING AS A REGULATED PRACTICE

The boundaries of practice of nursing, medicine, dentistry, law, and many others are established and regulated at the state level. This means that the legislative body in each state sets practice law and then assigns authority to implement the law to appropriate regulatory agencies and boards. These laws are in the form of professional practice acts, which set the licensing standards for various professions.

The purpose of licensing certain professions is to protect the public health, safety, and welfare. The statute that defines and controls nursing is called a nurse practice act. All 50 states, the District of Columbia, and several U.S. territories have nurse practice acts passed by their legislatures. These acts are administered and enforced through regulatory bodies known as SBNs.

Statutory Authority of State Nurse Practice Acts

Nurses, as health care providers, have certain rights, responsibilities, and recognitions through various state laws, or statutes. The nurse practice act in each state accomplishes at least four objectives:

1. Defines the practice of professional nursing
2. Sets the minimum educational qualifications and other requirements for licensure
3. Determines the legal titles and abbreviations nurses may use
4. Provides for disciplinary action of licensees for certain causes

In many states, nurse practice acts also define the responsibilities and authorities of the SBN (National Council of State Boards of Nursing, 2006). Thus the nurse practice act of the state in which nurses practice is the most important statutory law affecting nursing practice within the bounds of that state.

Once the law regarding nursing practice is established or amended by the legislature, the legislative branch delegates authority to enforce the law to an executive agency, usually the SBN. SBNs are responsible for enforcing the nurse practice acts in the various states. The SBN publicizes rules and regulations that expand the law. The statutory law plus the rules and regulations propagated by the SBN give full meaning to the nurse practice act in each state.

Nurse practice acts are revised from time to time to keep up with new developments in health care and changes in nursing practice. State nurses' associations are usually instrumental in lobbying for appropriate updating of nurse practice acts.

Because of the importance of practice acts to professional nurses, both the American Nurses Association (ANA) and the National Council of State Boards of Nursing (NCSBN) have developed suggested language for the content of state nurse practice acts. The ANA's *Model Practice Act* was published in 1996 to guide state nurses' associations seeking revisions in their nurse practice acts (ANA, 1996). The guidelines encourage consideration of the many issues inherent in a nurse practice act and the political realities of each state's legislative and regulatory processes. Through this document, the ANA recognizes the great importance of the nurse practice act and urges that the following content be included:

1. A clear differentiation between advanced and generalist nursing practice
2. Authority for boards of nursing to regulate advanced nursing practice, including authority for prescription writing
3. Authority for boards of nursing to oversee unlicensed assistive personnel (UAP)
4. Clarification of the nurse's responsibility for delegation to and supervision of other personnel
5. Support for mandatory licensure for nurses while retaining sufficient flexibility to accommodate the changing nature of nursing practice

The NCSBN *Model Nurse Practice Act* and *Model Nursing Administrative Rules* (2004) are comprehensive documents developed to guide individual states' development and revisions of their nurse practice acts. The NCSBN began development of model regulations in 1982. The NCSBN describes the current model, in its third major revision, as both a standard toward which states may strive and a reflection of the current and changing regulatory and health care system environments. Discussions over the past 20 years at the national level, facilitated by both the NCSBN and ANA, have brought a national perspective on nursing regulation to the state level, fostered dialogue and the development of more consistent standards across state lines, and provided increased protection for the public (Mikos, 2004).

Executive Authority of State Boards of Nursing

At both the federal and state government levels, the executive branch administers and implements law. The governor, who holds the state's highest executive office, generally delegates the responsibility for administering the nurse practice act to the State Board of Nursing (SBN), the agency charged with executing (carrying out) laws. In most states, the SBN consists of registered nurses (RNs), licensed practical nurses (LPNs), and consumers (members of the general public), all of whom are generally appointed to the board by the governor.

The SBN's authority is limited. It can adopt rules that clarify general provisions of the nurse practice act, but it does not have the authority to enlarge the law. Within these confines, SBNs have three functions that mirror those of the federal and state governments:

1. Executive, with the authority to administer the nurse practice act
2. Legislative, with authority to adopt rules necessary to implement the act
3. Judicial, with authority to deny, suspend, or revoke a license or to otherwise discipline a licensee or to deny an application for licensure

Each of these functions is as broad or as limited as the state legislature specifies in the nurse practice act and related laws.

SBNs may be independent agencies in the executive branch of state government or part of a department or bureau such as a department of licensure and regulation. Some state boards have authority to carry out the nurse practice act without review of their actions by other state officials. Others must recommend action to another department or bureau and receive approval of the recommendation before the decision is finalized.

Licensing Powers

Because nursing is a regulated practice, nurses must hold a valid license to practice. Getting to the point of being granted a license to practice nursing takes several years of hard work, and keeping one's license active and in good standing is a professional priority. Each state determines who is qualified to receive a license to practice nursing, and also determines the limits on the license. Licensure laws may be either mandatory or permissive. A mandatory law requires any person who practices the profession or occupation to be licensed. A permissive law protects the use of the title granted in the law but does not prohibit persons from practicing the profession or occupation if they do not use the title. All states now have a mandatory licensure law for the practice of nursing to safeguard the public. This means that only licensed nurses—RNs or LPNs—can call themselves nurses. UAP such as certified nursing assistants (CNAs) may not refer to themselves as nurses. It is not uncommon for patients to mistake the roles of various practitioners who are providing care; however, the CNA should correct the mistake if a patient refers to him or her as a nurse.

In most states, SBNs have the authority to set and enforce minimum criteria for nursing education programs. The practice act usually stipulates that an applicant for licensure must graduate from a state-approved nursing education program as a prerequisite to being admitted to the licensure examination. This means that schools of nursing must have state approval to operate. State approval requirements are generally less stringent than are national accreditation standards. Schools may voluntarily seek national accreditation to demonstrate that they meet higher than minimal standards. Although many other professions and occupations require graduation from a nationally accredited educational program as a prerequisite of licensure, only state approval is currently required in nursing. Some states are currently undertaking rule changes to require that nursing programs have national accreditation to achieve state approval.

Not only does the state, through the SBN, grant licenses, but it also has the power to discipline a licensee for performing professional functions in a manner that is dangerous to patients or the general public. Discipline may include sanctions such as temporary license suspension or revocation arising from unsafe, uninformed, or impaired practice by the nurse licensee. The most common reason nurses are disciplined by SBNs is for practicing while impaired (under the influence of alcohol or other substance).

Historically, the nursing profession has demonstrated a commitment to the rehabilitation of nurses whose practice is impaired by mental health issues or substance abuse. In 1990 the ANA published a recommendation that a Nursing Disciplinary Diversion Act be implemented by states through their boards of nursing (ANA, 1990). This included peer assistance programs to combat substance abuse as a voluntary alternative to divert traditional disciplinary actions of suspension or revocation of a license. In a NCSBN survey of boards of nursing (NCSBN, 2006), nearly all responding boards had disciplinary diversion processes in place to assist chemically impaired nurses to return to safe practice. More than half the boards also provided alternative programs for nurses with mental health problems, and one third had provisions for nurses with other health problems.

Licensure Examinations

Persons who have successfully completed their basic nursing education from a state-approved school of nursing are eligible to sit for the licensing examination. The nurse licensure examination for RNs is the National Council Licensure Examination for Registered Nurses (NCLEX-RN®). It is administered by computerized adaptive testing at various testing centers across each state, at a time scheduled by the test-taker. The NCLEX-RN, which is updated periodically, tests critical thinking and nursing competence in all phases of the nursing process. The test plan can be reviewed at the NCSBN website at https://www.ncsbn.org/1287.htm. Test-takers

who are not successful in passing the NCLEX typically may take the examination again after paying the examination fees. Passing rates of graduates of different schools of nursing are published online on SBNs' websites. Passing rates for first-time test-takers indicate something about the quality of the education that graduates of specific programs are receiving.

Until 1978 the national nursing licensing examination was developed by the ANA's Council of State Boards of Nursing, and the National League for Nursing served as the testing service. In 1978 the NCSBN was established and continued the activities of the ANA Council of State Boards. Through the NCSBN, each state participates in the licensing process through test plan and item development, periodic validation of the exam content with current practice, and adoption of a minimum passing score.

Mobility of Nurses: Licensure by Endorsement

Since 1944 most SBNs have participated in a cooperative effort to assist in the interstate mobility of nurses. The NCLEX is a national examination; therefore states recognize the licensure awarded in other states because nurses have passed the NCLEX. This is called licensure by endorsement. Endorsement means that RNs may practice in different states without having to take another licensing examination. To receive a license in a different state, nurses submit proof of licensure in another state and pay a licensure fee, and they receive a license in the new state by endorsement. Licensure by endorsement is not available to all practice disciplines. Nursing's plan serves as a national model for other licensed professions and occupations.

Nurse Licensure Compact

Because the United States is a mobile society, a new regulatory approach known as a mutual recognition model to licensure was developed by the NCSBN and has been adopted by a significant number of states. The Nurse Licensure Compact was developed to improve mobility of nurses, while still protecting the public health, safety, and welfare. Mobility occurs in travel nursing, in crossing state lines from one's home to one's workplace, in the telehealth practices (being physically present in one state while providing nursing care to a patient in another state through digital technology), and simply moving to another state for personal or career purposes. Nursing workforce mobility during national or regional disasters is also increased (Hellquist and Spector, 2004).

The Nurse Licensure Compact allows an RN to have one license (in the state of residency) yet practice in other compact member states without an additional license in the state of employment. Importantly, the nurse is subject to the nurse practice act in the state where she or he is practicing, not to that of the state of licensure. The concept of a single license for each nurse and the concomitant reduction of state barriers provide better protection for the public through improved tracking of nurses for disciplinary purposes and information sharing.

Each state that wishes to participate in the compact must pass legislation enabling the board of nursing to enter into the interstate Nurse Licensure Compact. Utah, Texas, and Wisconsin were the first states to implement the compact on January 1, 2000. By mid-2008, 23 states had enacted this legislation. Nurses licensed in any state that has implemented the compact can practice in their own states, as well as in any other compact state without applying for licensure by endorsement. A nurse who has changed permanent residence from one compact state to another may practice under the license from their former state of residence for up to 30 days, while waiting for licensure in the new state of residence. This means that a nurse moving between compact states does not have to delay working as a nurse until a new license is granted. Updated information about states participating in or seeking legislation to participate can be found at https://www.ncsbn.org/nlc.htm. Application of the compact model to advanced practice nurses is under discussion.

Exploration of the global perspective on nursing regulation is currently on the NCSBN agenda (Apple and Spector, 2005). On the basis of a demand from nurses educated abroad, the NCSBN began administering the NCLEX internationally to competent nurses applying for U.S. licensure in January 2005. The recruitment of nurses from outside the United States, particularly from poorer nations with their own high health care demands, is controversial (Dugger, 2006), with both legal and ethical considerations. Chapter 5 contains a fuller discussion of the significant issues surrounding recruiting nurses from other countries to practice in the United States.

LEGAL RISKS IN PROFESSIONAL NURSING PRACTICE

Nurses make decisions daily that affect the well-being of their patients. Because they have access to personal information about patients and interact with them during stressful times, they are in positions of great responsibility and trust. Several areas of nursing practice—in particular, delegation, informed consent, and confidentiality—are fraught with legal risk. Nurses may also be charged with malpractice or assault and battery. In this section, we will discuss these areas of concern.

Malpractice

Malpractice is the greatest legal concern of health care practitioners. Nurses are accountable for their own practice and are being named in malpractice suits more frequently than in the past (National Practitioner Data Bank, 2004). Malpractice suits are very complex legal entities. This discussion will give you some basic information about malpractice and, importantly, how to protect yourself from practices that make you susceptible to claims of malpractice.

Negligence is the central issue in malpractice. Negligence is the failure to act as a reasonably prudent person would have acted in the same circumstances. For example, if in burning yard debris on a windy day a man sets fire to his neighbor's garage, the neighbor may seek damages in a civil suit on charges of negligence. A reasonably prudent person would not have started a fire on a windy day, and an injury (the burned garage) can be shown to be a direct result of his failure to act reasonably.

Malpractice is negligence applied to the acts of a professional. In other words, malpractice occurs when a professional, for example a nurse or a physician, fails to act as a reasonably prudent professional would have acted under the same circumstances. Malpractice does not have to be intentional, that is, the professional did not mean to act in a negligent manner. Malpractice, that is, professional negligence, may occur in two ways: by commission—doing something that that should not have been done, and by omission—failing to do things that should have been done (Box 4-1).

A patient who brings a claim of malpractice against a nurse (or other professional) is known in the legal system as the plaintiff. The nurse becomes the defendant. Getting a malpractice case to be pleaded in front of a judge and jury is a very long process and is actually very unlikely to get this far. Many times malpractice cases are settled out of court, meaning that the outcome is negotiated between attorneys for the plaintiffs and defendant(s). (See Critical Thinking Challenge 4-1.)

The central question in any charges of malpractice is "Was the prevailing standard of care met?" The nursing standard of care is what the reasonably prudent nurse, under similar circumstances, would have done. Standard of care reflects a basic minimum level of prudent care based on the ethical principle of nonmaleficence ("do no harm"). Nurses are responsible for determining whether standard of care is met, not

Box 4-1   Malpractice: Professional Negligence

Malpractice is not limited to what a nurse *does* (commission), but what a nurse *fails to do* (omission) in a situation. The following is an example in which an RN is negligent in both ways.

A patient had surgery one morning for an abdominal mass. He was given morphine 8 mg intravenously (IV) at 5 PM. At 5:20, he was very drowsy, but, when the nurse woke him and asked about his pain, he complained that his "stomach still hurts some." She gave him a second dose of morphine 8 mg IV. When the nurse went back to check on him an hour later, he was in respiratory arrest.

The nurse was negligent by commission when she gave the patient a second dose of morphine. First, the nurse had to awaken the patient to ask him about his pain; the patient's complaint of "some pain" likely did not warrant a second dose of IV morphine so soon after the first dose. A reasonably prudent nurse in the same situation would not have given a relatively large dose of morphine so soon after the first, especially given that the patient was now drowsy and had to be awakened in order to assess his pain.

The nurse was negligent by omission when she failed to check on her patient for an hour after giving a second substantial dose of morphine. The first dose made him very drowsy after 20 minutes; this would indicate that he had a significant response to the first dose. The nurse also failed to assess the patient for causes of his continuing pain, such as examining his abdomen and checking his vital signs for evidence of a surgical complication.

CRITICAL THINKING *Challenge 4-1*

You hear nursing colleagues discussing prevention of malpractice, and you notice that some nurses are spending more time tending to patients' records than they are in providing care to patients. Think about how this emphasis on "defensive practice," that is, making sure that your patient's chart is perfect, may actually impede the delivery of safe care. As you think about this issue, consider what the purpose of charting is. How can you use the medical record to enhance the care of your patients? How might excessive charting harm you in a malpractice suit?

Box 4-2   Standards of Care: A Case Example

An 8-month-old infant was brought by his parents to the emergency department (ED) with significant fever and dehydration. The family with the infant was Spanish-speaking and included a family member trained in nursing in her home country. Intravenous (IV) fluids were ordered for rehydration. Because of the need for the infant to be able to move from bed to the arms of his caregivers, the IV was set up before needle insertion with both regular and extension length tubing. The ED RN, a new nurse in her second year in the ED, failed to flush the line to clear air from the tubing and then inserted the needle and began the infusion. This was noted by the family, and an unsuccessful attempt was made to alert the medical staff. The infant subsequently died of a significant air embolus, confirmed on autopsy. The family reported the event to the local district attorney, who investigated the incident. In considering whether charges were to be brought against the nurse, the following standards of care were considered:

1. Hospital policy indicated that an interpreter should have been called for communication with family.
2. Hospital policies and orientation competency guidelines, completed by this nurse, indicated that flushing of an IV line was a required step in the process.
3. Local schools of nursing indicated that flushing of an IV line was part of basic skills training, and current textbooks about fundamentals of nursing confirmed this content.
4. Other nurses in local EDs were interviewed, and all reported that flushing of an IV line before insertion was standard practice.
5. The company manufacturing the IV tubing had visual and written instructions on the box indicating proper use of the product, including flushing of the line.

practitioners from other disciplines. Nurse expert witnesses are hired by each side that will testify as to whether or not the prevailing standard of care was met. "Prevailing" is an important qualifier. As practice changes and develops, standards of care change accordingly. The issue in malpractice cases is the standard of care that prevailed—or was in effect—at the time the negligent act occurred. What may be considered negligent now may not have been considered negligent at the time. The standard of care that prevailed at the time is key and is ascertained through expert witness testimony; documents, including national standards of nursing practice; the patient record; and other pertinent evidence such as the direct testimony of the patient, the nurse, and others. Box 4-2 illustrates the presumed failure of an RN to meet the prevailing standard of care.

There are two requirements of a malpractice action. First, the defendant (nurse) has specialized knowledge and skills, and, second, through the practice of that specialized knowledge the defendant causes the plaintiff's (patient's) injury. All four elements of a cause of action for negligence must be proved. These elements are the same for any professional accused of malpractice:

1. The professional (nurse) has assumed the duty of care (responsibility for the patient's care).
2. The professional (nurse) breached the duty of care by failing to meet the standard of care.
3. The failure of the professional (nurse) to meet the standard of care was the proximate cause of the injury.
4. The injury is proved.

A high degree of proof is needed in each of these four elements. Monetary damages are awarded when a plaintiff prevails. These awards are based on proved economic losses, such as time missed from work or out-of-pocket health care costs, and on remuneration for pain and suffering caused by the injury. In the case of a death, the next of kin can become the plaintiff on behalf of the deceased patient.

In the past, some malpractice lawsuits involved nurses, but the physician or hospital defendants were typically sued for damages even when the substandard care was provided by nurses. In these instances, physicians were implicated through the "captain of the ship" doctrine. This outmoded doctrine implies that the physician is ultimately in charge of all patient care and thus should be responsible financially. Hospitals were implicated through the legal theory of *respondeat superior* (from Latin, meaning "let the master answer"), which attributes the acts of employees to their employer (Blumenreich, 2005). However, as nurses have obtained more credentials and their expertise, autonomy, and authority for nursing practice have increased, direct liability for nursing care has risen correspondingly.

Croke (2003) conducted a review of "more than 350 trial, appellate, and supreme court case summaries" (p. 56) from a variety of legal research sources and analyzed 253 cases that met the following criteria: A nurse was engaged in the practice of nursing as defined by his or her state's nurse practice act; a nurse was a defendant in a civil lawsuit as the result of an unintentional action (no criminal cases were considered); and a trial was held between 1995 and 2001.

Analysis revealed, not surprisingly, that the largest number of cases of reported negligence occurred in acute care hospitals (60%). Other settings included nursing homes/rehabilitation/transitional care units (18%), psychiatric settings (8%), home health settings (2%), and physician offices (2%); also included were cases involving care by advanced practice nurses (9%).

This review identified six major categories of negligence resulting in malpractice lawsuits against nurses: failure to follow standards of care, failure to use equipment in a responsible manner, failure to communicate, failure to document, failure to assess and monitor, and failure to act as a patient advocate. More details of Croke's analysis are presented in Box 4-3.

The key point is that professional nurses must carefully consider the legal implications of practice and be willing to and capable of conforming to prevailing professional standards and all legal expectations. Among factors leading to the increase in the number of malpractice cases against nurses is delegation.

Delegation

Delegation—that is, giving someone authority to act for another—is an issue that carries great legal and safety implications in nursing practice. The ability to delegate has generally been reserved for professionals because they hold licenses that sanction the entire scope of practice for a particular profession. Professional nurses, for example, may delegate independent nursing activities (as well as medical functions that have been delegated to them) to other nursing personnel. State nurse practice acts do not give LPNs or licensed vocational nurses the authority to delegate.

Professional RNs retain accountability for acts delegated to another person. This means that the RN is responsible for determining that the delegated person (delegatee) is competent to perform the delegated act. Likewise, the delegatee is responsible for carrying out the delegated act safely. The professional nurse remains legally liable, however, for the nursing acts delegated to others unless the delegatee is also a licensed professional whose scope includes the assigned act. For example, an RN can assign an unlicensed CNA who has been properly trained to take vital signs of all the patients under the RN's care. The nursing assistant cannot, however, reassign this responsibility to another person. The RN remains accountable for the data that the CNA collects, as it is not the CNA's responsibility, nor is it within his or her training, to interpret those data.

Delegation must also be considered in terms of ethical implications. The ANA's *Code of Ethics for Nurses* states, "The nurse is responsible and accountable for individual nursing practice and determines the appropriate delegation of tasks consistent with the nurse's obligation to provide optimum patient care" (ANA, 2001, section 4.4).

Delegation is an important liability and one not fully appreciated by many practicing nurses. The professional nurse's primary legal and ethical consideration must be the patient's right to safe, effective nursing care. Box 4-4 contains a list of "Five Rights" to ensure safe delegation of tasks to unlicensed assistive personnel (UAP). With the present nursing shortage, the use of UAP has expanded, further increasing the RN's liability

Box 4-3   Six Major Categories of Negligence That Result in Malpractice Lawsuits

1. Failure to follow standards of care, including failure to:
   - Perform a complete admission assessment or design a plan of care
   - Adhere to standardized protocols or institutional policies and procedures (for example, using an improper injection site)
   - Follow a physician's verbal or written orders
2. Failure to use equipment in a responsible manner, including failure to:
   - Follow the manufacturer's recommendations for operating equipment
   - Check equipment for safety before use
   - Place equipment properly during treatment
   - Learn how equipment functions
3. Failure to communicate, including failure to:
   - Notify a physician in a timely manner when conditions warrant it
   - Listen to a patient's complaints and act on them
   - Communicate effectively with a patient (for example, inadequate or ineffective communication of discharge instructions)
   - Seek higher medical authorization for a treatment
4. Failure to document, including failure to note in the patient's medical record:
   - A patient's progress and response to treatment
   - A patient's injuries
   - Pertinent nursing assessment information (for example, drug allergies)
   - A physician's medical orders
   - Information about telephone conversations with physicians, including time, content of communication between nurse and physician, and actions taken
5. Failure to assess and monitor, including failure to:
   - Complete a shift assessment
   - Implement a plan of care
   - Observe a patient's ongoing progress
   - Interpret a patient's signs and symptoms
6. Failure to act as a patient advocate, including failure to:
   - Question discharge orders when a patient's condition warrants it
   - Question incomplete or illegible medical orders
   - Provide a safe environment

Reprinted with permission from Croke EM: Nurses, negligence, and malpractice: an analysis based on more than 250 cases against nurses, *Am J Nurs* 103(9):54-63, 2003.

related to delegation. The NCSBN has developed a position paper on "Working with Others" (NCSBN, 2006), as well as model regulatory language. This paper and other additional information on delegation can be found on the NCSBN website at http://www.ncsbn.org.

In an attempt to further clarify issues of delegation, the ANA (2005a) also defined the responsibilities of the nurse when delegating to nursing assistive personnel. They reinforce the stance that the RN may delegate elements of care but cannot delegate the nursing process itself. Further, they reaffirm that the judgment of the nurse is primary in determining the patients, environments, and care situations for safe delegation; and that the nurse remains responsible for evaluating the outcomes of nursing care.

Currently the most debated area of delegation involves the delegation of medication administration to UAP. In an exploratory study of board of nursing executives and practice specialists about medication administration for older adults in

The following are standards that delineate responsibility for the staff RN who is delegating
responsibility to UAP.

1. Right task: Is the task appropriate for
   delegation in a specific care situation?
2. Right circumstances: Is delegation
   appropriate in this case? Consider the
   patient's health status, care delivery setting,
   complexity of the activity and delegate's
   competency, and available resources, and
   determine any other relevant factors.
3. Right person: Can the nurse can verify
   that the person delegated to do the task is
   competent to complete this task?
4. Right direction/communication: Has the
   RN given clear, specific instructions? These
   include identifying the patient clearly, the
   objective of the task, time frames, and
   expected results.
5. Right supervision/evaluation: Can the RN
   or other licensed nurse provide supervision
   and evaluation of the patient and the
   performance of the task? *and result accountability*

National Council of State Boards of Nursing: *The five
rights of delegation,* approved August 1997 by the Delegate
Assembly (http://www.ncsbn.org).

assisted living facilities, it was found that current practices vary across states, with 22 states
permitting nurses to delegate at least some type
of medication administration to assistive personnel. The majority of states that permit delegation
also addressed the nurses' accountability in the
relationship. In some states, however, UAP can
be trained to administer medications outside the
nurse delegation model (Reinhard, Young, Kane et
al, 2006). This is an unwelcome development that
bears close scrutiny from the nursing profession.

Assault and Battery

Assault and battery is occasionally the basis for legal
action against a nurse defendant. Assault is a threat
or an attempt to make bodily contact with another

person without the person's consent. Assault precedes battery; it causes the person to fear that battery is about to occur. Battery is the assault carried
out, the impermissible, unprivileged touching of
one person by another. Actual harm may or may
not occur as a result of assault and battery.

If, for example, a nurse threatens a patient with
a vitamin injection if he does not eat his meals,
the patient may charge assault. Actually giving
the patient a vitamin injection against his will
leaves the nurse open to charges of battery, even
if there is a physician's order. Patients have the
right to refuse treatment, even if the treatment
would be in their best interest. Both by common
law and by statute, informed consent is required
in the health care context as a defense to battery
(42 USC 1395 cc., 1990).

Informed Consent

All patients or their guardians (parents of minor
children, for instance) must be given an opportunity to grant informed consent before treatment unless there is a life-threatening emergency.
Three major conditions of informed consent are
the following:

1. Consent must be given voluntarily.
2. Consent must be given by an individual with
   the capacity and competence to understand.
3. The patient must be given enough information
   to be the ultimate decision maker.

Informed consent is a full, knowing authorization by the patient for care, treatment, and procedures and must include information about the
risks, benefits, side effects, costs, and alternatives.
Consumers of health care need a great deal of
information and should be told everything that
they would consider significant in making a treatment decision. This is a long-standing element of
health care law (*Canterbury* v. *Spence,* 464 F2 772,
1972).

For informed consent to be legally valid, elements of completeness, competency, and voluntariness are evaluated. Completeness refers to the
quality of the information provided. Competency
takes into account the capability of a particular patient to understand the information given
and make a choice. Voluntariness refers to the

freedom the patient has to accept or reject alternatives. In the case of patients who are minors, who are under the effects of drugs or alcohol (including preoperative medications), or who have other mental deficits, it is questionable that competency to consent exists. For example, a nurse was asked to obtain a signed consent for an endoscopic procedure from a patient with advanced dementia. In this situation, consent needs to be granted by the patient's spouse, next of kin, or court-ordered guardian or health care proxy (Garvis, 2005).

The role of nurses in informed consent, unless they are themselves primary providers, is to collaborate with the primary provider, most often a physician. A nurse may witness a patient's signing of informed consent documents but is not responsible for explaining the proposed treatment (Figure 4-2). The nurse is not responsible for evaluating whether the physician has truly explained the significant risks, benefits, and alternative treatments. However, professional nurses are responsible for determining that the elements for valid consent are in place, providing feedback if the patient wishes to change consent, and communicating the patient's need for further information to the primary provider.

CONFIDENTIALITY

Confidentiality is both a legal and an ethical concern in nursing practice. Confidentiality is the protection of private information gathered about a patient during the provision of health care services. The *Code of Ethics for Nurses* states, ". . . the nurse has a duty to maintain confidentiality of all patient information. . . . Only information pertinent to a patient's treatment and welfare is disclosed, and only to those directly involved with the patient's care. The nurse safeguards the client's right to privacy by judiciously protecting information of a confidential nature" (ANA, 2001, section 3.2).

The Code acknowledges exceptions to the obligation of confidentiality. These include discussing the care of patients with others involved in their direct care, quality assurance activities, legally mandated disclosure to public health authorities,

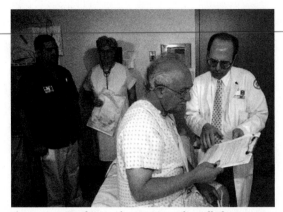

Figure 4-2 Professional nurses may be called on to witness a patient's signing of informed consent documents. The primary provider, however, is responsible for providing necessary information to the patient or legal guardian. (From Leahy JM, Kizilay PE: *Foundations of nursing practice,* Philadelphia, 1998, WB Saunders.)

and information required by third-party payers (ANA, 2001). The Code also recognizes the need to disclose information without the patient's consent when the safety of innocent parties is in question (*Tarasoff* v. *Board of Regents of the University of California,* 551 P2 334, 1976).

The principle of confidentiality is protected by state and federal statutes, but there are exceptions and limitations. Although some professions have statutorily protected privileged communication, such as attorneys and priests, nurses are usually not included in such statutes (Figure 4-3). Thus nurses may be ordered by a court to share information without the patient's consent. The professional nurse must understand these legal limitations to confidentiality.

On the basis of common, state, or municipal law, nurses have the duty to report or disclose certain information such as suspected abuse or neglect of a child (or elder, in some states), gunshot wounds, certain communicable diseases, and threats toward third parties. These laws vary by state and may be the responsibility of institutions providing health care services and not of an individual practitioner. Nurses should be aware of these requirements, however, and make sure the appropriate supervisory person is informed.

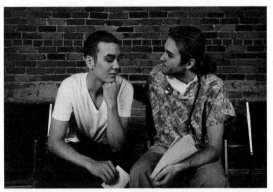

Figure 4-3 Nurses have an obligation for confidentiality, but are not protected by privileged communication statutes. In some cases, nurses are required to report what a patient has told them.

The Health Insurance Portability and Accountability Act of 1996

The Health Insurance Portability and Accountability Act of 1996 (HIPAA) is the first federal privacy standard governing protection of patients' medical records. The privacy provisions in the act began as a 337-word guideline, but as the final regulations were written, the provisions expanded to 101,000 words (Parker, 2003). HIPAA was designed, in part, to reinforce the protection of patient information as it is transmitted electronically, but the final act goes far beyond that goal. The regulations protect medical records and other individually identifiable health information, whether on paper, electronically, or communicated orally.

HIPAA requires all health care providers, including physicians, hospitals, health plans, pharmacies, public health authorities, insurance companies, billing agencies, information systems sales and service providers, and others, to ensure the privacy and confidentiality of patients. Although passed in 1996, the confidentiality regulations were not implemented until April 2003 to give providers time to prepare the necessary safeguards and documents and to train workers in their use.

HIPAA regulations require several major patient protections:

- Patients are able to see and obtain copies of their medical records, generally within 30 days of their request, and to request corrections if they detect errors. Providers may charge patients for the cost of copying and mailing the records.
- Providers must give patients written notice describing the provider's information practices and explaining patients' rights. Patients must be asked to agree to these practices by signing or initialing the notice.
- Limitations are placed on the length of time records can be retrieved, what information can be shared, where it can be shared, and who can be present when it is shared.

A number of other protections are provided in this comprehensive federal legislation. A summary of the complicated HIPAA regulations can be found online at http://www.hhs.gov/ocr/privacy/hipaa/understanding/summary/.

The struggle to integrate HIPAA into clinical practice continues and has prompted reflection on the impact on nursing (Flores and Dodier, 2005), causing an increase in repetitive paperwork (Kumekawa, 2005). For many nurses, however, HIPAA is also an affirmation of our long-standing responsibility to our patients (Erickson and Millar, 2006). Analysis of HIPAA 2 years into implementation supported its role in the protection of patient privacy but noted the tremendous impact on the clinical environment, including high implementation costs (Harman, 2005).

EVOLVING LEGAL ISSUES AND THE NURSE

You are entering nursing practice at a time of great change in the health care system. Because of the dynamic nature of nursing and health care, legal issues affecting nursing practice are also evolving. Specific legal issues that illustrate the changing nature of nursing practice are related to role changes, supervision of UAP, payment mechanisms, and issues associated with the implementation of the Patient Self-Determination Act (PSDA). Each of these issues is discussed briefly in the following sections.

Role Changes in Health Care

Just as a nurse's knowledge base and the nurse's accountability for nursing practice have increased over time, so has the need to expand the legal authority for nursing practice. Professional nurses realize that it is important for a state nurse practice act to reflect nursing practice accurately and to keep up with changes in health care delivery as they occur. In other words, states' nurse practice acts must reflect change in practice. Advanced practice nurses set the pace for evolving nursing practice, and the nurse practice act must support their ability to offer nursing services to consumers in various settings (Cady, 2003). Otherwise, nurses have questionable legal basis for practice and are open to litigation.

Historically, in some states, nurses in advanced practice such as nurse-midwives and nurse practitioners have not been supported by timely changes in the nurse practice act. For example, nurses in a women's health practice in Missouri were sued for practicing medicine without a license. After intense litigation, their practice was supported by the Missouri Supreme Court. The court found "legislative intent" in the nurse practice act not to limit nursing practice except to protect the public. The nurses in question were well credentialed and were practicing with the knowledge and support of the Missouri Board of Nursing and the Missouri Nurses Association, so the safety of the public was not in question (*Sermchief* v. *Gonzales*, 660 SW2 683, 1983).

This is only one example of the legal exposure nurses face when their state's nurse practice act is not updated periodically to support explicitly an expanded scope of practice. Working within the constituent member (state nurses) association to expand the evolving scope of nursing practice appropriately ensures the growth of the profession and increases the number of primary care providers needed by the public. Professional nurses must support their professional associations, which guide the development of legislation that accurately reflects current nursing practice at all levels. Your practice is directly affected by the work of professional organizations at the legislative levels.

Prescriptive authority

An important role expansion for advanced practice nurses is prescriptive authority. Prescriptive authority is defined as the legal acknowledgment of prescription writing as an appropriate act of nursing practice. The ANA, the American Academy of Nurse Practitioners, and others support prescriptive authority for advanced practice nurses, as distinguished from generalist RNs.

Nurses should consider several questions about prescriptive authority: Does the state recognize prescriptive authority for nurses? If so, is the SBN the state regulatory authority for this practice? Does the law require physician collaboration or supervision or written protocols? What are the parameters for prescribing controlled substances, if any?

In 2006 advanced practice nurses had some type of prescriptive authority in all 50 states. This authority ranged from completely independent authority with no collaborative requirements in 13 states and districts (Alaska, Arizona, Iowa, Maine, Montana, New Hampshire, New Mexico, Oregon, Utah, Washington, Wisconsin, Wyoming, and the District of Columbia), to 5 states (Alabama, Florida, Kentucky, Missouri, and Texas) where nurse practitioners can prescribe (excluding controlled substances) with some degree of physician involvement or delegation of prescription writing (Phillips, 2006). In the remaining states, nurse practitioners can prescribe (including controlled substances) with some degree of physician involvement or delegation of prescription writing (Phillips, 2006). Variation among states regarding physician involvement in advanced practice nurse practice has prompted nurses in Georgia to sustain a 15-year battle for more autonomy (Nelson, 2006). This is an evolving area of practice, and advanced practice nurses must be aware of the boundaries on prescriptive authority given to them in the state where they are practicing.

Both generalist and advanced practice nurses must understand prescriptive authority of advanced practice in their states. Generalist nurses must know from whom they can accept medication orders, and advanced practice nurses must stay within their legal scope of practice.

Supervision of unlicensed assistive personnel

Another evolving legal issue is the continued role expansion of UAP or limited licensed (licensed practical/vocational nurses) personnel within health care institutions. Nurse aides (i.e., UAP) are increasingly being substituted for nurses, thus creating greater risks to patients and increasing the liability of nurses, who supervise their work. The important findings from a research study described in the Evidence-Based Practice Note indicate that lack of professional nurse supervision and the educational level of nurses themselves significantly affect patients, institutions, and nurses alike (Institute of Medicine, 1996; Buerhaus, Needleman, Mattke et al, 2002; Aiken, Clarke, Cheung et al, 2003).

The substitution of unlicensed personnel for RNs is a strategy used by health care facilities to hold down costs. Such substitution jeopardizes quality of care and places the RN at increased risk for patient injury liability because of acts performed or omitted by UAP. Over the long term, professional nursing care may actually be less expensive than care provided by unlicensed personnel, who are less likely to provide patient teaching and recognize complications.

The licensure or state approval of UAP is a complex issue that has relevance for RNs because professional nurses are legally responsible for the tasks delegated to UAP. Nationally standardized education and training for these workers would assure nurses that their coworkers have a minimum level of competence. The NCSBN has developed the National Nurse Aide Assessment Program (NNAAP) examination, a test of both cognitive and skill performance to certify nurse aide competency. The Medication Aide Certification Examination (MACE), also administered by

---

☀ EVIDENCE-BASED PRACTICE NOTE

An interdisciplinary group of Pennsylvania researchers, led by Linda Aiken, PhD, FAAN, RN at the University of Pennsylvania, was concerned about nurse understaffing and the resulting threats to patient safety in hospitals. The group members decided to study the educational composition of RNs in relation to patient outcomes. Their objective was "to examine whether the proportion of hospital RNs educated at the baccalaureate level or higher is associated with risk-adjusted mortality and failure to rescue (deaths in surgical patients with serious complications)" (p. 1617).

The researchers analyzed outcome data for 232,342 general, orthopedic, and vascular surgery patients discharged from 168 nonfederal adult general Pennsylvania hospitals between April 1, 1998, and November 30, 1999. These figures were linked to data on educational composition, staffing, and other characteristics.

The percentage of RNs with a bachelor's or higher degree ranged from 0 percent to 77% in the various hospitals in the study.

After adjusting for patient characteristics and hospital structural characteristics (size, teaching status, level of technology), as well as for nurse staffing, nurse experience, and whether the patient's surgeon was board-certified, a 10 percent increase in the proportion of bedside nurses holding a bachelor's degree was associated with a 5 percent decrease in both the likelihood of patients dying within 30 days of admission and the odds of failure to rescue (p. 1617).

These researchers concluded that significantly lower mortality and failure to rescue rates were found in hospitals with higher proportions of baccalaureate-prepared nurses. They recommended that investments in public funds be made to increase the number of baccalaureate nurses to substantially improve the quality of care in the nation.

Aiken LH, Clarke SP, Cheung RB et al: Educational levels of hospital nurses and surgical patient mortality, *JAMA* 290(12): 1617-1623, 2003.

the NCSBN, certifies competency in administration of simple medications by UAP. Regardless of certifications by UAP, it remains the responsibility of professional nurses to know the limitations of the particular assistive personnel under their supervision.

Payment mechanisms for nurses

Nurses are increasingly practicing in nontraditional roles and settings. Many professional nurses are both capable of and interested in offering nursing services as private practitioners, but payment mechanisms may limit such activities. Nurses are concerned about offering services for which consumers are unable to obtain reimbursement from their insurance carriers, and third-party reimbursement has traditionally been limited to care provided by physicians.

Over the years, nurses and their professional associations have supported state and federal legislation to provide direct and indirect payments to nurses for nursing services rendered. A major legislative victory in the 8-year fight to obtain direct reimbursement of advanced practice nurses came with the passage of the 1997 Balanced Budget Act. This legislation authorized nurse practitioners and clinical specialists, beginning in January 1998, to bill the Medicare program directly for nursing services furnished in any setting. It remains a regulatory challenge to devise a fair and equitable payment system for advanced practice nurses, whose scopes of practice vary from state to state. Nurses are concerned that these changes are often not implemented or that advanced practice nurses are paid less for services similar to those provided by other health care professionals who are paid at a higher rate.

Laws are passed that are sometimes not implemented. This occurs when the group affected by the law (for example, the insurance industry) is unwilling to implement the changes and no "watchdog" agency is created to ensure that changes occur. For example, federal legislation was enacted requiring state Medicaid agencies to pay certain nurses (nurse practitioners, nurse-midwives, and nurse anesthetists) directly for services provided to Medicaid recipients. As with the laws affecting private insurers, these requirements have not been implemented in every state. Nurses may need to seek legal remedies to require implementation of policies mandated by federal law (*Nurse Midwifery Associates* v. *Hibbett,* 918 Fed2 605, 1990).

The need for health care reform was one of the key discussions during the 2008 presidential campaign. President Barack Obama campaigned on a platform of health insurance for all Americans. The debate about health care over the course of the campaign brought health care inequities, high costs, and poor access to preventive care into the spotlight. Health care reform is one of the Obama administration's highest priorities, although the specifics of this reform have yet to be determined at the time of this writing. As a result of these new priorities, the ANA and constituent member (state) associations are working to ensure that nurses are included in discussions and roundtables addressing health care reform in the United States.

Patient Self-Determination Act

Although the Patient Self-Determination Act (PSDA) became effective in 1991, almost 20 years later there remain many problems in its implementation. Nurses are in a position to help patients and families understand this law and how it can assist them to have the end-of-life care they prefer. The PSDA applies to acute care and long-term care facilities that receive Medicare and Medicaid funds. It encourages patients to consider which life-prolonging treatment options they desire and to document their preferences in case they should later become incapable of participating in the decision-making process. Written instructions recognized by state law that describe an individual's preferences in regard to medical intervention should the individual become incapacitated are called an advance directive. Additional details about the PSDA are included in Chapter 5.

This act was passed partly in response to the U.S. Supreme Court's decision in *Cruzan* v. *Director Missouri Department of Health* (110 Supreme Court 2841, 1990), which was viewed as limiting an individual's ability to direct health care when unable to do so. The PSDA requires the health care facility to document whether the patient has completed an advance directive.

The PSDA's basic assumption is that each person has legal and moral rights to informed consent about medical treatments with a focus on the person's right to choose (the ethical principle of autonomy). The act does not create any new rights, and no patient is required to execute an advance directive.

According to the PSDA, acute care (hospitals) and long-term care facilities must:

1. Provide written information to all adult patients about their rights under state law
2. Ensure institutional compliance with state laws on advance directives
3. Provide for education of staff and the community on advance directives
4. Document in the medical record whether the patient has an advance directive

The Agency for Health Care Policy Research reported that even when patients had advance directives in place, the directives were not guiding end-of-life care as legislators and advocates had anticipated. This was attributable to several factors: the patients were not considered hopelessly ill; the family members were not available, were too overwhelmed to implement the patient's wishes, or disagreed with the patient's wishes; and the advance directive itself was not specific enough or did not cover pertinent clinical issues (Ditto, Danks, and Smucker, 2001). The nursing role with advance directives can often become a tangle of state and federal laws, hospital policies, and conflicting family desires (Ryan, 2004). Documentation of the existence of advance directives and use of them in planning care is an important patient advocacy role for nurses and is a legal requirement that needs careful implementation in clinical settings.

PREVENTING LEGAL PROBLEMS IN NURSING PRACTICE

Although the discussion about legal issues related to nursing practice has covered many topics, it is probably a good time to remind you that the vast majority of nurses never encounter the legal problem during their professional careers. This is because there are a number of effective strategies that professional nurses can use to limit the possibility of legal action.

Practice in a Safe Setting

To be truly safe, facilities in which nurses work must be committed to safe patient care. The safest situation is one in which the agency:

1. Employs an appropriate number and skill mix of personnel to care adequately for the number of agency patients at all levels of acuity
2. Has policies, procedures, and personnel practices that promote quality improvement
3. Keeps equipment in good working order
4. Provides comprehensive orientation to new employees, supervises all levels of employees, and provides opportunities for employees to learn new procedures consistent with the level of health care services provided by the agency. Note that a comprehensive orientation is not "on the job training."

In addition to an active quality improvement program, each health care organization should have a risk management program. Risk management seeks to identify and eliminate potential safety hazards, thereby reducing patient and staff injuries. Common areas of risk include patient falls, failure to monitor, failure to ensure patient safety, improper performance of a treatment, failure to respond to a patient, medication errors, failure to follow agency procedure, improper technique, and failure to supervise treatment (Aiken, 2004).

In a nonrandom survey of nearly 5000 practicing nurses regarding patient safety in their worksites, 80 percent of the nurses believed that bedside nurses contribute to a culture of safety, while voicing concern that chronic understaffing impeded safe care (Manno, Hogan, Heberlein et al, 2006). In a desire to promote improvements in patient safety, the Joint Commission on Accreditation of Healthcare Organizations (2005) adopted patient safety goals in 2005. These 14 goals identify significant ways in which patient safety can be enhanced through environmental, educational, practice, and policy changes. They can be reviewed online at http://www.jointcommission.org/PatientSafety/NationalPatientSafety Goals.

Communicate With Other Health Professionals, Patients, and Families

The professional nurse must have open and clear communication with nurses, physicians, and other health care professionals. Safe nurses trust their own assessments, inform physicians and others of changes in patients' conditions, and question unclear or inaccurate physicians' orders. A key aspect of communication essential in preventing legal problems is keeping good patient records. This written form of communication is called documentation (Figure 4-4).

The clinical record, particularly the nurse's notes, provides the core of evidence about each patient's nursing care. No matter how good the nursing care, if the nurse fails to document it in the clinical record, in the eyes of the law the care did not take place. Be sure to document accurately, in a timely manner, and concisely. Know the charting policies of your agency and your unit, particularly the acceptable abbreviations.

Current and descriptive documentation of patient care is essential, not only to provide quality care but also to protect the nurse. Assessments, plans, interventions, and evaluation of the patient's progress must be reflected in the

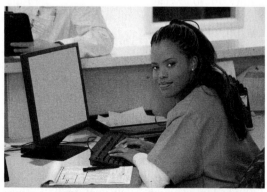

Figure 4-4 Documentation is the written form of communication among various disciplines providing care to patients. Many health care settings use electronic charting.

patient's clinical record if malpractice is alleged. Nurses must also document telephone calls with patients, family members, physicians, and other health care providers.

If a patient is angry, noncompliant, or complaining, nurses should be even more careful to document thoroughly. Professional nurses recognize that establishing and maintaining good communication and rapport with patients and their families not only is an aspect of best practice but also is a means of protection from lawsuits.

Accountability for accurate documentation has increased in recent years because of the advent of electronic documentation and multiple uses of recorded data, such as reimbursement, research, and quality assurance audits. The importance of the patient record as basis for safe practice remains (ANA, 2005b). Common documentation pitfalls to avoid include leaving gaps in data or entries, including subjective bias in notes, and deviating from agency policies and procedures for recording (Austin, 2006).

Meet the Standard of Care

The most important protective strategy for the nurse is to be a knowledgeable and safe practitioner and to meet the standard of care with all patients. Meeting the standard of care involves being technically competent, keeping up-to-date with health care innovations, being aware of peer expectations, and participating as an equal on the health care team.

Nurses must familiarize themselves with the policies and procedures of the agency in which they work and must not deviate from those policies. They must know how to use equipment properly and know when that equipment is malfunctioning. They must keep up with trends in their practice area by reading the professional literature and attending continuing education conferences and workshops. Professional nurses must use national standards of practice, care planning, and care evaluation. The ANA has developed generic and specialty standards of nursing practice and published these in the document *Nursing: Scope and Standards of Practice* (2004). These national standards can be used by quality improvement programs in individual hospitals in establishing their own "local" standards of nursing care.

Continued competence is an issue the nursing profession has not uniformly addressed. At this time, different states have differing requirements for continuing education as a prerequisite for license renewal. The efficacy of continuing education mandates has been challenged (Smith, 2004). An example of using creative methods of maintaining competency can be found on the North Carolina Board of Nursing's website: http://www.ncbon.org/content.aspx?id=664. The wise nurse recognizes that continuing education and maintaining competence are essential to safe practice, whether or not they are state requirements.

In the final analysis, the best protection a nurse can have is to know the limits of his or her own education and expertise and the provisions of the nurse practice act. Staying within those limits may sometimes require nurses to enlist assistance from more experienced nurses to be able to meet the standard of care. This should be viewed as a learning opportunity and an indication of maturity rather than as a failure or evidence of incompetence. Box 4-5 contains information about documents that all professional nurses should own, read, understand, and keep in their professional libraries to ensure that they meet the standard of care.

Box 4-5   Four Documents You Should Own

Professional nurses are accountable for practicing within their scope of practice. To stay abreast of changes that may affect the scope of nursing practice, you should always have the latest revision of the following four documents. You must read and understand them and be mindful of their provisions as you practice.

1. A copy of the nurse practice act of the state in which you practice. These are generally available for downloading from states' board of nursing websites. Familiarity with the law in your state is a key safeguard against inadvertently overstepping your limits of practice while understanding the full set of responsibilities that your state requires you to fulfill as a professional RN.

2. *Nursing's Social Policy Statement.* Available from the ANA (http://www.nursingworld.org), this short but important document lays out in concise language the most current definition of nursing; the knowledge base for nursing, including specialization and advanced practice roles; and the regulation of practice. It represents "an expression of the social contract between society and professional nursing" (p. v) in this country. The ANA has taken the position that the scope of nursing practice should flow from the definition of nursing that is contained in this document. It therefore has considerable impact on the national scope of practice.

3. *Nursing: Scope and Standards of Practice.* Also published by the ANA, this document expands on the Social Policy Statement. It focuses on defining and delimiting clinical practice and its safe implementation. Scope and Standards' statements, in conjunction with other documents, are widely used in legal cases to determine whether a nurse has met the "standard of care" in a particular case. In addition to this general document, the ANA has published standards for 21 specialized areas of practice, such as hospice and palliative care and gerontological, pediatric, neuroscience, vascular, and psychiatric–mental health nursing, among others.

4. ANA's *Code of Ethics for Nurses with Interpretive Statements.* This document is available for viewing only (http://www.nursingworld.org/ethics/code/protected_nwcoe303.htm) and may be purchased even if you are not yet a member of the ANA. It describes the nine ethical provisions that cover all aspects of nursing practice, found inside the back cover of this text. In addition, it adds a number of clarifying statements for each of the nine provisions. Knowledge of your professional organization's code of ethics is an important protection for you as you begin or continue your nursing practice.

The three ANA documents are available as a "Foundational Package" on the ANA website http://www.nursingworld.org.

Box 4-6   Basic Types of Professional Liability Insurance Policies

OCCURRENCE POLICIES

Cover injuries that occur during the period covered by the policy, whether or not the policy is still in effect at the time the suit is brought

CLAIMS-MADE POLICIES

Cover injuries only if the injury occurs within the policy period and the claim is reported to the insurance company during the policy period or during the "tail." A tail is an uninterrupted extension of the policy period and is also known as the extending reporting endorsement.

Box 4-7   Guidelines for Preventing Legal Problems in Nursing Practice

- Practice safely in a safe setting.
- Communicate with other health professionals, patients, and—with patient's permission—family members. Document fully, carefully, and in a timely manner.
- Delegate wisely, remembering the five "rights" of delegation.
- Meet or exceed the standard of care by staying on top of new developments and skills.
- Carry professional liability insurance, and know the specifics of the policy.
- Promote positive interpersonal relationships and a nondefensive manner while practicing caring, compassionate, holistic nursing care.

Carry and Understand Professional Liability Insurance

Despite the efforts of dedicated professionals, sometimes mistakes are made and, unfortunately, patients are injured. It is essential for nurses to carry professional liability insurance to protect their assets and income in case they are required to pay monetary compensation to an injured patient. Nursing students should also carry insurance, and most nursing education programs require that they do so. In addition to carrying the insurance, nurses must read and understand the provisions of their malpractice coverage.

Professional liability insurance policies vary. Generally, they provide up to $2 million coverage for a single incident and up to $4 million total. The amount of coverage depends on the nurse's specialty. Nurse-midwives, for example, pay much higher liability insurance premiums than do psychiatric nurses because a nurse-midwife's potential for being sued is greater. Look for a policy that has portable coverage and make sure that it covers court judgments, out-of-court settlements, legal fees, and court costs. Furthermore, a good policy covers incidents occurring anytime—as long as the incident took place while the policy was in force, even if you no longer carry the insurance (occurrence policy).

Professional liability insurance is available through most state nurses' associations, nursing students' associations, and private insurers.

Group policies, such as those available through professional associations, are usually less expensive than individual policies and are an important benefit of association membership. Box 4-6 provides information about the two main types of professional liability policies.

Promote Positive Interpersonal Relationships

Even in the face of untoward outcomes from a health care provider, it is usually only the disgruntled patient that sues. Therefore the best strategy for the professional nurse is prevention of legal actions through positive interpersonal relationships.

Prevention includes giving personalized, concerned care; including the patient and the family in planning and implementing care; and promoting positive, open interpersonal relationships that communicate caring and compassion. When confronted with angry patients or family members, wise nurses avoid criticizing or blaming other health care providers and maintain a concerned and nondefensive manner.

The professional nurse who is clinically competent and caring, communicates openly with patients, and acknowledges the holism of the patient is likely to prevent most legal problems. Box 4-7 summarizes the important steps nurses can take to avoid legal problems in professional practice.

Summary of Key Points

Nurses must recognize that the law is a system of rules that governs conduct and attaches consequences to certain behavior.

- Consequences include civil or criminal action or both.
- Nursing practice is limited by the definition of practice in the state nurse practice act and the qualifications for licensure to practice nursing in that state.
- The law is dynamic and must be responsive to society's needs.
- Broadening the scope of nursing practice has increased the possibility for legal actions involving nurses.
- Technologic advances have increased concern about informed consent and patients' rights to direct the care they choose to receive or refuse.
- Many nurses possess inadequate knowledge of legal issues that affect nursing practice every day. These issues deserve increased attention by nurses in all areas of practice.

Critical Thinking Questions

1. Using your state's nurse practice act, describe the scope of practice of the RN. When was the last time the law was modified? Does it accurately reflect current nursing practice?
2. Read the section of the nurse practice act relating to advanced practice. What differences are identified between the scope of practice of the general RN and that of the advanced practice nurse?
3. If a physician writes an order for an unusually high dose of a medication, what steps should the nurse take to ensure patient safety?
4. What are the liability issues for a nurse who fails to raise the side rails on a postoperative patient's bed if the patient is injured in a fall?
5. Explain the PSDA to your family and friends. What questions do they have about an advance directive? Find out what the laws regarding advance directives are in your state.
6. When you are interviewing for a position, what questions should you ask to determine whether it is a legally safe setting in which to practice?

7. In your state, under what circumstances can a nurse who administers a medication causing an allergic reaction be found negligent?
8. Discuss the legal and ethical issues for a nurse who is asked by a nurse manager to help clear up a backlog of paperwork by postdating forms and signing off on equipment inspections that were not performed as required.

The author wishes to thank Beverly Foster, PhD, RN, for her previous contributions to this chapter.

⊖volve *To enhance your understanding of this chapter, try the Student Exercises on the Evolve site at http://evolve.elsevier.com/Chitty/professional.*

REFERENCES

Aiken LH, Clarke SP, Cheung RB, et al: Educational levels of hospital nurses and surgical patient mortality, *JAMA* 290(12):1617-1623, 2003.

Aiken T: *Legal, ethical and political issues in nursing,* Philadelphia, 2004, FA Davis.

American Nurses Association: *Suggested state legislation: nurse practice act, nursing disciplinary diversion act, prescriptive authority act,* Kansas City, Mo, 1990, American Nurses Association.

American Nurses Association: *Model practice act,* Washington, DC, 1996, American Nurses Publishing.

American Nurses Association: *Code of ethics for nurses with interpretive statements,* Washington, DC, 2001, American Nurses Publishing.

American Nurses Association: *Nursing: scope and standards of practice,* Washington, DC, 2004, American Nurses Publishing.

American Nurses Association: *Principles for delegation,* Silver Spring, Md, 2005a, American Nurses Publishing.

American Nurses Association: *Principles for documentation,* Silver Spring, Md, 2005b, American Nurses Publishing.

Apple K, Spector N: Global initiatives in regulation at National Council of State Boards of Nursing, *JONAS Healthc Law Ethics Regul* 7(4):112-113, 2005.

Austin S: Ladies of the jury I present the nursing documentation, *Nursing2006* 36(1):56-64, 2006.

Blumenreich GA: Doctrine of corporate liability, *AANA J* 73(4):253-257, 2005.

Buerhaus PI, Needleman J, Mattke S, et al: Strengthening hospital nursing, *Health Affairs* 21(5):123-132, 2002.

Cady RF: *Advanced practice nurse's legal handbook*, Philadelphia, 2003, Lippincott Williams & Wilkins.

Croke EM: Nurses, negligence and malpractice: an analysis based on more than 250 cases against nurses, *Am J Nurs* 103(9):54-63, 2003.

Ditto PH, Danks JH, Smucker WD: Advance directive as acts of communication, *Arch Intern Med* 161:421-430, 2001.

Dugger CW: US plan to lure nurses may hurt poor nations, *New York Times*, May 24, 2006.

Erickson JI, Millar S: Caring for patients while respecting their privacy: renewing our commitment, *Online J Issues Nurs* 10(2):2, 2005:downloaded 2006.

Flores JA, Dodier A: HIPAA: past, present and future implications for nurses, *Online J Issues Nurs* 10(2), 2005.

Garvis MS: Getting informed consent when competence is at issue, *RN* 68(8):68, 2005.

Harman LB: HIPAA: a few years later, *Online J Issues Nurs* 10(2), 2005.

Hellquist K, Spector N: A primer: the National Council of State Boards of Nursing nurse licensure compact, *JONAS Healthc Law Ethics Regul* 6(4):86-89, 2004.

Helm A: *Nursing practice: sidestepping legal minefields*, Philadelphia, 2003, Lippincott Williams & Wilkins.

Institute of Medicine: *Nursing staff in hospitals and nursing homes: is it adequate?* Washington, DC, 1996, National Academies Press.

Joint Commission on Accreditation of Healthcare Organizations: *National patient safety goals*, 2005 (website): http://www.jointcommission.org/Patient Safety.

Kumekawa J: Overview and summary: HIPAA: how our health care world has changed, *Online J Issues Nurs* 10(2), 2005.

Leahy JM, Kizilay PE: *Foundations of nursing practice*, Philadelphia, 1998, WB Saunders.

Manno M, Hogan P, Heberlein V, et al: *Nursing2006* patient-safety survey report, *Nursing2006* 36(5):54-63, 2006.

Mikos CA: Inside the nurse practice act, *Nurs Manag* 35(9):20-24, 2004.

National Council of State Boards of Nursing: *Model nurse practice act*, 2004 (website):http://www.ncsbn.org/regulation/nursingpractice_nursing_practice_model_act_and_rules.asp.

National Council of State Boards of Nursing: *The five rights of delegation*, approved August 1997 by the Delegate Assembly (website): http://www.ncsbn.org.

National Council of State Boards of Nursing: *Working with others: a position paper*, 2006 (website): http://www.ncsbn.org/pdfs/Working_with_Others.pdf.

National Practitioner Data Bank: *Annual report*, 2004 (website): http://www.npdb-hipdb.com/annualrpt.html.

Nelson R: The politics of prescribing, *Am J Nurs* 106(3):25-26, 2006.

Parker L: Medical-privacy law creates wide confusion, *USA Today* 17:1A-2A, 2003:Oct.

Phillips SJ: Eighteenth annual legislative update: a comprehensive look at the legislative issues affecting advanced nursing practice, *Am J Prim Health Care* 31(1):6-8, 2006:11.

Reinhard SC, Young HM, Kane RA, et al: Nurse delegation of medication administration for older adults in assisted living, *Nurs Outlook* 54:74-80, 2006.

Ryan B: Advance directives: your role, *RN* 67(5):59-62, 2004.

Smith JE: Exploring the efficacy of continuing education mandates, *JONAS Healthc Law Ethics Regul* 6(1):22-31, 2004.

Ethics: Basic Concepts for Nursing Practice

Beth Perry Black

After studying this chapter, students will be able to:

- Differentiate between values, morals, ethics, and bioethics
- Explain the difference between Kohlberg's and Gilligan's approaches to moral reasoning
- Identify and define basic ethical principles
- Discuss the concept of justice as an ethical principle in health care delivery
- Discuss the relevance of a code of ethics for the profession of nursing
- Understand how professional ethics override personal ethics in professional settings
- Describe ethical dilemmas resulting from conflicts between patients, health care professionals, family members, and institutions
- Identify a model for ethical decision making and discuss the steps of the model
- Discuss the impact of ethical issues on nurses and other health care professionals
- Recognize the ethics behind paperless documentation and computer use
- Understand the important ethical issues related to immigration, migration, and health care

Scholars have devoted their entire careers to the study of ethics, the examination of questions of right and wrong, how values are determined, and how morals are applied in specific situations. Ethics are also known as moral philosophy. There are three general types of ethics: (1) metaethics, which focus on universal truths, and where and how ethical principles are developed; (2) normative ethics, which focus on the moral standards that regulate behaviors; and (3) applied ethics, which focus on specific difficult issues such as euthanasia, capital punishment, abortion, and health disparities. In a practice profession such as nursing, ethical issues arise frequently, created by the very nature of the work of nursing. The purpose of this chapter is to give you a basic introduction to the very complex issues of ethics so that you will be better prepared to recognize and work through situations with ethical implications.

Common situations with ethical implications for nurses include making decisions about the allocation of time and resources, what and how much information to share with patients and their families, how to manage and deal with colleagues professionally, and how to resolve problems when desires and needs of patients and families conflict with institutional policies. More dramatic ethical issues for nurses include assisting families making end-of-life decisions, triaging patients in emergency settings, managing excruciating pain with large doses of narcotics, and advocating for a patient even when the nurse does not agree with the patient. To manage the complex ethical issues they face, nurses need an understanding of the theoretical basis for ethical decision making. Throughout their education and practice, nurses are called on to exercise judgment when making clinical decisions. However, when nurses encounter ethical dilemmas, they need an ethical decision-making model to apply to the situation and one that works for individual nurses in the context of their own value system. Box 5-1,

Box 5-1   To Be Guardians of the Ethical Treatment of Patients

Anne Bavier, PhD, RN, FAAN, Dean of the University of Connecticut School of Nursing, recently wrote to nursing students and their faculty in an editorial about the high standards of integrity for themselves and for all who serve patients.

To become the guardians of patients' well-being and of the nursing profession, nurses must learn more than technical skills, even more than just critical thinking or ethical criteria . . . . The topic is timely: If recent headlines are any indication, professional ethics are in critical condition. We are all familiar with reports of financial dishonesty that have contributed to a contracted global economy, and we have seen recent surveys about student cheating and plagiarism. It seems that a chronic ailment, human frailty, is the underlying disorder.

For nurses and nurse faculty, the outcomes of dishonesty are, without hyperbole, a matter of life and death. When a math student or an English student cheats without learning, society is impaired, to be sure. However, if a nursing student cheats without learning, patients may sicken or die . . . . When the NLN adopted its core values, it included integrity, "evident when organizational principles of communication, ethical decision-making, and humility are encouraged, expected, and demonstrated consistently." The NLN states that "not only is doing

the right thing simply how we do business, but our actions reveal our commitment to truth telling and to how we always see ourselves from the perspective of others in a larger community" (http://www.nln.org/aboutnln/corevalues.htm). Most schools and universities have similar codes of conduct that stress the greater good of individual actions and the pursuit of truth.

Nurses and nurse faculty must be the guardians of the ethical treatment of patients. Aristotle's deceptively simple rationale for living well and doing good seems exquisitely suited to nursing education: "Every art and every inquiry, and similarly every action and choice, is thought to aim at some good; and for this reason the good has rightly been declared to be that at which all things aim." Nursing, as both art and inquiry, action and choice, must always reflect on its aims. That is what Aristotle called phronesis, practical wisdom, change for good by planning an effective route to a desirable goal. Thus, a nurse educator (whether in classroom or clinic) is not just a master of skills conveyed to the student, but a teacher of practical wisdom: ethical action . . . .

Deeply mentored by nurse faculty, they must become confident, autonomous health care professionals who have high standards of integrity for themselves and for all who serve patients.

"To Be Guardians of the Ethical Treatment of Patients," describes the importance of the role of nurses and nursing faculty in achieving high standards of integrity to provide ethical care for our vulnerable patients.

BASIC DEFINITIONS

To understand ethics and its relationship to health care, the terms *values, morals, ethics,* and *bioethics* must first be defined. **Values** are

attitudes, ideals, or beliefs that an individual or a group holds and uses to guide behavior. Values are usually expressed in terms of right and wrong, hierarchies of importance, or how one should behave. Values are freely chosen and indicate what the individual considers important, such as honesty and hard work. *Morals* and *ethics* are often used interchangeably, although we make a distinction for purposes of this book. Philosophers and scholars have conflicting views on how to define these terms. **Morals** are established rules of conduct to be used in situations where a decision about right and wrong must be made. Morals provide standards of behavior that guide the actions of an individual or social group. An example of a moral standard is "One should not lie." Morals are learned over time and are influenced by life experiences and culture.

Ethics is a term used to reflect what actions an individual should take and may be "codified," as in the ethical code of a profession. *Ethics* is derived from the Greek word *ethos*, which means habits or customs. Ethics are process oriented and involve critical analysis of actions. If ethicists (persons who study ethics) reflected on the moral statement "One should not lie," they would clarify definitions of lying and explore whether or not there are circumstances under which lying might be acceptable.

Bioethics is the application of ethical theories and principles to moral issues or problems in health care. Bioethics (also referred to as biomedical ethics) as an area of ethical inquiry came into existence around 1970, as the health care system began to give attention not only to treating and curing disease but also to patients' rights and a holistic view of the patient. Bioethics is concerned with determining what should be done in a specific situation by applying ethical principles. For instance, discussions about genetic testing often have a strong bioethical component surrounding use of knowledge from this type of testing.

Advances in science and medical technologies have allowed health care providers to sustain lives under circumstances that once would have caused a patient's death. On one hand, these technologies solve some problems, such as assisting with ventilation until a patient is able to breathe without assistance. On the other hand, these advances sometimes create ethical dilemmas for health care providers. For example, a patient may be "kept alive" even when there is no discernible brain activity or hope for the return of spontaneous respiration. Nurses struggle with situations such as these, asking questions whether or not a patient should be sustained ("kept alive") under these circumstances. These situations sometimes raise serious questions for nurses about the meaning of life and what constitutes being "alive."

Nurses need to think carefully about their own personal values and morals. Being clear on where one stands personally on a situation will help the nurse make good choices about work environment and types of patients with whom he or she would like to work. For instance, if a nurse has a very strong personal belief that abortion is wrong under any circumstances, he or she would not do well with the requirements of a setting in which pregnancy terminations were done for genetic disorders. Similarly, if a nurse believes that drug addiction is a moral problem, choosing to work on an infectious disease unit where many patients have addiction problems would be a poor choice. It is very important that nurses understand their own personal values so that they can recognize where their personal morals and professional ethics may be in conflict. In a professional setting, professional ethics override personal morals and values.

The American Nurses Association's (ANA's) Code of Ethics for Nurses is printed on the inside back cover of this text. Provision 2 describes the nurse's primary commitment to the patient; provision 5 describes the responsibility of nurses to maintain their own integrity. These two provisions are not in conflict, but they do underscore the importance of understanding nursing's primary ethical obligations to the care of patients. A wise nurse who is aware of deep personal values and moral standards will make decisions regarding practice setting so that the nurse's own personal integrity remains intact, while putting patients and their needs first. In any complex ethical situation, nurses should analyze their own actions so that they can reduce inner conflicts between their personal values and morals and their professional ethics. This critical analysis of one's morals, beliefs, and actions is "moral reflection"—a process through which a person develops and maintains moral integrity. Moral integrity in a professional setting is a goal in which one's professional beliefs and actions are assessed and analyzed (reflected on) so that professional ethics continue to mature and respond to changes in practice (Hardingham, 2001).

When nurses are faced with ethical dilemmas but also encounter constraints that limit their actions, they may experience **moral distress** (Hardingham, 2004). Moral distress is the pain or anguish affecting the mind, body, or relationships in response to a situation in which the person is aware of a moral problem, acknowledges moral responsibility, and makes a moral judgment about the correct action; however, as a result of real or perceived constraints, participates in perceived moral wrongdoing (Nathaniel, 2002, p. 4). The following situation has several important ethical implications that cause a moral dilemma for the health care team and the family. Examine this scenario for various ethical issues, and think about what parts of this situation might pose a moral dilemma or moral distress for you.

A newborn infant was admitted to the neonatal intensive care unit (NICU). She was born very prematurely and weighs only 520 grams (about 1 pound). The parents want "everything done" for the infant to ensure her survival; the infant, however, has multiple setbacks including serious infections, feeding problems, and then a grade IV intraventricular hemorrhage, which is severe bleeding into the ventricles of the brain. The neonatologists are convinced that the infant will have profound physical, cognitive, and developmental problems if she even survives and ask for a meeting with the parents to discuss discontinuing the infant's life support. The parents want life support to be continued and for the infant to be a "full code" meaning that all effort will be made to resuscitate her in case her heart stops. The nurse understands the parents' deep desire to give their child every chance to live; however, he also understands the severe physical and neurologic complications of extreme prematurity. He is concerned about pain and suffering the infant may be experiencing because of her numerous treatments and extensive supportive technology. He thinks about the resources in terms of time and money that continuing support of this infant requires, and although

he does not like thinking about patient care in those terms, he recognizes the tension he feels about the effort the infant is requiring. The nurse realizes that he dreads going in to work every day to take care of this infant and finds himself dwelling on the situation when he is not at work. After a long shift one night, he goes home and blurts out to his wife, "This just isn't right, and I don't know what to do about it."

This example demonstrates numerous aspects of moral dilemmas and resulting moral distress. The nurse experienced moral distress, a sense of being unable to act in a way that he believes is moral in this situation. The nurse recognized the parents' desire for their child to live; the possibility of pain and suffering of the infant; the real possibility of severe, long-term problems if she lives; the expense in terms of time and money; the emotional toll of care of the infant; and his own discomfort and sense of helplessness. This nurse also demonstrated that he was reflecting on his own practice and beliefs, which will help maintain his moral integrity. He will also use the lessons from this patient situation as he matures as a nurse, so that similar situations in the future may not be so distressful for him. Critical Thinking Challenge 5-1 refers to this patient situation; once you have studied the remainder of this chapter, you will have additional knowledge, tools and perspective with which to consider the complexities of this scenario.

To function effectively in today's complex health care arena, nurses need to understand approaches to moral reasoning, theories of ethics, basic ethical principles, and ethical decision-making models. A significant advance in the professionalization of a traditional occupation such as nursing is the adoption of a formal code of ethics (Baker, 2009). Professional ethical codes such as that of the ANA provide substantial guidance in determining how to respond and act in practice settings when faced with an ethical dilemma. The remainder of this chapter will provide a basic orientation to these complex topics.

CRITICAL THINKING *Challenge 5-1*

Think back to the clinical example on page 102 about the nurse's moral distress related to the prematurely born infant in the NICU. Now that you have some basic knowledge about ethics, consider these questions:

1. What would a deontologist's position be with regard to the sustaining of the infant's life?
2. What would a utilitarian's position be in this case?
3. What virtues of the nurse do you see at work in this case?
4. What basic ethical principles do you think the nurse may be using in analyzing this moral dilemma?

5. What are your own personal beliefs and values regarding the sustaining of a very premature infant on extensive life support?
6. What are alternative ethical viewpoints that someone else may hold regarding this situation?
7. Who holds the primary responsibility for determining what should happen in this case? The parents? The health care providers? Defend your response from an ethical perspective.

APPROACHES TO MORAL REASONING

Similar to other forms of human development, moral reasoning is a process in which maturation occurs over time as persons become more abstract in their thinking and understanding of the world. Moral development describes how a person learns to handle moral dilemmas from childhood through adulthood. Two important theorists in moral development and reasoning are Lawrence Kohlberg and Carol Gilligan.

Kohlberg's Stages of Moral Reasoning

Kohlberg (1976, 1986) proposed three levels of moral reasoning as a function of cognitive development: (1) preconventional, (2) conventional, and (3) postconventional. Each of these three levels is then considered in terms of stages. In the preconventional level, the individual is inattentive to the norms of society when responding to moral problems. Instead, the individual's perspective is self-centered. At this level, what the individual wants or needs takes precedence over right or wrong. A person in stage 1 of the preconventional level responds to punishment. In stage 2 the person responds to the prospect of personal reward. Kohlberg observed the preconventional level of moral development in children under 9 years of age, as well as in some adolescents and adult criminal offenders. A more typical example, however, is that of a toddler for whom the word

"no" has yet to have meaning as she persists in reaching for a breakable object on a table.

The conventional level is characterized by moral decisions that conform to the expectations of one's family, group, or society. The person making moral choices based on what is pleasing to others characterizes stage 3 within this level. An individual in stage 4 of the conventional level makes moral choices based on a larger notion of what is desired by society. When confronted with a moral choice, people functioning at the conventional level follow family or cultural group norms. According to Kohlberg, most adolescents and adults generally function at this level. "Because it's the law" is a common explanation of persons operating at a conventional level of moral reasoning.

The postconventional level consists of stage 5 and stage 6 and involves more independent modes of thinking than previous stages. The individual has developed the ability to define his or her own moral values. Individual who apply moral reasoning at the postconventional level may ignore both self-interest and group norms in making moral choices. For example, they may sacrifice themselves on behalf of the group. Part of their moral reasoning and behavior is based on a socially agreed-on standard of human rights (Haynes et al, 2004). In this highest level of moral development, people create their own morality, which may differ from society's norms. Kohlberg believed that only a minority of adults achieves this level.

Progression through Kohlberg's levels and their corresponding stages occurs over varying lengths of time for different individuals. The stages are sequential, they build on each other, and each stage is characterized by a higher capacity for moral reasoning than the preceding stage.

Kohlberg (1976) suggested that certain conditions might stimulate higher levels of moral development. Intellectual development is one necessary characteristic. Individuals at higher levels intellectually generally operate at a higher stage of moral reasoning than those with lower levels of intellect. An environment that offers people opportunities for group participation, shared decision-making processes, and responsibility for the consequences of their actions also promotes higher levels of moral reasoning. Moral development is stimulated by the creation of conflict in settings in which the individual recognizes the limitations of present modes of thinking. For example, students have been stimulated to higher levels of moral reasoning through participating in courses on moral discussion and ethics (Kohlberg, 1973).

Gilligan's Stages of Moral Reasoning

Gilligan (1982) was concerned that Kohlberg did not adequately recognize women's experiences in the development of moral reasoning. She noted that Kohlberg's theories had largely been generated from research with men and boys, and when women were tested by using Kohlberg's stages of moral reasoning, they scored lower than men. Gilligan believed that women's and girls' relational orientation to the world shaped their moral reasoning differently from that of men and boys. Women do not have inadequate moral development but different development because of their gender. Kohlberg's inattention to gender differences meant that his theory was inadequate in explaining women's moral development.

Gilligan described a moral development perspective focused on care. In Gilligan's view, the moral person is one who responds to need and demonstrates a consideration of care and responsibility in relationships. This perspective differed from the orientation toward justice described by Kohlberg (1973, 1976). In Gilligan's research on moral reasoning, women most often exhibited a focus on care, whereas men more often exhibited a focus on justice. Gilligan described the differences between women and men's moral reasoning not as a matter of better or worse, or mature or immature, but simply as a matter of having "a different voice" in moral reasoning.

Gilligan (1982) suggested that women view moral dilemmas in terms of conflicting responsibilities. She described women's development of moral reasoning as a sequence of three levels and two transitions, with each level representing a more complex understanding of the relationship between self and others. Each transition resulted in a critical reevaluation of the conflict between selfishness and responsibility. Gilligan's levels of moral development are (1) orientation to individual survival, (2) a focus on goodness with recognition of self-sacrifice, and (3) the morality of caring and being responsible for others, as well as self. The focus of nursing on care as a moral attribute is congruent with Gilligan's assertion that the dynamics of human relationships are "central to moral understanding, joining the heart and the eye in an ethic that ties the activity of thought to the activity of care" (p. 149). Critical thinking within a caring professional relationship is a sound basis for nursing practice.

Nurses at times combine the care/justice perspective when forced to make ethical decisions (Chally, 1995). Nurses have shifted from the moral perspective of care to a justice orientation where universal rules and principles are used in moral decision making (Zickmund, 2004). Caring may be devalued as the profession of nursing becomes more oriented toward technology (Zickmund). Moreover, as economics and scarcity of resources shape the delivery of health care, nurses may find themselves less able to use critical thinking, reflection, and higher stages of moral reasoning in their practice setting. This article described in this chapter's Evidence-Based Practice Note demonstrates that this problem exists across nursing internationally.

EVIDENCE-BASED PRACTICE NOTE

A growing concern exists regarding nurses' ethical competence. Barriers to ethical practice compromise nurses' ability to care for patients in a manner that they consider to be moral. De Casterlé, Izumi, Godfrey, and Denhaerynck, an international team of nurse researchers, conducted a meta-analysis using data from nine different studies in four countries to determine how nurses became involved in ethical decision making and action in their daily practice. A meta-analysis is a means of using similar data from different studies that address similar hypotheses and research questions to get results from a larger sample. By combining data, these researchers were able to pool the responses of 1592 registered nurses who completed the Ethical Behaviour Test, which is based on an adaptation of Kohlberg's theory of moral development.

De Casterlé, Izumi, Godfrey, and Denhaerynck first reviewed the existing literature about nurses' ethical decision making in practice. They found in their review that nurses typically were often ill prepared to address ethical dilemmas and that nurses do not use critical thinking in making ethical decisions. Nurses were also found to experience conflicts between their personal values and professional ethics, and few nurses were able to express ethical problems to the health care team. In addition, nurses found that their work environment hindered their ability to practice nursing in a manner that they believed was ethical. Heavy workloads, time and financial constraints, and staffing problems all interfered with nurses' ability to make ethical decision making a priority.

Among the 1592 registered nurses included in the sample of this meta-analysis, 58 nurses were recruited specifically because they were known to demonstrate high-level ethical reasoning and practice. These nurses constituted the "expert group."

This strategy is known as "purposeful sampling," to include in a study a very specific group of participants as a comparison group.

The expert group exhibited a significantly higher likelihood to make ethical decisions from a postconventional level of moral reasoning, usually at Kohlberg's sixth stage. The nonexpert group (the other 1534 nurses) generally preferred moral decisions that corresponded to Kohlberg's fourth stage, the conventional level of moral reasoning. The nonexpert nurses were significantly more likely than expert nurses to prefer moral decisions from the preconventional level, at Kohlberg's second stage.

The findings suggested that nurses typically make ethical decisions at a conventional level and that this is an international phenomenon among nurses. The researchers referred to this as "conformist practice" that "excludes a critical and creative search for the best caring answer" to ethical dilemmas. The conventions of practice—medical prescriptions, rules of the nursing unit, and policies and procedures—serve as a framework for practice but should not preclude individualized patient care. The findings of this study confirmed much of what the researchers had seen from their review of the literature: that nurses often face ethical challenges, that workplace conditions hinder nurses from ethical practice, and that there is a growing concern about nurses' ability to practice ethically. In addition, de Casterlé, Izumi, Godfrey, and Denhaerynck found that nurses tend to conform to workplace rules and norms, rather than using creativity and reflecting critically on their practice. The researchers suggest that to provide the best care possible for patients, nurses must develop maturity in their moral reasoning, especially at a time when economic values tend to predominate in shaping workplace decisions.

De Casterlé BD, Izumi S, Godfrey NS, Denhaerynck K: Nurses' responses to ethical dilemmas in nursing practice: meta-analysis. *J Adv Nurs* 63(6):540-549, 2009.

ETHICAL THEORIES

Ethical theories, like all theories, are conceptual descriptions of phenomena. In ethics, the phenomena that are being described are understandings of behaviors in terms of their moral implications. Theories are broad descriptions, and no single ethical theory can be applied universally in health care situations. In this section, selected ethical theories that are useful to nurses—deontology, utilitarianism, virtue ethics, and principalism—are presented briefly.

Deontology

The term *deontology* has its origins from the Greek word *deon*, which means obligation or duty. German philosopher Immanuel Kant (1724-1804) was a preeminent deontologist. He believed that an act was moral if its motives or intentions were good, regardless of the outcome. Ethical action consists of doing one's duty or honoring one's obligations to human beings: to do one's duty was right; not to do one's duty was wrong. The outcomes or consequences of an action can be desired or deplored, but they are not relevant from the deontological perspective. For example, a nursing student was providing care to an elderly man who was dying and who had been estranged from his son for many years. From his wallet, he pulled out a tattered piece of paper with a phone number on it. Handing it to the nursing student, he asked her to promise him that she would call his son and ask him to come for a final visit. Although she was filled with dread, the nursing student felt an obligation to her patient to honor one of his dying wishes. With trembling hands, she called the number. The man who answered listened to her for a few moments; then he said, "I wouldn't go to see him if you paid me. Tell him I am glad he's dying." And then he hung up on her. The student was horrified and was very upset about what to tell her dying patient. From a deontological perspective, the nursing student acted in an ethical way, as she had a duty to respond to her patient's request, despite the outcome.

Deontology can be further divided into act deontology and rule deontology. Act deontologists determine the right thing to do by gathering all the facts and then making a decision. Much time and energy are needed to judge each situation carefully. Once a decision is made, there is commitment to universalizing it. In other words, if one makes a moral judgment in one situation, the same judgment will be made in any similar situation. Rule deontologists, on the other hand, emphasize that principles guide our actions. Examples of rules might be "Always keep a promise" or "Never tell a lie." In all situations, the rule is to be followed. Deontologists are not concerned with the consequences of adhering to certain rules or actions. If one's guiding principle is "Always keep a promise," a deontologist will keep promises, even if circumstances have changed. For the nursing student in the previous example, by judging that making a call under these circumstances was ethical, she set for herself a precedent—that she would act the same way in each circumstance like this one. Similarly, if she acted on the principle to never tell a lie, she would find a way to tell her patient how his son had responded when he asked.

Utilitarianism

Utilitarianism is based on a fundamental belief that the moral rightness of an action is determined solely by its consequence. Utilitarianism was first described by David Hume (1711-1776) and was developed further by many notable philosophers, including Jeremy Bentham (1748-1832) and John Stuart Mill (1806-1873). Mill had a significant influence on utilitarian ethics as it is known today.

Those who subscribe to utilitarian ethics believe that "what makes an action right or wrong is its utility, with useful actions bringing about the greatest good for the greatest number of people" (Guido, 2006, p. 4). In other words, maximizing the greatest good for the benefit, happiness, or pleasure of the greatest number of people is moral. Utilitarianism assumes that it is possible to balance good and evil with a goal that most people experience good rather than evil. Professional health care providers employ utilitarian theory in many situations. Consider, for example, the concept of triage, in which the sick or injured are classified by the severity of their condition to determine priority of treatment. Imagine that there is a plane crash in a remote area in which many of the survivors are severely burned. The local health care facility cannot manage all of the patients, and, although air transport is available from a large medical facility 3 hours away, only those with the possibility of surviving can be transported. Those with less serious burns can be managed at a smaller hospital. This means that someone must make the decision as to who will and will not be treated. The most gravely injured will not be treated until those with a reasonable chance of survival are taken care of, although this means that some of the more severely injured will die awaiting care. As a function of utilitarianism, triage is accepted worldwide as an ethical basis for determining treatment.

Frequently, utilitarianism is the basis for deciding how health care dollars should be spent. For example, money is more likely to be spent on research for diseases that affect large numbers of people than for research on diseases that affect relatively few. Some health care systems, such as the National Health Service in the United Kingdom, depend on utilitarian ethics as one determinant of who receives treatment. For example, inexpensive procedures that benefit large numbers of people, such as cataract surgeries, are easier to access than expensive ones, such as organ transplantations, that benefit a few. A difficulty inherent in utilitarianism is that in the interests of the benefiting of the majority, the interests of the individual or minority, who also deserve help, may be overlooked.

Virtue Ethics

Virtue ethics was first noted in the works of Plato, Aristotle, and early Christians. According to Aristotle, virtues are tendencies to act, feel, and judge that develop through appropriate training but come from natural tendencies. This suggests that individuals' actions are built from a degree of inborn moral virtue (Burkhardt and Nathaniel, 2002).

Recently, bioethics literature has emphasized the character of the decision maker. Virtues refer to specific character traits, including truth telling, honesty, courage, kindness, respectfulness, compassion, fairness, and integrity, among others. These virtues become obvious through one's actions and are expressions of specific ethical principles. Truthfulness, for example, embodies the principle of veracity, which will be discussed in the next section of this chapter. When virtuous people are faced with ethical dilemmas they will instinctively choose to do the right thing because they have developed character through life experiences (Butts and Rich, 2005).

Descriptions of character in terms of virtues portray an individual's way of being, rather than the process of decision making. One's actions in both personal and professional domains extend from this way of being (Davis et al, 1997). This does not guarantee right behavior, but it may predispose an individual to right behavior. Similarly, the development of a profession's code of ethics provides a framework of virtues and qualities of character that shape the behaviors of persons engaged in that profession; however, there is no guarantee that members of the profession will act in an ethical manner.

The ability to respond to ethical dilemmas or situations in the health care arena is dependent on the nurse's own integrity, honesty, courage, or other personal attributes. Practicing in an ethical manner requires a decision to act within the ethical code of the profession, demanding commitment, personal investment, and the intention and motivation to become a good nurse (Gallagher and Wainwright, 2005). Nurses' ways of being and acting are essential to the integrity of nursing practice and patient care. Nurses frequently practice in challenging circumstances in which they must rely on their own integrity to ensure that care is given conscientiously and consistently. Virtues may be what separate the competent nurse from the exemplary nurse.

Principalism

Ethical principles, rather than theories, have generally provided the means to analyze and act on ethical dilemmas in health care in the

United States. Principalism uses key ethical principles of beneficence (do good), nonmaleficence (do no harm), autonomy (respect for the person's ability to act in his or her own best interests), and justice in the resolution of ethical conflicts or dilemmas. Fidelity (faithfulness) and veracity (truth telling) are also important ethical principles that may be at work in managing ethical dilemmas. Nurses are more knowledgeable of ethical principles than ethical theories and are more likely to use a combination of ethical principles when critically analyzing ethical dilemmas. Further discussion of major ethical principles follows.

ETHICAL PRINCIPLES

Respect for humans as a function of human dignity is the primary ethical responsibility for nurses in practice. The *Code of Ethics for Nurses* states that "the nurse practices with compassion and respect for the inherent dignity, worth and uniqueness of every individual, unrestricted by considerations of social or economic status, personal attributes or the nature of health problems" (ANA, 2001). Respect for persons requires that each person be valued as a unique individual equal to all others and that every aspect of a person's life is valued. This can be difficult, because it is sometimes hard to value those parts of human lives that differ from our own. Human dignity and respect for persons are the foundation of the six ethical principles discussed in this section: autonomy, beneficence, nonmaleficence, justice, fidelity, and veracity.

Autonomy

The principle of autonomy asserts that individuals have the right to determine their own actions and the freedom to make their own decisions. Respect for the individual is the cornerstone of this principle. Autonomous decisions are based on (1) individuals' values, (2) adequate information, (3) freedom from coercion, and (4) reason and deliberation. Autonomous decisions lead to independent, autonomous actions. Autonomous actions by a patient would include deciding to refuse treatment; giving consent for treatment or

procedures; and obtaining information regarding results of diagnostic tests, diagnosis, and treatment options.

Disregard for autonomy, however, is often missing in the health care system. Health care professionals often take actions that affect patients' lives profoundly without adequate consultation with the patients themselves. Some health care providers, including physicians and nurses, may operate unknowingly in a paternalistic way that assumes that health care providers are better equipped than patients to make health care decisions for patients. Some patients, however, prefer to have decisions made for them, perhaps because of a lack of information or fears of making a poor choice.

Incorporating the principle of autonomy in all health care situations can be difficult. Autonomy poses a problem for health care workers when the patient is incompetent to make decisions because of physical condition, psychological or mental status, or developmental age. Examples of those unable to participate in decisions include infants or small children, mentally incompetent patients, and unconscious patients. Other patients may be unable to participate in decision making because of external constraints, such as the lack of necessary information, or the norms of their culture. Nevertheless, the principle of autonomy is an increasingly important one in health care and nursing.

Beneficence

Beneficence is commonly defined as "the doing of good" and is one of the critical ethical principles in health care. In essence, one should always consider one's actions in the context of promoting good for others (i.e., the patient). Although this sounds simple, health care providers are challenged daily when what is good for the patient may also cause harm to the patient or is in conflict with what the patient wants. Suppose, for example, that an elderly patient has become confused, especially at night, and is at high risk for falls. She has fallen at home twice. Now that she is confused, she is at even more risk for a fall, especially as confusion can become worse at night in the elderly. The health care team decides that the patient needs a sitter to stay with her in her room all night. The patient objects stridently, as she is very dignified and proud and enjoys her privacy. She complains that she "doesn't need a baby sitter" and cries for a long time. The patient is prevented from falling but is psychologically distressed because of limitations on her independence and freedom, privacy, and dignity.

Virtually everyone would agree that promoting good and avoiding harm are important to all human beings—and certainly to health care professionals. It may seem surprising, therefore, how often conflicts occur surrounding the principle of beneficence. A beneficent act may conflict with other ethical principles, most often autonomy. Even though a nurse or physician may understand that a particular treatment has a benefit for the patient, the patient may decide to forgo that treatment (autonomy) for a variety of reasons. In this instance, the health care provider should avoid acting paternalistically and recognize that the patient remains in a position of self-determination.

Nonmaleficence

Nonmaleficence is defined as the duty to do no harm. This principle is the foundation of the medical profession's Hippocratic Oath; it is likewise critical to the nursing profession. Inherent in the Code of Ethics for Nurses (ANA, 2001), the nurse must not act in a manner that would intentionally harm the patient. Although this point appears straightforward, the nature of health care dictates that some therapeutic interventions carry risks of harm for the patient, but the treatment will eventually produce great good for the patient. Classic examples of this are chemotherapy and bone marrow or stem cell transplantation procedures. Both interventions can make patients sicker for a time, posing a risk for complications such as opportunistic infections, but the possibility of achieving a cure or remission of disease may justify the temporary harm. The concept that justifies risking harm is referred to as the principle of double effect.

Double effect considers the intended foreseen effects of actions by the professional nurse. The doctrine states that as moral agents we may not intentionally produce harm. It is ethically permissible, however, to do what may produce a distressful or undesirable result if the intent is to produce an overall good effect (Beauchamp and Childress, 2001).

According to Guido (2006), four conditions must be present to justify the use of the double effect principle:
1. The action must be good or at least morally indifferent.
2. The health care provider must intend only the good effects.
3. The undesired effects cannot be a means to the end or good effect.
4. There is a favorable balance between desirable and undesirable effects (Guido, 2006, p. 6).

Justice

The principle of justice states that equals should be treated the same and that unequals should be treated differently (Beauchamp and Childress, 2001). In other words, patients with the same diagnosis and health care needs should receive the same care. Those with greater or lesser needs should receive different care. Also at issue with justice is who receives health care. Ongoing debates continue on whether health care is a right or a privilege.

In health care, the most common concern about justice relates to allocation of resources. How much of our national resources should be appropriated to health care? What health care problems should receive the most financial resources? What patients should have access to health care services? According to the principle of justice, the answer to these questions is based on treating all individuals equally.

Numerous models have been developed for distributing health care resources. These models include the following:
1. To each equally
2. To each according to merit (this may include past or future contributions to society)
3. To each according to what can be acquired in the marketplace
4. To each according to need (Jameton, 1984)

All of these suggestions for distribution have merit, but no single one is adequate in ensuring a just model for the distribution of health care resources. In an ideal world, all people would receive all available treatment and resources for their health needs, including disease prevention and health promotion. Unfortunately, this is not possible because of costs and limited supplies, such as transplantable organs. When persons with wealth have advantageous access to the best health care available, including lifesaving medical devices or innovations, how does one apply the concept of justice? Conversely, how does the issue of justice apply when access to care that is known to be cost-effective and simple, such as prenatal care, is difficult or impossible for working class women who are on the job during clinic hours? In addition, when disasters such as Hurricane Katrina strike and health care institutions are left with acutely ill patients and no electricity to operate medical devices that monitor or sustain patients, how does one decide what is just? Health disparities among ethnic minorities with regard to types of treatments and services that are available represent a difficult problem in terms of an ethic of justice. Research has demonstrated that allocation of resources in the health care system is not equitable among racial groups and that "racial disparity exists in health care access, treatment options and outcomes" (Harrison and Falco, 2005, p. 252). This chapter's Cultural Considerations Challenge describes lessons learned by nursing students who participate in international learning experiences, and how to continue one's growth of social consciousness and sense of justice.

Justice as a principle often leaves us with more questions than answers. It raises our consciousness in identifying unjust situations and in shaping resolutions to those situations, but applying the principle of justice does not determine what the answer should be. A single ethical principle cannot typically be used to resolve complex ethical dilemmas such as those encountered in health care settings.

Fidelity

The principle of fidelity refers to faithfulness or honoring one's commitments or promises. For nurses, this specifically refers to fidelity to patients. Through the process of licensure, nurses are granted the privilege to practice. The licensure process is intended to ensure that only a qualified nurse, appropriately trained and educated, can practice nursing. When nurses are licensed and become a part of the profession, they accept certain responsibilities as part of the contract with society. Nurses must be faithful in keeping their promises of respecting all individuals, upholding the Code of Ethics for Nurses (ANA, 2001), practicing within the scope of nursing practice, maintaining competence in nursing, abiding by the policies of the employing institution, and keeping promises to patients (Burkhardt and Nathaniel, 2002). Fidelity entails meeting reasonable expectations in all these areas. Fidelity is a key foundation for the nurse-patient relationship. When nurses receive patient assignments and accept reports on those patients, they are committed to provide care to those assigned to them. Failure to carry out the prescribed care is unethical (provided that the prescribed care is safe and consistent with good practice) and may constitute patient abandonment or neglect (Haynes, Boese, and Butcher, 2004). This is a serious charge that would likely require state board of nursing review of the particulars of the case to determine whether the nurse failed to carry out this responsibility ethically.

Fidelity suggests that one is faithful to the promises, agreements, and commitments made. This faithfulness creates the trust that is essential to any relationship. Most ethicists believe there is no absolute duty to keep promises, however. In every situation, the harmful consequences of the promised action must be weighed against the benefits of promise keeping (Burkhardt and Nathaniel, 2002).

Veracity

Veracity is defined as telling the truth, or not lying. Truth telling is fundamental to the development and continuance of trust among human

Cultural Considerations Challenge
"To Keep the Vision" of Social Justice

Nursing students often have a great deal of interest in and energy for international learning experiences. These experiences expose students to the huge gap in health care practices and availability between developed and undeveloped nations. In a recent article, Kirkham, Van Hofwegen, and Pankratz (2009) describe the challenge of "keeping the vision" for nursing students and their faculty as they return home—sustaining the social consciousness that is raised during these international experiences.

Kirkham, Van Hofwegen, and Pankratz (2009) defined social consciousness in terms of "personal awareness of social injustice," borrowed from Giddings (2005, p. 224). Specifically, they described social injustice as unfairness in the burdens and rewards of a society in which there is inequitable access to health care services. Social injustice is the foundation of health disparities, a serious ethical issue that challenges the human right to health and health care.

In their study of student learning that took place in international settings and the long-term benefits and effects of these experiences, Kirkham, Van Hofwegen, and Pankratz sought to describe students' experiences but also to find ways to integrate and maintain the students' learning once they returned home (in this case, Canada). Students had many experiences that opened their eyes to the health care practices and accessibility of care in an underdeveloped country (Guatemala). Students related the realization that "statistics . . . became faces of people I know" (p. 6) and that "people are the same everywhere" (p. 6). They also recognized the significant prosperity and power gradients that exist between North and Central America. From these realizations, the students began to have a deep sense of social injustice and the consequences of short-term international efforts that are not sustained. These insights challenged the students' worldview.

Despite the immense learning and intense reflection that resulted from these experiences, "keeping the vision" became hard as students returned home. Kirkham, Van Hofwegen, and Pankratz (p. 9) suggested four strategies that may help students in translating their learning and sustaining their new vision for social justice. Individually, students can write journals of their reflections and insights, read journals, and maintain contact with their host families. In formal groups, students can mentor new students who will go through the same experiences, participate in forums and focus groups, and become involved in other humanitarian projects. In informal groups, students can reflect on and share their experiences with other students and faculty who participated in the international experience. And last, nursing school curricula can be shaped to integrate themes of social justice.

Kirkham SR, Van Hofwegen L, Pankratz D: Keeping the vision: sustaining social consciousness with nursing students following international learning experiences, *International Journal of Nursing Education Scholarship* (online) 6(1)(article 3), 2009.

beings. Telling the truth is expected. It is necessary to basic communication, and societal relationships are built on the individual's right to know the truth, or not to be deceived. Inherent in nurse-patient relationships is the understanding that nurses will be honest with their patients. However, in some (rare) instances nurses are constrained in some health care systems that place limits on what a nurse can tell a patient. These situations, however, can pose an ethical dilemma for nurses who believe that it is unethical to withhold information from patients, especially when patients ask for information about their condition or diagnosis. A nurse can still remain truthful by telling the patient, "Dr. Samuels always prefers to discuss his findings with his patients directly. I will page him and ask him when you can expect him to make rounds tonight to talk to you." Intentional deception, however, is considered morally wrong.

Some health care providers attempt to justify deceiving their patients. For the most part, these justifications are related to the idea that patients would be better off not knowing certain information or that they are not capable of understanding the information. This reflects a posture toward patients known as "paternalism," in which someone believes that they know what is best for another person who is competent to make his or her own autonomous judgments about a course of action. Some justify not being truthful with a patient if they perceive that the patient might refuse medical treatment if he or she knew the "complete" truth. However, if both patient and health care provider are respectful of each other as individuals, it is difficult to accept that deception is ever justified. Two exceptions exist, however. If a patient asks *not* to be told the truth, the nurse can, under the ethical principles of beneficence and nonmaleficence, withhold the truth. This does not mean that the nurse must lie but that the nurse is released from obligation to report to the patient what he or she may know. Furthermore, if a patient is mentally incompetent, autonomy and the capacity for self-determination are diminished, thereby justifying withholding of health care information (Tuckett, 2004).

Hines (2008) made an interesting observation that true cultural humility (a posture that requires that clinicians make every effort to understand their patients' beliefs and how their patients want themselves and their illness to be treated) is tied to respecting patient preferences for information and for treatment. Although Hines was writing about care in an oncology setting, her observation that "goals of care can be established, refined, or refocused at any point in the trajectory of care, whether truth telling or not telling is occurring" (p. 415) holds true for any practice setting for nurses.

NURSING CODES OF ETHICS

A code of ethics is a hallmark of mature professions. A code of ethics is a social contract through which the profession informs society of the principles and rules by which it functions. Ethical codes shape professional self-regulation, serving as guidelines to the members of the profession, who then meet their responsibility as trustworthy, qualified, and accountable caregivers. Codes

of ethics, however, are useful only to the extent that they are known and upheld by the members of the profession in practice.

American Nurses Association's Code of Ethics for Nurses

Ethical practice has been a priority for nurses in America since the late nineteenth century. In 1893, the Nightingale Pledge (Box 5-2) became the first public evidence of an ethical code in nursing. In 1896, the Nurses' Associated Alumnae of the United States and Canada that later became the ANA was organized with the purpose to establish and maintain a code of ethics. A suggested code was developed in 1926 and published in the *American Journal of Nursing* (*AJN*) but was never formally adopted. Similarly, a "tentative" code was published in the *AJN* in 1940, but this version also was never formally adopted. Finally, in 1950, with the addition of 17 provisions, the 1940 version was formally adopted as the Code of Ethics for Nurses. Between 1950 and 1985, the Code was revised and refined six times; the ANA's House of Delegates adopted a complete revision of the Code in 2001.

The *Code of Ethics for Nurses With Interpretive Statements* is the nursing profession's expression of its ethical values and duties to the public (ANA, 2001). The Code has undergone no fewer than seven revisions, each clarifying meanings, defining terms, and making the Code more relevant to nursing practice at the time. Codes through the years have also reflected trends in social awareness issues, such as women's and patients' rights. The consequences of breaking the Code have become more specific with later versions.

The *Code of Ethics for Nurses With Interpretive Statements* (ANA, 2001) is the latest version of nursing's ethical code. The Code of Ethics for Nurses can be found on the inside back cover of this text. Interpretive statements can be found online in read-only format at http://nursingworld.org/ethics/code/protected_nwcoe813.htm. The ANA is responsible for the periodic review of the code to ensure that it reflects the contemporary issues of this dynamic profession and is consistent with the ethical standards of the society in which we live.

The ANA's *Nursing: Scope and Standards of Practice* is another very important document for professional nurses. It defines standards of practice and standards of professional performance. The current version of the *Scope and Standards of Practice* was published in 2004. Standard 12 of the Scope states, "the registered nurse integrates ethical provisions in all areas of practice" (ANA, 2004, p. 39). This standard attests to the importance of ethics in the profession and spells out eight measurement criteria to indicate achievement of the standard for the registered nurse. Examples of these criteria include "uses the Code of Ethics for Nurses with Interpretive Statements to guide practice" and "contributes to resolving ethical issues of patients, colleagues or systems as evidenced in such activities as participation on ethics committees" (ANA, 2004, p. 39). Chapter 4 contains more detailed information on the Scope and Standards of Practice.

International Council of Nurses Code of Ethics for Nurses

The International Council of Nurses (ICN) also has published a code of ethics for the profession. This document discusses the rights and responsibilities of nurses related to people, practice, society, coworkers, and the profession. The ICN first adopted a code of ethics in 1953. Its last revision, adopted in 2005, represents agreement by more than 80 national nursing associations that participate in the international association. Inherent in the ICN Code for Nurses is nursing's respect for the life, dignity, and rights of all people in a manner that is unmindful of nationality, race, creed, color, age, sex, political affiliation, or social status. The preamble of *The ICN Code of Ethics for Nurses* (Box 5-3) details the four fundamental responsibilities for nurses and describes the ethical foundations for nursing practice. The ICN's Code for Nurses can be viewed online (http://www.icn.ch/ethics.htm).

ETHICAL DECISION MAKING

Nurses encounter situations daily that require them to make professional judgments and act on those judgments. The judgments or decisions

---

Box 5-2   The Florence Nightingale Pledge

The Florence Nightingale Pledge was written in 1893 by Lystra Gretter at the Farrand Training School in Detroit, Michigan. It was modeled after the Hippocratic oath taken by physicians as they begin their medical careers. The oath is dated in its wording and gender references; however key ethical principles discussed in this chapter and elsewhere in this text are present in this early statement intended to hold nurses to a high standard of professional ethical behavior. These principles are noted parenthetically in *italics*.

I solemnly pledge myself before God and presence of this assembly; to pass my life in purity and to practice my profession faithfully (fidelity).

I will abstain from whatever is deleterious and mischievous and will not take or knowingly administer any harmful drug (nonmaleficence).

I will do all in my power to maintain and elevate the standard of my profession (beneficence)

and will hold in confidence all personal matters committed to my keeping and family affairs coming to my knowledge in the practice of my calling (confidentiality).

With loyalty will I endeavor to aid the physician in his work (fidelity),

and devote myself to the welfare of those committed to my care (justice).

---

are usually made in collaboration with other persons involved in the situation: patients, families, and other health care professionals. Ethical decision making requires that the nurse make judgments or decisions when two or more of their values are incongruent. When an ethical decision is made, respect and valuing of the perspectives held by others, even when all do

Box 5-3   International Council of Nurses Code of Ethics for Nurses: Preamble

Nurses have four fundamental responsibilities: to promote health, to prevent illness, to restore health and to alleviate suffering. The need for nursing is universal.

Inherent in nursing is respect for human rights, including cultural rights, the right to life and choice, to dignity and to be treated with respect. Nursing care is respectful of and unrestricted by considerations of age, colour, creed, culture, disability or illness, gender, sexual orientation, nationality, politics, race or social status.

Nurses render health services to the individual, the family and the community and co-ordinate their services with those of related groups.

ICN Code of Ethics for Nurses, 3, place Jean-Marteau, 1201 Geneva (Switzerland), 2005. Copyright 2006.

Table 5-1   Comparison of Nursing Process With Ethical Decision-Making Model

Nursing Process	Ethical Decision-Making Model
Assess	Clarify the ethical dilemma
	Gather additional data
Analyze	Identify options
Plan	Make a decision
Implement	Act
Evaluate	Evaluate

not agree on the resolution, is an important professional behavior. Through respectful collaboration, the best decision can be reached in even the most difficult dilemma. Note that "the best decision" will be made: in an ethical dilemma, there is usually not a clear-cut right or wrong answer. Instead, we search for the best answer.

Ethical Decision-Making Model

Whether involved in a collective or individual decision, nurses need to be knowledgeable about suggested steps in ethical decision making. Table 5-1 demonstrates the similarity in the processes required in ethical decision making and the nursing process, both of which are based in sound critical thinking. A variety of ethical decision-making models are available in published literature across many disciplines and share more similarities than differences. The steps are not always necessarily sequential nor are they intended to be rigid processes. Instead, ethical decision making is a process in which ideas are thoroughly examined to determine the best solution to a difficult situation.

The following steps can be used in ethical decision making:

1. Clarify the ethical dilemma.

   What is the specific issue in question? Who owns the problem and should actually make the decision? Who is affected by the dilemma? Determine the ethical principle or theory related to the dilemma. Are there value conflicts? What is the time frame for the decision?

2. Gather additional data.

   After clarifying the ethical dilemma, in most instances more information needs to be gathered. It is important to have as many facts as possible about the situation. Make sure you are up-to-date on any legal cases or precedents related to the situation because ethical and legal issues often overlap.

3. Identify options.

   Most ethical dilemmas have multiple solutions, some of which are more feasible than others. The more options that are identified, the more likely it is that an acceptable solution can be identified. Brainstorm with others and consider every possible alternative that you can come up with.

4. Make a decision.

   To make a decision, think through the options that are identified and determine each option's impact. Ethical principles and theories, as well as universal basic human values, may help determine the significance of each option. When confronted with an ethical dilemma, an active decision should be made. Refusing to make a decision (being nonactive) is not responsible professional behavior.

5. Act.

    Once a course of action has been determined, the decision must be carried out. Implementing the decision usually involves working collaboratively with others.

6. Evaluate.

    Unexpected outcomes are common in crisis situations that result in ethical dilemmas. Decision makers should consider the impact an immediate decision may have on future ones. Reflecting on a decision and action can help determine whether a different course of action might have resulted in a better outcome. If the action accomplished its purpose, the ethical dilemma should be resolved. If the dilemma has not been resolved, engage in additional deliberation and reexamine alternative options.

Consider the six suggested ethical decision-making steps in the context of Case Study 5-1.

1. Clarify the ethical dilemma. The specific issue is the patient's right of autonomy versus the nurse's professional ethics and personal morals.

2. Gather additional data. Is Daniel responding to something that happened before you even got to his home today, such as an argument or a confrontation? Is he becoming depressed?

3. Identify options. Options may include the following: (1) simply telling Daniel you will not help him die; (2) responding to his dire request with compassion and trying to determine what is behind his sudden sense that he wants to die; (3) determine whether there is better symptom management that you can implement to make him more comfortable; (4) consider what would happen if Daniel told his mother the truth about his sexual orientation and HIV; (5) with Daniel and his partner's support, enlist the assistance of other hospice services such as pastoral care to help him ease his spiritual distress. (NOTE: there are many choices available here. These are just some suggestions.)

4. Make a decision. Make sure that everyone, especially Daniel, agrees with the plan.

5. Act. This may include a number of interventions, both physical and psychoemotional.

6. Evaluate. Did Daniel continue to express his desire to die now? Is he more comfortable? Is

---

CASE STUDY 5-1

Your hospice patient wants to die . . . and he wants you to help him.

Daniel is a 55-year-old white man with advanced lung cancer and is HIV positive. He is miserable with the profuse secretions from his lungs and struggles with every breath. Yet despite his weakened physical condition, his mind is still very alert. He is getting oxygen via nasal cannula. He is very vain, and part of each of your visits is helping him groom himself and putting on fresh designer pajamas. His mother is staying with him and his partner, and his mother has never known that Daniel is a homosexual and has HIV. He confides to you that trying to maintain the secret that he has kept from his mother is exhausting and is becoming burdensome. In the middle of your visit, he asks for a mirror to see what he looks like. You hand him a small mirror, and he is shocked at what he sees—a gray, shrunken, emaciated image looking back at him. He sets the mirror down carefully on the bedside table and looks at you evenly and with all seriousness says, "I am ready to die, and I want you to help me."

As a new nurse, you are not ready for this. You know that in his bedside drawer there is enough oral morphine to stop his breathing. You know that his death is still probably days away, and you are very sad for him in his misery. When you say, "I can't do that, Daniel," he starts crying and says, "I trusted you to help me . . ."

What should you do in response to this situation? What does the ANA say about assisted suicide and euthanasia? What is your personal moral code in this situation?

---

his distress less troublesome? Is he at some level of peace with his partner, his mother, and his life? Did your actions enhance the nurse-patient relationship with mutual trust and caring?

NAVIGATING ETHICAL DILEMMAS IN NURSING

Ethical dilemmas are a common occurrence in nursing practice. Many ethical dilemmas arise in nursing because of conflicts between patients, their families, health care professionals, and institutions. The following section will explore the major issues involved in these conflicts: (1) personal value systems, (2) peers' and other professionals' behaviors, (3) patients' rights, (4) institutional and societal issues, (5) patient data access issues, and (6) global dilemmas.

Dilemmas Resulting From Personal Value Systems

Values are important preferences that influence the behavior of individuals. Values are learned beliefs that help people choose among difficult alternatives, even when there may not be a good choice.

Each person has a set of values that was shaped by the beliefs, purposes, attitudes, qualities, and objects of a child's early caregivers. In time, individuals develop their own value systems that are grounded in their culture and life experiences. Variations in value systems become highly significant when dealing with critical issues such as health and illness or life and death. Value systems enable people to resolve conflicts and decide on a course of action based on a priority of importance.

Professions have a "built-in" value system known as a code of ethics, discussed earlier in this chapter. A very difficult issue for nursing students to come to terms with on occasion is when their personal values are in conflict with their professional values, or, more specifically, when they are faced with a professional situation that has some elements that are not in keeping with the nurse's personal moral code or values. The overriding concern in this situation is that professional ethics outweigh personal ethics in a professional setting. It is incumbent on the nurse to find a work situation in which his or her personal ethics are not routinely challenged by situations that occur with patients.

Nurses must have a good sense of their own values and be able to identify clearly what they believe to be good or right. We each develop our own value systems based on a variety of messages that we received in our formative years from our parents, siblings, friends, teachers, and religious training. The "Childhood Value Messages" exercise (Box 5-4) can help you to identify values learned as a child that may still influence you today.

To understand how personal and professional values can conflict in nursing practice, consider the following situation:

Marta had been a nurse on a postpartum unit for a number of years. Over time, an increasing number of pregnant women (antepartum) with serious problems related to the pregnancy were admitted to the unit where Marta worked. Although Marta preferred to work with new mothers and their infants, she occasionally took care of antepartum patients. One day in report, she learned that there was a newly admitted patient, Mrs. Anderson, who was in early pregnancy with triplets. Mrs. Anderson had a history of serious heart disease, but her condition was thought to be stable. Marta agreed to take care of her, having very little information about her. Shortly after report, Marta went into Mrs. Anderson's room to do her usual assessment, only to find that she was crying, being comforted by her husband who was also crying. Mrs. Anderson related to Marta that the maternal-fetal medicine specialist and her cardiologist had recommended that they do what is known as a selective reduction, a form of pregnancy termination in which a multiple pregnancy is reduced to one or two remaining embryos. The woman was already having signs of cardiac decompensation early in the pregnancy, and remaining pregnant at all was risky. But it was clear that Mrs. Anderson was not going to be able to tolerate the demands on her heart of a multiple pregnancy. She and her husband, although sad, understood that the selective reduction was their only chance of having a child at all, and, without it, her own life was in danger.

Marta was very upset with this news. As a practicing Catholic, she had a very strong moral stance against abortion, and, as a nurse, she had worked specifically with mothers and their new infants to avoid issues related to pregnancy termination. The procedure was going to be done in

Box 5-4   Childhood Value Messages

By the time we are about 10 years old, most of our values have already been "programmed." Values are taught to us by family members and friends, through the media, in churches and schools, and by watching other people. What are the value messages you learned as a child?

Recall as many values as you can remember hearing as a child and write them in the blanks provided below. Here are a few examples to get you thinking:

"Nothing worthwhile ever comes easy."

"Life is fatal—you're eternal."

"You can accomplish almost anything you want to if you persevere."

"Clean your plate; there are starving children in China!"

"You are your brother's keeper—reach out to others."

"Tell me the truth, and I won't punish you!"

"Get your work done first; then you can play."

Now it's your turn to write some of your childhood values. How many of these values still influence the way you think and act today? Which ones influence you professionally? If you want to further explore your values, you may do the following:

1. Next to each value on your list, write the person's name who taught or modeled that value.

2. Put a star next to those messages that are still your values today.

3. Put a check mark next to those messages that you need to alter.

4. How are some of these values still influencing you today? Is this a positive or negative influence?

1. _____
2. _____
3. _____
4. _____
5. _____
6. _____
7. _____
8. _____

Reprinted with permission of Uustal DB: *Clinical ethics and values: issues and insights in a changing healthcare environment,* East Greenwich, RI, 1993, Educational Resources in HealthCare.

Mrs. Anderson's room under ultrasound guidance within the next few minutes. Marta faced a serious moral dilemma in determining what to do. She sought the advice and counsel of a colleague whose wisdom she admired and trusted. In a few moments, Marta decided that her responsibility was to her patient and that, although she was present during the termination, she was not participating in performing it in any way. She understood her patient's deep distress and sadness. Before reentering the room, Marta took a moment to calm herself to be in a better state of mind to provide care for her patient. After taking a deep breath, she went in to Mrs. Anderson, encouraged Mr. Anderson to sit near his wife where they could see each other, and then took Mrs. Anderson's hand.

"I will be with you through this." Mrs. Anderson whispered, "Thank you." Marta had set aside her personal values to take excellent care of her patient as a trained and caring professional nurse.

Dilemmas Involving Peers' and Other Professionals' Behavior

All practicing nurses participate as members of the health care team. This involves cooperation and collaboration with other professionals. As is true in all situations involving human beings, conflicts can easily develop, particularly in stressful circumstances. These conflicts may be between two nurses, the nurse and physician, the nurse and agency policies, or the nurse and any other health care professional (Box 5-5).

Box 5-5   Distress in an Expert Labor and Delivery Nurse

This is a true account of a moral dilemma and moral distress in a labor and delivery nurse, Mary Tilghman, RN, who had been in practice for 6 years at the time of this event. She asked to use a pseudonym in recounting this story, as she does not want anyone to identify her situation or location where this event happened. But the story itself is true and illustrates the very difficult ethical situations that nurses find themselves in and the lingering distress that these situations can cause. Here is Mary's story:

I was working on a slow evening in a labor and delivery unit. We got a call from our dispatcher that emergency medical services (EMS) was bringing in a pregnant patient who was 25 weeks pregnant and having some vaginal bleeding. This is not really unusual, but it can be serious. I notified the resident doctor and another nurse and I set about getting a labor room ready. In about 10 minutes, EMS arrived with a young woman who was extremely pale, and was crying loudly. Her young husband was with her.

When we moved her to the labor bed, it was obvious that "some bleeding" was an understatement. She was bleeding profusely; even her gums, nose and a small crack in her lip were also bleeding. I listened for fetal heart tones and when I couldn't hear them, I asked her when the last time was that she had felt the baby move. I suspected that she had DIC—disseminated intravascular coagulopathy—a severe problem that sometimes occurs when a fetus is dead but labor doesn't begin. She said it had been "two, maybe three weeks." Her husband was shocked, because she hadn't told him that she hadn't been feeling the baby move. I called for the doctor right away, and then I paged the anesthesiologist to come to labor and delivery STAT. This was a severe emergency. I started a large-gauge IV so that we could give her blood and fluids, and sent some labs including a type and cross-match.

The doctor confirmed the fetal death by doing a quick ultrasound examination. The doctor explained to the woman that this was an emergency and had her sign a consent form. We hurried the patient to the OR for an emergency dilatation and evacuation (D&E). At the time, I had seen a lot as an obstetric nurse in a high-risk unit, but I was horrified at her huge and rapid blood loss. The anesthesiologist ordered as many units of O-negative blood (universal donor) as we could get until donor blood could be matched to hers in the blood bank. Weakly but as firmly as she could, the woman declared, "No blood. No blood. I am a Jehovah's Witness. Please no blood. If I die, I will be all right. No blood. Please." Everyone in the room heard her. The anesthesiologist patted her shoulder and told her that she would "be okay."

Everybody in the room could tell that this woman was bleeding to death. The anesthesiologist prepared to give her medications to increase her blood pressure and perfusion. By then the senior resident doctor and the attending physician were working quickly to perform the D&E. The junior obstetric resident was appalled by the situation. He left the room in a hurry and found the woman's husband, who was pacing outside in the hallway. The resident asked him, "Were you planning to be with your wife when she gave birth to your baby?" The husband said yes. The resident then told him, "Your wife is going to die. I think that you might want to be with her as she dies."

He gave the husband some scrubs to put on over his clothes and started towards the OR. By then, the woman's blood had begun to run out from under the OR door and into the hallway. When the husband saw it, he threw up his hands, saying, "Just give her the blood. Give her the blood . . . ." The resident patted him on the back and told him it was a good decision. The husband left the OR, and the

Box 5-5   Distress in an Expert Labor and Delivery Nurse—cont'd

anesthesiologist began infusing unit after unit of blood and blood products into the woman. I objected strenuously to this, but the physicians agreed that her husband's verbal consent was enough for them. The junior resident said, "I just don't think they understand what it means to bleed to death. I thought he'd change his mind if I showed him."

The patient went to intensive care for many days but recovered. I never saw her again. But I was very distressed over what I thought—and still think—was coercion of the part of the resident physician, showing the husband

his wife's blood, and overriding the woman's clear and unmistakable pleas for no blood products. She was willing to die rather than break her deep religious conviction. No matter what I believed about her religious views, my role was to advocate on her behalf—to be her voice. This situation is still distressful to me many years after it happened. Sometimes ethical dilemmas in nursing are unforgettable. For me, this is the one that stands out most clearly, the one that still haunts me.

Mary Tilghman, RN

Contributed courtesy of Mary Tilghman, RN.

As discussed previously, conflicts can evolve because of differing value systems, cultures, education levels, or a variety of other factors. Like Marta in the previous example, a nurse may believe that abortions are wrong, whereas the institution in which he or she is employed routinely performs them. This creates a conflict between the nurse's value system and the institution's practices, which can be the source of distress. Conflicts relevant to human rights often center around one of the ethical principles discussed earlier: autonomy, beneficence, nonmaleficence, veracity, or justice.

A disturbing reality in health care is the presence of providers in all disciplines who fail to meet standards of care routinely, who may simply be incompetent, or who participate in actions that are considered unethical by other professionals. An incompetent worker may suffer from physical or mental impairment or may be indifferent to standards of care. Unethical actions result when health care workers break basic norms of conduct toward others, especially the patient, whatever the reason.

A serious issue today is the disturbingly large number of nurses and other health care professionals impaired by drug dependence or other addictions. Deciding how and when to confront a suspected drug user may result in an ethical

dilemma. This dilemma can be overwhelming. Nurses agonize over whether to report observed or suspected instances of unethical conduct or incompetent care including impairment caused by alcohol or drugs. Fortunately, some employers and state nurses associations have developed plans to assist impaired nurses in getting the help they need and make provisions for them to return to the profession once they are far enough along in their recovery process. The board of nursing in each state, as well as each state nurses association, can provide information on specific programs for impaired nurses in the state. However, the process must begin with a co-worker who follows the ANA standard of care that obligates professional nurses to "report illegal, incompetent, or impaired" colleagues (ANA, 2004, p. 39).

To understand the ethical dilemmas that can result from conflict between peers, consider the following situation:

Gloria is a registered nurse who works on a surgical floor. She has just assisted in the transfer of Mr. Hudson to his room from the postanesthesia care unit after surgery and noticed that he was resting comfortably. Gloria sees another nurse drawing up morphine, a narcotic, in a syringe and then leaving the medications room. Ten minutes later, she returns with an empty syringe. Gloria asks, "Who needed pain medication?" The other nurse replies, "Mr. Hudson. He was in pain after surgery." Confused, Gloria checks Mr. Hudson's room and learns from his wife that he has not asked for nor received pain medication.

What should Gloria do now? What are her options, and how should she best manage this situation?

Dilemmas Regarding Patients' Rights

As health care has changed over the years so has the nature of relationships between providers and patients. Years ago, health professionals, particularly physicians, were considered to have the final word on care decisions and treatment options. Now consumers of health care are increasingly demanding to have a voice in their health care decisions. A number of special interest groups have developed published lists of patient rights. In 1971, the United Nations passed a resolution known as the Declaration of the Rights of Mentally Retarded Persons, an early model that recognized the interests of a particular group of persons with disabilities. In 1990, the Congress of the United States passed the Americans with Disabilities Act, which was amended in 2008. This extensive act has provided significant improvement in the lives of persons with a variety of mental and physical disabilities, recognizing their rights to participate fully in all aspects of society. Other less formal interest groups have written guidelines such as the Dying Person's Bill of Rights, Pregnant Patient's Bill of Rights, and Rights of Senior Citizens. The health care system has responded to consumers' awareness of their rights. Many of the rights demanded by patients as consumers of health care are legal rights that have been upheld by the judicial system. The American Hospital Association has an extensive website (http://www.aha.org/aha/issues/Communicating-With-Patients/pt-care-partnership.html) that addresses the wide range of rights of patients in the hospital setting. Some of the rights described in these documents are the

right to privacy, the right to informed consent, the right to die, the right to confidentiality and respectful care, the right to care without discrimination, and the right to information concerning medical condition and treatment.

Patient Self-Determination Act

In 1990, Congress passed the Patient Self-Determination Act (PSDA) that was enacted in December 1991. The PSDA is a safeguard for patients' rights, giving patients the legal right to determine how vigorously they wish to be treated in life-or-death situations, and calls for hospitals to abide by patients' advance directives. The PSDA specifies that any organization receiving Medicare or Medicaid funds must inform patients of state laws regarding directives, document the existence of directives in the patient's medical record, educate staff regarding directives, and educate the community about directives. This act encourages individuals to think about the type of medical and nursing treatment they would want if they were to become critically injured or ill. At the time questions arise, the patient is often unconscious or too sick to make decisions or communicate personal wishes.

Advance directives are designed to ensure individuals the rights of autonomy, refusal of medical intervention, and death with dignity. Advance directives are legal documents that indicate the wishes of individuals in regard to end-of-life issues. Critically ill individuals can remain in charge of their own end-of-life decisions if their advance directives are carried out. Each time they access a health care institution patients should have in their possession their advance directives. In addition, copies should be given to significant others, primary care providers, and any legal counsel that may be involved with the patient. The best directive is one that has been notarized or developed in conjunction with a legal expert.

Families should talk about how each member wants critical situations to be handled. Individual preferences can then be understood. Ideally, family members, caregivers, and courts, in very extreme cases, will not need to make decisions for the patient. Too often the first time a patient

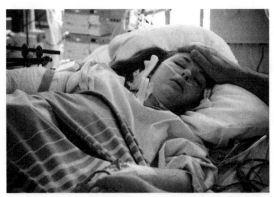

Figure 5-1 When families have made their wishes known through advance directives and planning, they can spend time together near the end of life that is peaceful, knowing that they are acting on the wishes of their dying family member.

learns about advance directives is on admission to a health care facility. The question then arises as to who is responsible for discussing this sensitive issue with the patient. The ideal time for patients to make difficult end-of-life decisions is well in advance of the need (Figure 5-1).

Advance directives have not been without controversy. One problem is that states have passed different legislation, and there is no guarantee that one state will honor another's advance directives. A trusted person may be appointed to make decisions on behalf of the patient when the patient cannot make them on his or her own. This is known as the assignment of the health care power of attorney. Rarely, persons have been designated by a family member to hold health care power of attorney without their prior knowledge. Ideally, the person making this designation and the trusted person being assigned this important responsibility should have a detailed discussion and prior understanding about what he or she is to do on behalf of the person. Holding health care power of attorney and making decisions based on the unambiguous wishes of the patient is a serious moral obligation, requiring that this designee act as the moral agent for the patient. Prior assignment of one's health care power of attorney can minimize, but in cases not altogether avoid, disagreements among family members. When

family members are left to make difficult treatment and end-of-life decisions, conflicts can occur at a time when families are already in distress and are vulnerable. Health care providers sometimes convene family meetings to work out these types of difficult situations.

Ethical Issues Related to Immigration and Migration

The movement of persons among nations—population migration—has become a topic of great interest across the world. The United States is no exception and faces a number of ethical issues that affect health care. We address two distinct issues here that affect nursing and have ethical implications: communication/language problems between patients and heath care providers, and the migration of nurses.

Communication is fundamental to safe, effective health care, the moral commitment to patients. Patients who do not speak English, and who hold a variety of health care beliefs and practices to which American health care workers may not be accustomed, pose a challenge. Many health care institutions, especially larger medical centers, have addressed the issue of language by hiring professional medical interpreters. Interpretation involves the spoken word, and translation refers to the written word.

Medical interpretation is a specialty that requires extensive knowledge of medical terminology, in addition to cultural humility and sensitivity to the needs of the patient. Many nursing students have some working knowledge of another language, often Spanish. The level of fluency needed for safe interpretation, however, is not typically achieved in language coursework. Nurses who are not bilingual or fluent in medical terminology should defer to a professional medical interpreter for explanations of procedures, diagnoses, obtaining informed consent, and other complex health care–related issues. Furthermore, although it is tempting to enlist the assistance of a patient's family member to interpret, this is not safe practice. Children of patients should never be asked to interpret under any circumstances. The International Medical Interpreters Association

(IMIA) is moving quickly toward establishing national certification standards for medical interpreters. IMIA's website (http://imiaweb.org/) addresses many issues of interest to nurses.

Another second issue with significant ethical implications for health care delivery is international nurse migration. As the nursing shortage intensifies and threatens to become worse as our population ages, some legislators have proposed changing American immigration laws to open the door to nurses from other countries (Dugger, 2006). The idea is endorsed by the American Hospital Association, which reported in April 2006 that there were 118,000 vacancies for registered nurses nationwide. The federal government has forecast a shortfall of 800,000 nurses by the year 2020. Removing the immigration cap for nurses would increase the flow of English-speaking foreign nurses, who may be drawn to practice in the United States by higher salaries and improved living and working conditions.

This poses two distinct ethical problems. First, this exacerbates nursing shortages in other countries. Countries particularly hard hit by this phenomenon include the Philippines, which already loses several thousand nurses a year to this country, India, South Africa, and, possibly, China. Leaders in these countries oppose the U.S. open-immigration policy for nurses. Importantly, the ANA is on record as opposing the measure, expressing support instead to increase appropriations to expand nursing programs in this country. This comes at a time when a majority of qualified applicants to American schools of nursing are not admitted because of inadequate numbers of faculty and facilities. The ANA was joined by Physicians for Human Rights in opposing the proposal. One physician member of this advocacy group described the open-immigration policy as having the potential to "undermine our multibillion-dollar effort to combat AIDS and malaria by potentially worsening the shortage of health workers in poor countries. We're pouring water in a bucket with a hole in it, and we drilled the hole" (Dugger, 2006).

The second ethical issue this raises is the documentation of competency to provide safe nursing care, which occurs in the passing of the National Council Licensure Examination (NCLEX) by graduates of approved American nursing schools. Nurses who may come to the United States expecting to find well-paying jobs as professional registered nurses may find that their education and skills may not be sufficient to practice as a registered nurse. English as a second language for nurses who migrate to the United States poses similar communication difficulties as described above, and cultural acclimation to the United States may pose particular challenges for these nurses. Moreover, there has been an increase in exploitative and highly unethical recruitment practices by companies that, after collecting huge fees for their services, mislead foreign nurses and/or misrepresent work opportunities in the United States available to these nurses (Jeans, 2006).

Dilemmas Created by Institutional Issues

Health care institutions must be in compliance with many governmental regulations that affect both workers and patients. In turn, hospitals and other health care institutions implement their own policies and procedures. Nurses may experience moral dilemmas when they disagree with the policies of their institutions. Health care organizations are subject to public scrutiny and accountability, and those that receive public funds through the Centers for Medicare & Medicaid Services are under particular scrutiny. Ethical dilemmas between nurses and the organizations that employ them may develop over policies dictated by the organizations or mandated by governmental agencies. Nurses experience great difficulty when the correct course of action is known but they are unable to implement the ethically or morally correct action because of the constraints of institutional policy (Austin, Lemermeyer, Goldberg et al, 2005). Ethics committees were created to assist with ethical dilemmas in institutional settings. These committees are multidisciplinary groups charged with the responsibility of providing consultation and emotional support in situations in which difficult ethical choices are necessary. Those desiring help, usually clinical caregivers such as physicians and nurses, refer cases to the committee for additional direction.

The following vignette illustrates an ethical conflict between a nurse and the employing institution:

Jennifer is a registered nurse working in a critical care unit. All beds in the unit are full. For the past 2 days, she has been assigned to care for a 81-year-old woman who is critically ill with heart failure. The patient is widowed. She has no financial resources of her own, and no family member has seen her since she was admitted, although her sister has been informed of her admission to the intensive care unit. She has no advance directives in her chart. Suddenly, orders come for the elderly woman to be transferred to a bed on a regular nursing unit. As she is being prepared to be transferred out of the critical care unit, word comes that a state senator's son with a non–life-threatening condition is to be admitted to the recently vacated bed. What are the ethical issues at stake in this situation? What action should the nurse take?

Dilemmas Created by Patient Data Access Issues

Electronic technologies and paperless documentation including hand-held devices are powerful sources of information about patients. These are useful tools in the sharing of information across health care specialties and disciplines. However, these technologies have created an electronic portal into patients' confidential medical information. Those in positions to access health care information share a great responsibility to protect this information from unauthorized use.

Curtin (2005) noted that information technology, particularly the computerized electronic medical record, places great power in the hands of health care workers and exacerbates basic ethical problems that exist. Computer ethics have been in existence since the 1970s, but in recent years there is renewed interest in scholarly inquiry in nursing informatics as the use of technology has

become standard in health care institution. The following example illustrates the type of ethical dilemma that can result from inappropriate use of paperless technologies:

Tom, a third-year nursing student, observed Susan, a first-year nursing student, sitting at the nurses' station reading patient information on a third student known to both who was hospitalized with a serious illness in the same facility. Neither Susan nor Tom was directly involved in the care of the third student. Considering Susan's inexperience, what steps should Tom take? Does Susan's inexperience factor into your thinking about this situation?

The safe practice of nursing is inextricable from moral and ethical challenges. We encourage you as students of nursing to become aware of your own values, morals, and ethics and to become sensitive to the values, morals, and ethics at work in every nursing situation.

Summary of Key Points

- The terms *morals* and *ethics* are often used interchangeably. Technically, however, morals reflect what is done in a situation, whereas ethics are concerned with what should be done. Values are beliefs, ideals, and attitudes that one uses to guide behavior.
- It is important that nurses are familiar with ethical theories and principles, moral development, and decision-making models to participate actively in resolving ethical dilemmas that occur frequently in health care settings. Two major theorists in moral development are Kohlberg and Gilligan.
- Codes of ethics, developed by the profession's members, are important to the development of the profession.
- The ANA's Code of Ethics for Nurses serves as a guideline for nurses regarding ethical behavior.
- The history of the Code of Ethics for Nurses is reflective of nursing's history as a profession.
- Ethical dilemmas occur in all areas of nursing practice.

- Respect for humans is the foundation for the six ethical principles of autonomy, beneficence, nonmaleficence, fidelity, veracity, and justice.
- Use of technology in health care institutions has compounded common ethical dilemmas and created new ones for health care workers.
- Dilemmas often occur because of conflicts between personal value systems, patients, families, health care professionals, institutions, and society.
- Ethical decision-making models are helpful in determining the best action to take when faced with an ethical dilemma.

Critical Thinking Questions

1. Explain the differences among morals, values, and ethics. Give an example of each from your own value system.
2. How can the ANA's Code of Ethics for Nurses be used by the bedside nurse, by the home health nurse, and by student nurses?
3. Compare the ANA's Code of Ethics for Nurses with the ICN's Code of Ethics for Nurses. How are they similar, and how are they different?
4. Select an ethical theory or principle that is most congruent with your approach to ethical dilemmas. Use it as a basis for resolving the ethical dilemmas in this chapter. How well does it hold up under these test conditions?
5. Discuss your reactions to the following scenarios and questions in a small group:
   a. Mrs. Otto has recently undergone extensive surgery for gynecologic cancer. The day after surgery, she asks for more pain medication than the physician has prescribed. You call for an order to increase the pain medication dosage, but she still complains every 2 hours that she cannot tolerate the pain. What should be done?
   b. Mrs. Loriz suffers from severe chronic pain, the cause of which has not been definitely diagnosed. Her husband has brought her into the emergency department for the fifth time this month asking for narcotic relief from the pain. In tears she states, "A shot of Demerol is the only thing that takes the edge off." She threatens suicide if she is sent home without some help. The physician has ordered a placebo. What is the nurse's responsibility?
   c. Mr. Nelson, aged 87 years, suffered a serious stroke. His wife of 65 years keeps a constant vigil at his bedside. After 4 weeks, he remains totally unresponsive, and pneumonia develops. A tracheotomy is performed and a feeding tube inserted. Mrs. Nelson feels that agreeing to a "do-not-resuscitate" order is letting her husband down but recognizes he has no quality of life. How should the nurse counsel Mrs. Nelson?
   d. Emily and Michael Mills are parents of a young child dying of Tay-Sachs disease. Emily recently found out she was pregnant and wants to know whether their second child is affected with the same disease. She undergoes genetic testing of the embryo, and, to the parents' extreme dismay, they find that their second child also has Tay-Sachs disease. How can the nurse assist these parents in making a decision regarding the second pregnancy?
6. Answer the following questions, basing your answers on identified ethical principles:
   a. When is it acceptable to refuse an assignment?
   b. What is the nurse's duty when a patient confides that he wants to harm himself?
   c. Is health care a right?
   d. What should the nurse do when her personal values are in conflict with those of the patient?

The author acknowledges the contributions of Shielda Rodgers in her previous preparation of this chapter.

⊖volve *To enhance your understanding of this chapter, try the Student Exercises on the Evolve site at http://evolve.elsevier.com/Chitty/professional.*

REFERENCES

American Nurses Association: *Code of ethics for nurses with interpretive statements*, Washington, DC, 2001, American Nurses Publishing.

American Nurses Association: *Nursing: Scope and standards of practice*, Washington, DC, 2004, American Nurses Association.

Austin W, Lemermeyer G, Goldberg L, et al: Moral distress in healthcare practice: the situation of nurses, *HEC Forum* 17(1):33-48, 2005.

Baker R: In defense of bioethics, *J Law Med Ethics* 37(1):83-92, 2009.

Bavier A: Holding students accountable when integrity is challenged, *Nurs Educ Perspect* 30(1):5, 2009.

Beauchamp TL, Childress JF: *Principles of biomedical ethics*, ed 4, New York, 2001, Oxford University Press.

Burkhardt MA, Nathaniel AK: *Ethics and issues in contemporary nursing*, ed 2, Albany, NY, 2002, Delmar.

Butts J, Rich K: *Nursing ethics: across the curriculum and into practice*, Sudbury, Mass, 2005, Jones and Bartlett.

Chally PS: Nursing research: moral decision making by nurses in intensive care, *Plast Surg Nurs* 15(2):120-124, 1995.

Curtin LL: Ethics in informatics, *Nurs Adm Q* 29(4):349-352, 2005.

Davis AJ, Aroskar MA, Liaschenko J, et al: *Ethical dilemmas and nursing practice*, ed 4, Stamford, Conn, 1997, Appleton & Lange.

de Casterlé BD, Izumi S, Godfrey NS, Denhaerynck K: Nurses' responses to ethical dilemmas in nursing practice: meta-analysis, *J Adv Nurs* 63(6):540-549, 2009.

Dugger CW: US plan to lure nurses may hurt poor nations, *The New York* Times, May 24, 2006.

Gallagher A, Wainwright P: The ethical divide, *Nurs Stand* 20(7):22-25, 2005.

Giddings L: A theoretical model of social consciousness, *Adv Nurs Sci* 28:224-239, 2005.

Gilligan C: *In a different voice: psychological theory and women's development*, Cambridge, Mass, 1982, Harvard University Press.

Guido GW: *Legal & ethical issues in nursing*, ed 4, Upper Saddle River, NJ, 2006, Pearson Education.

Hardingham LB: Ethics in the workplace: reflective practice, *Alberta RN* 57(3):28-29, 2001.

Hardingham LB: Integrity and moral residue: nurses as participants in a moral community, *Nurs Philos* 5:127-134, 2004.

Harrison E, Falco SM: Health disparity and the nurse advocate: reaching out to alleviate suffering, *Adv Nurs Sci* 28(3):252-264, 2005.

Haynes L, Boese T, Butcher H: *Nursing in contemporary society: issues, trends and transition to practice*, Upper Saddle River, NJ, 2004, Pearson Prentice Hall.

Hines PS: Truth-telling, not telling, and listening, *Cancer Nurs* 31(6):415-416, 2008.

International Council of Nurses: *The International Council of Nurses code for nurses*, Geneva, Switzerland, 2000, International Council of Nurses.

Jameton A: *Nursing practice: the ethical issues*, Englewood Cliffs, NJ, 1984, Prentice-Hall.

Jeans ME: In-country challenges to addressing the effects of emerging global nurse migration on health care delivery, *Policy Polit Nurs Pract* 7(3 Suppl):58S-61S, 2006.

Kirkham SR, Van Hofwegen L, Pankratz D: Keeping the vision: sustaining social consciousness with nursing students following international learning experiences, *International Journal of Nursing Education Scholarship* (online) 6(1)(article 3), 2009.

Kohlberg L: Continuities and discontinuities in childhood and adult moral development revisited. In Kohlberg L, editor: *Collected papers on moral development and moral education*, Cambridge, Mass, 1973, Moral Education Research Foundation.

Kohlberg L: Moral stages and moralization: the cognitive developmental approach. In Lickona T, editor: *Moral development and behavior*, New York, 1976, Holt, Rinehart & Winston, pp 31-53.

Kohlberg L: A current statement on some theoretical issues. In Modgil S, Modgil C, editors: *Lawrence Kohlberg: consensus and controversy*, Philadelphia, 1986, Falmer, pp 485-546.

Nathaniel A: Moral distress among nurses, *Ethics Human Rights Issues Update* 1(3):3-6, 2002.

Tuckett AG: Truth-telling in clinical practice and the arguments for and against: a review of the literature, *Nurs Ethics* 11(5):500-513, 2004.

Uustal DB: Clinical ethics and values: *issues and insights in a changing healthcare environment*, East Greenwich, RI, 1993, Educational Resources in HealthCare.

Zickmund SL: Care and justice: the impact of gender and profession on ethical decision making in the healthcare arena, *J Clin Ethics* 15(2):176-187, 2004.

Becoming a Nurse: Defining Nursing and Socialization Into Professional Practice

Beth Perry Black

After studying this chapter, students will be able to:
- Describe the benefits of defining nursing and how this is related to professional socialization
- Compare early definitions of nursing with contemporary ones
- Recognize the impact of historical, social, economic, and political events on evolving definitions of nursing
- Identify commonalities in existing definitions of nursing
- Develop personal definitions of nursing
- Discuss how students' initial images of nursing are transformed through professional education and experiences

- Differentiate between formal and informal socialization
- Identify factors that influence an individual's professional socialization
- Describe two developmental models of professional socialization and explain how they are used
- Differentiate between the elements of professional socialization that are the responsibility of nursing programs and those that are the individual's responsibility
- Describe strategies to ease the transition from student to professional nurse

Definitions of nursing and nursing's scope of practice seek to describe who nurses are and what they do. They answer questions such as the following: "What is nursing?" "What is the role of the nurse?" "What is unique about nursing?" and "What are the boundaries of nursing practice?" Although the answers for these questions seem quite simple, agreement on a single definition of nursing has been elusive.

In this chapter we will first examine definitions of nursing and explore how they have evolved over time. Once you have a clearer idea of definitions of nursing, we will discuss how you will make the move from student to nursing student, and then from nursing student to professional nurse through the process of socialization. Defining nursing is an important first step in becoming a professional nurse in practice. Having a clearer understanding of what nursing is, and, as Nightingale said, "what it is not," helps you move closer to incorporating the values of professional practice. This process of socialization takes

time but is enhanced when you have a clear idea of what your end point is: safe, informed, and professional nursing practice.

DEFINING NURSING: HARDER THAN IT SEEMS

You may be surprised to learn that finding a universally acceptable definition of nursing has been difficult. Ask almost anyone on the street what nursing is and you will get answers that range from "they take care of people in the hospital" to "they help doctors." Few persons outside of the health care setting have a clear idea of what nurses are and what they do.

Even nurses themselves have been unable to agree on one definition. For more than 150 years, individuals, starting with Florence Nightingale, and organizations around the world such as the International Council of Nurses (ICN), the United Kingdom's Royal College of Nursing (RCN), and the American Nurses Association (ANA) have attempted to achieve a consensus on a definition of nursing. Some efforts have been more successful than others.

Most of the definitions reviewed in this chapter have some terms in common. Considering the variations in knowledge and technology during the different points in history when these definitions were written, the similarities are remarkable. All the definitions are rooted in history and were affected by significant political, economic, and social events that shaped nursing.

Why Define Nursing?

Why is it important to spend time trying to define nursing? Having an accepted definition of nursing is essential in a variety of ways and provides a framework for nursing practice. A definition establishes the parameters (or boundaries) of the profession and clarifies the purposes and functions of the work of nursing. In addition, a definition guides the educational preparation of aspiring practitioners and guides nursing research and theory development. Importantly, a clear definition makes the work of nursing visible and valuable to the public and to policy makers who determine when, where, and how nurses can practice. Norma Lang, an influential contemporary nursing leader, put it succinctly by stating, "If we cannot name it, we cannot control it, finance it, research it, teach it, or put it into public policy. It's just that blunt!" (Styles, 1991).

Definitions clarify purposes and functions

Nursing is a complex enterprise that is often confusing to its own practitioners, as well as to the public. Defining nursing assists people to grasp its nuances, many of which are not readily observable. Nursing benefits when people such as journalists, public policy makers, insurers, other health care professionals, and the public understand what it is that nurses do.

Definitions differentiate nursing from other health occupations

More than 200 different allied health occupations have been developed in the past several decades. Each new advance in technology bred

a new "technician" who needed to be educated, hired, oriented, and paid with limited health care dollars, a trend that continues today. The resulting cost was a major factor leading to significant redesign of the health care system during the 1990s and required the redefining of roles within the system. In response to these changes, defining nursing became even more important to manage the overlap of nursing with other fields without losing the core identity of nursing. Furthermore, with health care reform as a priority for the Obama administration, nurses can expect to see other significant changes that will require that nursing is clearly defined and its importance within the health care system is unmistakable. The ability to articulate the impressive abilities of nurses to address a wide variety of health issues is crucial in keeping nurses in key places of influence as health care reform takes shape in the next few years.

Definitions influence health policy at local, state, and national levels

Policy makers, such as legislators and regulators, need to understand the role and scope of nursing. Without that understanding, they cannot institute good health care policy that maximizes use of nurses' particular skills to improve the health of the public.

A key reason to define nursing is that nursing practice is regulated at the state level. Nurse practice acts of each state need to reflect the widening expertise and autonomy of nurses. When the roles of professional registered nurses (RNs), advanced practice nurses, licensed or vocational nurses, and nursing assistants are well defined, legislators can pass progressive laws regulating and expanding nursing practice. Otherwise, nurse practice acts may restrict nursing practice and inhibit professional growth.

Definitions aid in developing educational curricula and research agendas

When nursing faculty plan the curriculum of a school of nursing, one of the major determinants of the design is their definition of nursing. Without the foundation of a definition, what to include and how to prioritize the huge array of information today's nurses need to know would be extremely difficult and unwieldy. A definition of nursing provides a good starting point for curriculum development. In much the same way, nurse researchers cannot easily determine phenomena of interest for nursing unless they are clear about the boundaries and purposes of nursing actions that a definition of nursing sets in place.

Evolution of Definitions of Nursing

In the last century and a half as nursing was progressing as a more formal academic discipline and practice profession, a number of attempts have been made to define nursing that reflect the profession's evolution over the years.

Nightingale defines nursing

Florence Nightingale was the first person to recognize the complexities of nursing that led to difficulty in defining it. Considering how relatively undeveloped nursing was during her time, Nightingale's definitions contain surprisingly contemporary concepts. Remember that during Nightingale's day, formal schooling in nursing was just beginning. In *Notes on Nursing: What It Is and What It Is Not* (originally published in 1859), she became the first person to attempt a written definition of nursing, stating, "And what nursing has to do. . . is put the patient in the best condition for nature to act upon him" (Nightingale, 1946, p. 75). She also wrote:

> I use the word nursing for want of a better. It has been limited to signify little more than the administration of medicines and the application of poultices. It ought to signify the proper use of fresh air, light, warmth, cleanliness, quiet, and the proper selection and administration of diet—all at the least expense of vital power to the patient (Nightingale, 1946, p. 6).

Although Nightingale lived in a time when little was known about disease processes and available treatments were extremely limited, these definitions foreshadowed contemporary nursing's focus on the therapeutic milieu (environment), as well as the modern emphasis on health promotion and health maintenance. She accurately observed that although simply possessing observational skills does not make someone a good nurse, without these skills a nurse is ineffective. Indeed, informed observation has always been an integral part of the process of nursing. Nightingale was also the first person to differentiate between nursing provided by a professional nurse using a unique body of knowledge and nursing care provided by a layperson such as a mother caring for a sick child.

Early twentieth-century definitions

Fifty years after Nightingale wrote *Notes on Nursing*, the search for a definition began in earnest. Following the English model, many schools of nursing had been established in the United States, and numbers of "trained nurses" were in practice. These nurses sought to develop a professional identity for their rapidly expanding discipline. Shaw's *Textbook of Nursing* (1907) defined nursing as an art: "It properly includes, as well as the execution of specific orders, the administration of food and medicine, the personal care of the patient" (pp. 1-2). Harmer's *Textbook of the Principles and Practice of Nursing* (1922) elaborated on Shaw's bare-bones definition: "The object of nursing is not only to cure the sick . . . but to bring health and ease, rest and comfort to mind and body. Its object is to prevent disease and to preserve health" (p. 3). The fourth edition of the Harmer text, which showed the influence of coauthor and visionary Virginia Henderson, redefined nursing: "Nursing may be defined as that service to an individual that helps him to attain or maintain a healthy state of mind or body" (Harmer and Henderson, 1939, p. 2). Henderson's perceptions represented the emergence of contemporary nursing and were so inclusive that they remained useful for many years. We will see her influence again in the next section.

Post–World War II definitions

World War II helped advance the technologies available to treat people, which, in turn, influenced nursing. The war also made nurses aware of the influential role emotions play in health, illness, and nursing care. Hildegard Peplau (1952), widely regarded as a pioneer among contemporary nursing theorists and herself a psychiatric nurse, defined nursing in interpersonal terms: "Nursing is a significant, therapeutic, interpersonal process . . . . Nursing is an educative instrument . . . that aims to promote forward movement of personality in the direction of creative, constructive, productive, personal and community living" (p. 16). Peplau reinforced the idea of the patient as an active collaborator in his or her own care.

During the late 1950s and early 1960s, the number of master's programs in nursing rapidly increased. As more nurses were educated at the graduate level and learned about the research process, they were eager to test new ideas about nursing. Nursing theory was born. (See Chapter 13 for an in-depth discussion of nursing theory.)

One of the theorists who began work during this early period of theory development was Dorothea Orem. Her 1959 definition captures the flavor of her later, more completely elaborated self-care theory of nursing: "Nursing is perhaps best described as the giving of direct assistance to a person, as required, because of the person's specific inabilities in self-care resulting from a situation of personal health" (Orem, 1959, p. 5). Orem's belief that nurses should do for a person only those things the person cannot do without assistance emphasized the patient's active role.

By 1960 Henderson's earlier definition had evolved into a statement that had such universal appeal that it was adopted by the ICN:

> The unique function of the nurse is to assist the individual, sick or well, in the performance of those activities contributing to health or its recovery (or to a peaceful death) that he would perform unaided if he had the necessary strength, will or knowledge. And to do this in such a way as to help him gain independence as rapidly as possible (Henderson, 1960, p. 3).

Never before or since has one definition of nursing been so widely accepted both in the United States and throughout the world.

Many believe it is still the most comprehensive and appropriate definition of nursing in existence.

Another pioneer nursing theorist, Martha Rogers, included the concept of the nursing process in her definition: "Nursing aims to assist people in achieving their maximum health potential. Maintenance and promotion of health, prevention of disease, nursing diagnosis, intervention, and rehabilitation encompass the scope of nursing's goals" (Rogers, 1961, p. 86).

Professional association definitions

Nursing organizations worldwide have also struggled with defining nursing. Definitions to be reviewed here include those of the ANA, the RCN, and the ICN. As you read these definitions, notice that some new concepts and terms are introduced in the more recent American definitions. In the United States, nursing has defined itself as the health discipline that "cares," although recent discussion suggests that limiting nursing to "caring" only overlooks the significant role that nurses have in the curative processes of health care (Gordon, 2005).

American Nurses Association. The ANA has published several definitions of nursing over the years. The second edition of *Nursing's Social Policy Statement* defined nursing comprehensively. This definition included six essential features of contemporary nursing practice (ANA, 2003, p. 5):

- Provision of a caring relationship that facilitates health and healing
- Attention to the range of human experiences and responses to health and illness within the physical and social environments
- Integration of objective data with knowledge gained from an appreciation of the patient or group's subjective experience
- Application of scientific knowledge to the processes of diagnosis and treatment through the use of judgment and critical thinking
- Advancement of professional nursing knowledge through scholarly inquiry
- Influence on social and public policy to promote social justice

The wide focus of the practice of nursing is described in the preface to the *Code of Ethics for Nurses* (2001): "Nursing encompasses the prevention of illness, the alleviation of suffering, and the protection, promotion, and restoration of health in the care of individuals, families, groups, and communities" (p. 4).

Royal College of Nursing. The RCN is the United Kingdom's voice of nursing and is the largest professional union of nurses in the world. This organization embarked on an 18-month-long initiative to define nursing, culminating in the April 2003 publication of the document titled *Defining Nursing* (RCN, 2003).

The RCN definition of nursing has a core statement supported by six defining characteristics. The core statement is this:

Nursing is the use of clinical judgment in the provision of care to enable people to improve, maintain, or recover health, to cope with health problems, and to achieve the best possible quality of life, whatever their disease or disability, until death.

The six defining characteristics are too lengthy to reprint here; however, the entire document is worthy of examination and reflection because of its comprehensiveness and thoughtfulness. You can locate it at http://www.rcn.org.uk/downloads/definingnursing/definingnursing-a5.pdf.

International Council of Nurses. The ICN is a federation of national nurses associations representing nurses in more than 120 countries. Although ICN's membership is diverse, its definition of nursing is quite similar to that of single-nation organizations such as the ANA and RCN. According to the ICN:

Nursing encompasses autonomous and collaborative care of individuals of all ages, families, groups, and communities, sick or well, and in all settings. Nursing includes the promotion of health, prevention of illness, and the care of ill, disabled, and dying people. Advocacy, promotion of a safe environment,

research, participation in shaping health policy and in patient and health systems management, and education are also key nursing roles (ICN, 2003).

You can learn much more about the ICN online at http://www.icn.ch.

Definitions Developed by State Legislatures

One of the most significant definitions of nursing is contained in the nurse practice act of the state in which a nurse practices. Regardless of how restrictive or permissive it may be, this definition constitutes the legal definition of nursing in a particular state, and the professional nurse maintains familiarity with the latest version of the act. Ohio's nurse practice act contains wording typical of many states' acts (State of Ohio Board of Nursing, 2009):

"Practice of nursing as a registered nurse" means providing to individuals and groups nursing care requiring specialized knowledge, judgment, and skill derived from the principles of biological, physical, behavioral, social, and nursing sciences. Such nursing care includes:

1. Identifying patterns of human responses to actual or potential health problems amenable to a nursing regimen
2. Executing a nursing regimen through the selection, performance, management, and evaluation of nursing actions
3. Assessing health status for the purpose of providing nursing care
4. Providing health counseling and health teaching
5. Administering medications, treatments, and executing authorized by an individual who is authorized to practice in this state and is acting within the course of the individual's professional practice
6. Teaching, administering, supervising, delegating, and evaluating nursing practice

It is no accident that the language in these nurse practice acts sounds like familiar nursing language. State nurses associations and boards of nursing are actively involved with legislators to assist them in drafting laws that accurately reflect the nature and scope of nursing. The current nurse practice act in each state can be obtained by calling or writing the state board of nursing. The addresses of the boards of nursing can be found on the Evolve website (http://evolve.elsevier.com/Chitty/professional/).

Before moving on to the next discussion on socialization, take time to look at the accompanying Critical Thinking Challenge 6-1. How would you define nursing?

BECOMING A NURSE: SHAPING YOUR PROFESSIONAL IDENTITY

Defining nursing means that you have determined the most salient elements of what it means to be a nurse: what a nurse is and what a nurse does. When you first decided to become a nurse, you had certain preconceived notions about what nursing was and how you saw yourself as a nurse. Your desire to be a nurse may have been shaped by an illness experience of your own or a family member. Becoming a nurse may simply be something that you have always wanted to do without a specific event that spurred this desire. Or you may be pragmatic in your career choice by selecting a profession in which demand is high and the risk of unemployment is low. Whatever the reason you elected to pursue a career in nursing, your image of nursing and what it entails is almost certainly going to be changed while in nursing school. Your thinking about nursing should change, develop, and mature over the course of your education.

Although many students enter the profession of nursing with the worthy goal of "taking care of people," how this goal is translated into practice remains something of a mystery until you begin your studies as a nursing student. Being a student of nursing is the first of many steps in socializing you into professional practice: the goal of socialization is the development of professionalism. The goal of your nursing education is not simply teaching you the tasks of nursing, although they are important elements of your practice. The overriding goal of your education is to teach you to think like a nurse, to see the world of health care through the lens of nursing, and to respond to the effects of both educational and clinical experiences by developing professionalism.

This process requires that students internalize, or take in, new knowledge, skills, attitudes, behaviors, values, and ethical standards and make these a part of their own professional identity. For the RN returning to school for a bachelor of science in nursing (BSN) degree, a modification of an already-formed professional identity occurs. This process of internalization and development or modification of an occupational identity is known as professional socialization; it begins during the period students are in formal nursing programs and continues as they practice in "the real world."

EDUCATION AND PROFESSIONAL SOCIALIZATION

Nursing faculty are concerned with creating educational experiences that encourage and facilitate the transition from student to professional nurse. How does a student make the transition from a novice struggling to understand what is going on to a person who thinks and feels like a nurse?

CRITICAL THINKING *Challenge 6-1*

Nursing is . . .

Instructions: *Using your thoughts, as well as elements of others' definitions, write your own definition of nursing. Explain it to a classmate, giving your* *rationale for what you included and excluded. Keep it among your professional papers to refer to in later years. See how it evolves over time.*

Learning any new role is derived from a mixture of formal and informal socialization. We have all been socialized into a variety of roles over the course of our lives. One that is so familiar to you now is the role of student in a generic sense. You learned in kindergarten that there are particular ways to behave in class, times to sit quietly and times to play, ways to get the teacher's attention, and, definitely, ways that you did not want to get the teacher's attention! You learned the "rules" of being a student and, unless you were particularly incorrigible, you learned your role as a student early and well.

In nursing, formal socialization includes classroom lectures, assignments, and laboratory experiences taught by faculty, such as planning nursing care, writing a paper on professional ethics, learning steps of a physical examination of a healthy child, starting an intravenous line, or practicing communication with a psychiatric patient (Figure 6-1). Formal socialization proceeds in an orderly, building-block fashion, such that new information is based on previous information. For that reason, advanced nursing students are often encouraged to manage a larger number of patients than they did as novice students when their skills were fewer and less tested.

Informal socialization includes lessons that occur incidentally, such as the unplanned observation of a nurse teaching a young mother how to care for her premature infant, participating in a student nurse association, or hearing nurses discuss patient care in the nurses' lounge. Part of

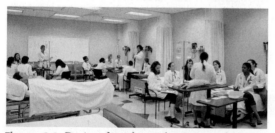

Figure 6-1 During formal socialization, students internalize the knowledge, skills, and beliefs of nursing in planned educational experiences and interactions with faculty and other nurses. (Courtesy Emory University/ Nell Hodgson Woodruff School of Nursing.)

professional socialization is simply absorbing the culture of nursing, that is, the rites, rituals, and valued behaviors of the profession. This requires that students spend enough time with nurses in work settings for adequate exposure to the nursing culture to occur. Most nurses agree that informal socialization experiences were often more powerful and memorable than formal socialization in their own development.

Learning a new vocabulary is also part of professional socialization. Each profession has its own jargon that is generally not well understood by outsiders. Professional students in any field usually enjoy acquiring the new vocabulary and practicing it among themselves. Although the vocabulary of any profession can be confusing and complex, the student quickly becomes fluent as a function of both formal and informal socialization. The student should be aware, however, that certain informal vocabulary overheard on nursing units is not always appropriate in professional settings and may actually be denigrating to patients or their families. A wise student will decide early to forgo these sorts of negative characterizations.

Learning any new role creates some degree of anxiety. Many of us remember the distress we felt when going to school for the first time as a young child. Some new students may find themselves particularly anxious as clinical experiences begin—the uncertainty of the situation, the unfamiliar language, the presence of patients with serious medical diagnoses, and a keen sense of the importance of the work of nursing can all contribute to this anxiety. This is not uncommon and may conjure up memories of our early days of formal education.

Once the initial nerves and excitement of entering nursing school have worn off, students may find themselves dealing with disappointment and frustration when their learning expectations come into conflict with educational realities. Students' ideas of what they need to learn, when they need to learn it, and what might be the best way to learn it may differ from how their education actually unfolds. Students sometimes become disillusioned when they observe nurses behaving in ways that conflict with their ideas and ideals about how nurses should behave. Knowing in advance that these things may happen can help students accurately assess the sources of their anxiety and manage it more effectively.

Factors Influencing Socialization

As students progress through nursing programs, a variety of factors challenge their customary ways of thinking. These include personal feelings and beliefs, some of which may conflict with professional values. For example, if students have strong religious beliefs, they may be uncomfortable working with patients who have no such belief or whose beliefs are different from their own. Yet the very first statement in the *Code of Ethics for Nurses* (ANA, 2001) requires that nurses work with all patients regardless of their beliefs. However, if you have a strong moral objection to a particular belief system of a patient or a negative reaction to a patient based on some characteristic of the patient, you should seek out your clinical faculty or other professional mentor to discuss your reaction and determine how to handle your conflicted feelings in an appropriate and professional way. This is not an uncommon response in nursing students as their sphere of contact with others different from themselves grows.

When children are growing up, they are first influenced by the values, beliefs, and behaviors of the significant adults around them. Later, peers become a significant influence. These influences also shape ideas about health, health care, and nursing. A common issue in nursing practice revolves around negative health behaviors of patients. If a nurse's family valued fitness, for example, it may be difficult for that nurse to empathize with an obese patient with heart disease who refuses to exercise even though there are clear health benefits. In this example, a family value (fitness) comes into conflict with a professional value (nonjudgmental acceptance of patients). Other patient issues that sometimes challenge students' values are substance abuse; self-destructive behaviors; abortion; issues related to sexuality, such as sexual identity, infertility, and end-of-life issues.

All people have biases; however, unexamined biases are more likely to influence behavior than examined ones. Nurses need to be aware of their biases and discuss them with peers, instructors, and professional role models. Failure to do so may adversely affect the nursing care provided to certain patients. Professional nurses make every effort to avoid imposing their personal beliefs on others (see Chapter 9 for further discussion of self-awareness and nonjudgmental acceptance as necessary attributes of professional nurses). Becoming a professional nurse requires learning how to deal with values conflicts such as these while respecting patients' differing viewpoints. This cannot be taught but is the responsibility of each aspiring professional. The key point here is that you should begin to identify those "hot button" issues that seem to affect you negatively, so that you can understand your own responses and how to set them aside while still providing excellent care of your patients.

As seen from this brief overview, socialization is much more than the transmission of knowledge and skills. Socialization serves to develop a common nursing consciousness and is the key to keeping the profession vital and dynamic while preserving its fundamental focus on human responses in health and illness.

A New Factor Influencing Socialization: Distance Learning

Distance learning in nursing is a fast-growing phenomenon. More nursing schools are using technology to deliver education to nurses who do not have access to traditional on-campus programs. Initially, single courses or continuing education short courses were offered by distance education. Today, entire nursing curricula are offered by distance learning, and the amount of on-campus time may be very limited. Many programs today routinely use highly technologic resources such as video teleconferencing and online courses. This trend is expected to increase as demand and technologic developments continue. Even within traditional nursing curricula, some content is taught online with infrequent classroom sessions.

Questions about whether students could achieve educational outcomes through distance learning have been answered: they can and do pass their courses, some with distinction, using these methodologies (Anderson, 2004; Hurst, 2005). Questions then arose about whether professional attitudes and values—in other words, professional socialization—could be effectively achieved through distance education. Although more study is needed, initial indicators were positive (Cragg, Plotnikoff, Hugo et al, 2001; Nesler, Hanner, Melburg et al, 2001).

MODELS OF PROFESSIONAL SOCIALIZATION

The transition from student to professional is a topic of importance to nurse researchers interested in creating effective means of professional socialization. During the 1970s and 1980s, a number of models of professional socialization of basic and RN students were developed. Cohen (1981) and Hinshaw (1976) described developmental models appropriate for beginning nursing students. Bandura (1977) described a type of socialization he called modeling, which is useful when learning any new behavior. Benner (1984) identified five stages nurses pass through in the transition from "novice to expert." Two of these models, Cohen's and Benner's, are presented in more detail below. Although these models were developed in the early 1980s, they serve to describe processes of transition and socialization that many faculty have come to recognize as almost universal among nursing students.

Cohen's Model of Basic Student Socialization

Cohen (1981) proposed a model of professional socialization consisting of four stages. Basing her work on developmental theories and studies of beginning students' attitudes toward nursing, she asserted, "Students must experience each stage in sequence to feel comfortable in the professional role" (p. 16). She believed that a positive outcome in all four stages is necessary for satisfactory socialization to occur. Readers may wish to compare themselves and nursing classmates against these four stages. A reminder, however: although it is interesting and potentially useful, this model has not been subjected to rigorous testing or scientific validation. However, this model does appear to fit the behaviors that experienced faculty note in the development of students' socialization into professional practice.

Cohen identified the first stage in her model, stage I, as unilateral dependence. Because they are inexperienced and lack knowledge, students at this stage rely on external limits and controls established by authority figures such as teachers. During stage I, students are unlikely to question or analyze critically the concepts teachers present because they lack the necessary background to do so. An example of a student operating in a unilateral dependent stage would be the student who agrees to a clinical assignment without questioning the clinical faculty's thinking about the appropriateness of the assignment or what the student may gain from the assignment. The student "soaks in" the faculty's direction and discussion about the patient without yet making linkages of his or her own in thinking about the patient's condition. Fundamentally, students at this stage do as they are told because they lack the experience and knowledge to question.

In stage II (negativity/independence) students' critical thinking abilities and knowledge bases expand. They begin to question authority figures. Cohen called this occurrence cognitive rebellion. Much as young children learn that they can say no, students at this level begin to free themselves from external controls and to rely more on their own judgment. They think critically about what they are being taught. This is a stage when students begin to question, "Why do I have to learn about this? This isn't nursing!" or complain, "I will never learn to give an injection to a patient if I have to sit here reading about the nursing process!" This can be a stage where a student's fledgling independence may cause some lack of judgment in the clinical setting, much as a toddler may overestimate his or her own powers of mobility or dexterity. In addition, students at this stage may begin to demand "more difficult" patient situations to manage and resist faculty's (more informed) judgment that the student is not yet ready for complex patients.

Stage III (dependence/mutuality) is characterized by what Cohen described as students' more reasoned evaluation of others' ideas. They develop an increasingly realistic appraisal process and learn to test concepts, facts, ideas, and models objectively. Students at this stage are more impartial; they accept some ideas and reject others. This is a time when students begin to appreciate the usefulness of the nursing process in organizing care and begin to use more sophisticated critical thinking skills.

In stage IV (interdependence) students' needs for both independence and mutuality (sharing jointly with others) come together. Students develop the capacity to make decisions in collaboration with others. The successfully socialized student completes stage IV with a self-concept that includes a professional role identity that is personally and professionally acceptable and compatible with other life roles. Faculty appreciates the maturity and trustworthiness that students exhibit when they reach this stage in their professional development. These students are often highly self-directed, seeking out learning experiences to maximize their knowledge before the completion of their formal education. Table 6-1 summarizes the key behaviors associated with each of Cohen's stages.

Benner's Stages of Nursing Proficiency (Basic Student Socialization)

Patricia Benner, a nurse, was curious about how nurses made the transition from inexpert beginners to highly expert practitioners. She described a process consisting of five stages of nursing practice, on which she based her 1984 book, *From Novice to Expert*. The stages Benner described are "novice," "advanced beginner," "competent practitioner," "proficient practitioner," and "expert practitioner." Advancing from stage to stage occurs gradually as nurses gain more experience in patient care. Clinical judgment is stimulated when the nurse's "preconceived notions and

Table 6-1 Cohen's Model of Basic Student Socialization

Stage	Key Behaviors
I: Unilateral dependence	Reliant on external authority; limited questioning or critical analysis
II: Negativity/ independence	Cognitive rebellion; diminished reliance on external authority
III: Dependence/ mutuality	Reasoned appraisal; begins integration of facts and opinions following objective testing
IV: Interdependence	Collaborative decision making; commitment to professional role; self-concept now includes professional role identity

Data from Cohen HA: *The nurse's quest for professional identity,* Menlo Park, Calif, 1981, Addison-Wesley.

expectations" (p. 3) collide with, or are confirmed by, the realities of everyday practice.

In 2000, many years after she generated this model, Benner's work was one of several theories presented to a group attempting to demonstrate how learning theories apply to adult skill acquisition. They tested and confirmed that Benner's model was valid, and they suggested that her stages apply to any adult learning situation (Hom, 2003).

Benner's novice stage, or stage I, begins with students entering nursing school. Because they generally have little background on which to base their clinical behavior, they must depend rather rigidly on rules and expectations established for them. Their practical skills are limited. For example, a novice nurse is faced with the request of a mother to let her 2-year-old child take "just a peek" at his newborn sister, even though it is against hospital protocol to allow children to visit when the newborn is in the room with the mother. The novice is very uncomfortable with the request because it is against the rules. The novice denies the request, citing the hospital rules.

By the time learners enter the advanced beginner period, or stage II, they have discerned that a particular order exists in clinical settings (Benner,

Tanner, and Chesla, 1996). Their performance is marginally competent. They can base their actions on both theory and principles but tend to experience difficulty formulating priorities, viewing many nursing actions as equally important. When faced with the same situation as the novice nurse and the mother of a 2-year-old, the advanced beginner is still likely to deny the mother's request, but the nurse also has an understanding of the needs of the mother to see her 2-year-old in addition to spending time with the new infant. The advanced beginner suggests that the mother send the infant to the nursery and then have an uninterrupted visit with her older child.

Competent practitioners, or stage III learners, usually have 2 to 3 years' experience in a setting. As a result, they feel competent, organized, and efficient most of the time. These feelings of mastery are a result of planning and goal-setting skills and the ability to think abstractly and analytically. These learners can coordinate several complex demands simultaneously. For example, the competent nurse spends a few moments at the start of his or her shift, examining the needs of each patient and planning fundamental care. At this stage, the competent nurse understands that situations change quickly and that planning is the best way to ensure that care gets implemented even when emergencies or unexpected events arise. This nurse may or may not allow the 2-year-old child to visit with his new sister; however, the nurse will examine the needs of everyone carefully and many of the exigencies involved before making a final decision about allowing the toddler "a peek" at his baby sister.

Proficient practitioners (stage IV) have typically been in practice 3 to 5 years. These nurses are able to see patient situations holistically rather than in parts, to recognize and interpret subtleties of meaning, and to easily recognize priorities for care. They can focus on long-term goals and desired outcomes. These experienced nurses are likely to be leaders on their units, having a wealth of experience and commitment to nursing. Concerned with patient outcomes rather than institutional rules, the proficient nurse would likely understand in a holistic way the needs of the mother and her 2-year-old son and their desire to incorporate the new infant into their family. This nurse is likely to allow the "rules" to be broken in deference to the needs of the family.

Expert practitioner, or stage V, status is reached only after extensive practice experience. These nurses perform intuitively, without conscious thought, automatically grasping the significance of the patient's complete experience. They move fluidly through nursing interventions, acting on the basis of their feeling of "rightness" of nursing action. They may find it difficult to express verbally why they selected certain actions, so integrated are their responses. Both to themselves and to observers, their expertise seems to "come naturally." Expert nurses on occasion have difficulty deconstructing their work, that is, being able to describe what they experience clinically, because it comes so naturally to them. The expert nurse might even initiate a suggestion to the newborn's mother that the 2-year-old "take a peek" at his baby sister because this nurse recognizes the complexities of incorporating a new member into the family.

Table 6-2 summarizes Benner's stages from novice to expert. Box 6-1 contains a nurse's experience as a student that demonstrated the clear difference between novice and expert nursing.

Actively Participating in One's Own Professional Socialization

Many schools of nursing have programs for RNs with associate degrees or diplomas to return for completion of their BSN degree. These students have special socialization needs as they return to the classroom, sometimes after many years of practice. Davidhizar, Gigen, and Reed (1993) recommended some strategies for RNs to decrease the stress they experience on returning to school. Although written for returning students, these strategies could apply to all students:

- Actively involve yourself in the learning process.
- Keep your eye on the prize. You are temporarily uncomfortable but will ultimately get something you want (such as certification, promotion, sense of self-confidence, personal growth, or graduate school).

Table 6-2 Benner's Stages of Nursing Proficiency (Basic Student Socialization)

Stage	Nurse Behaviors
I: Novice	Has little background and limited practical skills; relies on rules and expectations of others for direction
II: Advanced beginner	Has marginally competent skills; uses theory and principles much of the time; experiences difficulty establishing priorities
III: Competent practitioner	Feels competent, organized; plans and sets goals; thinks abstractly and analytically; coordinates several tasks simultaneously
IV: Proficient practitioner	Views patients holistically; recognizes subtle changes; sets priorities with ease; focuses on long-term goals
V: Expert practitioner	Performs fluidly; grasps patient needs automatically; responses are integrated; expertise comes naturally

Data from Benner P: *From novice to expert: excellence and power in clinical nursing practice*, Menlo Park, Calif, 1984, Addison-Wesley.

- Keep your perspective. You are in school by choice. No one is doing this to you.
- Set aside preconceived ideas, prejudices, and habits. Give yourself and the school experience a chance.
- Open up your creative side, your abstract thinking, and your willingness to engage in hypothetical thinking. Everything need not be immediately applicable in the work setting to be of value.
- Be receptive to feedback, even if it is critical. If you were perfect, you would not need to be here.
- Develop your time management skills.
- Get a mentor for emotional support—another nurse, older friend, relative, or faculty member.
- Use faculty members as resources. They want to be helpful but need to ask for their guidance.

For other ideas about how to become an active participant in your own socialization process, use the checklist in Box 6-2.

SOCIALIZATION TO THE WORK SETTING

When nurses graduate, professional socialization is not over. In fact, the intensity of their socialization is likely to increase as their exposure to nursing and the culture of nursing increases. Most experts believe that socialization, similar to learning, is a lifelong activity. The transition from student to professional nurse is another of life's challenges and, similar to most challenges, is one that helps people grow.

It can seem that just as students become well socialized to the culture of the educational setting, they graduate and must become socialized to a work setting. Most new nursing graduates feel somewhat unprepared and overwhelmed with the responsibilities of their first positions. Although agencies that employ new graduates realize that the orientation period will take time, graduates may have unrealistic expectations of themselves and others.

During the early days of practice, most graduate nurses quickly realize that the ideals taught in school are not always possible to achieve in everyday practice. This is largely a result of time constraints and produces feelings of conflict and even guilt. In school, students are taught to spend time with patients and to consider their emotional, as well as physical, needs. In practice, the emphasis may seem to be on finishing tasks or completing checklists and flow sheets. Talking with patients, engaging in patient teaching, or counseling family members may be viewed as an unproductive use of time. In the early days of professional practice, having time to do comprehensive, individualized nursing care planning, a staple of life for nursing students, may seem like an unrealistic luxury. Establishing positive relationships with your new colleagues can have a long-lasting effect on your effectiveness in your work setting (Kopp, 2008). An interesting suggestion offered by Kopp (2008) is to "listen to gossip." This can help you determine who is "plugged

Box 6-1   From Novice to Expert: "How Did You Know That?"

The difference between a novice and an expert nurse was demonstrated to me in a very stark way when I was in my first semester of nursing school. I was assigned to a surgical unit with other junior students. Our clinical instructor, Janie, had 8 years of surgical intensive care unit experience as an RN and had been a faculty member for several years. The fact that she was 7 months pregnant never deterred her or slowed her down in any way. Janie just always seemed to know when we needed her, even when we didn't know we needed her.

I had finished my patient's morning care, a kind elderly man who was going to be transferred to a long-term care facility later that morning. Because I was not busy, I asked one of the other students on the unit if she needed any help. Her patient was fairly complex, having been transferred from the surgical ICU the night before. He had a deep sacral decubitus ulcer that needed to be assessed, in addition to gangrene in his lower extremities. She asked me to help turn him so she could assess his sacral area. Using our best communication skills, we told the patient exactly what we were going to do, that we were going to turn him on his side and assured him that we were not going to hurt him.

Being the two novices that we were, we were fascinated by the size and depth of the ulcer and spent what seemed like several minutes staring at it. The patient never complained about the position we were holding him in. We continued to try to figure out what to do with regard to his pressure sore. I finally took a look at his face and began to reassure him that we were almost done. Then I realized that he was not responding. My novice assessment: "He looks funny" ("funny" in an odd way, not in a humorous way).

Thank goodness Janie, the expert nurse and clinical faculty, was walking past the patient's door. She heard my novice assessment and immediately understood the severity of "looking funny" to a new student. In my memory she became airborne as she dashed into the room; in reality she simply walked in, made an immediate and correct assessment of the patient and called a code. He was in a full cardiac arrest. My novice classmate and I stood cowering in the corner as the room was quickly filled with persons responding to the emergency. I wondered how Janie knew what to do with so little effort and so much intuition. I envied her calmness and leadership in the resuscitation effort, the placement of a pacemaker in the patient, and coordination of his transfer back to the ICU.

My novice assessment: "He looks funny." Her expert assessment: "New students, can't describe patient. Complex patient. Risk for variety of complications due to prolonged bed rest and post-op infection, unresponsive, cyanotic, eyes open, not breathing, no heart rate. Call code, lower head of bed, start CPR, make sure IV is patent, make sure oxygen is available, etc., etc. . . ."

To her credit, Janie took my classmate and me to lunch that day, encouraging us to discuss what had happened and reassuring us that nothing we did caused him to have an arrest. She allowed us to work through our own considerable distress. And I knew that I wanted to be "just like her" when I became an RN. Thirty years later, I am still grateful for her example of expert nursing and compassionate mentoring.

• *Beth Black, PhD, RN*
University of North Carolina at Chapel Hill School of Nursing

in" to the culture of the unit and give you insight into the idiosyncratic behaviors or responses of coworkers. Participating in malicious gossip is unprofessional and hurtful to others, but being aware of comments that give you insight into your new colleagues can help you understand the culture of the unit more quickly.

Speed of functioning is another area in which new nurses vary widely. By the end of a

well-planned orientation, new graduates should be able to manage an average patient load without too much difficulty. Time management is a skill that is closely related to speed of functioning. Managing your time well means managing yourself well and requires self-discipline. The ability to organize and prioritize nursing care for a group of patients is the key to good time management. (It is also an asset to students!) Box 6-3 and

Box 6-2   A Do-It-Yourself Guide to Professional Socialization

Listed below are 20 possible behaviors demonstrated by students who take responsibility for their own professional socialization. Place a check next to the behaviors you regularly exhibit. Be honest with yourself.

1. I interact with other students in and out of class.
2. I participate in class by asking intelligent questions and initiating discussion occasionally.
3. I have formed or joined a study group.
4. I use the library, labs, and teachers as resources.
5. I organize my work so that I can meet deadlines.
6. If I have a conflict with another student or a teacher, I take the initiative to resolve it.
7. I do not let minor personality problems distract me from my goals.
8. I seek out new learning experiences and sometimes volunteer to demonstrate new skills to others.
9. I have chosen professional role models.
10. I am realistic about my performance.
11. I try to accept constructive criticism without becoming defensive.
12. I recognize that trying to do good work is not the same as doing good work.
13. I recognize that each teacher has different expectations, and it is my responsibility to learn what is expected by each.
14. I demonstrate respect for my teachers' time by making appointments whenever possible.
15. I demonstrate respect for my classmates, patients, and teachers by never coming to class or clinical unprepared.
16. I recognize my responsibility to help create an interactive learning environment and am not satisfied to be merely an academic spectator.
17. I participate in the student nurse association and encourage others to do the same.
18. I represent my school with pride.
19. I project a professional appearance.
20. One of my goals is to become a self-directed, lifelong learner.

Scoring: 1-10 checks—You need to examine your behavior and think about taking more responsibility for your own socialization; 11-15 checks—you are active in your own behalf; try to begin using some of the remaining behaviors on the list or come up with your own; more than 15 checks—you are a role model of positive action in your own professional socialization process.

Box 6-3   Time Management Self-Assessment

Effective time management is a skill that can be developed. Listed are principles reflecting good time management. For each of statements A through J, circle the answer that most closely characterizes how you manage your time.

Scoring: Give yourself 2 points for each "Frequently," 1 point for each "Sometimes," and 0 points for each "Rarely." If your score is 0-10, you need to improve your time management skills; 11-15, you are doing fine but can still improve; 16-18, you have very good time management skills; and 19-20, your time management skills are superior!

A. I spend some time each day planning how to accomplish school and other responsibilities.
   0. Rarely
   1. Sometimes
   2. Frequently
B. I set specific goals and dates for accomplishing tasks.
   0. Rarely
   1. Sometimes
   2. Frequently

(Continued)

Box 6-3   Time Management Self-Assessment—cont'd

C. Each day I make a "to do" list and prioritize it. I complete the most important tasks first.
   0. Rarely
   1. Sometimes
   2. Frequently
D. I plan time in my schedule for unexpected problems and unanticipated delays.
   0. Rarely
   1. Sometimes
   2. Frequently
E. I ask others for help when possible.
   0. Rarely
   1. Sometimes
   2. Frequently
F. I take advantage of short but regular breaks to refresh myself and stay alert.
   0. Rarely
   1. Sometimes
   2. Frequently
G. When I really need to concentrate, I work in a specific area that is free from distractions and interruptions.
   0. Rarely
   1. Sometimes
   2. Frequently

H. When working, I turn down other people's requests that interfere with completing my priority tasks.
   0. Rarely
   1. Sometimes
   2. Frequently
I. I avoid unproductive and prolonged socializing with fellow students or employees during my workday.
   0. Rarely
   1. Sometimes
   2. Frequently
J. I keep a calendar of important meetings, dates, and deadlines and carry it with me.
   0. Rarely
   1. Sometimes
   2. Frequently

Figure 6-2 provide guidance on how to keep poor time management from becoming a problem while you are a student. Once you have established good time management skills, they will carry over to the work setting.

New nurses also must adapt to collaborating with other nursing care personnel, such as nursing assistants, patient care technicians, and other unlicensed assistive personnel who help them in caring for patients. This is a difficult adjustment for some nurses who are unaccustomed to delegating, are unsure of the abilities of others, or believe only they can provide quality care.

An overlooked aspect of stress in new graduates is the sheer physical fatigue caused by 8- to 12-hour shifts accompanied by the standing, walking, lifting, bending, and stooping that patient care requires. Many new graduates have never spent an entire shift on a unit during schooling. When physical fatigue combines with the mental and emotional stress of decision making, efforts to become integrated into a peer group, uncertainty about policies or procedures, and lack of role clarity, sensory overload is almost certain to occur.

With all of this talk of fatigue, gossip, demands of the job, and mental and emotional stress of decision making, it is no wonder that sometimes nursing units become difficult places to maintain one's good humor, much less create a culture of civility. Lower (2007) described the issues facing nurses in terms of incivility that they face from a variety of sources. Civil conduct is defined as "conduct that consistently shows respect for others, makes them feel valued, and contributes to effective communication" (p. 49). Although

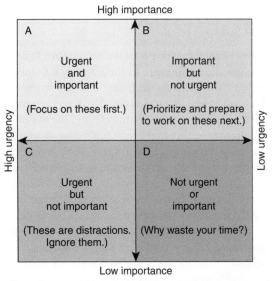

High importance

A | B
Urgent and important | Important but not urgent
(Focus on these first.) | (Prioritize and prepare to work on these next.)

C | D
Urgent but not important | Not urgent or important
(These are distractions. Ignore them.) | (Why waste your time?)

High urgency ← → Low urgency

Low importance

Figure 6-2 Setting priorities is an important aspect of time management. Use this grid to determine whether a task should go to the top, middle, or bottom of your daily "to do" list or whether it is a time-waster and should be ignored.

many hospital settings may face incivility to some degree, Lower described ways of turning the culture into one of civility. This starts with the recognition of the civility issue; developing a framework at the institutional level that sets behavioral standards and operationalizes them; and being patient but persistent in watching the culture turn from one that is "toxic" to one that promotes the civil behavior.

This chapter's Cultural Considerations Challenge contains the description of one nurse's early adjustment to nursing practice. Still in practice after 25 years, this man entered and remained in nursing at a time when few men considered nursing as a profession.

"Reality Shock": When Ideals and Reality Collide

A reality of nursing today is the shortage of nurses to provide care in a complex health care system with an aging population and more persons living with chronic illness. Working conditions are sometimes very difficult, especially when acuity (severity of illness) of the patients is high and staffing is low. Despite the rewards of a career spent in nursing, nursing can be difficult at times. A current challenge in nursing is retention: keeping nurses in nursing. Replacing nurses who leave is extremely expensive for hospitals (Atencio, Cohen, and Gorenberg, 2003). Many of the difficulties faced by nurses now are not very different from other times of shortage when the needs of the health care system were greater than the profession could provide. This section is intended to leave you in a more powerful position to understand some of the negative feelings you may experience as you make the transition into professional nursing. Because as the saying goes, "forewarned is forearmed," we are including some discussion of not only how to recognize these feelings but also how to manage them so that you will remain an involved, well-prepared, and productive professional nurse.

"Reality shock" (Kramer, 1974) was a term used to describe the feelings of powerlessness and ineffectiveness experienced by new graduates, a term that is still relevant more than 30 years later. Psychological stresses generated by reality shock decrease the ability of individuals to cope effectively with the demands of the new role. Causes of reality shock include the following:

- Absence of positive reinforcement (such as coaching) and frequent communication
- Lack of support, such as faculty availability
- The gap between the ideals taught in school and the actual work setting
- The inability to implement desired nursing care because of circumstances such as a heavy case load or time constraints

Unfortunately, some new nurses "drop out" at this point, rather than taking steps to resolve reality shock. Kramer identified several ways nurses may drop out:

- Disengaging mentally and emotionally
- Driving oneself and others to the breaking point by trying to do it all
- "Job hopping"—looking for the perfect, non-stressful job that is completely compatible with professional values

Cultural Considerations Challenge
A Look Back at a Man's Career in Nursing in a Small Rural Setting

I "fell into" the nursing profession by chance, not planning to become a nurse at first. At the time I made my decision to become a nurse, I was working in construction and took a part-time job as a nursing assistant at the small 40-bed community hospital in my home town. The male assistants were called "orderlies" back then. I think we were called "orderlies" because we were expected to keep order when patients became "unruly," which they sometimes did. The biggest change for me when I became a licensed professional was assuming responsibility for my actions. In working as an orderly/assistant, I had someone else take responsibility. That was fun. I could leave my worries at work. When I became an RN, I realized that "the buck stops here," so to speak. As an RN, it became *my* responsibility to make a decision. I looked forward to my work every evening, because every day it was always something new and interesting. Twenty-five years later, it still is.

I selected my BSN program because I felt that it was the best program in the state. I still think that. The nursing program was tough but I don't recall feeling out of place, even though I was one of very few males in my class, maybe 3 or 4 of more than 100 students. I had good friends in school and we supported each other through clinicals, exams, and complaints about all those things nursing students complain about. After graduation, I had to decide whether to go back to the small community hospital where I had worked as an orderly or stay at the large university teaching hospital where I had trained. I find myself occasionally wondering how my life would have been different had I stayed at the teaching hospital. But now, I don't think I'd trade my experiences in a small community hospital with fewer than 100 beds.

In this beautiful setting near the mountains, I grew to know a lot of people in the small community. I knew their histories, their families, and many of their individual idiosyncrasies. I still see some of these patients in the community from time to time, and they remember that I was their nurse. Working in a small community hospital gave me experiences like these that I wouldn't have had in a large referral hospital. I look back on my early days in nursing rather fondly at times. From a "male" perspective, it did seem that I was called on quite a bit to do a lot of the heavy labor of the unit! I recall only one other male RN in the little community hospital. He worked in the ER and I didn't have a lot of contact with him, other than taking report on a patient from time to time.

I left the small hospital 11 years ago to work in a larger hospital, forcing me to grow professionally because the patients are more acutely ill in the cardiac care unit where I now work. Another substantial difference is that there are a lot of men who are RNs. Occasionally, I'll even work a shift where all of the nurses are men. I have always felt like I fit in as a nurse because my values are the same as other nurses that I know, males and females.

Twenty-five years after graduation, I am still glad I made the decision to become a nurse. I have many interests outside of nursing which keep me busy. But the challenges of nursing never grow old. As a nurse, no two days are alike. I think that's what holds me in this position in spite of the stress of working in a cardiac care unit. That's what I liked about it in the beginning, and that's what I still like about it today.

• *Kim Elder, BSN, RN*
University of North Carolina at Chapel Hill
School of Nursing, 1981

- Prematurely returning to school
- Burning out—a condition of unresolved reality shock with subsequent emotional exhaustion
- Leaving the nursing profession entirely, which neither nursing nor society can afford

Much can be done to reduce reality shock in the transition from student to professional. Students must recognize that schools cannot provide enough clinical experience to make graduates comfortable on their first day as new nurses. They can take responsibility for obtaining as much practical experience as possible outside of school. Working in a health care setting during summers, on school breaks, and on weekends may be helpful. They should avoid work during the school week, if at all possible, or keep it to an absolute minimum because academic responsibilities take priority during that time, and exhausted students make poor learners.

Some schools offer programs in which students are paired with practicing nurses (preceptors) and work closely with them to experience life as an RN. If your school offers such a program, take advantage of it. If not, seek out information about similar programs at area hospitals. Many agencies, including hospitals and the military, are now providing excellent opportunities for students nearing graduation to function in expanded roles.

Talking with other new graduates about your feelings is one of the best ways to combat reality shock. Take the initiative to form a group for mutual support—others need it too! Another interpersonal strategy is to seek a professional mentor. A mentor is an experienced nurse who is committed to nursing and to sharing knowledge with less experienced nurses to help advance their careers. A mentor can be a great source of all types of knowledge, as well as another source of support. Having a mentor is different from having a preceptor. Mentoring involves the formation of a long-term relationship through which ideas, experiences, and successful behavior patterns are shared.

Ask a nurse whose work you admire to be your mentor and identify what he or she can offer. Some inexperienced nurses are fearful of approaching potential mentors with this request. They should remember that this process is not a one-way street; it has benefits to both parties because it complements and validates the mentor's knowledge and self-esteem, as well as provides important information and support to the nurse being mentored. To get the most from a mentoring relationship, first understand your professional and personal needs and select a mentor who seems to share your values and beliefs. Set up specific times to meet and be willing to communicate openly with your mentor. A mentoring relationship is a powerful tool by which a new nurse can benefit from the experience, wisdom, and feedback from someone who has "been there"—who understands your experience because he or she has experienced the same thing.

The Internet provides opportunities for nursing students to learn more about the profession of nursing and to assist with socialization into practice. One excellent website for student nurses is http://www.nursingnet.org. This website was created and is maintained by practicing nurses who seek to improve professionalization in nursing.

Care of self is an important activity as you begin your career in the care of others. Have you ever noticed that when you are traveling on a plane the flight attendants instruct you, in the case of an emergency, to put on your own oxygen mask first? Then you are prepared to help those around you. The same principle applies here. You will provide better care to others if you care for yourself first, such as eating nutritiously, exercising regularly, avoiding tobacco and excessive alcohol use, seeking spiritual support if that is important to you, and having friends outside of work—all of those things that you know are "good for you." The stronger and healthier you are physically, psychologically, and spiritually, the better prepared you are to face the demands of your transition into the important work of nursing.

In the final analysis, you—and only you—are responsible for your own lifelong professional socialization. Those nurses who maintain a good balance between their work and personal lives and who have reasonable expectations of the work of nursing without sacrificing their own values and ideals have great potential to be effective nurses over a long career.

Summary of Key Points

- Although attempts to define nursing have been under way since the days of Nightingale, efforts have generally fallen short of capturing the diversity and richness that constitutes nursing.

- Definitions reviewed in this chapter have more commonalities than differences.
- Definitions change over time as society and nursing change and as each individual's perceptions about, and experiences in, nursing change.
- The dynamic nature of the nursing profession, society, and health care will likely prevent us from ever developing one eternal, universally accepted definition of nursing.
- Professional socialization is a critical process that turns novices into fully functioning professionals.
- Two major components of socialization to professional nursing are socialization through education and socialization in the workplace.
- Conceptual models of professional socialization that identify stages in the process and key behaviors occurring at each stage are applicable to nursing.
- Individuals have responsibility for actively participating in their own professional socialization. They should identify needed learning experiences and seek opportunities that provide these experiences.
- Reality shock is a stressful period that new nurses may experience when entering nursing practice. Understanding the stages of reality shock and how to resolve them can assist new graduates through this transition.
- Mentors can be valuable resources in enhancing and enriching the professional socialization experience.

Critical Thinking Questions

1. Obtain your school's definition of nursing. How is it similar to or different from definitions in this chapter?
2. From the definitions of nursing presented in this chapter, select the one you most prefer and explain your choice.
3. How might new technologies, economic factors, social trends, and new practice options for nurses affect future definitions of nursing? How might these factors affect the scope of nursing?

4. If you are already a practicing nurse, how has your personal definition of nursing changed over time? How have you seen the scope of nursing change since you entered practice?
5. Obtain a copy of the nurse practice act for your state. Find the legal definition of nursing and compare it with other definitions found in this chapter. How are they alike and how are they different? How does your state define the scope of nursing practice?
6. Describe how both formal and informal socialization experiences in school are modifying your image of nursing.
7. Examine one of the two models of socialization discussed in this chapter and place yourself in one of the stages. Give your rationale for that placement. If none of the models or stages fits your experience, create your own model (or stage) and share it with the class.
8. List five things you can do to take active responsibility for your own professional socialization.
9. Interview a new nurse and discuss his or her experience with reality shock. How is this individual handling the transition from student to practicing nurse? What can you learn from his or her experience?
10. Identify several personal and professional areas in which a mentor might be helpful to you. Select a potential mentor and talk with him or her about your needs.

⊖volve *To enhance your understanding of this chapter, try the Student Exercises on the Evolve site at http://evolve.elsevier.com/Chitty/professional.*

REFERENCES

American Nurses Association: *Code of ethics for nurses,* Washington, DC, 2001, American Nurses Publishing.

American Nurses Association: *Nursing's social policy statement,* ed 2, Washington, DC, 2003 (website): http://www.nursebooks.org.

Anderson ET: Impact of community health content on nurse practitioner practice: a comparison of classroom and web-based teaching, *Nurs Educ Perspect* 25(4):171-175, 2004.

Atencio BL, Cohen J, Gorenberg B: Nurse retention: is it worth it?, *Nurs Econ* 21(6):262-268, 2003:299.

Bandura A: *Social learning theory*, Englewood Cliffs, NJ, 1977, Prentice-Hall.

Benner P: *From novice to expert: excellence and power in clinical nursing practice*, Menlo Park, Calif, 1984, Addison-Wesley.

Benner P, Tanner CA, Chesla CA: *Expertise in nursing practice: caring, clinical judgment, and ethics*, New York, 1996, Springer.

Cohen HA: *The nurse's quest for professional identity*, Menlo Park, Calif, 1981, Addison-Wesley.

Cragg CE, Plotnikoff RC, Hugo K, et al: Perspective transformation in RN-to-BSN distance education, *J Nurs Ed* 40(7):317-322, 2001.

Davidhizar R, Gigen JN, Reed C: RN to BSN: avoiding the pitfalls, *Health Care Supervisor* 12(1):48-56, 1993.

Gordon S: *Nursing against the odds: how health care cost cuts, media stereotypes and medical hubris undermine nurses and patient care*, Ithaca, NY, 2005, Cornell University Press.

Harmer B: *Textbook of the principles and practice of nursing*, New York, 1922, Macmillan.

Harmer B, Henderson V: *Textbook of the principles and practice of nursing*, ed 4, New York, 1939, Macmillan.

Henderson V: *Basic principles of nursing care*, London, 1960, International Council of Nurses.

Hinshaw AS: *Socialization and resocialization of nurses for professional nursing practice*, New York, 1976, National League for Nursing.

Hom EM: Coaching and mentoring new graduates entering perinatal nursing practice, *J Perinat Neonatal Nurs* 17(1):35-49, 2003.

Hurst J: EDTNA/ERCA, *J Renal Care* 31(3):160-163, 2005.

Kopp G: How to fit in fast at your new job, *American Nurse Today* 3(1):40-41, 2008.

Kramer M: *Reality shock: why nurses leave nursing*, St Louis, 1974, Mosby.

International Council of Nurses: *The ICN definition of nursing*, 2003 (website): http://www.icn.ch/definition.htm.

Lower J: Creating a culture of civility in the workplace, *American Nurse Today* 2(9):49-52, 2007.

Nesler MS, Hanner MB, Melburg V, et al: Professional socialization of baccalaureate nursing students: can students in distance nursing programs become socialized?, *J Nurs Educ* 40(7):293-302, 2001.

Nightingale F: *Notes on nursing: what it is and what it is not*, Philadelphia, 1946, JB Lippincott, reprint (originally published in 1859).

Orem D: *Guidelines for developing curricula for the education of practical nurses*, Washington, DC, 1959, Government Printing Office.

Peplau H: *Interpersonal relations in nursing: a conceptual frame of reference for psychodynamic nursing*, New York, 1952, GP Putnam's Sons.

Rogers M: *Educational revolution in nursing*, New York, 1961, Macmillan.

Royal College of Nursing: *Defining nursing*, 2003 (website): http://www.rcn.org.uk/downloads/defining nursing/definingnursing-a5.pdf.

Shaw CW: *Textbook of nursing*, ed 3, New York, 1907, Appleton.

State of Ohio Board of Nursing: *Law and rule information*, 2009 (website): http://codes.ohio.gov/orc/4723.

Styles MM: Bridging the gap between competence and excellence, *ANNA J* 18(4):353-366, 1991.

The Education of Nurses*

Kay Kittrell Chitty

7
CHAPTER

LEARNING OUTCOMES

After studying this chapter, students will be able to:
- Trace the development of basic and graduate education in nursing
- Discuss the influence of early nursing studies on nursing education
- Describe traditional and alternative ways of becoming a registered nurse
- Discuss program options for registered nurses and students with nonnursing baccalaureate degrees
- Differentiate between licensed practical/vocational nurses and registered nurses
- Differentiate between associate degree and baccalaureate degree education
- Explain the difference between licensure and certification
- Define accreditation and analyze its influence on the quality and effectiveness of nursing education programs
- Discuss recommendations of the Institute of Medicine and major nursing organizations regarding transforming nursing education
- Identify current and future challenges in nursing education

Diversity is the major characteristic of nursing education today. Influenced by a variety of factors—societal changes, periodic shortages, historical factors, public expectations, professional standards, legislation, national studies, and constant changes in the health care system—many different types of nursing education programs currently exist.

In 2006, the latest date for which figures are available, there were 1547 state-approved programs preparing registered nurses (RNs) in the United States (Figure 7-1). Of these, 58.8% were associate degree programs, 37.2% were baccalaureate programs, and 4% were diploma programs (National League for Nursing, 2006a).

More current figures are available for graduate programs in nursing. In 2008, there were 458

master's programs and 166 doctoral programs (Fang, Htut, and Bednash, 2008). Also included in the educational system of nursing are a large number of practical nursing programs (licensed practical nurse [LPN]/licensed vocational nurse [LVN] programs), continuing education programs, and advanced practice certification programs.

This chapter provides an orientation to the multiple and sometimes confusing nursing educational pathways in existence today. This coverage includes the history behind educational programs, descriptions of the various programs, and trends and future issues.

DEVELOPMENT OF NURSING EDUCATION IN THE UNITED STATES

Florence Nightingale is credited with founding modern nursing and creating the first educational system for nurses. After hospitals came into existence in Western Europe, and before the influence of Florence Nightingale, nurses had no formal preparation in giving care, because there

---

*Educational terms and definitions used in this chapter are congruent with those used by the American Association of Colleges of Nursing, as defined in *2007-2008 Enrollment and Graduations in Baccalaureate and Graduate Programs in Nursing* (Fang, Htut, and Bednash, 2008).

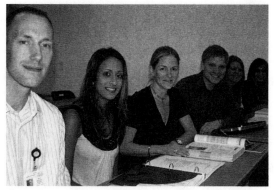

Figure 7-1 In 2009 there were more than 1500 programs preparing RNs in the United States and its territories. Students entering nursing today are diverse in terms of age, sociocultural background, and gender.

were no organized programs to educate nurses until the late 1800s. Before this time, nursing care was administered either by the patient's relatives, by individuals affiliated with religious or military nursing orders, or by self-trained persons who were often held in low regard by society.

Nightingale revolutionized and professionalized nursing by stressing that nursing was not a domestic, charitable service but a respected occupation requiring advanced education. In 1860 she opened a school of nursing at St. Thomas's Hospital in London and established the following principles, which were considered highly innovative at the time:

1. The nurse should be trained in an educational institution supported by public funds and associated with a medical school.
2. The nursing school should be affiliated with a teaching hospital but also independent of it.
3. The curriculum should include both theory and practical experience.
4. Professional nurses should be in charge of administration and instruction and should be paid for their instruction.
5. Students should be carefully selected and should reside in "nurses' houses" that form discipline and character [Nightingale envisioned nursing as a profession only for women].
6. Students should be required to attend lectures, take quizzes, write papers, and keep diaries. Student records should be maintained (Notter and Spalding, 1976).

Nightingale also believed that nursing schools should be financially and administratively separate from the hospitals in which the students trained. This was not the case, however, when nursing schools were first established in the United States.

The first training schools for nurses in the United States were established in 1872. Located at Bellevue Hospital in New York, the New England Hospital for Women and Children in New Haven, Connecticut, and Massachusetts General Hospital in Boston, the course of study was 1 year in length. These schools became known as the "famous trio" of nursing schools. In October 1873, Melinda Anne (Linda) Richards became the first "trained nurse" educated in the United States. By 1879 there were 11 U.S. nursing training schools. Other schools rapidly developed, and by 1900 there were 432 hospital-owned and hospital-operated programs in the United States (Donahue, 1985). These early training programs differed in length from 6 months to 2 years, and each school set its own standards and requirements. On graduation from these programs, students were awarded a diploma. The term *diploma program* was, and still is, used to identify hospital-based nursing education programs. The primary reason for the schools' existence was to staff the hospitals that operated them. The education of student nurses was not always the primary concern.

Early Studies of the Quality of Nursing Education

Nursing leaders of the early 1900s were concerned about the poor quality of many of the recently formed nurse training programs. They initiated studies about nursing and nursing education to prompt changes. October 1899 marked the culmination of some 4 years of work by the American Society of Superintendents of Training Schools for Nurses. Isabel Hampton Robb chaired a Society-selected committee to investigate a means to prepare nurses better for leadership in schools of nursing. Teachers College, which had opened in New York 10 years earlier for the training of teachers, seemed the logical location for the leadership training of nurses. A program, originally designed to prepare administrators of nursing service and nursing education, began as an 8-month course in hospital economics (Donahue, 1985).

Mary Adelaide Nutting came to Teachers College in 1907 as the first nursing professor the world had ever known. Under her direction, the department progressed and became a pioneer in nursing education. The school became known as the "Mother House" of collegiate education because it fostered the initial movements toward undergraduate and graduate degrees for nurses (Donahue, 1985). In 1912 Nutting conducted a nationwide investigation of nursing education, *The Educational Status of Nursing*, that focused on the living conditions of students, the material being taught, and the teaching methods being used (Christy, 1969).

Another major study of nursing education was published in 1923. Titled *The Study of Nursing and Nursing Education in the United States* and referred to as the Goldmark Report, the study focused on the clinical learning experiences of students, hospital control of the schools, the desirability of establishing university schools of nursing, the lack of funds specifically for nursing education, and the lack of prepared teachers (Kalisch and Kalisch, 1995).

The year 1924 marked another first in nursing education when the Yale School of Nursing was opened as the first nursing school to be established as a separate university department with an independent budget and its own dean, Annie W. Goodrich. The school demonstrated its effectiveness so well that in 1929 the Rockefeller Foundation ensured the permanency of the school by awarding it an endowment of $1 million (Kalisch and Kalisch, 1995).

In 1934 a study entitled *Nursing Schools Today and Tomorrow* reported the number of schools in existence, gave detailed descriptions of the schools, described their curricula, and made recommendations for professional collegiate education (National League of Nursing Education, 1934). In 1937 *A Curriculum Guide for Schools of Nursing* was published, outlining a 3-year curriculum and influencing the structure of diploma schools for decades after its publication (National League of Nursing Education, 1937).

Although published over a 30-year period and undertaken by different groups, these early studies consistently made five similar recommendations:

1. Nursing education programs should be established within the system of higher education.
2. Nurses should be highly educated.
3. Students should not be used to staff hospitals.
4. Standards should be established for nursing practice.
5. All students should meet certain minimum qualifications on graduation.

These studies set the stage for the development of the educational programs that exist today.

EDUCATIONAL PATHWAYS TO BECOMING A REGISTERED NURSE TODAY

Today, preparation for a career as an RN usually begins in one of three ways: in a hospital-based diploma program, a baccalaureate degree program, or an associate degree program. These basic programs vary in the courses offered, length of study, and cost. After the completion of a basic program for RNs, graduates are eligible to take the National Council Licensure Examination for Registered Nurses (NCLEX-RN®). On successful completion of the licensing examination, graduates may legally practice as RNs and use the credential RN. Employment and career advancement vary depending on the type of basic program attended (Figure 7-2).

Having three different educational routes to achieve RN licensure is confusing to the public—and even to many nurses themselves. In the following sections, each type of basic program is described, along with its history, unique characteristics, and special issues. These basic programs are discussed in the chronological order in which they were developed.

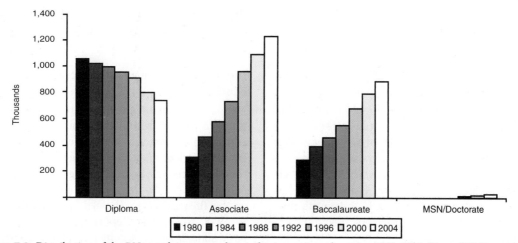

Figure 7-2 Distribution of the RN population according to basic nursing education, 1980-2004. (From U.S. Department of Health and Human Services: *The registered nurse population, March 2004: findings from the National Sample Survey of Registered Nurses,* Washington, DC, 2006, Government Printing Office, p 10.)

Diploma Programs

The hospital-based diploma program was the earliest form of nursing education in the United States. At the peak of diploma education in the 1920s and 1930s, approximately 2000 programs existed, with numerous programs in almost every state. Since their numbers peaked in the first third of the twentieth century, the number of diploma programs has decreased, with a dramatic decline since the mid-1960s when nursing education moved rapidly into collegiate settings. In 1960 there were approximately 800 diploma programs in the United States. Today there are only 62 (National League for Nursing, 2006a). This decline in the number of diploma programs is attributable to several factors: the growth of associate degree and baccalaureate degree programs in nursing, which moved the education of nurses into the mainstream of higher education; the inability of hospitals to continue to finance nursing education; accreditation standards that have made it difficult for diploma programs to attract qualified faculty; and the increasing complexity of health care, which has required nurses to have greater academic preparation.

Despite the significant decrease in the number of diploma programs, many outstanding nurses practicing today received their basic nursing education in these programs. In the early days of formal nurses' "training" in this country—that is, during the late 1800s and early 1900s—diploma programs provided one of the few avenues for women to obtain formal education and jobs. Most of the early programs followed a modified apprenticeship model. Lectures were given by physicians, and clinical training was supervised by head nurses and nursing directors. Nursing courses paralleled medical areas and included surgery, obstetrics, pediatrics, operating room experience, and, somewhat later, psychiatry. Students were sometimes sent to affiliated institutions where they could obtain experiences that were not available at the home hospital.

The schedule was demanding, with classes being held after patient care assignments were completed. Critics charged that students were used as inexpensive labor to staff the hospitals and that education was given a lower priority. The truth of those charges varied, depending on which hospital was scrutinized, but there is no question that early nursing students virtually ran the hospitals. Programs lasted 3 years, and, at graduation, students were awarded diplomas in nursing. Today, most diploma programs are about 24 months in duration.

A problem that many diploma program graduates faced was that hospitals were not part of the higher education system in the United States. Therefore most colleges and universities did not recognize the nursing diploma as an academic credential and often refused to give college credit for courses taken in diploma programs, regardless of the quality of the courses, students, and faculty. Most diploma programs today have established agreements with colleges and universities that allow students to earn college credit in courses such as English, psychology, and the sciences, thereby enabling them to attain advanced standing in a baccalaureate program on completion of the diploma program.

Baccalaureate Programs

Armed with the early studies of nursing education, nursing leaders continued to push for nursing education to move into the mainstream of higher education, that is, into colleges and universities where other professionals were educated. They believed that nurses needed a baccalaureate degree, the bachelor of science in nursing (BSN), to qualify nursing as a recognized profession and to provide leadership in administration, teaching, and public health.

By the time the first baccalaureate nursing program was established in 1909 at the University of Minnesota, diploma programs were numerous and firmly entrenched as the system for educating nurses. This first baccalaureate program was part of the University's School of Medicine and followed the 3-year diploma program structure. Despite its many limitations, it was the start of the movement to bring nursing education into the recognized system of higher education.

Seven other baccalaureate programs in nursing were established by 1919 (Conley, 1973). Most of the early baccalaureate programs were 5 years in duration. This structure provided for 3 years of nursing education and 2 years of liberal arts. The growth in the numbers of these programs was slow both because of the reluctance of universities to accept nursing as an academic discipline and because of the power of the hospital-based diploma programs. The theoretical, scientific orientation of the baccalaureate program was in sharp contrast to the "hands-on" skill and service orientation that was the hallmark of hospital-based diploma education.

Influences on the growth of baccalaureate education

National studies of nursing and nursing education stated and restated the need for nursing education and practice to be based on knowledge from the sciences and humanities. Chief among these studies was Esther Lucille Brown's report *Nursing for the Future,* more commonly known as the Brown Report (Brown, 1948). Published in 1948, the Brown Report recommended that basic schools of nursing be placed in universities and colleges, with effort made to recruit men and minorities into nursing education programs. This report, sponsored by the Carnegie Foundation, was widely reviewed, discussed, and debated.

In 1965 the American Nurses Association (ANA) published a position paper entitled *Educational Preparation for Nurse Practitioners and Assistants to Nurses.* Although not all nursing historians agree, this paper, which subsequently created conflict and division within nursing, had a significant influence on the growth of baccalaureate education in nursing. In preparing the position paper, the ANA studied nursing education, nursing practice, and trends in health care. It concluded that baccalaureate education should become the basic foundation for professional practice. The ANA position paper made four major recommendations:

1. Education for all those who are licensed to practice nursing should take place in institutions of higher learning.
2. Minimum preparation for beginning professional nursing practice should be the baccalaureate degree in nursing.
3. Minimum preparation for beginning technical nursing practice should be the associate degree in nursing.
4. Education for assistants in the health service occupations should consist of short, intensive preservice programs in vocational education institutions rather than on-the-job training programs (ANA, 1965).

Despite tremendous opposition from proponents of diploma and associate degree programs, in 1979 the ANA further strengthened its resolve by proposing three additional positions:

1. By 1985 the minimum preparation for entry into professional nursing practice should be the baccalaureate degree in nursing.
2. Two levels of nursing practice should be identified (professional and technical) and a mechanism to devise competencies for the two categories established by 1980.
3. There should be increased accessibility to high-quality career mobility programs that use flexible approaches for individuals seeking academic degrees in nursing (ANA, 1979).

The controversy created by the 1965 ANA position paper and the additional 1979 resolutions continued for many years. Practicing nurses across the United States, who were mainly diploma program graduates, as well as hospitals that supported diploma programs, vehemently protested the recommendations.

In 1970 the National Commission for the Study of Nursing and Nursing Education published a report entitled *An Abstract for Action* (Lysaught, 1970). Also known as the Lysaught Report, it made recommendations concerning the supply and demand for nurses, nursing roles and functions, and nursing education. Among the priorities identified by this study were (1) the need for increased research into both the practice and education of nurses and (2) enhanced educational systems and curricula (Lysaught, 1970).

In the early 1980s the National Commission on Nursing published two reports suggesting that the major block to the advancement of nursing was the ongoing conflict within the profession about educational preparation for nurses. These studies recommended establishing a clear system of nursing education, including pathways for educational mobility and development of additional graduate education programs.

Another major national nursing group supporting the baccalaureate as the entry credential was the National League for Nursing (NLN). The organization's membership consists of nurses, faculty members, health care agencies, all types of nursing programs, and nonnursing citizens who are supportive of nursing. After much debate, in 1982 the NLN board of directors approved the *Position Statement on Nursing Roles: Scope and Preparation,* which affirmed the nursing baccalaureate degree as the minimum educational level for professional nursing practice and the associate degree or diploma as the preparation for technical nursing practice (NLN, 1982).

In 1996 the American Association of Colleges of Nursing (AACN) board approved a position statement, *The Baccalaureate Degree in Nursing as Minimal Preparation for Professional Practice.* This document supports, among other things, articulated programs, which enable associate degree nurses to attain the baccalaureate degree. This document was updated in 2000. It can be found online: http://www.aacn.nche.edu/Publica tions/positions/baccmin.htm.

Regardless of the many position statements issued by nursing organizations, the minimum educational requirement for entry into practice is unlikely to change until safeguards are devised that ensure that all nurses currently in practice continue to feel that they are valued members of the profession.

Baccalaureate programs today

Today, baccalaureate programs provide education for both basic students who are preparing for licensure and RNs returning to school to obtain a baccalaureate degree in nursing. This section focuses on the program characteristics of prelicensure baccalaureate education, also known as basic programs. Baccalaureate programs for RNs are discussed later in this chapter.

Basic baccalaureate programs combine nursing courses with general education courses in a 4-year curriculum in a senior college or university. Students may be admitted to the nursing program as entering freshmen or after completing certain liberal arts and science courses. Students meet the same admission requirements to the university as other students and often must meet even more stringent requirements to be admitted to the nursing major. Courses in the nursing major focus on nursing science, communication,

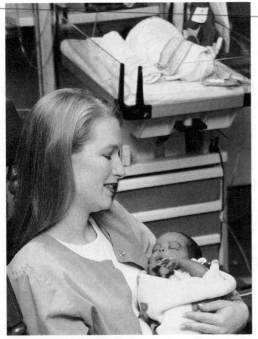

Figure 7-3 Clinical experience is a vitally important aspect of every basic nursing program, providing confidence in the application of knowledge and skills acquired in the classroom and laboratory.

decision making, leadership, and care to persons of all ages in a wide variety of settings (Figure 7-3).

Faculty qualifications in baccalaureate programs are usually higher than in other basic nursing programs. A minimum of a master's degree for clinical faculty and a doctorate in nursing or a related field is required for permanent, tenure-track faculty. The requirement of a doctorate ensures that nursing faculty members are able to meet the teaching, research, and service requirements expected of all faculty in universities.

Baccalaureate graduates are prepared to take the National Council Licensure Examination for Registered Nurses (NCLEX-RN) and, after licensure, assume beginning practice and ultimately leadership positions in any health care setting, including hospitals, community agencies, schools, clinics, and homes. Graduates with baccalaureate degrees are also prepared to move into graduate programs in nursing and advanced practice

certification programs. Programs granting a baccalaureate are the most costly of the basic programs in terms of time and money, but such an investment results in long-term professional advancement. Today, there is great demand for baccalaureate graduates, and they enjoy the greatest career mobility of all basic program graduates in nursing.

According to the AACN's 2008 publication, *The Essentials of Baccalaureate Education for Professional Nursing Practice,* nurses who graduate from bachelor's degree programs are prepared "to practice within complex healthcare systems and assume the roles: provider of care; designer/manager/coordinator of care/ and member of a profession" (AACN, 2008, p. 3). The AACN document also stressed the concepts of patient-centered care, interprofessional teams, evidence-based practice, quality improvement, patient safety, informatics, clinical reasoning/critical thinking, genetics and genomics, cultural sensitivity, professionalism, and practice across the lifespan in an ever-changing and complex health care environment (AACN, 2008, p. 3). Content relating to all these concepts can be found in this textbook and will be built on as you continue your studies.

Associate Degree Programs

Associate degree in nursing (ADN) education is the newest form of basic preparation for RN practice. Begun in 1952 as a result of a post–World War II nursing shortage, based on a model developed by Dr. Mildred Montag, and fueled by the post–World War II community college movement of the 1950s, associate degree programs are now the most common type of basic nursing education program in the United States and graduate the most RN candidates of all the basic programs.

The popularity of ADN programs is attributable to several features: accessibility of community colleges, low tuition costs, part-time and evening study opportunities, shorter duration of programs, and graduates' eligibility to take the licensure examination for RNs.

When first envisioned by Dr. Montag as part of her doctoral dissertation, associate degree programs were proposed as a solution to a nursing shortage. She suggested a shorter program

Box 7-1   Landmarks in the History of Nursing Education

1860 Florence Nightingale founded the first organized program to educate nurses at St. Thomas's Hospital in London.

1872 The "famous trio," the first year-long training schools for nurses, was established in the United States, founded at Bellevue Hospital, the New England Hospital for Women and Children, and Massachusetts General Hospital.

1873 Melinda Anne (Linda) Richards became the first "trained nurse" to graduate in the United States.

1899 Teachers College, Columbia University, offered the first postgraduate course in hospital economics for nurses.

1907 Mary Adelaide Nutting became the first nursing professor at Teachers College, Columbia University.

1909 The first baccalaureate program in nursing was established at the University of Minnesota.

1923 The Goldmark Report was published, the first such report focusing on hospital control of schools of nursing and lack of proper teacher preparation.

1924 Yale University established the first nursing school as a separate university department with its own dean, Annie W. Goodrich.

1932 The first doctoral degree in nursing education (EdD) was granted by Teachers College.

1934 The first PhD program in nursing was initiated by New York University.

1948 Esther Lucille Brown's report *Nursing for the Future* was published, recommending that basic nursing programs be situated in colleges and universities rather than in hospitals.

1952 The first associate degree in nursing program, based on Dr. Mildred Montag's model, was established to prepare nurse technicians.

1965 The ANA issued a position paper advocating the baccalaureate degree as the minimum educational preparation for entry into nursing practice.

designed to prepare nurse technicians who would function under the supervision of professional nurses. Associate degree nurses were to work at the bedside, performing routine nursing skills for patients in acute and long-term care settings. The original associate degree program, as outlined by Montag (1951), offered general education courses in the first year and nursing courses in the second year. Montag originally viewed the associate degree as a final, end-point degree, not a stepping stone to the baccalaureate degree in nursing.

In practice, Montag's original conceptions of associate degree programs have been greatly modified. Associate degree curricula now offer more nursing credits than she suggested. They also include content on leadership and clinical decision making, abilities that Montag did not foresee in technical nurses. Because of additions to the curriculum, it is now virtually impossible for students to complete an associate degree in only 2 years. Associate degree graduates are employed in a wide variety of settings and usually function autonomously alongside baccalaureate and diploma graduates. In the educational system of nursing today, the associate degree can be a step in the progression to the baccalaureate degree or master's degree.

Since 1990 the NLN Council of Associate Degree Programs has sought to differentiate the competencies of the associate degree nurse from those of the baccalaureate nurse. The original document, first written in 1990, was revised in 2000 in response to a changing health care delivery system. Entitled *Educational Competencies for Graduates of Associate Degree Nursing Programs,* the revised document identified eight core competencies of ADN education: professional behaviors, communication, assessment, clinical decision making, caring interventions, teaching and learning, collaboration, and managing care (NLN, 2000). Box 7-1 reviews landmarks in the history of nursing education.

External Degree Programs

External degree programs in nursing are different from traditional basic nursing education in that students attend no classes. Learning is independent and is assessed through highly standardized and validated competency-based outcomes assessments, leading to the description, "virtual university." Students are responsible for arranging their own clinical experiences in accordance with established standards.

Excelsior College, formerly known as the New York Regents External Degree Nursing Program, is as well recognized external degree model. Beginning in 1970 with an associate degree program, Excelsior College now offers associate degree, baccalaureate, and master's degrees in nursing. All the nursing programs are accredited by the National League for Nursing Accreditation Commission (NLNAC).

Since 1981 the California State University Consortium has offered a statewide external degree baccalaureate program in nursing. The California program is for RNs already holding current licenses to practice in the state.

There are numerous external degree programs in existence today, many of which are marketed online and by direct mail. Prospective students must exercise caution to choose only bona fide accredited programs that are affiliated with recognized colleges and universities.

Articulated Programs

In response to the demand for educational mobility, articulation (mobility) between programs has become much more common in today's nursing education system. The purpose of articulation is to facilitate opportunities for nurses to move up the educational ladder. An example of a fully articulated system is the licensed practical nurse/associate degree in nursing/bachelor of science in nursing/master of science in nursing (LPN/ADN/BSN/MSN) program in which students spend the first year preparing to be an LPN and the second year completing the associate degree. If desired or necessary, students can "stop out" of the program at the end of the first year, take the licensure examination for practical nursing, and return to the associate degree program at a later time. On the other hand, they may continue study in the program after the initial 2 years to earn a baccalaureate degree and even continue for a master's or doctoral degree.

Multiple-entry, multiple-exit programs are difficult to develop. A tremendous amount of joint institutional planning is needed to work out equivalent courses and to keep the programs congruent with one another. A change in one curriculum dictates changes in all the others. These challenges explain why fully articulated programs have been slow to develop. In increasing numbers, however, articulation agreements between baccalaureate and ADN programs and between ADN and LPN programs are being established that facilitate student movement between programs and accept transfer credit between institutions. These requirements often result in acceleration or advanced placement within the higher-degree school.

In spite of the difficulties in developing them, several state legislatures have mandated their public institutions to create articulation programs to facilitate upward educational mobility for nurses. Other states have statewide voluntary articulation plans, and still others have individual school-to-school agreements in place. For a list of the types of articulation agreements for all 50 states and the District of Columbia, refer to the Evolve website: http://evolve.elsevier.com/Chitty/professional.

ALTERNATIVE EDUCATIONAL PROGRAMS IN NURSING

In addition to the basic programs leading to entry-level nursing practice, several types of alternative educational programs exist.

Baccalaureate Programs for Registered Nurses

After nursing organizations of the 1960s and 1970s publicly advocated for the baccalaureate degree to be the minimum education level for professional practice, the demand for the nursing bachelor's degree increased. Employers of nurses recognized that broadly educated nurses matched well with the complexities of health care. As a result, many supported the baccalaureate as a requirement for career mobility. Diploma and associate degree graduates returned to school in increasing numbers. Today, many students enter ADN programs with plans to earn a baccalaureate degree ultimately. Baccalaureate programs for RNs allow them, as well as diploma nurses, to accomplish this goal.

RNs with diplomas and associate degrees were not always welcomed into baccalaureate programs. In the early years of baccalaureate education for RNs, many schools required these students to take courses in areas the students believed they had already mastered. For a number of years, there were barriers for these nurses in completing their baccalaureate degrees. Now, however, the majority of baccalaureate programs have recognized the legitimacy and importance of RN-to-baccalaureate in nursing education and have developed alternative tracks to accommodate the unique learning needs of the RN student.

Baccalaureate programs for RNs are most often offered by universities that also offer basic nursing education in baccalaureate programs. The RN students may be integrated with the basic students, or they may be enrolled in a separate or partially separate sequence. Some baccalaureate programs for RNs are freestanding; that is, they are offered by colleges that do not have a basic baccalaureate nursing program or in single-purpose institutions.

Most 4-year colleges and universities allow the transfer of general education credits from associate degree nursing programs. With increasing frequency, transfer credit is given for nursing courses as well, or there is the option of receiving credit for previous nursing courses through a variety of advanced placement methods such as examinations, demonstrations, and portfolios.

For diploma graduates, transfer credit is usually given for previous college courses, such as English, if they were included as part of the diploma program and taught by college faculty. Options for advanced placement of diploma graduates into baccalaureate programs are extremely variable, and prospective RN students should seek detailed information to select a program that fits individual needs and goals.

The demand for the baccalaureate degree by large numbers of associate degree and diploma graduates continues to be strong. More nurses are returning to school to prepare for the wider opportunities offered by the baccalaureate degree. With broad preparation in clinical, scientific, community health, and patient education skills, the baccalaureate nurse is well positioned to move across community-based settings such as home health care, outpatient centers, and neighborhood clinics, where opportunities are fast expanding.

Programs for Second-Degree Students

A noteworthy trend is the significant increase in the number of students with baccalaureate degrees in other fields making a career change to nursing. The educational system in nursing has responded to this group of students by offering options to the traditional basic baccalaureate education. Increasingly, baccalaureate programs offer these students an accelerated or fast track sequence, awarding either a second baccalaureate degree or, in some cases, a master's degree in nursing. Accelerated master's degree programs in nursing for individuals with bachelor's degrees in another field are known as generic master's degree programs. They usually require about 3 years to complete, depending on the number of prerequisite courses needed. Graduates take the RN licensure examination (NCLEX-RN) after completing the generic master's program.

Another educational track for students with baccalaureate degrees in other fields was the generic nursing doctorate (ND). This degree is discussed later in this chapter (see History of Doctoral Education in Nursing).

Online and Distance Learning Programs

The vast majority of nursing programs, particularly entry-level programs, are still offered in the traditional way with in-person course work. Technologic advances, however, have made it possible for students to take courses online, and some colleges are now offering some or all of their courses online. This is often referred to as distance learning (DL). Originally intended to improve educational access for nurses from rural areas, students enrolled in Web-based courses today often live in the same town as the educational institution but have significant demands on their time and prefer the flexibility of online offerings.

Master's and doctoral programs in nursing have been at the forefront in the development of online programs with up to 30% of MSN programs and up to 50% of doctor of nursing practice (DNP) programs now offering half or more of their courses online. According to the AACN, less than 1% of entry-level baccalaureate programs offer half or more of their courses online and 64.4% offer no online courses. In contrast, RN-to-BSN programs are often offered online with nearly 37% offering at least half their courses online (Fang, Htut, and Bednash, 2008).

As more colleges of nursing offer coursework and entire degrees through distance learning, the issue of adequate and properly supervised clinical experience arises. Technology may again provide at least a partial answer to this dilemma through the use of virtual reality. Virtual reality "employs computers and other multimedia peripherals to produce a simulated (i.e., virtual) environment that users perceive as comparable to real-world objects and events" (Simpson, 2003). DL students validate their clinical competence in a number of traditional ways, including preceptorships, clinical examinations, demonstrations, and clinical portfolios. Preliminary research findings on the outcomes of these courses indicate that when they are properly structured, well monitored, and offered to carefully selected students, achievement levels of DL students are comparable with those of traditional students (Zucker and Asselin, 2003).

There have been reports of fraudulent online programs in which large fees are charged for "mail-order degrees." Other programs look good at the outset but enrolled students find serious flaws in the delivery and evaluation processes. Students contemplating taking courses toward entry-level or advanced nursing degrees should be educated consumers and consider several factors when evaluating options (Trossman, 2007):

1. Does the program have legitimate accreditation from a regional accrediting body and from one of the two legitimate nursing accreditation bodies?
2. What is the pass rate on the licensing exam?
3. How are clinical experiences planned and supervised? Does your state board of nursing approve of the type of experiences offered?
4. What is the reputation of the program and its faculty?
5. Do you have the self-discipline needed to keep up with assignments outside a traditional classroom setting?
6. Do you learn best when you can interact with other learners and faculty? As a distance learner, how much access will you have to faculty members?
7. Do distance students have access to student support services just as if they were students-in-residence on campus?

Clearly, selecting a Web-based program is a serious matter requiring much research and thought. To assist students in evaluating their readiness for online learning, a faculty member in the School of Nursing at Indiana University–Purdue University Indianapolis has devised a 20-item assessment instrument entitled "Readiness Index for Learning Online (RILO)." You can find this useful assessment tool online: http://nursing.iupui.edu/students/rilo.shtml.

PRACTICAL NURSING PROGRAMS (LICENSED PRACTICAL NURSE OR LICENSED VOCATIONAL NURSE)

Nursing education includes a large number of programs preparing practical nurses. Practical nurses (LPNs/LVNs) are differentiated from RNs by education and licensure and have a limited scope of practice. LPNs or LVNs are considered technical workers in nursing.

Practical nursing programs became a significant component of the nursing field during World War II. These programs were created to satisfy the demand for nurses and programs that could produce nurses quickly. The first planned curriculum for practical nursing was developed in 1942. Although national accreditation is available for practical nursing programs, the majority of LPN/LVN programs have state approval rather than national accreditation.

Practical nursing education typically lasts 12 months and takes place in a variety of settings: vocational/technical schools, community colleges, and high schools. Many LPN/LVN programs now offer credit for prior learning to health care workers such as hospital aides, orderlies, paramedics, emergency medical technicians, and military corps personnel. These individuals often enter nursing through practical nursing programs.

Graduates of practical nursing programs must pass the National Council Licensure Examination for Practical Nurses (NCLEX-PN) to become licensed. The scope of their practice focuses on meeting basic patient needs in hospitals, long-term care facilities, and homes. They must practice under the supervision of a physician or RN and are not a substitute for RNs, although they are valuable members of the nursing team.

Many newly licensed practical nurses plan to become RNs, with the majority of these individuals either taking courses or planning to begin RN courses in 1 to 2 years. National statistics from 2004, the last year for which figures are available, show that 16.6% of all licensed RNs have practiced previously as LPNs or LVNs, indicating that many are achieving their goal of becoming RNs (U.S. Department of Health and Human Services, 2006).

ACCREDITATION OF EDUCATIONAL PROGRAMS

The concept of accreditation of educational programs in nursing is important. Although all nursing programs must be approved by their respective state boards of nursing for graduates to take the licensure examination, nursing programs may also seek accreditation, which goes beyond minimum state approval. Accreditation refers to a voluntary review process of educational programs by a professional organization. The organization, called an accrediting agency, compares the educational quality of the program with established standards and criteria. Accrediting agencies derive their authority from the U.S. Department of Education. Two agencies, the NLNAC and the Commission on Collegiate Nursing Education, are responsible for accrediting nursing educational programs today, as described below.

Accreditation of nursing schools grew out of concerns repeatedly expressed in reports and by leaders of the profession about the lack of quality and standards for nursing education. An accredited program voluntarily adheres to standards that protect the quality of education, public safety, and the profession itself. Accreditation provides both a mechanism and a stimulus for programs to initiate periodic self-examination and self-improvement. It assures students that their educational program is accountable for offering quality education.

Accrediting bodies establish standards by which a program's effectiveness is measured. Programs under review prepare reports, known as self-studies, that show how the school meets each standard. The self-study is reviewed by a volunteer team composed of nursing educators from the type of program being reviewed, and an on-site program review is conducted by the same team. After the site visit, the visitors' report and the program's self-study are reviewed by the accrediting organization, and a decision is made about the accreditation status of each nursing program.

Prospective nursing students should inquire about the accreditation status of any nursing program they are considering. Qualifying for certain scholarships, loans, and military service usually depends on being enrolled in an accredited program. Acceptance into graduate programs in nursing may also depend on graduation from an accredited baccalaureate program. Employers of nurses are usually interested in hiring only nurses who are graduates of accredited programs.

From 1952 through 1996, the NLN was the only official professional accrediting organization for master's, baccalaureate, associate degree, diploma, and practical nursing programs in the United States. In 1997, as a result of a mandate from the U.S. Department of Education, a separate division of the NLN was created. The new division, the National League for Nursing Accreditation Commission (NLNAC), assumed responsibility for all NLN national program accreditation activity. Accreditation is conducted through four NLNAC councils: the Council of Associate Degree Programs, the Council of Diploma Programs, the Council of Baccalaureate and Higher Degree Programs, and the Council of Practical Nursing Programs. Each council develops its own accreditation program and criteria and revises them periodically.

Once a program is accredited and in good standing, continuing accreditation reviews take place every 8 to 10 years. Programs that do not meet standards may be placed on warning and given a specific time period to correct deficiencies. Accreditation can be withdrawn if deficiencies are not corrected within the specified time.

In 1996 the American Association of Colleges of Nursing (AACN) organized the Commission on Collegiate Nursing Education (CCNE) and began the process of acquiring recognition from the U.S. Department of Education as the national accrediting body for baccalaureate and higher degree nursing programs. CCNE began operation in 1998 and has subsequently established an organizational structure, policies and procedures, and accreditation standards and criteria. In December 1999 CCNE received a recommendation from the National Advisory Committee on Institutional Quality and Integrity, a panel of the U.S. Department of Education, that the Secretary of Education grant initial recognition of CCNE as a national agency for the accreditation of baccalaureate and graduate nursing education programs. This status was renewed in 2002. The establishment of a second national accrediting body for nursing education represented a significant development in the evolution of the nursing profession. Practical nursing programs, diploma programs, and associate degree programs continue to be accredited by the NLNAC,

and baccalaureate and higher degree programs may choose which of the two accrediting bodies they wish to use.

GRADUATE EDUCATION IN NURSING

A variety of economic, educational, and professional trends are fueling the demand for RNs with advanced degrees (master's or doctorates). The rapidly changing health care system requires nurses to possess increasing knowledge, clinical competency, greater independence, and autonomy in clinical judgments. Trends in community-based nursing centers, case management, complexity of home care, sophisticated technologies, and society's orientation to health and self-care are rapidly causing the educational needs of nurses to expand, thereby requiring graduate education. Health care reforms anticipated during the Obama administration are expected to increase the demand for master's and doctorally prepared nurses.

Nurses who have advanced education can become researchers, nurse practitioners (NPs), clinical specialists, educators, and administrators. Some open their own clinics, where they provide direct care and serve as consultants to businesses and health care agencies. Chapter 1 describes some of the opportunities open to nurses with advanced degrees. Certainly, having a workforce of highly educated nurses will further strengthen the profession.

Master's Education

The purpose of master's education is to prepare persons with advanced nursing knowledge and clinical practice skills in a specialized area of practice. Teachers College, Columbia University, is credited with initiating graduate education in nursing. As mentioned, beginning in 1899, the college offered a postgraduate course in hospital economics, which prepared nurses for positions in teaching and hospital administration. From this beginning, there has been consistent growth in the number of master's nursing programs in the United States.

Over the last 40 years, the growth in numbers of master's programs in nursing has been dramatic. In 1970 there were 70 programs. In 2007 there were 458. Enrollment in master's nursing degree programs grew from 19,958 in 1986 to 62,451 in 2007. A majority of these students were attending school part-time (Fang, Htut, and Bednash, 2008).

Most nurses in the 1950s and 1960s viewed the master's degree in nursing as a terminal (final) degree. The master's degree was considered the highest degree nurses would ever need. Early master's programs were longer and more demanding than master's programs in other disciplines. Master's programs in the 1950s and 1960s prepared students for careers in nursing administration and nursing education.

With the rapid development of doctoral programs for nurses during the 1970s, however, the master's degree could no longer be considered a terminal degree. Programs were shortened from as long as 2 years to the approximate 1-year length of master's study in most other disciplines. Advanced practice through clinical specialization became the emphasis. Master's programs in nursing are most often found in senior colleges and universities that have basic baccalaureate programs in nursing. These programs may also seek voluntary accreditation from either the NLNAC or the CCNE.

Entrance requirements to master's programs in nursing usually include the following: a baccalaureate degree from an accredited program in nursing, licensure as an RN, completion of the Graduate Record Examination (GRE) or other standard aptitude test, a minimum undergraduate grade point average (GPA) of 3.0, recent work experience as an RN in an area related to the desired area of specialization, and specific goals for graduate study.

The average traditional program length is 18 to 24 months of full-time study, although part-time study and fast-track curricula are far more common today than in the past. The curriculum includes theory, research, clinical practice, and courses in other disciplines. Master's students generally select both an area of clinical specialization, such as adult health or gerontology, and an area of role preparation,

such as informatics, administration, or teaching. Students may be required to write a comprehensive examination and/or to complete a thesis or research project.

Major areas of role preparation include administration, case management, informatics, health policy/health care systems, teacher education, clinical nurse specialist, NP, nurse-midwifery, nurse anesthesia, and other clinical and nonclinical areas of study.

As illustrated in Figure 7-4, all other role preparation fields trail NP preparation in popularity. Nearly 48.5% of all master's level students enrolled in 2007-2008 were pursuing the NP credential. Other role preparation majors included 7.1% preparing for clinical specialist roles, 7.6% for administration/management, 6.5% for nurse anesthesia, and 14.7.8% for teaching. The remaining master's students were specializing in various other majors or were undeclared (Fang, Htut, and Bednash, 2008). The top six clinical track choices for NP enrollees in 2007 included (in descending order of popularity) family NP, adult NP, pediatric NP, adult acute care NP, NP dual tracks, and women's health NP (Fang, Htut, and Bednash, 2008).

With the increasing demand for NPs, master's programs have expanded their practitioner tracks. Master's programs offering NP options increased from 108 in 1992 to 344 in 2007 (Berlin et al, 2005; Fang, Htut, and Bednash, 2008).

The master of science (MS) and the master of science in nursing (MSN) are the two most common graduate degrees offered. A more recent option in master's education is the RN/MSN track, which allows RNs who are prepared at the associate degree or diploma level and who meet graduate admission requirements to enter a program leading to a master's degree rather than a baccalaureate degree. Other recent graduate program options are combined degrees such as the master of science in nursing/master of business administration (MSN/MBA) for nurse administrators or the master of science in nursing/juris doctor (MSN/JD) for nurse attorneys. Clearly, diversity in nursing education extends to the graduate, as well as the basic, level.

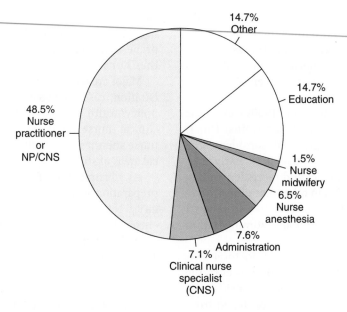

NOTE: Percents may not total 100.0 due to rounding.

Figure 7-4 By a large margin, master's graduates in 2007-2008 selected role preparation as nurse practitioners. The smaller number of students choosing teacher education is cause for concern about the future supply of nursing faculty. (Data from Fang D, Htut A, and Bednash GD: *2007-2008 Enrollment and graduations in baccalaureate and graduate programs in nursing,* Washington, DC, 2008, American Association of Colleges of Nursing.)

Doctoral Education

Doctoral programs in nursing prepare nurses to become faculty members in universities, administrators in schools of nursing or large medical centers, researchers, theorists, and advanced practitioners. Doctoral programs in nursing offer several degree titles. These can be divided into two categories, research-focused degrees such as the doctor of nursing science (DNSc) and the doctor of philosophy (PhD) and practice-focused degrees such as the nursing doctorate (ND) and the doctor of nursing practice (DNP).

History of doctoral education in nursing

Formal doctoral education for nurses began at Columbia University's Teachers College in 1910 with the creation of the Department of Nursing and Health. The first student completed work for the doctor of education (EdD) in nursing education and was awarded the doctoral degree in 1932. Seventy-seven years later, in 2002, Teachers College was still granting EdDs in nursing education.

In 1934 New York University initiated the first PhD program for nurses. The programs at Teachers College and New York University provided many of the profession's early leaders, who worked over the years for improvements in nursing education (Parietti, 1990).

From 1934 through 1953, no new nursing doctoral programs were opened. In 1954 the University of Pittsburgh opened the first PhD program in clinical nursing and clinical research in the United States. As the 1950s drew to a close, a total of only 36 doctoral degrees had been awarded in nursing (Parietti, 1990).

Because of the limited number of nursing doctoral programs, most nurses in the 1950s and 1960s earned doctorates in nonnursing fields, such as education, sociology, and physiology. Doctoral education for nurses moved into a new phase when the federal government initiated nurse scientist programs in 1962. These programs were created to increase the research skills of nurses and provide faculty for the development of doctoral programs in nursing. The nurse scientist programs were discontinued in 1975 after more universities began offering doctoral programs in nursing.

A program offering the nursing doctorate (ND) to students as their first nursing degree was begun at Case Western Reserve University in 1979. The ND program was designed for students with baccalaureate degrees in fields other than nursing. The program, which has been phased out, was based on that school's philosophy that professional nursing education should begin at the postbaccalaureate level. After completion of 900 clinical hours, ND graduates were eligible to take the RN licensure examination before continuing to the postlicensure portion of the program. Graduates were prepared for leadership positions in practice, business, management, research, and education. All programs currently offering the doctor of nursing (ND) are transitioning to the doctor of nursing practice (DNP) discussed later (AACN, 2004).

The 1970s saw a major increase in the number of doctoral programs in nursing. In that decade alone, 15 new doctoral programs were established. Between 1970 and 1980, the number of programs increased to 22, and between 1980 and 1990, the number more than doubled, from 22 to 48 (Parietti, 1990). In 1996 the number of doctoral programs stood at 66 (NLN, 1997). By 2007 that number had risen to 166, 68% of which were research focused and 32% of which were practice focused (Fang, Htut, and Bednash, 2008).

Current status of doctoral education in nursing

Research-focused doctoral degrees for students with prior degrees in nursing include the doctor of nursing science (DNSc) and the doctor of philosophy (PhD). Both of these degrees build on master's preparation in nursing. The DNSc is an advanced practice degree with an emphasis on clinical research. The DNSc is intended to bridge the gap between practice and research (Allen, 1990). The PhD is considered an academic degree and prepares nurse scholars for research and the development of theory.

In October 2004, the members of the AACN debated and passed a resolution calling for a new doctoral degree, the doctor of nursing practice (DNP). Designed to replace the master's degree, the DNP would be required to be completed by nurses who wished to practice in advanced roles, such as NP or nurse-midwife. Proponents of this change suggest that it would put nursing on an even footing with other health care disciplines, several of which are moving in the same direction. Conversely, the proposed change could increase confusion within and outside of the profession about the qualifications of nurses prepared at the doctoral level. It could also discourage nurses from seeking the PhD in nursing and thereby further deepen the shortage of nurse faculty prepared in the manner of other professors on campus (Dracup and Bryan-Brown, 2005). In spite of early concerns, the degree has proved to be popular, and increasing numbers of universities are offering the DNP. In 2007 there were 53 DNP programs in existence with a total of 122 graduates completing their degrees in that year. The number of programs and graduates is expected to grow rapidly. Proponents of national health reform see DNPs as a solution to the shortage of primary-care physicians that will add to the profession's credibility (Landro, 2008; Croasdale, 2008). Care must be taken, however, to standardize the education and certification of DNPs nationwide. To that end, in July 2008, the AACN issued a report that resulted from the work of numerous nursing organizations. Entitled, "Consensus Model for APRN Regulation: Licensure, Accreditation, Certification & Education," it sets forth a uniform model of regulation of advanced practice registered nurse (APRN) practice across the nation. As of October 2009, 72 certifying bodies, associations, and boards had endorsed the model. The entire document is available online: http://www.aacn.nche.education/pdf/APRNReport.pdf.

Enrollment trends indicate that there is continued demand for all types of doctoral education in nursing. The number of programs, as well as the number of requests for admission to these programs, continues to increase. This trend has

partially stemmed from the requirement of a doctorate for academic advancement and tenure for
university nursing faculty. A doctorate is required
to become a competent researcher who can compete for grants and develop nursing science. This
advances the profession as a whole. Doctoral
programs that prepare nurses predominantly for
research and teaching reported 3949 students
enrolled in 2007. Far fewer students complete
their doctoral programs, however, with 54% of
students enrolled part-time. For example, in 2007
only 531 students (13.5%) actually completed
research-focused doctorates in 113 reporting
programs (Fang, Htut, and Bednash, 2008). This
low completion rate further aggravates the nursing faculty shortage, discussed later in this chapter. It is projected that large numbers of nurses
with doctoral degrees will continue to be needed
in the future as positions requiring this degree
expand in universities and throughout the health
care system.

CERTIFICATION PROGRAMS

Licensure and certification are both forms of
credentialing of nurses. Licensure refers to state
regulation of the practice of nursing. Licensure
is required of individuals at the entry point to
practice and must be renewed periodically. It
is a legal designation that assures public safety
by assessing basic and continuing competence.
Certification goes beyond licensure by validat-
ing a high level of knowledge and proficiency
in a particular practice area. It is voluntarily
pursued by individual nurses and is therefore
a credential that has professional but not legal
status.

Certification means that a certificate is awarded
by a certifying body as validation of specific qualifications demonstrated by an RN in a defined
area of practice. A comprehensive examination
is required to become certified, as well as documentation of experience, letters of reference, and
other documents. Currently, 48 organizations
offer certification (Yoder-Wise, 2009). Box 7-2
lists examples of the professional associations that
currently grant certification.

**Box 7-2 A Sample of Certifying Organiza-
tions in Nursing***

- AACN Certification Corporation (critical care)
- American Association of Diabetes Educators
- American Association of Spinal Cord Injury Nurses
- American Board for Occupational Health Nurses, Inc.
- American College of Nurse-Midwives
- American Nurses Credentialing Center (40 areas of certification)
- American Organization of Nurse Executives
- American Psychiatric Nurses Association
- Board of Certification for Emergency Nursing
- Council on Recertification of Nurse Anesthetists
- National Association of Neonatal Nurses
- National Association of Nurse Practitioners
- National Certification Corporation for Obstetric, Gynecologic, and Neonatal Specialties
- National Board for Certification of School Nurses
- Pediatric Nursing Certification Board
- Rehabilitation Nursing Certification Board

*A complete list of certifying boards can be obtained by
writing to the *Journal of Continuing Education in Nursing*,
Slack, Inc., 6900 Grove Drive, Thorofare, NJ 08086. Ask for
the Annual Continuing Education Survey. Also available
online (http://www.jcenonline.com/survey.asp).

Certified nurses may have greater earning
potential; wider employment opportunities; a
broader scope of practice; validation of their
skills, knowledge, and abilities; public recognition; a sense of personal satisfaction; and prestige
that sets them apart from noncertified nurses.
Increasingly, they are eligible for insurance reimbursement for their services. Requirements for
admission to certification programs vary, with
some requiring only RN licensure and others
requiring either a baccalaureate or a master's
degree. The American Nurses Credentialing Center (ANCC), a subunit of the ANA, is the largest
of the certification bodies, providing 40 different

certification programs for RNs at the associate degree, baccalaureate, and advanced practice levels. Advanced practice nurses (APNs) certified by the ANCC must have master's degrees and demonstrate successful completion of a certification examination based on nationally recognized standards of nursing practice and designed to test their special knowledge and skills. For most specialties, candidates also must show evidence of specified clinical practice experience. Once granted, certification is effective for 3 to 5 years, whereupon the individual must apply for recertification either based on retesting or by demonstrating continuing education credits and evidence of ongoing clinical practice.

In response to the need to create uniformity in the numerous certification programs, the ANCC and more than a dozen other certification boards formed the American Board of Nursing Specialties (ABNS) in 1991. Membership is open to certifying bodies that have met the standards and principles of ABNS. There are currently 31 regular members of ABNS. The organization's stated aims are to promote standards of excellence in nursing certification and to increase public awareness of the value of certification.

Nurses holding certification at the associate degree/diploma level use the initials RN, C (Registered Nurse, Certified) after their names. Certified baccalaureate nurses are entitled to use RN, BC (Registered Nurse, Board Certified). Those certified as clinical specialists use APRN, BC (Advanced Practice Registered Nurse, Board Certified). Box 7-3 lists the areas in which the ANCC offers certification.

Although certification is a desirable concept, a major challenge must be overcome in regard to the current methods of certification. With so many different organizations offering certification, the lack of uniformity of programs, testing, and practice requirements must be examined. How the profession can ensure certification standards and who should be responsible for certification of nurses are continuing concerns.

Many in the nursing profession believe that nurses should be certified in a standardized manner by nationally recognized certifying boards only and that having multiple standards of certification is confusing and disadvantageous to the profession. The AACN has been particularly vocal in this regard and issued position statements in 1994, 1998, and 2008. As discussed above, the 2008 Consensus Model emphasized standardization goals focusing on APRNs (APRN Consensus Work Group & the National Council of State Boards of Nursing APRN Advisory Committee, 2008). This could become a model for nursing certifications at all levels, thereby unifying certification processes and rendering them more understandable by both employers and the public and thereby benefiting nursing.

CONTINUING EDUCATION

Continuing education (CE) is a term used to describe non–degree-seeking ways in which nurses maintain expertise during their professional careers. It is also known as "lifelong learning." It differs from staff development, which refers to how an agency or institution assists its employees in maintaining competence. CE opportunities are those pursued by individual nurses themselves. CE for nurses takes place in a variety of settings: colleges, universities, hospitals, community agencies, professional organizations, and professional meetings. CE is available in many formats, such as workshops, institutes, conferences, short courses, evening courses, telecourses, and instructional modules offered in professional journals and by professional organizations online.

The ANCC is responsible for standards of CE, accreditation of programs offering CE, transferability of CE credit from state to state, and development of guidelines for recognition systems within states.

The contact hour is the measure of CE credit. Generally, nurses receive 1 contact hour of CE credit for each 50 or 60 minutes they spend in a CE course.

A major nationwide need is for mandatory CE as a prerequisite for license renewal. Before renewing their licenses in states and territories with mandatory CE, nurses must provide evidence

Box 7-3   Areas of Certification Offered by the American Nurses Credentialing Center (ANCC) in 2009

NURSE PRACTITIONER (NP) CERTIFICATION AREAS

- Acute Care NP
- Adult NP
- Adult Psychiatric and Mental Health NP
- Diabetes Management—Advanced
- Family NP
- Family Psychiatric and Mental Health NP
- Gerontological NP
- Pediatric NP
- School NP

CLINICAL NURSE SPECIALIST (CNS) CERTIFICATION AREAS

- Adult Health CNS
- Adult Psychiatric and Mental Health CNS
- Child/Adolescent Psychiatric and Mental Health CNS
- CNS Core Exam
- Diabetes Management—Advanced
- Gerontological CNS
- Home Health CNS
- Pediatric CNS
- Public/Community Health CNS

OTHER ADVANCED-LEVEL CERTIFICATION AREAS

- Diabetes Management—Advanced
- Nurse Executive—Advanced
- Public Health Nursing—Advanced

SPECIALTY CERTIFICATIONS

- Ambulatory Care Nursing
- Cardiac Rehabilitation Nursing
- Cardiac Vascular Nursing
- Case Management Nursing
- College Health Nursing
- Community Health Nursing
- Gerontological Nursing
- High-Risk Perinatal Nursing
- Home Health Nursing
- Informatics Nursing
- Maternal-Child Nursing
- Medical-Surgical Nursing
- Nurse Executive
- Nursing Professional Development
- Pain Management
- Pediatric Nursing
- Perinatal Nursing
- Psychiatric and Mental Health Nursing
- School Nursing

From American Nurses Credentialing Center: Accessed October 1, 2009, from http://www.nursecredentialing.org/certification.aspx.

that they have met contact hour requirements. The requirement for mandatory continuing education is a government's way of ensuring that nurses remain up-to-date in their profession and is required in most professions including medicine, the law, pharmacy, and accounting, among others. In 2008 mandatory CE credit as a prerequisite for license renewal was required in only 33 states and U.S. territories. There is wide variation in the requirements for CE. The number of CE hours required ranged from a low of 10 hours in 2 years in Rhode Island to a high of 30 hours annually in Alaska (Yoder-Wise, 2009). Box 7-4 lists mandatory CE states and territories.

CHALLENGES IN NURSING EDUCATION

A number of challenges face nursing education. Two major challenges are discussed in this section: the inability of nursing programs to produce enough nurses to meet society's needs because of faculty and other resource shortages and the need to transform nursing education to meet the complex health care needs of the nation for the future.

Faculty and Other Resource Shortages Threaten Nation's Supply of Nurses

Despite the fact that enrollments in associate and baccalaureate degree programs across the nation have increased in recent years, the number of ng Continuing Education for License Renewal in 2008*

- New Hampshire
- New Jersey
- New Mexico
- North Carolina
- North Dakota
- North Mariana Islands
- Ohio
- Pennsylvania
- Puerto Rico
- Rhode Island
- South Carolina
- Texas
- U.S. Virgin Islands
- Utah
- West Virginia
- Wyoming

ng continuing education for license renewal can be obtained by writing to
g, Slack, Inc., 6900 Grove Drive, Thorofare, NJ 08086. Ask for a reprint of the
vailable online (http://www.jcenonline.com/survey.asp).

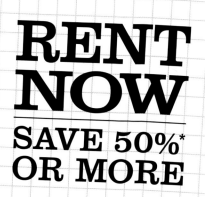
rrent needs
pulation ages
ere was a lev-
05 and 2006
a suspected
ents in nurs-
nd nearly one
turned away
fman, 2008).
alified appli-
y-level bacca-
alone. When
er, it was often
ficient clinical
s.

s, so does the
ally, the mean
years in 1993.
51.1 years, and
ll-time nursing
ears old (NLN,
dicate that the
average age of nursing professors was 59 years

and the average age of associate professors was 52 years (Fang, Htut, and Bednash, 2008). This trend will result in increasing numbers of faculty retirements in the next decade; as many as 75 percent of current nursing faculty are expected to retire by 2019 (NLN, 2005). The faculty shortage, already affecting many areas of the country, is predicted to become severe in the majority of the nation's schools of nursing as early as 2010 (AACN, 2005).

Recognizing that the shortage of faculty would soon reach critical proportions, the AACN issued an official report, known as a white paper, outlining the problem (AACN, 2005). Among their findings were the following:

- A 2000 national sample of schools reported 7.4% faculty vacancies, with only 20 of 220 schools reporting no vacancies. Although this may not seem like a large vacancy rate, it has a considerable impact because of teacher/student ratios mandated by nursing accreditation bodies. Accredited schools are required to limit the size of a faculty member's clinical supervision responsibilities to 10 students at any one time.

- Reasons for faculty shortages include age and retirement time lines; an inadequate pool of younger faculty for replacement; resignations for nonacademic jobs; decrease in the overall number of graduates from both master's and doctoral programs; average age of doctoral graduates (46.2 years) as compared with graduates of all professions (33.7 years), meaning that the number of productive work years for these older faculty members is curtailed; plans of new doctoral graduates to work outside education; average academic salaries lower than those in clinical areas and continuing budgetary constraints within most higher education systems, making salary increases unlikely; and expanding expectations of the faculty role. Furthermore, faculty members are challenged more and more by nontraditional students who demand more individual attention—at the same time as they are increasingly required to do research, service, and publishing.

The AACN (2005) white paper suggested numerous additional strategies for dealing with the faculty shortage (see the entire 2005 report at http://www.aacn.nche.edu/Publications/White Papers/FacultyShortages.htm). Faculty shortages are severe and seriously affect the nation's supply of RNs. Interest in nursing careers is strong, but access to professional nursing programs is increasingly difficult and is expected to become even more so for the foreseeable future. This represents a formidable challenge for the profession's continued vitality.

Need to Transform Nursing Education

In any practice-based profession, educational programs preparing new professionals are challenged to stay current with the rapidly changing technologies in the practice arena. During the last decade of the twentieth century, nursing organizations turned their attention to the future. A number of organizations issued reports identifying changes needed in nursing education to prepare nurses for practice in the twenty-first century. The reports included the NLN's *A Vision for Nursing Education* (1993; see also NLN, 1995), the AACN's *Nursing Education's Agenda for the 21st Century* (AACN, 1993, 1999), and the report from the Pew Health Professions Commission entitled *Health Professions Education for the Future: Schools in Service to the Nation* (O'Neil, 1993). Although the three organizations advocated somewhat different approaches and strategies, several common themes emerged in their reports. Common emphases included the following eight points:

1. Schools should recruit diverse students and faculties that reflect the multicultural nature of society.
2. Curricula and learning activities should develop students' critical thinking skills.
3. Curricula should emphasize students' abilities to communicate, form interpersonal relationships, and make decisions collaboratively with patients, their families, and interdisciplinary colleagues.
4. The number of advanced practice nurses should be increased, and curricula should emphasize health promotion and health maintenance skills for all nurses.
5. Emphasis should be placed on community-based care, increased accountability, state-of-the-art clinical skills, and increased information management skills (Figure 7-5).
6. Cost-effectiveness of care should be a focus in nursing curricula.

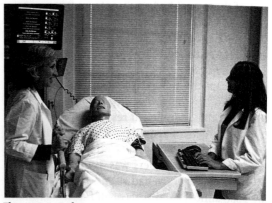

Figure 7-5 Information management is more important than ever in nursing. This nursing student is developing information technology skills to manage multiple sources of patient information successfully.

7. Faculty should develop programs that facilitate program articulation and career mobility.
8. Continuing faculty development activities should support excellence in practice, teaching, and research.

These eight areas of emphasis remain as relevant today as they were when first identified in the 1990s.

In April 2002 the ANA issued a document entitled *Nursing's Agenda for the Future: The Future Vision for Nursing*. The vision for nursing education articulated in this paper included the valuing of nursing education by the public; education programs that are accessible, affordable, and flexible; adequate faculty with high qualifications who engage in innovative teaching, clinical practice, and research; learning environments conducive to the creativity of faculty and students; evidence-based education; safe, quality care; and partnerships to enhance clinical experiences, meet the needs of special populations, and promote professional involvement. The following five strategies were outlined for achieving the vision: (1) establish congruence between the educational enterprise and societal needs; (2) enrich the high caliber of nursing faculty; (3) attain clarity in education about nursing roles and scopes of practice; (4) work for universal excellence in nursing education; and (5) promote the value of nursing education to the profession and the public. In 2008 when health care reform was again the focus of the presidential campaigns, the ANA prepared an updated *Health System Reform Agenda*. You can read both of these reports in full online. Go to the following website, and scroll down to the links to pdf files for both documents. Website: http://www.nursingworld.org/MainMenuCategories/HealthcareandPolicyIssues/HealthSystemReform/Agenda.aspx.

Some experts believe that education of all health professions is in need of systemic change. A notable example is the 2003 report of the Institute of Medicine (IOM), *Health Professions Education: A Bridge to Quality*. This report built on the 2001 IOM report, *Crossing the Quality Chasm: A New Health System for the 21st Century*, which recommended a complete restructuring of clinical education across all health professions. As a follow-up to the initial report, a multidisciplinary summit of health profession leaders met in 2002; this high-level panel composed of 150 participants recommended the goal of "an outcome-based education system that better prepares clinicians to meet both the needs of patients and the requirements of a changing health system" (IOM, 2003). Five major problems were identified in all health professions' education. They were the following (IOM, 2003):

1. Students are not being educated to care for the increasingly diverse, elderly, and chronically ill patient populations.
2. Students are not being prepared to work in teams, but once in practice, they are usually expected to work in interdisciplinary teams.
3. Students are not consistently educated in how to find, evaluate, and use the rapidly expanding scientific evidence on which practice should be based.
4. There is little opportunity to learn how to identify, analyze, and eliminate the root causes of errors and other quality problems in health care delivery systems.
5. Students often are not provided basic informatics training to enable them to access information and use computerized order entry systems.

They recommended that all the health professions develop and share a set of core competencies that would result in better educational quality and relevance. This comprehensive report can be read in its entirety online (http://www.nap.edu/catalog.php?record_id=10681#toc).

In 2005 the NLN issued a position statement entitled *Transforming Nursing Education*. This statement promoted evidence-based education, that is, educational practices based on research into best educational practices rather than "tradition, past practices, and good intentions" (NLN, 2005, p. 1). For a number of years several professions, including nursing, have emphasized evidence-based practice. This statement calls on faculty to follow suit in designing and implementing educational practices.

The NLN in 2008 issued another position statement that focused on new models of nursing education. *Preparing the Next Generation of Nurses to Practice in a Technology-rich Environment: An Informatics Agenda* called on nursing programs to prepare graduates to use electronic health records (EHRs), as recommended by the IOM and others. The report (NLN, 2008) pointed out that a new federal office, the Office of the National Coordinator for Health Information Technology, was created to lead the way in developing EHRs. EHRs, designed to connect clinicians so that patient data can be shared and health care personalized, will certainly be a part of a reformed health system. Both the NLN's 2005 and 2008 position statements can be found in their entirety online (http://www.nln.org/aboutnln/PositionStatements/index.htm).

The important thing for students of nursing to recognize about all these reports is that nursing organizations and leaders are constantly analyzing the changes in the health care system and working to set standards by which high-quality education nursing programs can be designed, implemented, and evaluated. The complexity of health care delivery systems and the dynamic nature of the patient populations served, the shortage of faculty, and the lack of human and financial resources make this a challenging task. However, there is no question that the transformation of nursing education over the next two decades will be significant.

Other Challenges

In addition to the two major challenges discussed above, nursing education must address a variety of other issues, including job market fluctuations, increasing competition for clinical learning sites by all health profession schools, diminishing resources in institutions of higher education and the high cost of operating nursing education programs, and the inability of some nursing programs to meet accreditation standards. Nursing organizations and nursing advocates are increasingly working together to overcome these and other challenges and to promote nursing as a vibrant, flexible, and exciting profession.

Summary of Key Points

- The development of nursing education has been influenced by a number of factors, leading to a diverse array of program offerings.
- First provided in hospitals, entry-level nursing education has evolved into three major types of basic programs: diploma, baccalaureate, and associate degree, each of which has a range of features.
- Alternatives such as baccalaureate degree programs for RNs, external degree programs, accelerated options for postbaccalaureate students, and online programs contribute to a rich, yet complex educational picture for RNs.
- Voluntary accreditation is designed to ensure the quality of nursing education programs.
- Schools have found it necessary to restrict enrollments because of faculty shortages, lack of clinical sites, and budget constraints.
- Lifelong learning through continuing education is considered essential for all professionals, particularly in practice-based disciplines such as nursing. CE is now mandated as a prerequisite for relicensure in 33 states and U.S. territories, and this number is expected to increase.
- The problem of reduced resources in nursing education may soon reach crisis proportions, and weaker schools may close. This is a result of underfunding of higher education in general and, in particular, diminishing sources of federal and state funding for schools of nursing.
- Graduate programs in nursing are not preparing adequate numbers of nursing educators to meet current and future needs. Faculty shortages are already developing, and a severe faculty shortage is expected nationwide in the next decade.
- In response to changes in higher education and the health care system, national organizations have suggested initiatives to revise educational requirements and program emphases for the twenty-first century that will enable future RNs at all levels to meet the changing health care needs of society.

Critical Thinking Questions

1. What factors did you use to determine the type of basic nursing program you entered? Knowing what you know now, what changes, if any, would you make in your choice?
2. How would you advise a high school student interested in nursing to select a program?
3. Should nursing have only one basic program type that leads to entry into the profession? Discuss the pros and cons of a single program. In what part of the higher education system should this basic program be located? What academic credential should be awarded at the completion of the program? In what ways would the unification of nursing education strengthen the profession? What are the drawbacks to this approach?
4. What content areas and skills should be included in basic nursing programs to prepare graduates for contemporary nursing practice? What should be eliminated to make room for this content?
5. Offering complete articulation of all types of nursing education from practical nursing through doctoral study seems like a logical course of action. Should all states mandate program articulation? Why or why not?
6. Discuss the merits and drawbacks of mandatory CE from viewpoints of both nurses and consumers of nursing care.
7. What unique contributions to nursing are possible by nurses with master's-level education? With doctoral-level degrees?
8. Find out which of the national accrediting bodies, NLNAC or CCNE, accredits your school or college. Research their standards online (visit Evolve for WebLinks related to the content of this chapter: http://evolve.elsevier.com/Chitty/professional/), and analyze how your school meets those standards.

⊖volve *To enhance your understanding of this chapter, try the Student Exercises on the Evolve site at http://evolve.elsevier.com/Chitty/professional.*

REFERENCES

Allen J, editor: *Consumer's guide to doctoral degree programs in nursing*, New York, 1990, National League for Nursing.

American Nurses Association: *Educational preparation for nurse practitioners and assistants to nurses, Position paper*, Kansas City, Mo, 1965, American Nurses Association.

American Nurses Association: *A case for baccalaureate preparation in nursing*, Kansas City, Mo, 1979, American Nurses Association.

American Association of Colleges of Nursing: *Nursing education's agenda for the 21st century, Position statement*, Washington, DC, 1993, American Association of Colleges of Nursing, revised 1999.

American Association of Colleges of Nursing: *Certification and regulation of advanced practice nurses, Position statement*, Washington, DC, 1994, American Association of Colleges of Nursing, revised 1998.

American Association of Colleges of Nursing: *The baccalaureate degree in nursing as minimal preparation for professional practice, Position statement*, Washington, DC, 1996, American Association of Colleges of Nursing.

American Nurses Association: *Nursing's agenda for the future: the future vision for nursing*, Washington, DC, 2002, American Nurses Association.

American Association of Colleges of Nursing: *The practice doctorate in nursing: a position statement*, Washington, DC, 2004, American Association of Colleges of Nursing.

American Association of Colleges of Nursing: *Faculty shortages in baccalaureate and graduate nursing programs: scope of the problem and strategies for expanding the supply, a working paper*, Washington, DC, 2005, American Association of Colleges of Nursing.

American Association of Colleges of Nursing: *The essentials of baccalaureate education for professional nursing practice*, Washington, DC, 2008, American Association of Colleges of Nursing.

American Nurses Credentialing Center: Accessed October 1, 2009, from http://www.nursecredentialing.org/certification.aspx.

APRN Consensus Work Group & the National Council of State Boards of Nursing APRN Advisory Committee: *Consensus model for APRN regulation: licensure, accreditation, certification & education*, 2008. Online: http://www.aacn.nche.edu/education/pdf/APRNReport.pdf.

Berlin LE, Wilsey SJ, Bednash GD: *2004-2005 enrollment and graduations in baccalaureate and graduate programs in nursing*, Washington, DC, 2005, American Association of Colleges of Nursing.

Brown EL: *Nursing for the future*, New York, 1948, Russell Sage Foundation.

Christy T: Portrait of a leader: M. Adelaide Nutting, *Nurs Outlook* 17(1):20-24, 1969.

Conley V: *Curriculum and instruction in nursing*, Boston, 1973, Little, Brown.

Croasdale M: *Medical testing board to introduce doctor of nursing certification*, American Medical Association, June 16, 2008. Online: http://www.ama-assn.org/amednews/2008/06/16/prl10616.htm.

Donahue MP: *Nursing: the finest art: an illustrated history*, St Louis, 1985, Mosby.

Dracup K, Bryan-Brown CW: Doctor of nursing practice: MRI or total body scan, *Am J Crit Care* 14(4):278-281, 2005.

Fang D, Htut A, Bednash GD: *2007-2008 Enrollment and graduations in baccalaureate and graduate programs in nursing*, Washington, DC, 2008, American Association of Colleges of Nursing.

Institute of Medicine: *Crossing the quality chasm: a new health system for the 21st century*, Washington, DC, 2001, National Academies Press.

Institute of Medicine: *Health professions education: a bridge to quality*, Washington, DC, 2003, National Academies Press.

Kalisch P, Kalisch B: *The advance of American nursing*, ed 3, Boston, 1995, Little, Brown.

Kaufman K: Executive summary from the Nursing Data Review, academic year 2005-2006, *Nurs Educ Perspect* 29(3):182-184, 2008.

Landro L: *Making room for 'Dr. Nurse'*, New York, April 2, 2008, Wall Street Journal, D-1.

Lysaught J: *An abstract for action*, New York, 1970, McGraw-Hill.

Montag M: *The education of nursing technicians*, New York, 1951, Putnam.

National League of Nursing Education: *Nursing schools today and tomorrow*, New York, 1934, National League of Nursing Education.

National League of Nursing Education: *A curriculum guide for schools of nursing*, New York, 1937, National League of Nursing Education.

National League for Nursing: *Position statement on nursing roles: scope and preparation*, New York, 1982, National League for Nursing.

National League for Nursing: Council of Associate Degree Programs: *Educational outcomes of associate degree nursing programs: roles and competencies*, New York, 1990, National League for Nursing.

National League for Nursing: *A vision for nursing education*, New York, 1993, National League for Nursing.

National League for Nursing: *Emerging environment for nursing education and practice examined during two-year vision campaign: news from the National League for Nursing*, New York, 1995, National League for Nursing.

National League for Nursing: Center for Research in Nursing Education and Community Health: *NLN guide to undergraduate RN education*, ed 5, Sudbury, Mass, 1997, NLN Press and Jones and Bartlett.

National League for Nursing: *Educational competencies for graduates of associate degree nursing programs*, New York, 2000, National League for Nursing.

National League for Nursing: *Transforming nursing education*, New York, 2005, National League for Nursing. Online: http://www.nln.org/aboutnln/Position Statements/index.htm.

National League for Nursing: *A guide to state approved schools of nursing 2006 RN*, ed 58, New York, 2006a, National League for Nursing.

National League for Nursing: *Nurse educators 2006*, New York, 2006b, National League for Nursing.

National League for Nursing: *Preparing the next generation of nurses to practice in a technology-rich environment; an informatics agenda*, New York, 2008, National League for Nursing. Online: http://www.nln.org/aboutnln/PositionStatements/index.htm.

Notter L, Spalding E: *Professional nursing: foundations, perspectives and relationships*, ed 9, Philadelphia, 1976, JB Lippincott.

O'Neil EH: *Health professions education for the future: schools in service to the nation*, San Francisco, 1993, Pew Health Professions Commission.

Parietti E: The development of doctoral education in nursing: a historical overview, In Allen J, editor: *Consumer's guide to doctoral degree programs in nursing*, New York, 1990, National League for Nursing, p 1532.

Simpson R: Welcome to the virtual classroom, *Nurs Adm Q* 27(1):83-86, 2003.

Trossman S: Virtual learning: nurse leaders offer strategies for choosing online programs, *American Nurse Today* 2(9):37-38, 2007.

U.S. Department of Health and Human Services: *The registered nurse population, March 2004: preliminary findings from the National Sample Survey of Registered Nurses*, Washington, DC, 2006, Government Printing Office.

Yoder-Wise PS: Annual CE survey: state certifying board/associations: CE and competency requirements, *J Contin Educ Nurs* 40(1):5-13, 2009.

Zucker DM, Asselin M: Migrating to the web: the transformation of a traditional RN to BS program, *J Contin Educ Nurs* 34(2):86-89, 2003.

Critical Thinking, the Nursing Process, and Clinical Judgment

8

Beth Perry Black

LEARNING OUTCOMES

After studying this chapter, students will be able to:
- Define critical thinking
- Describe the importance of critical thinking in nursing
- Contrast the characteristics of "novice thinking" with those of "expert thinking"
- Explain the purpose and phases of the nursing process
- Differentiate between nursing orders and medical orders

- Explain the differences between independent, interdependent, and dependent nursing actions
- Describe evaluation and its importance in the nursing process
- Define clinical judgment in nursing practice and explain how it is desveloped
- Devise a personal plan to use in developing sound clinical judgment

---

Almost every encounter a nurse has with a patient is an opportunity for the nurse to assist the patient to a higher level of wellness or comfort. Whether or not this actually happens depends in large measure on the nurse's ability to think critically about the patient's particular needs and how best to meet them. It also depends on the nurse's ability to use a reliable cognitive approach that leads to sound clinical decisions about what the patient's priority nursing needs are. This chapter explores several important and interdependent aspects of thinking and decision making in nursing: critical thinking, the nursing process, and clinical judgment.

DEFINING CRITICAL THINKING

Defining critical thinking is a complex task that requires an understanding of how people think through problems. Educators and philosophers struggled with definitions of critical thinking for several decades. In 1990 the American Philosophical Association's Committee on Pre-College Philosophy published an expert consensus statement (Box 8-1) describing critical thinking and the ideal critical thinker. This expert statement was the culmination

of 3 years of work by Facione and others who synthesized the work of numerous persons who had defined critical thinking. In his essay "Critical Thinking: What It Is and Why It Counts," Facione (2006) suggested that giving a definition of critical thinking that can be memorized by the learner is actually antithetical to critical thinking! This means that the very definition of critical thinking does not lend itself to simplistic thinking and memorization. Paul and Elder's (2005) definition of critical thinking is similar: "Critical thinking is a process by which the thinker improves the quality of his or her thinking by skillfully taking charge of the structures inherent in thinking and imposing intellectual standards upon them." They go on to describe a "well-cultivated critical thinker" as one who does the following:

- Raises questions and problems and formulates them clearly and precisely
- Gathers and assesses relevant information, using abstract ideas for interpretation
- Arrives at conclusions and solutions that are well-reasoned and tests them against relevant standards
- Is open-minded and recognizes alternative ways of seeing problems, and has the ability to

Box 8-1   Expert Consensus Statement Regarding Critical Thinking and the Ideal Critical Thinker

We understand critical thinking (CT) to be purposeful, self-regulatory judgment that results in interpretation, analysis, evaluation, and inference, as well as explanation of the evidential, conceptual, methodological, criteriological, or contextual considerations upon which that judgment is based. CT is essential as a tool of inquiry. As such, CT is a liberating force in education and a powerful resource in one's personal and civic life. While not synonymous with good thinking, CT is a pervasive and self-rectifying human phenomenon. The ideal critical thinker is habitually inquisitive, well-informed, trustful of reason, open-minded, flexible, fair-minded in evaluation, honest in facing personal biases, prudent in making judgments, willing to reconsider, clear about issues, orderly in complex matters, diligent in seeking relevant information, reasonable in the selection of criteria, focused in inquiry, and persistent in seeking results that are as precise as the subject and the circumstances of inquiry permit. Thus educating good critical thinkers means working toward this ideal. It combines developing CT skills with nurturing those dispositions that consistently yield useful insights and that are the basis of a rational and democratic society.

From American Philosophical Association: *Critical thinking: a statement of expert consensus for purposes of educational assessment and instruction, The Delphi report: research findings and recommendations prepared for the committee on pre-college philosophy,* 1990, ERIC Document Reproduction Services, pp 315-423.

assess the assumptions, implications, and consequences of alternative views of problems
• Communicates effectively with others as solutions to complex problems are formulated

The similarities are evident between Facione's and Paul and Elder's definitions: critical thinking is a process that requires disciplined engagement of the intellect to solve problems most effectively.

You may be asking, "What does this have to do with nursing?" The answer is very simple. Making good clinical judgments requires excellent critical thinking skills. For you as a practitioner of professional nursing responsible and accountable for your own decisions, the development of critical thinking skills is crucial as you provide nursing care for patients with increasingly complex conditions. Critical thinking skills provide the nurse with a powerful means of determining patient needs, interpreting physician orders, and intervening appropriately. Box 8-2 presents an example of the importance of critical thinking in the provision of safe care.

CRITICAL THINKING IN NURSING

You may be wondering at this point, "How am I ever going to learn how to make connections among all of the data I have about a patient?" This is a common response for a nursing student who is just learning some of the most basic psychomotor skills in preparation for practice. You need to understand that, just like learning to give injections safely and maintaining a sterile field properly, you can learn to think critically. This involves paying attention to how you think and making thinking itself a focus of concern. A nurse who is exercising critical thinking asks the following questions: "What assumptions have I made about this patient?" "How do I know my assumptions are accurate?" "Do I need any additional information?" and "How might I look at this situation differently?"

Nurses just beginning to pay attention to their thinking processes may ask these questions after nurse-patient interactions have ended. This is known as **reflective thinking**. This is the same process described in Chapter 5 about reflecting on ethical dilemmas that you encounter in practice. Reflective thinking is an active process valuable in learning and changing behaviors, perspectives, or practices. Nurses can also learn to examine their thinking processes during an interaction as they learn to "think on their feet." This is a characteristic of expert nurses. As you move from novice to expert, your ability to think critically will improve with practice. In Chapter 6 you read about Dr. Patricia Benner (1984, 1996), who studied the differences in expertise of nurses at different stages in their careers, from novice to expert. So it is with critical thinking; novices think differently than experts. Box 8-3 summarizes the differences in novice and expert thinking.

Box 8-2   Using Critical Thinking Skills to Improve a Patient's Care

Mr. Smith is a 77-year-old man admitted to your general medicine unit with several problems, including dehydration secondary to severe nausea and vomiting and a urinary tract infection. His medication orders include hydrochlorothiazide 50 mg q AM for mild hypertension, ampicillin 2 g q6 hours. His IV order is D_5LR at 125 mL/hour. His laboratory values show a serum potassium level of 2.6 mEq/L. You recognize that this is low. Mr. Smith seems weak and lethargic; his urine output has been 35 mL/hour for the past 2 hours. You are concerned about him and his condition.

A nurse using good critical thinking skills will note the following: the source of his dehydration, his antibiotic order for his UTI, his low potassium level, his IV rate, his low urinary output, and his daily use of a diuretic known to be associated with potassium loss. His lethargy and weakness could be a product of his age and general condition, but you also know that they are signs of hypokalemia. Critical thinking does not stop at noting these issues, however. Critical thinking requires making a judgment about what to do with your concerns. A nurse not using critical thinking may simply follow physician orders with the expectation that Mr. Smith will feel better once his dehydration is reversed and his UTI is adequately treated. Using your good critical thinking skills, however, you come to the conclusion that Mr. Smith may be better supported with a different approach to his care. You call his physician to discuss your concerns, describing in detail the "big picture." The specific, detailed information that you communicate clearly allows the physician to reconsider Mr. Smith's medical regimen and proceed from a more informed position. The next day you are pleased to see Mr. Smith walking in the hall when you come onto the unit at the beginning of your shift. He says that he feels "like a new person."

Box 8-3   Novice Thinking Compared With Expert Thinking

NOVICE NURSES

- Tend to organize knowledge as separate facts. Must rely heavily on resources (e.g., texts, notes, preceptors). Lack knowledge gained from actually doing (e.g., listening to breath sounds).
- Focus so much on actions that they tend to forget to assess before acting
- Need clear-cut rules
- Are often hampered by unawareness of resources
- Are often hindered by anxiety and lack of self-confidence
- Must be able to rely on step-by-step procedures. Tend to focus more on procedures than on the patient response to the procedure.
- Become uncomfortable if patient needs preclude performing procedures exactly as they were learned
- Have limited knowledge of suspected problems; therefore they question and collect data more superficially
- Tend to follow standards and policies by rote
- Learn more readily when matched with a supportive, knowledgeable preceptor or mentor

EXPERT NURSES

- Tend to store knowledge in a highly organized and structured manner, making recall of information easier. Have a large storehouse of experiential knowledge (e.g., what abnormal breath sounds sound like, what subtle changes look like).
- Assess and think things through before acting
- Know when to bend the rules
- Are aware of resources and how to use them
- Are usually more self-confident, less anxious, and therefore more focused
- Know when it is safe to skip steps or do two steps together. Are able to focus on both the parts (the procedures) and the whole (the patient response).
- Are comfortable with rethinking a procedure if patient needs require modification of the procedure

(Continued)

Box 8-3   Novice Thinking Compared With Expert Thinking—cont'd

• Have a better idea of suspected problems, allowing them to question more deeply and collect more relevant and in-depth data • Analyze standards and policies, looking for ways to improve them	• Are challenged by novices' questions, clarifying their own thinking when teaching novices

From Alfaro-LeFevre R: *Critical thinking in nursing: a practical approach*, ed 2, Philadelphia, 1999, WB Saunders. Reprinted with permission.

Box 8-4   Self-Assessment: Critical Thinking

Directions: Listed below are 15 characteristics of critical thinkers. Mark a plus sign (+) next to those you now possess, mark IP (in progress) next to those you have partially mastered, and mark a zero (0) next to those you have not yet mastered. When you are finished, make a plan for developing the areas that need improvement. Share it with at least one person, and report on progress weekly.

CHARACTERISTICS OF CRITICAL THINKERS: HOW DO YOU MEASURE UP?

_____ Inquisitive/curious/seeks truth
_____ Self-informed/finds own answers
_____ Analytic/confident in own reasoning skills
_____ Open-minded
_____ Flexible
_____ Fair-minded
_____ Honest about personal biases/self-aware
_____ Prudent/exercises sound judgment
_____ Willing to revise judgment when new evidence warrants
_____ Clear about issues
_____ Orderly in complex matters/organized approach to problems
_____ Diligent in seeking information
_____ Persistent
_____ Reasonable
_____ Focused on inquiry

Critical thinking in nursing, however, involves more than good problem-solving strategies. It is a complex, purposeful, disciplined process that has specific characteristics that make it different from run-of-the-mill problem solving. Consciously developed to improve patient outcomes, critical thinking by the nurse is driven by the needs of the patient and family. Critical thinking in nursing is undergirded by the standards and ethics of the profession. Nurses who think critically seek to build on patients' strengths while honoring patients' values and beliefs (Alfaro-LeFevre, 1999). They are engaged in a process of constant evaluation, redirection, improvement, and increased efficiency. Be aware that critical thinking involves far more than stating your opinion. You must be able to describe how you came to a conclusion and support your conclusions with explicit data and rationales. This is a different way of thinking for most people and requires practice. Dimensions of critical thinking include both cognitive skills and "habits of the mind" (Scheffer and Rubenfeld, 2000). Box 8-4 summarizes these characteristics and offers an opportunity for you to evaluate your progress as a critical thinker.

An excellent continuing education self-study module designed to improve your ability to think critically can be found online (http://www.nurse.com/ce/CE168-60/Improving-Your-Ability-to-Think-Critically/). Continuing one's education through lifelong learning is an excellent way to maintain and enhance your critical thinking skills. The website http://www.nurse.com has more than 500 continuing education opportunities available online and may be helpful to you as you seek to increase your knowledge base and

CRITICAL THINKING *Challenge 8-1*

Six Caps

This is an hour-long group activity designed to clarify the various types of thinking that constitute critical thinking. For every six participants, you will need six pieces of colored paper (one white, one red, one black, one yellow, one green, and one blue). You will also need six straight pins. Divide the group into smaller groups of six and give each group member a pin and piece of colored paper. Each person draws a cap on the paper and pins it to his or her shirt in plain view. These represent the six "thinking caps," that is, the various types of thinking to be explored:

White cap—Information. Asks the questions, "What information do we have, what is needed, and how can we get it?"

Red cap—Feelings, intuition, and emotion. Asks the questions, "What are we, the patient, and the family feeling, and how do we know?"

Black cap—Policies, codes, standards, protocols, laws. Asks the questions, "What are the standards we should consider, and what are the risks?"

Yellow cap—Optimism. Asks the questions, "What are the benefits, who benefits, and what are the values being expressed?"

Green cap—Growth. Asks the questions, "Why don't we try it this way?" and "What are some different alternatives?"

Blue cap—Focuses on thinking. Asks the questions, "How are we going to proceed in thinking through this situation?" and "What have we achieved and what do we want to achieve?"

Read the case study below (or one prepared by your teacher), and discuss it from the viewpoint of each "cap." Identify issues for reflection. Then switch "thinking caps." Discuss the case study again. How easy or difficult was it to change your type of thinking? Do some types of thinking come more naturally to you than others? Which ones will you have to work to develop? Do you see value in each type of thinking? When the group reconvenes, summarize what you have learned on a flip chart.

CASE STUDY FOR SIX CAPS

Marianne is a 79-year-old woman who was admitted to the emergency department yesterday with a severe headache. Shortly after admission, she became unresponsive; a brain scan revealed she had experienced a hemorrhagic stroke. Marianne's pupils are dilated and do not respond to light; she is breathing with the assistance of a respirator. Her elderly husband and three adult children are all assembled. The physician has recommended surgery to remove the blood clot but cannot offer much assurance that she will recover function. She has no advance directives, but her husband wants to "try everything." The children believe that she would not want to undergo this surgery only to be kept alive with poor quality of life, which they agree is the likely outcome. The ethics committee is assembled to assist the family in making the decision. Before meeting with the family, the committee meets to discuss the situation.

Modified from De Bono E: *Edward de Bono's mind pack,* London, 1995, Dorling-Kindersley; Kenney LJ: Using Edward de Bono's six hats game to aid critical thinking and reflection in palliative care, *Int J Palliat Nurs* 9(3):105-112, 2003.

improve your clinical judgment. In addition, you can also begin to learn about the many facets of critical thinking by participating with classmates in the Critical Thinking Challenge, Six Caps, below. This exercise will allow you to practice thinking through the various questions that need to be asked in response to very complex patient and family issues.

THE NURSING PROCESS: AN INTELLECTUAL STANDARD

Critical thinking requires systematic and disciplined use of universal intellectual standards (Paul and Elder, 2005). In the practice of nursing, the **nursing process** represents a universal intellectual standard by which problems are addressed and solved. The nursing process is a method of critical thinking focused on solving patient problems in professional practice. The nursing process is "a designated series of actions intended to fulfill the purposes of nursing" (Yura and Walsh, 1983).

A simple example of using a process approach to problem solving is illustrated by examining a daily decision that you and most other people face: how to dress for the day. Before putting on your clothes, there are several factors you need to consider. What is the expected temperature? Will it be clear, raining, or snowing? How much time will be spent outdoors? Are there any activities planned that require special dress? Next, you probably look at the possible clothing choices. Some clothes may be out of season, and others need repairs, are too dressy or casual, or do not fit quite right. After considering the environmental factors, the day's activities, and your mood, you select the day's clothing. After dressing, you may look in a mirror to evaluate how you look. You may then modify your outfit on the basis of your image in the mirror. At this point, you have solved the problem of clothing yourself. You have identified a problem, considered various factors related to the problem, identified possible actions, selected the best alternative, evaluated the success of the alternative selected, and made adjustments to the solution based on the evaluation. This is the same general process nurses use in solving patient problems through the nursing process.

For individuals outside the profession, nursing is commonly and simplistically defined in terms of tasks nurses perform (e.g., give injections). Many students get frustrated with activities and courses in nursing school that are not focused on these tasks, believing themselves that the tasks of nursing are nursing. Even within the profession, the intellectual basis of nursing practice was not articulated until the 1960s, when nursing educators and leaders began to identify and name the components of nursing's intellectual processes. This marked the beginning of the nursing process.

In the 1970s and 1980s, debate about the use of the term *diagnosis* began. Until then, diagnosis was considered to be within the scope of practice of physicians only. Although nurses were not equipped to diagnose medical conditions in patients, nurses recognized that there were human responses amenable to independent nursing intervention. These responses could be identified (diagnosed) through the careful application of specific defining characteristics. In 1973, the National Group for the Classification of Nursing Diagnosis published its first list of nursing diagnoses. This organization is now known as **NANDA International** (NANDA-I; NANDA is the acronym for North American Nursing Diagnosis Association). Its mission is to "facilitate the development, refinement, dissemination and use of standardized nursing diagnostic terminology" with the goal to "improve the health care of all people" (http://www.nanda.org). In December 2008, NANDA-I published its 2009-2011 edition of *Nursing Diagnoses: Definitions and Classifications*. Currently, NANDA-I has 206 diagnoses approved for clinical testing and has recently added 21 new diagnoses and 9 revised diagnoses. Some of the new diagnoses include "impaired comfort," "dysfunctional gastrointestinal motility," and "ineffective peripheral tissue perfusion." Diagnoses are also retired if it becomes evident that their usefulness is limited or outdated, such as the newly retired diagnosis "disturbed thought processes."

Here is a simple example of how one of the newly approved nursing diagnoses may be used:

> *Two days after a surgery for a large but benign abdominal mass, Mr. Pierce has not yet been able to tolerate solid food and has diminished bowel sounds. His abdomen is somewhat distended. Your diagnosis is that Mr. Pierce has dysfunctional gastrointestinal motility. This diagnosis is based on NANDA-I's (2008) taxonomy because you have determined that the risk factors and physical signs and symptoms associated with this diagnosis apply to him.*

A more detailed discussion of nursing diagnosis is located in the next section of this chapter.

The nursing process as a method of clinical problem solving is taught in schools of nursing across the United States, and many states refer to it in their nurse practice acts. The nursing process has sometimes been the subject of criticism among nurses. In recent years some nursing leaders have questioned the use of the nursing process, describing it as linear, rigid, and mechanistic. They believe that the nursing process contributes to linear thinking and stymies critical thinking. They are concerned that the nursing process format, and rigid faculty adherence to it, encourages students to copy from published sources when writing care plans, thus inhibiting the development of a holistic, creative approach to patient care (Mueller, Johnston, and Bligh, 2002). Certainly the nursing process can be taught, learned, and used in a rigid, mechanistic, and linear manner. Ideally, the nursing process is used as a creative approach to thinking and decision making in nursing. Because the nursing process is an integral aspect of nursing education, practice, standards, and practice acts nationwide, learning to use it as a mechanism for critical thinking and as a dynamic and creative approach to patient care is a worthwhile endeavor. Despite reservations among some nurses about its use, the nursing process remains the cornerstone of nursing standards, legal definitions, and practice and, as such, should be well understood by every nurse.

PHASES OF THE NURSING PROCESS

Like many frameworks for thinking through problems, the nursing process is a series of organized steps, the purpose of which is to impose some discipline and critical thinking on the provision of excellent care. Identifying specific steps makes the process clear and concrete but can cause nurses to use them rigidly. Keep in mind that this is a process, that progression through the process may not be linear, and that it is a tool to use, not a road map to follow rigidly. More creative use of the nursing process may occur by expert nurses who have a greater repertoire of interventions from which to select. For example, if a newly hospitalized patient is experiencing a great deal of pain, a novice nurse might proceed by asking family members to leave so that he or she can provide a quiet environment in which the patient may rest. An expert nurse would realize that the family may be a source of distraction from the pain or may be a source of comfort in ways that the nurse may not be able to provide. The expert nurse, in addition to assessing the patient, is willing to consider alternative explanations and interventions, enhancing the possibility that the patient's pain will be relieved.

Phase 1: Assessment

Assessment is the initial phase or operation in the nursing process. During this phase, information or data about the individual patient, family, or community are gathered. Data may include physiologic, psychological, sociocultural, developmental, spiritual, and environmental information. The patient's available financial or material resources also need to be assessed and recorded in a standard format; each institution usually has a slightly different method of recording assessment data.

Types of data

Nurses obtain two types of data about and from patients: subjective and objective. Subjective data are obtained from patients as they describe their needs, feelings, strengths, and perceptions of the problem. Subjective data are frequently referred to as symptoms. Examples of subjective data are statements such as, "I am in pain" and "I don't have much energy." The only source for these data is the patient. Subjective data should include physical, psychosocial, and spiritual information. Subjective data can be very private. Nurses must be sensitive to the patient's need for confidence in the nurse's trustworthiness.

Objective data are the other types of data that the nurse will collect through observation, examination, or consultation with other health care providers. These data are measurable, such as pulse rate and blood pressure, and include observable patient behaviors. Objective data are frequently called signs. An example of objective data that a nurse might gather includes the observation that the patient, who is lying in bed, is diaphoretic, pale, and tachypneic, clutching his hands to his chest.

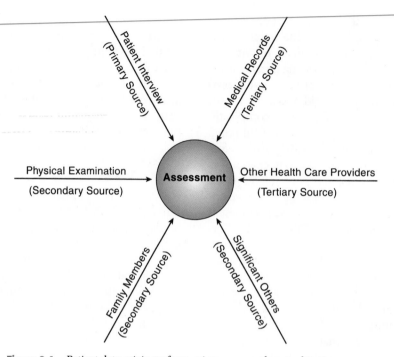

Figure 8-1   Patient data originate from primary, secondary, and tertiary sources.

Objective data and subjective data usually are congruent; that is, they usually are in agreement. In the situation just mentioned, if the patient told the nurse, "I feel like a rock is crushing my chest," the subjective data would substantiate the nurse's observations (objective data) that the patient is having chest pain. Occasionally subjective and objective data are in conflict. A stark example of incongruent subjective and objective data well-known to labor and delivery nurses is when a pregnant woman in labor describes ongoing fetal activity (subjective data); however, there are no fetal heart tones (objective data), and the infant is stillborn. Incongruent objective and subjective data require further careful assessment to ascertain the patient's situation more completely and accurately. Sometimes incongruent data reveal something about the patient's concerns and fears. To get a clearer picture of the patient's situation, the nurse should use the best communication skills he or she possesses to increase the patient's trust, which will result in more openness.

Sources of patient data

Patient data can be obtained from many sources (Figure 8-1). The patient is considered the only **primary source**. Sources of data such as the nurse's own observations or reports of family and friends of the patient are considered **secondary sources**. **Tertiary sources** of data include medical records and information gathered from other health care providers such as physical therapists, physicians, or dietitians.

Methods of collecting patient data

A number of methods are used when collecting patient data. The patient interview is a primary means of obtaining both subjective and objective data. The interview typically involves a face-to-face interaction with the patient that requires the nurse to use the skills of interviewing, observation, and listening (Figure 8-2). Many factors influence the quality of the interview, including the physical environment in which the interaction occurs. If the patient is not in a private room,

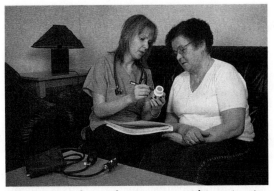

Figure 8-2 A face-to-face interview with a patient is a primary means of collecting data and requires good interviewing skills, observation, and listening.

the open exchange of information may not occur easily. Sometimes the presence of family members constrains the flow of information from a patient, especially when dealing with sensitive or private issues. Similarly, if an interview takes place in a cold, noisy, or public place, the type of data obtained may be affected by environmental distractions. Internal factors related to the patient's condition may influence the amount and the type of data obtained. For example, when interviewing a patient who is having difficulty breathing, the verbal data obtained by the interview may be limited, but careful observation and attentive listening can yield much information about the patient's condition.

Physical examination is the second method for obtaining data. Nurses use physical assessment techniques of inspection, auscultation, percussion, and palpation to obtain these data. A third method of obtaining data is through consultation. Consultation is discussing patient needs with health care workers and others who are directly involved in the care of the patient. Nurses also consult with patients' families to obtain background information and their perceptions about the patients' needs.

Organizing patient data

Once patient data have been collected, they must be sorted or organized. A number of methods have been developed to assist nurses in organizing

patient data. Abdellah's 21 nursing problems, Henderson's 14 nursing problems, Yura and Walsh's human needs approach, and Gordon's 11 functional health patterns are commonly used frameworks for collecting and organizing patient data. Contemporary nursing theorists continue to develop other organizing frameworks, including those of Madeleine Leininger, Sister Callista Roy, Dorothy Orem, and others you will read about in Chapter 13. Nurses choose different methods of organizing patient data depending on personal preference and the method used in the agencies where they are employed.

Confidentiality of patient data

A word of caution is needed in regard to patient data. Earlier, it was mentioned that patients confide personal information to nurses only if they believe the nurse is trustworthy. Patients need to know and trust that nurses share such information only with the other treatment team members. Nurses must respect patients' privacy rights and should never discuss patient information with anyone who does not have a work-related need to know. This is not only an ethical issue but also a legal issue. Patients' privacy is now protected by Federal law (see Health Insurance Portability and Accountability Act [HIPAA] on page 89).

Ensuring patients' privacy is complicated in that vast amounts of patient data may be stored digitally and retrieved relatively easily. Although the issues of confidentiality and access to electronically stored data have yet to be fully resolved, each nurse should be entrusted never to violate a patient's privacy by revealing patient information except to other members of that patient's treatment team.

Phase 2: Analysis and Identification of the Problem

During the data-gathering phase of the nursing process, nurses obtain a great deal of information about their patients. These data must first be validated and then compared with norms to sort out data that might indicate a problem or identify a pattern. Next, the data must be clustered or grouped so that problems can be identified and their cause discerned. Knowledge from the science of nursing, biologic sciences, and social sciences enables nurses to observe relationships among various pieces of patient data. This process is known as data analysis and results in the identification of one or more problems that are amenable to nursing intervention. The problems are often characterized as nursing diagnoses. In 1976, Gordon defined nursing diagnosis as "actual or potential health problems which nurses, by virtue of their education and experience, are capable and licensed to treat" (p. 1299). In 1990, NANDA defined nursing diagnosis as making "a clinical judgment about individual, family, or community responses to actual or potential health problems/life processes (which) provide the basis for selection of nursing interventions to achieve outcomes for which the nurse is accountable."

Distinctions between medical and nursing diagnosis

Nursing diagnosis is different from medical diagnosis and was never intended to be a substitute for it. Rather than focusing on what is wrong with the patient in terms of a disease process, a nursing diagnosis identifies the problems the patient is experiencing as a result of the disease process, that is, the human responses to the illness, injury, or threat.

An important difference between nursing diagnosis and medical diagnosis is that nursing diagnoses address patient problems that nurses can treat within their scope of practice. Proponents of nursing diagnosis argue that it does little good for nursing diagnoses to include "appendicitis" because appendicitis is a medical diagnosis requiring surgery, and nurses may not perform surgery. A nursing diagnosis for a patient after an appendectomy might be "ineffective airway clearance related to incisional pain." Because it is within the scope of practice in all states for nurses to provide comfort measures and to assist patients to cough and deep breathe, this would be an appropriate nursing diagnosis that is remedied by nursing interventions. The medical diagnosis becomes a platform from which nursing diagnoses are developed: a patient with a new medical diagnosis of diabetes will have some very specific

nursing diagnoses and interventions based on the requirements of the medical condition (diabetes) that caused the patient to seek care.

Although nursing diagnosis is still used in nursing, it does not have universal support among various constituencies of the discipline and profession. Critics believe that the language of nursing diagnosis obscures rather than clarifies patient problems. This causes confusion between disciplines involved in care of patients. For instance, Mr. Pierce, in the earlier example, may have a simple postoperative ileus. This is a medical diagnosis, but its management has important implications for nursing. The nursing diagnosis "dysfunctional gastrointestinal motility related to decreased motor activity status post abdominal surgery," with its accompanying "impaired comfort related to intolerance of medications" is a very long way of saying that Mr. Pierce has an ileus, has not been moving around, is in pain and not tolerating his medications. This more streamlined description of Mr. Pierce's clinical condition is recognizable across disciplines, and the implications for nursing management remain the same. In 2008, the American Association of Colleges of Nursing (AACN) issued an executive summary, "The Essentials of Baccalaureate Education for Professional Nursing Practice," which is described in Chapter 7. This summary emphasizes patient-centered care in interprofessional teams, which requires excellent communication across disciplines. Particular emphasis is placed on the translation of evidence into practice. Nursing diagnosis is not mentioned among the nine essentials. The complete summary can be found on the AACN website (http://www.aacn.nche.edu/Publications/positions/index.htm).

Despite a new focus on evidence-based practice, the need for interdisciplinary collaboration, and interprofessional teamwork, many schools of nursing still teach NANDA-I nursing diagnoses, and many advanced practice nurses use them in their own practices. NANDA-approved nursing diagnoses consist of five components (NANDA, 2003, pp. 263-264):

1. *Label:* Concise term or phrase that names the diagnosis

2. *Definition:* Term or phrase that clearly delineates meaning and helps differentiate from similar diagnoses
3. *Defining characteristics:* Clusters of observable cues or inferences
4. *Risk factors:* Factors that increase vulnerability to an unhealthful event
5. *Related factors:* Factors that precede, are associated with, or relate to the diagnosis

All nursing diagnoses must be supported by data, which NANDA-I refers to as defining characteristics, also known as signs and symptoms. Remember that a sign is observable and is objective, whereas a symptom is reported by the patient and is subjective. An easy way to understand the difference is to remember the difference between the words in the commonly used phrase "nausea and vomiting." Nausea is a subjective report of a specific feeling by a patient but is not directly observable by the nurse. Vomiting, on the other hand, is objective, verifiable, and quantifiable. It is a clear sign that the patient's report of nausea (a symptom) was correct.

Accurate diagnosis of human responses is very important. All nursing actions flow from the diagnosis, and inaccurate diagnoses can lead to lost time and wasted resources and may endanger the patient. Accuracy of diagnosis is a professional behavior, one of nursing's accountabilities (Lunney, 2001). Lunney (2008) wrote an appeal to nurses in practice and education to address this issue of diagnostic accuracy based on research findings that there is a need for more diagnostic consistency among nurses, that the issue of accuracy will always be present because of the complexities of nursing, and that electronic health records make the issue of accuracy of diagnosis even more broad-based.

Writing NANDA-I nursing diagnoses. A format used to write the diagnostic statement, called the PES format (Box 8-5), was developed by Gordon (1987). In this format, the *P* stands for the concise description of the problem, using the NANDA-I diagnostic label, for example, "ineffective breathing pattern."

Box 8-5   Writing Nursing Diagnoses

P = Problem (NANDA-I diagnostic label)
E = Etiology (causal factors)
S = Signs and symptoms (defining characteristics)

The *E* part of the statement stands for etiology, or cause, and begins with the words "related to." These related factors are conditions or circumstances that can cause or contribute to the development of the problem. To extend the previous example, "ineffective breathing pattern related to anxiety," explains the cause of the ineffective breathing pattern as the patient's high anxiety level. The etiology part of the statement is important, because if the cause were decreased energy or fatigue rather than anxiety, the nurse would need to select different nursing actions to solve the problem. A diagnosis may be technically correct, but, if the etiology is incorrect, interventions are likely to be ineffective. In early 2009, NANDA-I issued a position statement that the "related to" field in nursing diagnosis is an effective teaching strategy but may be too complex to be practical in clinical practice. Hence its new position is that just the diagnostic label may be acceptable. NANDA-I also notes in this statement that some electronic care plan systems may not be amenable to the inclusion of "related to" factors (http://www.nanda.org).

The last part of the diagnostic statement is *S*, which stands for signs and symptoms, or as NANDA-I refers to them, "defining characteristics." Thus the complete diagnostic statement for our sample diagnosis might be "ineffective breathing patterns related to anxiety as manifested by dyspnea, nasal flaring, use of accessory muscles to breathe, and respiratory rate of 24/minute." Some nurses use the phrase "as evidenced by" or "AEB" to preface to the list of defining characteristics.

Prioritizing nursing diagnoses

After diagnoses are identified, the nurse must put them in order of priority. Two common frameworks are used to establish priorities. One of these considers the relative danger to the patient.

With use of this framework, diagnoses that are life threatening are the nurse's first priority. Next are those that have the potential to cause harm or injury. Last in priority are those diagnoses that are related to the overall general health of the patient. Thus a diagnosis of "ineffective airway clearance" would be dealt with before "sleep pattern disturbance," and "sleep pattern disturbance" could have priority over "knowledge deficit."

Another framework used to prioritize diagnoses is Maslow's (1970) hierarchy of needs (refer to Chapter 12, Figure 12-2). When this framework is used, there is an inverse relationship between high-priority nursing diagnoses and high-level needs. In other words, highest priority is given to diagnoses related to basic physiologic needs. Diagnoses related to higher-level needs such as love and belonging or self-esteem, although important, have priority only after basic physiologic needs are met.

Except in life-threatening situations, nurses should take care to involve patients in identifying priority diagnoses. Because varied sociocultural factors have a great impact on the manner in which patients prioritize problems, nurses must be aware of these factors and take them into consideration when planning patient care. The nurse's own cultural perspective must not take priority over that of the patient in determining priorities. For example, many maternity nurses are very strong proponents of breast-feeding and consider it one of their priorities in assisting new mothers to establish effective breast-feeding patterns. However, for some women, breast-feeding is not a cultural norm or a desirable outcome of new motherhood. Although it may be difficult to understand for the maternity nurse who has expertise in the benefits of breast-feeding, imposing the nurse's cultural and professional perspective on the patient is unacceptable and can lead to diminished effectiveness of nursing care in other domains in which the new mother needs assistance.

Box 8-6 Bloom's Taxonomy

A taxonomy is a classification system. Bloom, an educator, described types of learning in terms of domains of educational activities. This taxonomy is helpful for nursing:

- **Psychomotor domain:** Involves physical movement and increasingly complex activities in the motor-skill arena. Learning in this domain can be assessed by measures such as distance, time, and speed.
  - **Nursing goal:** Patient will move from bed to chair 3 times today without assistance.
- **Cognitive domain:** Involves knowledge and intellectual skills. Cognitive skills range from simple recall to complex tasks such as synthesis and evaluation.
  - **Nursing goal:** Patient will list five signs of illness in her newborn infant by the date of hospital discharge.
- **Affective domain:** Involves the emotions, such as feelings, values, and attitudes.
  - **Nursing goal:** Patient will describe feeling more accepting of new colostomy within 1 week of providing ostomy self-care.

Setting nursing goals using Bloom's taxonomy is a simple way to address three important domains of the patient's needs. A single patient is likely to have goals in each of these domains.

Modified from Facione PA: Critical thinking: a statement of expert consensus for purposes of educational assessment and instruction, "The Delphi Report," Milbrae, Calif, 1990, The California Academic Press.

Phase 3: Planning

Planning is the third phase in the nursing process. Planning begins with identification of patient goals and determination of ways to reach those goals. Goals are used by the patient and the nurse to guide the selection of interventions and to evaluate patient progress. Bloom's taxonomy (as described by Clark, 2001) (Box 8-6) provides a simple description of domains of learning that drive the development of patient goals: psychomotor, cognitive, and affective goals. This taxonomy identified domains of educational activities that are well suited to nursing.

Just as nursing diagnoses are written in collaboration with the patient, goals should also be agreed on by both nurse and patient unless collaboration is impossible, such as when the patient has an altered mental status, is a young child, or is incapacitated in some way. In that event, family members or significant others can collaborate with the nurse. Goals give the patient, family, significant others, and nurse direction and make them active partners.

Writing patient goals and outcomes

The terms *goal* and *objective* are frequently used interchangeably. Note that the word *objective* is used differently here than its earlier use, when it was used as an adjective describing observable and measurable data. In terms of outcomes, the word *objective* is a noun and means a goal or specific aim of intervention. Goals or objectives are statements of what is to be accomplished and are derived from the diagnoses. Because the problem or diagnosis is written as a patient problem, the goal should also be stated in terms of what the patient will do rather than what the nurse will do. The goal begins with the words "the patient will" or "the patient will be able to." The goal sets a general direction, includes an action verb, and should be both attainable and realistic for the patient.

Outcome criteria are specific and make the goal measurable. Outcome criteria define the terms under which the goal is said to be met, partially met, or unmet. Each diagnosis has at least one patient goal, and each patient goal may have several outcome criteria. Effective outcome criteria state under what conditions, to what extent, and in what time frame the patient is to act. For the postoperative patient who had an abdominal procedure, a sample patient goal with outcome criteria might be, "The patient will have effective bowel elimination as evidenced by having one soft, formed stool every other day without the use of laxatives or enemas within 2 weeks." It is easy to see that this goal is written in terms of what the patient will do (have a bowel movement at least every other day), is measurable (one soft, formed stool), gives conditions (without the use of laxatives or enemas), and has a specified time frame for accomplishment (2 weeks).

Establishing a time frame for patient goals to be met is important. Short-term goals may be attainable within hours or days. They are usually specific and are small steps leading to the achievement of broader, long-term goals. For example, "The patient will lose 2 pounds" is a short-term goal, and the time limit for accomplishment can be brief, perhaps a week or 10 days. Long-term goals, however, usually represent major changes or rehabilitation. A goal such as "The patient will lose 75 pounds" may take months or perhaps even years to accomplish, and the time frame should be set accordingly. Setting realistic goals in terms of both outcomes and time is extremely important. Frustration and discouragement can occur when goals are unrealistic in outcomes or time.

The nurse can be a good resource for helping patients in determining accessible goals. For example, assume that your patient is a young man with a severely injured thigh and knee from a single-car automobile accident. The injury will require several orthopedic surgeries. To complicate matters, he has a nosocomial (hospital-acquired) infection in his surgical site. One day, he mentions to you that his goal is to run a marathon within a year. Running a marathon is a worthy goal and is reachable eventually for this young man. However, as his nurse, you recognize the importance of setting some short-term goals right now that will improve his health and better the chances of achieving his goal of running a marathon. Your care plan should reflect the short-term, attainable goals (such as walking with a walker the length of the hallway twice a day) that he needs to reach in the meantime that will move him toward his long-term, personal goal.

Cultural congruency is an important consideration in setting patient goals and selecting interventions. A culturally congruent intervention is one that is developed within the broad social, cultural, and demographic context of the patient's life. The patient is more likely to benefit from an intervention that is tailored to his or her specific sociocultural needs and interests. Although cultural congruency is an important element to effective intervention, the nurse must take care not to stereotype patients or assume that "all _____" (fill in the blank) like the same things, will react the same way, or respond to the same intervention. The Cultural Considerations Challenge on p. 184

✳ Cultural Considerations Challenge
Impact of Culture on Nursing Interventions

From the Association of Black Nursing Faculty website (http://www.abnf.net):

"The purpose of the Association of Black Nursing Faculty, Inc, (ABNF) is to form and maintain a group whereby Black professional nurses with similar credentials, interests and concerns may work to promote certain health-related issues and educational interests for the benefit of themselves and the Black community."

An example of the interests and work that have developed from the ABNF is found in The ABNF Journal, published six times each year. Volume 17 (1) in 2006 was dedicated to the issue of breast cancer in African-American women. The research article "Getting Ready: Developing an Educational Intervention to Prepare African American Women for Breast Biopsy" describes the efforts to produce intervention materials for African-American women preparing to undergo breast biopsies. African-American women are more likely to die of breast cancer than are white American women, although fewer black women than white women have a diagnosis of breast cancer. This is a source of great concern in the African-American

community and among researchers, who are trying to determine why this is the case. Theresa Swift-Scanlan, PhD, RN, whose research is highlighted in Chapter 11, is examining the epigenetics of breast cancer. It is her hope that this health disparity can be eliminated completely through research to determine why African-American women have a worse prognosis in breast cancer.

In the Implications section at the end of the article, the authors refer to the cultural appropriateness of study materials to be used in an intervention. As you read this article, consider these questions:

1. In addition to ethnicity, can you think of other ways that interventions should be made culturally appropriate?
2. What might happen if an intervention is not culturally appropriate?
3. Who determines what is and is not culturally appropriate?

You can find the article here:

Bradley PK, Berry A, Lang C, Myers RE: Getting ready: developing an educational intervention to prepare African American women for breast biopsy, The ABFN Journal (17)1:15-19, 2006.

describes a research report explaining the importance of having culturally appropriate educational materials to prepare African American women for their breast biopsies.

Selecting interventions and writing nursing orders

After short-term and long-term goals are identified through collaboration between nurse and patient, the nurse writes nursing orders. **Nursing orders** are actions designed to assist the patient in achieving a stated goal. Every goal has specific nursing orders, which may be carried out by a registered nurse (RN) or delegated to other members of the nursing staff.

Nursing orders and medical orders differ. Nursing orders refer to interventions that are designed to treat the patient's response to an

illness or medical treatment, whereas medical orders are designed to treat the actual illness or disease. An example of a nursing order is "Teach turning, coughing, and deep-breathing exercises prior to surgery." These activities are designed to prevent postoperative respiratory problems caused by immobility. They are appropriate nursing orders because prevention of complications due to immobility is a nursing responsibility. Nursing orders may include instructions about consultation with other health care providers, such as the dietitian, physical therapist, or pharmacist.

Types of nursing interventions. Nursing interventions are of three basic types: independent, dependent, or interdependent. **Independent interventions** are those for which the nurse's intervention requires no supervision or direction by others. Nurses are expected to possess the knowledge and skills to carry out independent actions safely. An example of an independent nursing intervention is teaching a patient how to examine her breasts for lumps. The nurse practice act of each state usually specifies general types of independent nursing actions.

Dependent interventions do require instructions, written orders, or supervision of another health professional with prescriptive authority. These actions require knowledge and skills on the part of the nurse but may not be done without explicit directions. An example of a dependent nursing intervention is the administration of medications. Although a physician or advanced practice nurse must order medications in inpatient settings, it is the responsibility of the nurse to know how to administer them safely and to monitor their effectiveness. The nurse also must question orders that he or she feels are incongruent with safe care or are not within accepted standards of care.

The third type, interdependent interventions, includes actions in which the nurse must collaborate or consult with another health professional before carrying out the action. One example of this type of action is the nurse implementing orders that have been written by a physician in a protocol. Protocols define under what conditions and circumstances a nurse is allowed to treat the patient, as well as what treatments are permissible. They are used in situations in which nurses need to take immediate action without consulting with a physician, such as in an emergency department, a critical care unit, or a home setting.

Writing the plan of care

Once interventions are selected, a written plan of care is devised. Some health care agencies use individually developed plans of care for their patients. The nurse creates and develops a plan for each patient. Others use standardized plans of care that are based on common and recurring problems. The nurse then individualizes these standard plans of care. An advantage of using standardized plans is that they can decrease the

time spent in generating a completely new plan each time a patient is seen. These plans are easily computer generated, with the nurse making selections from menus to individualize the plan to the particular patient. The amount of time needed to update and document these plans is then vastly decreased. Computer use also facilitates data collection for research.

Because of the decreasing average length of stay for patients in health care facilities, the increasing focus on achieving timely patient outcomes in the specific time frame permitted by reimbursement systems, and the emphasis by accrediting bodies on multidisciplinary care, many agencies adopted the use of multidisciplinary plans of care known as critical paths, care tracks, or care maps. Critical paths have been replaced with other types of multidisciplinary care plans in some settings. Multidisciplinary care plans are written in collaboration with physicians and other health care providers and establish a sequence of short-term daily outcomes that are easily measured. This type of care planning facilitates communication and collaboration among all members of the health care team. It also permits comparisons of outcomes between treatment plans, as well as among health care facilities. As with the nursing process, unyielding adherence to the critical path without taking a patient's idiosyncratic responses into consideration can negatively affect patient outcomes and is a detriment to successful nursing care.

The development of appropriate plans of care depends on the nurse's ability to employ critical thinking. Nurses must be able to analyze information and arguments, make reasoned decisions, recognize many viewpoints, and question and seek answers continuously. At the same time, nurses must be logical, flexible, and creative and take initiative while considering the holistic nature of each patient.

Phase 4: Implementation of Planned Interventions

Implementation, the fourth phase or operation of the nursing process, occurs when nursing orders are actually carried out. Most people think of nursing as "doing something" for or to a patient. Notice, however, that in using the nursing process, nurses do a great deal of thinking, analyzing, and planning before the first actual nursing action takes place.

Professional nurses understand the crucial nature of the first three phases of the nursing process in ensuring that safe and appropriate care occurs. Nurses who forgo these essential phases and move immediately into action are not providing care in a responsible, professional manner. Patients feel a greater sense of trust in nurses who are providing care when dependent, independent, and interdependent orders are planned and carried out in an orderly, competent manner. Common nursing interventions include such actions as managing pain, preventing postoperative complications, educating patients, and performing procedures (such as wound care and catheter insertion) that are ordered by other health care providers. As the nurse carries out planned interventions, he or she is continually assessing the patient, noting responses to nursing interventions, and modifying the care plan or adding nursing diagnoses as needed. Documentation of nursing actions is an integral part of the implementation phase.

Phase 5: Evaluation

Evaluation is the final phase of the nursing process. In this phase, the nurse examines the patient's progress in relation to the goals and outcome criteria to determine whether a problem is resolved, is in the process of being resolved, or is unresolved. In other words, the outcome criteria are the basis for evaluation of the goal. Evaluation may reveal that data, diagnosis, goals, and nursing interventions were all on target and that the problem is resolved.

Evaluation may also indicate a need for a change in the plan of care. Perhaps inadequate patient data were the basis for the plan, and further assessment has uncovered additional needs. The nursing diagnoses may have been incorrect or placed in the wrong order of priority. Patient goals may have been inappropriate or unattainable within the designated time frame. It is

possible that nursing actions were incorrectly implemented.

Evaluation is a critical phase in the nursing process and one that is often slighted. The best nursing care plan is one that is evaluated frequently and changed in response to the patient's condition. Sometimes a care plan will reflect all of the most common nursing interventions used to treat specific diagnoses; it is not enough, however, to continue to do the "right things" if the patient is not improving in the expected manner. If, on evaluation, the problem is not resolving in a timely way or will not resolve at all, the nursing care plan must be revised to reflect the necessary changes.

DYNAMIC NATURE OF THE NURSING PROCESS

Although the phases in the nursing process are discussed separately here, in practice they are not so clearly delineated nor do they always proceed from one to another in a linear fashion. The nursing process (Figure 8-3) is dynamic, meaning that nurses are continuously moving from one phase to another and then beginning the process again. Often a nurse performs two or more phases at the same time, for instance, observing a wound for signs of infection (assessment) while changing the dressing on the wound (intervention) and asking the patient the extent

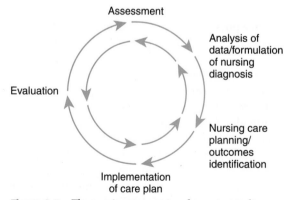

Figure 8-3 The nursing process is a dynamic, nonlinear tool for critical thinking about human responses.

to which pain has been relieved by comfort measures (evaluation).

Now that you have read about the phases of the nursing process, we will look back at the opening scenario. The problem that was identified was the necessity to wear appropriate clothing. Data, both objective (the temperature outdoors) and subjective (the mood one is in), were gathered. Selection was made and implemented, and an evaluation of the implementation was carried out by looking in the mirror. This comparison reveals that problem solving is something each person does every day. The use of the nursing process simply provides professional nurses with a patient-oriented framework with which to solve clinical problems.

An example of using the nursing process in a high-priority clinical situation is described in Box 8-7. This case study demonstrates how using the nursing process becomes so natural

---

Box 8-7   Nursing Process Case Study of a High-Priority Diagnosis

You have just received a report from the day shift about Mr. Burkes. You were told that he had been admitted with a diagnosis of cancer of the tongue and that he had a radical neck dissection yesterday. He has a tracheostomy and requires frequent suctioning of his secretions. He is alert and responds by nodding his head or writing short notes.

When you enter his room, you note that he is apprehensive and tachypneic and is gesturing for you to come into the room. You auscultate his lungs and note coarse crackles and expiratory wheezes. You can see thick secretions bubbling out of his tracheostomy. He has poor cough effort.

On the basis of these data, you realize that a priority nursing diagnosis is ineffective airway clearance. You immediately prepare to perform tracheal suctioning. As you are suctioning, you watch the patient's nonverbal responses and note that he is less apprehensive when the suctioning is completed. You also auscultate the lungs and note that there are decreased crackles and that the expiratory wheezes are no longer present. Mr. Burkes writes "I can breathe now" on his note pad.

I. Assessment
   A. Subjective data
      1. None because of inability to speak
   B. Objective data
      1. Tracheostomy with copious, thick secretions
      2. Tachypnea
      3. Gesturing for help
      4. Coarse crackles and expiratory wheezes
      5. Poor cough effort

II. Analysis
   A. Ineffective airway clearance related to copious, thick secretions
III. Plan
   A. Short-term goal: Patient will maintain patent airway as evidenced by absence of expiratory wheezes and crackles, decreased signs of anxiety and air hunger.
   B. Long-term goal: Patient will have patent airway as evidenced by his ability to clear the airway without the use of suctioning by the time of discharge.
IV. Implementation
   A. Assess lung sounds every hour for crackles and wheezes.
   B. Suction airway as needed.
   C. Elevate head of bed to 45 degrees.
   D. Teach patient abdominal breathing techniques.
   E. Encourage patient to cough out secretions.
V. Evaluation
   A. Short-term goal: Achieved as evidenced by decreased crackles and absent wheezes when auscultating the lungs; patient appears less anxious, indicated by writing that he "can breathe now"
   B. Long-term goal: Will be evaluated before discharge

that experienced nurses go through the phases fluidly and automatically. Although no responsible nurse would take the time to write out this care plan in advance of acting on a diagnosis of "ineffective airway clearance," you should understand that the nursing process is exactly the same for those high-priority nursing situations that require immediate action and those that will evolve over time.

DEVELOPING CLINICAL JUDGMENT IN NURSING

Becoming an effective nurse involves more than critical thinking and the ability to use the nursing process. It depends heavily on developing excellent clinical judgment. Clinical judgment consists of informed opinions and decisions based on empirical knowledge and experience. Nurses develop clinical judgment gradually as they gain a broader, deeper knowledge base and clinical experience. Extensive direct patient contact is the best means of developing clinical judgment.

Critical thinking and clinical reasoning used in the nursing process are both important aspects of clinical judgment. A nurse who has developed sound clinical judgment knows what to look for (e.g., elevation of temperature in a surgical patient), draws valid conclusions about possible alternative meanings of signs and symptoms (e.g., postoperative infection, atelectasis, dehydration), and knows what to do about it (e.g., listen to breath sounds, assess for dehydration, check incision for redness and drainage, seek another opinion, notify the physician). Developing sound clinical judgment requires recalling facts, recognizing patterns in patient behaviors, putting facts and observations together to form a meaningful whole, and acting on the resulting information in an appropriate way.

Knowing the limitations of your expertise is an important aspect of clinical judgment. Most nurses have an instinctive awareness of when they are approaching the limits of their expertise and will seek consultation with other professionals as needed. Your state's nurse practice act, health agency policies, school policies, and the professions' standards of practice all provide guidance in making the decision about nursing actions within your scope of practice. Nursing students, whether new to nursing or RNs in baccalaureate programs, must consider policies and standards in determining their scope of practice in any given nursing situation.

Box 8-8   **Clinical Judgment: Nine Key Questions**

1. **What major outcomes (observable beneficial results) do we expect to see in this particular person, family, or group when the plan of care is terminated?** Example: The person will be discharged without complications, able to care for himself, 3 days after surgery. Outcomes may be addressed on a standard plan, or you may have to develop these outcomes yourself. Make sure any predetermined outcomes in standard plans are appropriate to your patient's specific situation.
2. **What problems or issues must be addressed to achieve the major outcomes?** Answering this question will help you prioritize. You may have a long list of actual or potential health problems needing to be structured to set your priorities.
3. **What are the circumstances?** Who is involved (e.g., child, adult, group)? How urgent are the problems (e.g., life threatening, chronic)? What are the factors influencing their presentation (e.g., when, where, and how did the problems develop)? What are the patient's values, beliefs, and cultural influences?
4. **What knowledge is required?** You must know problem-specific facts (e.g., how problems usually present, how they are diagnosed, what their common causes and risk factors

Box 8-8   Clinical Judgment: Nine Key Questions—cont'd

are, what common complications occur, and how these complications are prevented and managed); nursing process and related knowledge and skills (e.g., ethics, research, health assessment, communication, priority setting); related sciences (e.g., anatomy, physiology, pathophysiology, pharmacology, chemistry, physics, psychology, sociology). You must also be clearly aware of the circumstances, as addressed in question 3 above.

5. **How much room is there for error?** In the clinical setting, there is usually minimal room for error. However, it depends on the health of the individual and the risks of interventions. A healthy, young postoperative patient with no chronic illnesses may tolerate early mobility after surgery better than an elderly person with a history of multiple chronic problems requiring numerous medications. Although their orders for postoperative ambulation may be identical and your commitment to their safe care exactly the same for these two patients, excellent clinical judgment based on your assessments allows you to conclude that the young patient is safe walking in the hallway with a family member, whereas the elderly patient needs your assistance and guidance during early ambulation.

6. **How much time do I have?** Time frame for decision making depends on (1) the urgency of the problems (e.g., there is little time in life-threatening situations, such as cardiac arrest) and (2) the planned length of contact (e.g., if your patient will be hospitalized only for 2 days, you have to be realistic about what can be accomplished, and key decisions need to be made early).

7. **What resources can help me?** Human resources include clinical nurse educators, nursing faculty, preceptors, experienced nurses, advanced practice nurses, peers, librarians, and other health care professionals (such as pharmacists, nutritionists, physical therapists, physicians). The patient and family are also valuable resources (usually they know their own problems best). Other resources include texts, articles, other references, computer databases, decision-making support, national practice guidelines, and facility documents (e.g., guidelines, policies, procedures, assessment forms).

8. **Whose perspectives must be considered?** The most significant perspective to consider is the patient's point of view. Other important perspectives include those of the family and significant others, caregivers, and relevant third parties (e.g., insurers).

9. **What is influencing my thinking?** Identify your personal biases and any other factors influencing your critical thinking and therefore your clinical judgment.

From Alfaro-LeFevre R: *Critical thinking in nursing: a practical approach,* ed 2, Philadelphia, 1999, WB Saunders. Reprinted with permission.

Alfaro-LeFevre (1999) developed a list of nine key questions (Box 8-8) to consider as you seek to improve your clinical judgment. Because the goal of nursing is to provide the best care to patients based on research and clinical evidence, the development of excellent clinical judgment is a professional responsibility. As you work to gain clinical experience and improve your own clinical judgment, these questions will help focus your thinking.

Nurses are responsible for developing sound clinical judgment and are accountable for their decisions and nursing practice that arises from those decisions. Your current level of clinical judgment can always be improved. It would be wise for you to devise a personal plan for improving your own clinical decision making. Working thoughtfully through the self-assessment in Box 8-9 will help you begin.

Box 8-9   Self-Assessment: Developing Sound Clinical Judgment

Answer the following questions honestly. When finished, make a list of the items you need to work on in your quest to develop sound clinical judgment. Keep the list with you and review it frequently. Seek opportunities to practice needed activities.

1. Use references.
   - Do I look up new terms when I encounter them to make them part of my vocabulary?
   - Do I familiarize myself with normal findings so that I can recognize those outside the norm?
   - Do I use research findings and base my practice on scientific evidence?
   - Do I learn the signs and symptoms of various conditions, what causes them, and how they are managed?
2. Use the nursing process.
   - Do I always assess before acting, stay focused on outcomes, and make changes as needed?
   - Do I always base my judgments on fact, not emotion or hearsay?
3. Assess systematically.
   - Do I have a systematic approach to assessing patients to decrease the likelihood that I will overlook important data?
4. Set priorities systematically.
   - Do I evaluate both the problem and the probable cause before acting?
   - Am I willing to obtain assistance from a more knowledgeable source when indicated?
5. Refuse to act without knowledge.
   - Do I refuse to perform an action when I do not know the indication, why it works, and what risks there are for harm to this particular patient?
6. Use resources wisely.
   - Do I look for opportunities to learn from others, such as teachers, other experts, or even my peers?
   - Do I seek help when needed, being mindful of patient privacy issues?
7. Know standards of care.
   - Do I read facility policies, professional standards, school policies, and state board of nursing rules and regulations to determine my scope of practice?
   - Do I know the clinical agency's policies and procedures affecting my particular patients?
   - Do I attempt to understand the rationales behind policies and procedures?
   - Do I follow policies and procedures carefully, recognizing that they are designed to help me use good judgment?
8. Know technology and equipment.
   - Do I routinely learn how to use patient technology such as intravenous pumps, patient monitors, computers?
   - Do I learn how to check equipment for proper functioning and safety?
9. Give patient-centered care.
   - Do I always remember the needs and feelings of the patient, family, and significant others?
   - Do I value knowing my patients' health beliefs and values within their own cultural contexts?
   - Do I "go the extra mile" for patients?
   - Do I demonstrate the belief that every patient deserves my very best efforts?

Modified from Alfaro-LeFevre R: *Critical thinking in nursing: a practical approach,* ed 2, Philadelphia, 1999, WB Saunders, pp 88-92. Used with permission.

Summary of Key Points

- Critical thinking is a skill that can be learned. In nursing, critical thinking is a purposeful, disciplined, active process that improves clinical judgment and thereby improves patient care.
- Thinking by novice nurses is different from that of expert nurses in identifiable ways.
- The nursing process is a systematic problem-solving framework that ensures that care is developed in an organized, analytic way.
- The phases of the nursing process are assessment, analysis and diagnosis, planning, implementation, and evaluation.
- Properly used, the nursing process is cyclic and dynamic rather than rigid and linear.
- Nurses may initially find that using the nursing process feels awkward or slow. With experience, however, most find it becomes a natural, organized approach to patient care.
- Consistent, comprehensive, and coordinated patient care results when all nurses use the nursing process effectively.
- Through the use of the nursing process, nurses are able to work toward resolving patient problems in a systematic and thorough manner, thus advancing both the scientific basis of nursing and professionalism.
- Sound clinical judgment is created by using critical thinking, applying the nursing process, staying current with developments in practice and research, understanding your scope of practice, and acquiring substantial clinical experience.

Critical Thinking Questions

1. Describe the characteristics of critical thinkers and explain why critical thinking is important in nursing.
2. List at least four ways in which novice thinking and expert thinking differ and give an example that illustrates each.
3. Describe the phases in the nursing process and explain the activities of each phase.
4. List a short-term career goal for yourself and a long-term career goal using all the essential elements of effective goals. Evaluate your progress toward these goals.
5. Explain the difference between independent, dependent, and interdependent nursing interventions and give an example of each.
6. List the pros and cons related to the use of nursing diagnosis.
7. Explain the difference between medical and nursing diagnoses.
8. Describe what is meant by the statement, "The nursing process is a cyclic process."
9. Using what you learned about yourself from Self-Assessment: Developing Sound Clinical Judgment (Box 8-9), set short-term goals for improvement in each of the nine areas. Make a checklist to take to your next clinical experience and consciously work on improving your clinical judgment.

⊝volve *To enhance your understanding of this chapter, try the Student Exercises on the Evolve site at http://evolve.elsevier.com/Chitty/professional.*

REFERENCES

Alfaro-LeFevre R: *Critical thinking in nursing: a practical approach*, ed 2, Philadelphia, 1999, WB Saunders.

American Philosophical Association: *Critical thinking: a statement of expert consensus for purposes of educational assessment and instruction, The Delphi report: research findings and recommendations prepared for the committee on pre-college philosophy*, 1990, ERIC Document Reproduction Services, pp 315-423.

Benner P: *From novice to expert*, Menlo Park, Calif, 1984, Addison-Wesley.

Benner P, Tanner CA, Chesla CA: *Expertise in nursing practice: caring, clinical judgment, and ethics*, New York, 1996, Springer.

Bradley PK, Berry A, Lang C, Myers RE: Getting ready: developing an educational intervention to prepare African American women for breast biopsy, *The ABFN Journal* (17)1:15-19, 2006.

Clark D: *Learning domains or Bloom's taxonomy*, 2001 (website): http://www.nwlink.com/~donclark/hrd/bloom.html.

De Bono E: *Edward de Bono's mind pack*, London, 1995, Dorling-Kindersley.

Facione PA: *Critical thinking: a statement of expert consensus for purposes of educational assessment and instruction, "The Delphi Report,"* Milbrae, Calif, 1990, The California Academic Press.

Facione PA: *Critical thinking: what it is and why it counts,* 2006 (website): http://www.insightassessment.com/pdf_files/what&why2006.pdf.

Gordon M: Nursing diagnosis and the diagnostic process, *Am J Nurs* 76(5):1298-1300, 1976.

Gordon M: *Nursing diagnosis: process and application,* ed 2, New York, 1987, McGraw-Hill.

Kenney LJ: Using Edward de Bono's six hats game to aid critical thinking and reflection in palliative care, *Int J Palliat Nurs* 9(3):105-112, 2003.

Lunney M: *Critical thinking and nursing diagnosis: case studies and analyses,* Philadelphia, 2001, North American Nursing Diagnosis Association.

Lunney M: Critical need to address accuracy of nurses' diagnoses, *Online J Issues Nurs* 13(3), 2008 (website): http://www.nursingworld.org/MainMenuCategories/ANAMarketplace/ANAPeriodicals/OJIN/TableofContents/vol132008/No1Jan08/ArticlePreviousTopic/AccuracyofNursesDiagnoses.aspx.

Maslow AH: *Motivation and personality,* New York, 1970, Harper & Row.

Mueller A, Johnston M, Bligh D: Joining mind mapping and care planning to enhance student critical thinking and achieve holistic nursing care, *Nurs Diagn* 13(1):24-27, 2002.

NANDA International: *Nursing diagnoses: definitions and classification, 1989-1990,* Philadelphia, 1990, NANDA International.

NANDA International: *Nursing diagnoses: definitions and classification, 2003-2004,* Philadelphia, 2003, NANDA International.

NANDA International: *Nursing diagnoses: definitions and classification, 2009-2011,* Philadelphia, 2008, Wiley-Blackwell.

Paul R, Elder L: *The miniature guide to critical thinking: concepts and tools,* Dillon Beach, Calif, 2005, Foundation for Critical Thinking.

Scheffer BK, Rubenfeld MG: A consensus statement on critical thinking, *J Nurs Educ* 39:352-359, 2000.

Yura H, Walsh MB: *The nursing process: assessing, planning, implementing, evaluation,* ed 4, Norwalk, Conn, 1983, Appleton-Century-Crofts.

Communication and Collaboration in Nursing

Kay Kittrell Chitty

LEARNING OUTCOMES

After studying this chapter, students will be able to:
- Describe therapeutic use of self
- Identify and describe the phases of the traditional nurse-patient relationship
- Differentiate between social and professional relationships
- Explore the role self-awareness plays in the ability to use nonjudgmental acceptance as a helping technique
- Explain the concept of professional boundaries
- Discuss factors creating successful or unsuccessful communication
- Evaluate helpful and unhelpful communication techniques
- Identify own communication strengths and challenges
- Demonstrate components of active listening
- Identify key aspects of collaboration
- Explain the impact of gender, cultural, and generational diversity on nurse-patient and nurse-colleague relationships

Interpersonal skills are very important to professional nurses. Regardless of the settings in which they work and the roles they assume within those settings, most nurses interact with many people every day. The way in which they relate to patients, families, colleagues, and other professionals and nonprofessionals determines the level of comfort and trust others feel and, ultimately, the success of their interactions. All the clinical skills in the world cannot overcome poor interpersonal relationships. This chapter includes information that can enhance the development of self-awareness, nonjudgmental acceptance of others, communication skills, and collaboration skills, all of which are essential components of effective interpersonal relationships in nursing.

THERAPEUTIC USE OF SELF

Hildegard Peplau, a pioneer in nursing theory development, first focused on the importance of the nurse-patient relationship in her 1952 book *Interpersonal Relations in Nursing.* She called using one's personality and communication skills to help patients improve their health status "therapeutic use of self" (Peplau, 1952).

The ability to use oneself therapeutically can be developed. Nurses develop this ability by acquiring certain knowledge, attitudes, and skills that assist them in relating effectively to patients, patients' families, coworkers, and other health care professionals.

The Traditional Nurse-Patient Relationship

The nursing process can begin only after the nurse and patient establish their initial therapeutic **nurse-patient relationship**. Awareness of the three identifiable phases of the nurse-patient relationship helps nurses to be realistic in their expectations of this important relationship. Each of three phases—orientation, working, and termination—is sequential and builds on previous phases.

The orientation phase

The orientation phase, or introductory phase, is the period often described as "getting to know you" in social settings. Relationships between nurses and their patients have some commonalities with other types of relationships. The chief similarity is that there must be trust between the two parties for the relationship to develop. Nurses cannot expect patients to trust them automatically and to reveal their innermost thoughts and feelings immediately.

During the orientation phase, nurse and patient assess one another. Early impressions made by the nurse are important. Some people have difficulty accepting help of any kind, including nursing care. Putting the patient at ease with a pleasant, unhurried approach is important during the early part of any nurse-patient relationship.

During the orientation phase, the patient has a right to expect to learn the nurse's name, credentials, and extent of responsibility. The use of simple orienting statements is one way to begin: "Good morning, Mr. Davis. I am Jennifer Carter, and I am your nurse until noon today. I am responsible for your care while I am here."

Developing trust. The orientation phase includes the beginning development of trust. Notice the use of the term "beginning development." Full development of trust is slow and may take months of regular contact. A fact of contemporary nursing practice is that patient interactions may be brief, sometimes lasting only minutes. However, even in the most abbreviated contacts, nurses must orient patients and help them feel comfortable and as trusting as possible.

Certain behaviors help patients develop trust in the nurse. A straightforward, nondefensive manner is important. Answering all questions as fully as possible and admitting to the limits of your knowledge also facilitate trust. Promise to find out the answers to all questions, and report the information to the patient as soon as possible. Meet with patients at the designated times, or make arrangements to let them know of a change in plans. Use active listening, and accept the patient's thoughts and feelings without judgment.

Congruence between verbal and nonverbal communication is a key factor in the development of trust. Communicating in a congruent manner requires that nurses be aware of their own thoughts and feelings and be able to share those with others in a nonthreatening manner. Developing an initial understanding of the patient's problem or needs also starts in the orientation phase. Because patients themselves often do not clearly understand their problems or may be reluctant to discuss them, nurses must use their communication skills to elicit the information needed to make a nursing diagnosis. Communication skills useful in nurse-patient interactions are discussed later in this chapter.

Tasks of the orientation phase. By the end of a successful orientation phase, regardless of its length, several things will have happened. First, the patient will have developed enough trust in the nurse to continue to participate in the relationship. Second, the patient and nurse will see each other as individuals, unique from all others and worthy of one another's respect. Third, the patient's perception of major problems and needs will have been identified. And fourth, the approximate length of the relationship will have been estimated, and the nurse and patient will have agreed to work together on some aspect of the identified problems. This agreement, whether formalized in writing or informally agreed on, is sometimes called a "contract." An example of a contract that might emerge from the orientation phase of the relationship with a patient in whom diabetes has been newly diagnosed is an agreement to work together on his ability to calculate and inject his daily insulin requirement.

The working phase

The second phase of the nurse-patient relationship is called the working phase, because it is during this time that the nurse and patient tackle tasks outlined in the previous phase. Because the participants now know each other to some extent, there may be a sense of interpersonal comfort in the relationship that did not exist earlier.

Nurses should recognize that in the working phase patients may exhibit alternating periods of intense effort and of resistance to change. Continuing the example of the patient with diabetes, the nurse can anticipate that he will experience some degree of difficulty in accepting the life changes the illness causes. He may show progress in learning to give himself insulin one week but not be able to demonstrate injection technique the next week. Nurses who become frustrated when a patient's progress toward self-care is not smooth and sustained must realize that regression is an ego defense mechanism that occurs as a reaction to stress and that regression often precedes periods of positive behavioral change.

It is difficult to make and sustain change. Patience, self-awareness, and maturity are required of nurses during the working phase. Continued building of trust, use of active listening, and other helpful communication responses facilitate the patient's expression of needs and feelings during the working phase.

The termination phase

The termination phase includes those activities that enable the patient and the nurse to end the relationship in a therapeutic manner. The process of terminating the nurse-patient relationship begins in the orientation phase when participants estimate the length of time it will take to accomplish the desired outcomes. This is part of the informal contract.

As in any relationship, positive and negative feelings often accompany termination. The patient and nurse feel good about the gains the patient has made in accomplishing goals. They may feel sadness about ending a relationship that has been open and trusting. People tend to respond to the end of relationships in much the same way they have responded to other losses in life. Feelings of anger and fear may surface, in addition to sadness.

Feelings evoked by termination should be discussed and accepted. Summarizing the gains the patient has made is an important activity during this phase. The importance of the relationship to both patient and nurse can be shared in a caring manner.

The giving and receiving of gifts at termination has different meanings for different people. The meaning of such behavior should be explored in a sensitive manner with the patient. Both the agency's policy on gifts and your instructor should also be consulted.

Because termination is often painful, participants are sometimes tempted to continue the relationship on a social basis, and requests for addresses, phone numbers, and e-mail addresses are not uncommon. The nurse must realize that professional relationships are different from social relationships. It is not helpful to stay in touch with patients after termination of a professional nurse-patient relationship. Other differences between social and professional relationships are outlined in Box 9-1.

Box 9-1   Differences in Social and Professional Relationships

SOCIAL RELATIONSHIPS
- Evolve spontaneously
- Not time-limited
- Not necessarily goal-directed; broad purpose is pleasure, companionship, sharing
- Centered on meeting both parties' needs
- Problem solving is rarely/occasionally a focus
- May or may not include nonjudgmental acceptance
- Outcome is pleasure for both parties

PROFESSIONAL RELATIONSHIPS
- Evolve through recognized phases; interactions are planned and purposeful
- Limited in time with termination date often predetermined
- Goal-directed; systematic exploration of identified problem areas
- Centered on meeting patient's needs; do not address nurse's needs
- Problem solving is a primary focus
- Includes nonjudgmental acceptance
- Outcome is improved health status of patient

During the course of a professional career, every nurse will experience countless nurse-patient relationships, each with its own meaning and duration. If nurses can view each new relationship both as an opportunity to assist another human being to grow and change in a positive, healthful way and as a challenge to grow and change themselves, the rewards of nursing will be rich indeed.

Developing Self-Awareness

Awareness of oneself, called self-awareness, is basic to effective interpersonal relationships, especially the nurse-patient relationship. Robert Burns, the eighteenth-century Scottish poet, described the rarity of true self-awareness in his poem "To a Louse": "Oh wad some Power the giftie gie us/To see oursels as ithers see us!" (Barke, 1955).

As Burns knew, few people have the innate capacity to recognize their own emotional needs, biases, and blind spots, as well as their impact on others. With practice, however, most can become more effective in doing so, thus improving self-awareness.

An important guideline in professional nursing is this: nurses should get their own emotional needs met outside of the nurse-patient relationship. When nurses' strong unmet needs for acceptance, approval, friendship, or even love enter into their relationships with patients, professionalism is lost, and relationships become social in nature. Becoming aware of one's needs and making conscious efforts to meet those needs in private life make professional, therapeutic relationships with patients possible. As discussed earlier and summarized in Box 9-1, there are important differences in social and therapeutic or professional relationships. When the nurse-patient relationship strays from the therapeutic, it can go beyond professional boundaries and result in role confusion that can be damaging to both patient and nurse.

Professional boundaries

Boundary issues are everywhere in nursing. They were first addressed by Florence Nightingale in the Nightingale Pledge (refer to Box 3-1 on p. 68 to review this statement). The American Nurses Association's *Code of Ethics for Nurses* (2001) also addressed boundaries. The subject of professional boundaries was comprehensively explored in a brochure published by the National Council of State Boards of Nursing (NCSBN) (1996). It defined professional boundaries as "the spaces between the nurse's power and the client's vulnerability. The power of the nurse comes from the professional position and the access to private knowledge about the client" (p. 1). Patient vulnerability arises from dependency on caregiving provided by the nurse (Holder and Schenthal, 2007). Boundary violations occur when "there is confusion between the needs of the nurse and those of the client" (p. 2).

According to the NCSBN brochure, nurse-patient relationships can be plotted on a continuum of professional behavior that ranges from underinvolvement (such as distancing, disinterest, neglect) through a zone of helpfulness to overinvolvement (such as excessive personal disclosure by the nurse, secrecy, role reversal, touching, gestures, money or gifts, special attention, social contact, getting involved in a patient's personal affairs, or sexual misconduct). Both underinvolvement and overinvolvement can be detrimental to patient and nurse (p. 3). Box 9-2 describes a case in which a nurse was disciplined by his state board of nursing for failing to honor the professional boundaries between a nurse and patient.

Because getting too personal with a patient is an offense reportable to your employer or state board of nursing, as well as violating nursing's code of ethics, nurses should have a thorough understanding of professional boundaries (Wright, 2007). Box 9-3 contains seven "guiding principles to determining professional boundaries and the continuum of professional behavior" (p. 4) from the NCSBN brochure. The brochure was so often requested that the NCSBN has now developed an entire continuing educational module about professional boundaries. It is offered online for continuing education credit (http://www.learningext.com/files/0d4372fd7f/respecting_syllabus0909.pdf).

Box 9-2   Legal Note: Nurse's Relationship With Patient Results in Disciplinary Action

Tapp v. Board of Registered Nursing, 2002 WL 31820206 P2d-CA

This case involved a California registered nurse at a psychiatric facility in Fresno who was accused of having sexual relations with his former patient after her discharge. The patient was hospitalized for emotional problems related to sex. She was hospitalized on a unit where the nurse worked the night shift. They became friendly; he brought her small gifts, gave her his telephone number, and called her during his off-work hours. After she was discharged, they spoke often by telephone, and he began to visit her at her apartment. On one occasion, the nurse gave her a tablet of a controlled substance.

One week after her discharge, they began a sexual relationship that lasted for 2 weeks. Shortly after the relationship ended, the patient was readmitted, "suffering adverse effects from the affair" (p. 4). The California Board of Registered Nursing initiated disciplinary proceedings for "acts of unprofessional conduct." An administrative law judge heard testimony, made a determination of misconduct, and recommended that the nurse's license be revoked, but stayed the revocation and recommended that the nurse be placed on probation for 5 years on multiple conditions. The California Board of Registered Nursing disagreed and ordered the revocation of his license. There were subsequent appeals, dismissals, and further appeals.

Nurses must realize that there can be no socialization between themselves and patients, particularly sexual in nature. Not only was this nurse's behavior with this patient during her hospitalization "highly improper, but his socialization with the patient after her discharge from the hospital, not to mention the fact that he provided the patient with a controlled substance, was ample reason to impose strict disciplinary action" (p. 5).

Abstracted from Nurse's relationship with patient results in disciplinary action, *Nurs Law Regan Rep* 43(8):4-5, 2003.

Box 9-3   Principles for Determining Professional Boundaries

1. The nurse, not the patient, is responsible for delineating and maintaining boundaries.
2. The nurse should work within the "zone of helpfulness," which is neither aloof nor too intense/emotionally involved.
3. The nurse should examine any boundary crossing, be aware of its potential implications, and avoid repeated crossings.
4. Variables such as the care setting, community influences, client needs, and the nature of therapy affect the delineation of boundaries.
5. Actions that overstep established boundaries to meet the needs of the nurse are boundary violations.
6. The nurse should avoid dual relationships in which the nurse has a personal or business relationship with a patient, as well as the professional one.
7. Posttermination relationships are complex because the client may need additional services, and it may be difficult to determine when the nurse-client relationship is truly terminated.

Modified from National Council of State Boards of Nursing: *Professional boundaries: a nurse's guide to the importance of appropriate professional boundaries,* Chicago, 1996, National Council of State Boards of Nursing.

Reflective practice

Nurses care for a diverse array of patients whose values, beliefs, and lifestyles may challenge the nurses' own. Nurses sometimes are attracted to patients and, conversely, may be repelled by them. Sometimes nurses find themselves meeting their own needs to be liked or needed through relationships with patients. Nurses who have emotional reactions to patients, positive or negative, sometimes feel disturbed or guilty about these feelings. Part of self-awareness is recognizing one's feelings and understanding that, although feelings cannot be controlled, behaviors can. Effective nurses control their behavior to prevent their own prejudices, beliefs, and needs from intruding into nurse-patient relationships. First they must be self-aware.

Developing self-awareness requires individuals to take time away from their tasks, to stop the "busyness," and to focus on their own thoughts, feelings, actions, and beliefs. In short, they must engage in personal reflection. Finding the time and space for reflective practice can be a challenge to busy students and practicing nurses alike. Reflection can produce discomfort as nurses become aware of the tensions and anxieties within themselves about their everyday activities. Perhaps their personal values are challenged by the realities of practice, or perhaps they experience desensitization to the needs of their patients because of time pressures. Whatever the reason, few students of nursing set aside the time to reflect on their experiences and interactions required to develop insight into self. Self-awareness empowers nurses and frees them to behave assertively on their own behalf and on behalf of their patients and is well worth the time required to develop and sustain it.

To make good use of your time, Johns (2002) has suggested a model for structured reflection depicted in Box 9-4. Perhaps you will use this model to reflect on your practice and become more self-aware.

Avoiding Stereotypes

Stereotypes are prejudices and attitudes developed through interactions with family, friends, and others in each individual's social and cultural system. It is not uncommon for even well-educated professionals to have stereotypical expectations of groups of people different from themselves. These stereotypes are established through childhood experiences and affect relationships with people in the stereotyped group. Because stereotypes and prejudices tend to persist despite contrary experiences, they are irrational, or illogical, beliefs.

The subtle intrusion of stereotyped expectations into the nurse-patient relationship can

---

Box 9-4   Model for Structured Reflection

- Bring the mind home.
- Write a description of an experience that seems significant in some way.
- What issue seemed significant to pay attention to?
- How was I feeling and what made me feel that way?
- What was I trying to achieve?
- Did I respond effectively and in tune with my values?
- What were the consequences of my actions on the patient, others, and myself?
- How were others feeling?
- What made them feel that way?
- What factors influenced the way I was feeling, thinking or responding?
- What knowledge did or might have informed me?
- To what extent did I act for the best?
- How does this situation connect with previous experiences?
- How might I respond more effectively given this situation again?
- What would be the consequences of alternative actions for the patient, others and myself?
- How do I now feel about this experience?
- Am I now more able to support myself and others as a consequence?
- Am I now more available to work with patients/families and staff to help them meet their needs?

Johns C: *Guided reflection: advancing practice,* Oxford, 2002, Blackwell Science, p. 10. Reprinted with permission of Wiley-Blackwell.

---

cause disturbed patterns of relating. For example, the expectation that elderly people are irritable and demanding may cause the nurse to avoid elderly patients or to treat their complaints as unimportant: "just another grumpy old person." Even worse, some nurses "talk down" to the elderly, as this chapter's News Note describes.

news note   In "Sweetie" and "Dear," a Hurt for the Elderly

Professionals call it elderspeak, the sweetly belittling form of address that has always rankled older people: the doctor who talks to their [adult] child rather than to them about their health; the store clerk who assumes that an older person does not know how to work a computer, or needs to be addressed slowly or in a loud voice. Then there are those who address any elderly person as "dear."

"People think they're being nice," said Elvira Nagle, 83, of Dublin, Calif., "but when I hear it, it raises my hackles."

Now studies are finding that the insults can have health consequences, especially if people mutely accept the attitudes behind them, said Becca Levy, an associate professor of epidemiology and psychology at Yale University, who studies the health effects of such messages on elderly people.

"Those little insults can lead to more negative images of aging," Dr. Levy said. "And those who have more negative images of aging have worse functional health over time, including lower rates of survival."

In a long-term survey of 660 people over age 50 in a small Ohio town, published in 2002, Dr. Levy and her fellow researchers found that those who had positive perceptions of aging lived an average of 7.5 years longer, a bigger increase than that associated with exercising or not smoking. The findings held up even when the researchers controlled for differences in the participants' health conditions.

In her forthcoming study, Dr. Levy found that older people exposed to negative images of aging, including words like "forgetful," "feeble," and "shaky," performed significantly worse on memory and balance tests; in previous experiments, they also showed higher levels of stress.

Despite such research, the worst offenders are often health care workers, said Kristine Williams, a nurse gerontologist and associate professor at the University of Kansas School of Nursing.

To study the effects of elderspeak on people with mild to moderate dementia, Dr. Williams and a team of researchers videotaped interactions in a nursing home between 20 residents and staff members. They found that when nurses used phrases like "good girl" or "How are we feeling?" patients were more aggressive and less cooperative or receptive to care. If addressed as infants, some showed their irritation by grimacing, screaming, or refusing to do what staff members asked of them.

The researchers, who will publish their findings in The American Journal of Alzheimer's Disease and Other Dementias, concluded that elderspeak sent a message that the patient was incompetent and "begins a negative downward spiral for older persons, who react with decreased self-esteem, depression, withdrawal and the assumption of dependent behaviors."

Dr. Williams said health care workers often thought that using words like "dear" or "sweetie" conveyed that they cared and made them easier to understand. "But they don't realize the implications," she said, "that it's also giving messages to older adults that they're incompetent."

"The main task for a person with Alzheimer's is to maintain a sense of self or personhood," Dr. Williams said. "If you know you're losing your cognitive abilities and trying to maintain your personhood, and someone talks to you like a baby, it's upsetting to you."

She added that patients who reacted aggressively against elderspeak might receive less care.

[The article went on to describe the equally negative effect of elderspeak on healthy older adults without cognitive problems.]

—John Leland

Professional nurses deliver high-quality care to all patients regardless of ethnicity, age, gender, religion, lifestyle, or diagnosis. The Code of Ethics for Nurses (see inside back cover of this text) calls on nurses to do this. Nurses are not without stereotypes and prejudices, however, and must strive to be aware of their own irrational feelings toward patients. Every professional nurse's goal is to accept all patients as individuals of dignity and worth who deserve the best nursing care possible.

Becoming Nonjudgmental

Acceptance is not always easy, because prejudices are strong and are often outside our awareness. This means that judging others as "good" or "bad," "right" or "wrong," may occur automatically, usually unconsciously. It is important to remember that acceptance conveys neither approval nor disapproval of patients and their personal beliefs, habits, expressions of feelings, or chosen lifestyles. Nonjudgmental acceptance means that nurses acknowledge all patients' rights to be different and to express their uniqueness.

Therapeutic use of self begins with the ability to convey acceptance to patients and requires self-awareness and nonjudgmental attitudes on the part of nurses. Ongoing examination of attitudes toward others is both a lifelong process and an essential part of self-awareness and interpersonal growth.

Reconceptualizing the Nurse-Patient Relationship: Theory of Human Relatedness

The type of nurse-patient relationship discussed in the previous section is the traditional model taught and practiced since the middle of the twentieth century. It is based on several assumptions that no longer hold true in many settings where nurses practice in today's fast-paced health care system. These assumptions are as follows (Hagerty and Patusky, 2003):

- The nurse-patient relationship is linear and proceeds through several phases, each building on the preceding one.
- Building trust is essential during early phases of the nurse-patient relationship.

- Time and repeated contacts are required to establish an effective nurse-patient relationship.
- Patients desire relationships with nurses, wish to receive services from them, and will cooperate and comply with those nurses.

Although the traditional, time-honored nurse-patient relationship is still appropriate in many settings, the assumptions on which it is based are being challenged by today's health care realities. The reality is that patients today are more acutely ill, nurses' workloads have increased, and the time nurses spend with patients may be quite limited, sometimes to only one or two contacts. Are these more limited nurse-patient contacts therefore meaningless, or can we rethink the nurse-patient relationship and find ways to modify it to suit today's streamlined caregiving contexts?

Hagerty and Patusky (2003) proposed reconceptualizing the nurse-patient relationship using the theory of human relatedness as a framework. They recommended approaching each nurse-patient contact as an opportunity for connection and goal achievement rather than as one step in a lengthy relationship-building process. They also recommended that nurses approach their patients with a sense of the patient's autonomy, choice, and participation (p. 147), putting the relationship on a more equitable basis than the traditional nurse-patient relationship, which gives much of the power to the nurse. Research into these concepts continues.

These ideas can form the basis for classroom discussion and provide "new insights and opportunities for assessment, intervention, and research toward positive, hopeful, and efficacious nursing care" (Hagerty and Patusky, 2003, p. 149).

COMMUNICATION THEORY

Communication is the exchange of thoughts, ideas, or information and is at the heart of all relationships. Communication is a dynamic process that is the primary instrument through which change occurs in nursing situations. Nurses use their communication skills in all phases of the nursing process. These skills are vital to effective nursing care and to effective interaction with others in health care.

Jurgen Ruesch (1972), a pioneer communications theorist, defined communication as "all the modes of behavior that one individual employs, conscious or unconscious, to affect another: not only the spoken and written word, but also gestures, body movements, somatic signals, and symbolism in the arts" (p. 16).

Communication begins the moment two people become aware of each other's presence. It is impossible not to communicate when in the presence of another person, even if no words are spoken. Even when alone, people routinely engage in "self-talk," which is an internal form of communication.

Levels of Communication

Communication exists simultaneously on at least two levels: verbal and nonverbal. Verbal communication consists of all speech and represents the most obvious aspect of communication. As much as 65 percent of a message, however, consists of nonverbal communication (Gordon, 1992). Nonverbal communication includes grooming, clothing, gestures, posture, facial expressions, eye contact, tone and volume of voice, and actions, among other things (Figure 9-1). Words can be

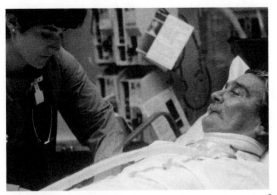

Figure 9-1 Nonverbal communication consists of grooming, clothing, gestures, posture, facial expressions, tone and volume of voice, and actions. Nonverbal communication is particularly important to patients using mechanical ventilation or whose ability to speak is otherwise impaired. (Courtesy Medical University of South Carolina.)

used to mask feelings, but individuals are less able to exercise conscious control over nonverbal communication than verbal communication. Therefore the nonverbal component is considered a more reliable expression of feeling. Certainly nurses must pay as much attention to nonverbal messages as they do to verbal ones.

Consider this example: A nurse who is preparing a patient for a breast biopsy notices that the patient keeps her head turned away, has tears in her eyes, and will not look at the nurse. When the nurse says, "Is there anything you want to talk about or ask?" the patient responds, "No, I'm fine." The wise nurse would pay more attention to her nonverbal communication than to the spoken word. If the nurse pays attention only to the patient's words, her underlying feelings would be ignored. The nurse's job in evaluating this patient's needs is made more difficult by the incongruence between her verbal and nonverbal messages.

When congruent communication occurs, the verbal and nonverbal aspects match and reinforce each other. In incongruent communication, the words and nonverbal communication do not match. Incongruent communication creates confusion in receivers, who are unsure to which level of communication they should respond. Nurses should be alert to incongruent communication for clues to patients' unexpressed feelings.

Elements of the Communication Process

Ruesch (1972) identified five major elements that must be present for communication to take place: a sender, a message, a receiver, feedback, and context. The sender is the person sending the message, the message is what is actually said plus accompanying nonverbal communication, and the receiver is the person receiving the message. A response to a message is termed feedback. The setting in which an interaction occurs—including the mood, relationship between sender and receiver, and other factors—is known as the context. All of these elements are necessary for communication to occur.

Consider the classroom situation. During a lecture, the professor is the sender, the lecture is the message, and students are the receivers. The professor (sender) receives feedback from the students (receivers) through their facial expressions, alertness, posture, attentiveness, and comments. The atmosphere in the classroom is the context. If the atmosphere is a relaxed one of give-and-take discussion between students and professor, the feedback is quite different from feedback in a more formal context of professor as lecturer and students as note takers. Figure 9-2 shows the relationships among the elements of communication.

Operations in the Communication Process

In addition to the five elements of communication, Ruesch (1972) also identified three major operations in communication: perception, evaluation, and transmission.

Perception

Perception is the selection, organization, and interpretation of incoming signals into meaningful messages. In the classroom situation just described, students select, organize, and interpret various pieces of the professor's message or lecture. Each student perceives the information differently, on the basis of factors such as personal experience, previous knowledge, alertness, sensitivity to subtleties of meaning, and sociocultural background. This is sometime referred to as an individual's perceptual screen, through which all incoming messages are filtered.

Evaluation

Evaluation is the analysis of information received. Is the content of the professor's lecture useful? Is it important or relevant to the students' needs? Does it build on previously learned information? Is it likely to be on the next test? Each student evaluates the message in a different manner.

Transmission

Transmission refers to the expression of information, verbal or nonverbal. While the professor is transmitting his verbal message to the students, his or her nonverbal behavior of excitement, uncertainty, confusion, or boredom with the subject matter also transmits a message to the class.

Factors influencing perception, evaluation, and transmission

Perception, evaluation, and transmission are influenced by many factors. The gender, age, and culture of the sender and receiver; the interest and mood of both parties; the value, clarity, and length of the message; the presence or absence of feedback; and the atmosphere of the context all are powerful influences. Also involved are individuals' needs, values, self-concepts, sensory and

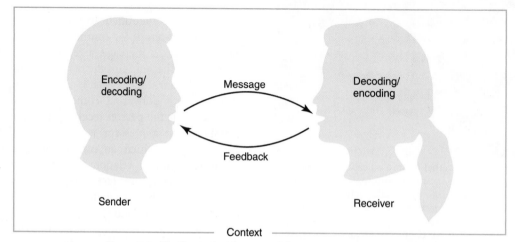

Figure 9-2 The five major elements of the communication process.

intellectual abilities or deficits, and sociocultural conditioning. Given the variety of factors involved, it is clear that communication is a complex human activity worthy of nurses' attention.

HOW COMMUNICATION DEVELOPS

Humans learn to communicate through a certain developmental sequence, which begins in infancy. Infants use somatic language to signal their needs to caretakers. Somatic language consists of crying; reddening of the skin; fast, shallow breathing; facial expressions; and jerking of the limbs. The sequence progresses to action language in older infants. Action language consists of reaching out, pointing, crawling toward a desired object, or closing the lips and turning the head when an undesired food is offered. Last to develop is verbal language, beginning with repetitive noises and sounds and progressing to words, phrases, and complete sentences.

If a child's development is normal, any one or combination of these forms of communication can be used. Somatic language usually decreases with maturity, but, because it is not under conscious control, some somatic language may persist past childhood. A familiar example is facial blushing when embarrassed or angry. The development of communication is determined by inborn and environmental factors. The amount of verbal stimulation an infant receives can enhance or retard the development of language skills. The extent of a caretaker's vocabulary and verbal ability is therefore influential. Some families engage in lengthy discussions on a variety of issues, thereby providing intense verbal stimulation, whereas others are quieter and less verbal.

Nonverbal communication development is similarly influenced by environment. Some families communicate through nonverbal gestures such as touch or facial expressions, which children learn to "read" at young ages. Other families ascribe to the adage "Children should be seen and not heard," thus discouraging verbal expression and increasing dependence on nonverbal cues for communicating. The ability to communicate effectively is dependent on a number of factors.

Primary among these are the quantity and quality of verbal and nonverbal stimulation received during early developmental periods.

CRITERIA FOR SUCCESSFUL COMMUNICATION

Everyone has had the experience of being the sender or receiver of unsuccessful communication. A simple example is arriving for an appointment with a friend at the wrong time or wrong place because of a communication mix-up. Unsuccessful communication creates little harm when done under social circumstances. In nursing situations, however, accurate, complete communication is vitally important. Nurses can achieve successful communication on most occasions if they plan their communication to meet four major criteria: feedback, appropriateness, efficiency, and flexibility.

Feedback

When a receiver relays to a sender the effect of the sender's message, feedback has occurred. Feedback was identified as one of Ruesch's five elements necessary for communication (see Figure 9-2). It is also a criterion for successful communication. In making the social appointment mentioned previously, if the receiver of the message had said, "Let's make sure I understand you. We'll meet at 12:30 on Tuesday at Café Al Fresco," that feedback could have led to successful communication.

In a nurse-patient interaction, a nurse can give feedback to a patient by saying, "If I understand you correctly, you have pain in your lower abdomen every time you stand up." The patient can then either agree or correct what the nurse has said: "No, the pain is there only when I arise in the morning." Effective nurses do not assume that they fully understand what their patients are telling them until they feed the statement back to the patient and receive confirmation.

Appropriateness

When a reply fits the circumstances and matches the message, and the amount is neither too great nor too little, appropriateness has been achieved.

In day-to-day conversation among acquaintances passing on the street, most people recognize the question "How are you?" as a social nicety, not a genuine question. The individual who launches into a lengthy, detailed description of how his morning has gone has communicated inappropriately. The reply does not fit the circumstances, and the quantity is too great. An appropriate response is, "Fine, and how are you?"

If a patient asks, "When is my doctor coming?" just after having seen her doctor, the nurse will be alert to other inappropriate messages by this patient that may signal a variety of problems. In this instance, the inappropriate message does not match the context.

Efficiency

Efficiency means using simple, clear words that are timed at a pace suitable to participants. Explaining to an adult that she will have "an angioplasty" tomorrow morning may not result in successful communication. Telling her she will have "an angioplasty, a procedure in which a small balloon is threaded into an artery and inflated to open up the vessel so more blood can flow through," will more likely ensure her understanding. This message would not be an efficient one for a small child, however. Messages must be adapted to each patient's age, verbal level, and level of understanding.

Some examples of patients who require special assistance in evaluating and responding to messages are young children, the mentally ill, some people with neurologic deficits, the developmentally disabled, and those recovering from anesthesia or receiving pain medication. For efficient communication to occur, nurses must recognize patients' needs and adjust messages accordingly.

Flexibility

The fourth criterion for successful communication is flexibility. The flexible communicator bases messages on the immediate situation rather than preconceived expectations. When a student nurse who plans to teach a patient about diabetic diets enters the patient's room and finds the patient crying, the student must be flexible enough to change gears and deal with the feelings the patient is expressing. Pressing on with the lesson plan in the face of the patient's distress shows a lack of compassion, as well as inflexibility in communicating.

Nurses can learn to use these four measures of successful communication to enhance their effectiveness with patients. The continuing absence or malfunction of any of these four criteria can create disturbed communication and hamper the implementation of the nursing process.

BECOMING A BETTER COMMUNICATOR

People are not born as good communicators. Communication skills can be developed if you are willing to put forth a moderate amount of time and energy. Becoming a better listener, learning a few basic helpful responding styles, and avoiding common causes of communication breakdown can put you on the path to becoming a better communicator. To begin evaluating your communication skills, refer to the Communication Patterns Self-Assessment in Box 9-5.

Listening

Listening has become a forgotten art, yet it is the only way to get to know patients and understand what is important to them. A requirement of successful communication is listening, but too often we hear without listening or engage in a task while listening with half an ear. Active listening involves focusing solely on a person and acknowledging feelings in a nonjudgmental manner. It is a method of communicating interest and attention and is best accomplished without a television or other distraction playing in the background. Fostering an unrushed manner and using such signals as good eye contact, nodding, and "mumbles" ("mm-hmm") and encouraging the speaker ("Go on" or "Tell me more about this") also help to communicate interest. Facing the speaker squarely with an inviting facial expression and using an open posture (leaning forward; relaxed; arms uncrossed) also communicate interest (Calcagno, 2008). Sit, bend, or

Box 9-5 Communication Patterns Self-Assessment

Directions: Answer the following true-or-false questions as honestly as possible; then review your answers and draw at least two conclusions about your habitual communication patterns that you need to work to improve. Check your conclusions for accuracy with a friend who knows your style of communicating well. Then score yourself using the key below.

1. I find it easier to start conversations by talking about myself.
2. I usually listen about as much as I talk.
3. I tend to be long-winded.
4. I rarely interrupt others.
5. When people hesitate or speak slowly, I try to complete their sentences for them.
6. I pay close attention to what others say, as well as to bodily cues.
7. I find it difficult to make eye contact with the person I am talking with.
8. I can usually tell if someone is angry or upset.
9. I find it difficult to express myself assertively.
10. I expect others to read my mind.
11. I hesitate to interrupt someone to ask for clarification.
12. People often tell me personal things about themselves.
13. I find it is best to change the subject if someone gets too emotional.
14. If I can't "make things better" for a friend with a problem, I feel uncomfortable.
15. I am comfortable talking with people much older or much younger than I am.
16. I have difficulty saying no.
17. I speak to others the way I like to be spoken to.
18. I fly off the handle easily.
19. I tend to withdraw from conflict or remain silent.
20. I try to evaluate when someone will be most receptive to my message.

Key: If you answered True to questions 2, 4, 6, 8, 12, 15, 17, and 20, you are on your way to becoming an effective communicator. If you answered True to other questions, select several to improve. Set a realistic goal and seek help from a trusted friend or faculty member.

---

stoop to place your eye level at that of the patient and repeat (reflect) what you hear, including feelings, checking to be sure you heard correctly. These indications of interest and active listening will help you focus on patients and tune into the meanings behind their words (listening with the "third ear").

Having someone listen to concerns, even if no problem solving takes place, may be therapeutic. Venting is the term used to describe the verbal "letting off steam" that occurs when talking about concerns or frustrations. The experience of feeling "listened to" is becoming rare in contemporary American society as individuals pay more attention to their cell phones and PDAs than to people.

Nurses may have difficulty listening for a variety of reasons. They may be intent on accomplishing a task and be frustrated by the time it takes to be a good listener. They may be planning their own next question or response and not hear what the patient is saying. They may be distracted by a vibrating pager or cell phone. Similar to other people, nurses have their own personal and professional problems that sometimes preoccupy them and interfere with effective listening. Nurses must remember that no verbal message can be received if the receiver (the nurse) is not listening.

Three common listening faults include interrupting, finishing sentences for others, and lack of interest. It is important for nurses to remember that what the patient is saying is just as important as what the nurse wishes to say.

Being listened to meets the patient's emotional need to be respected and valued by the nurse. Listening can help avert problems by letting people vent about the pressures they feel.

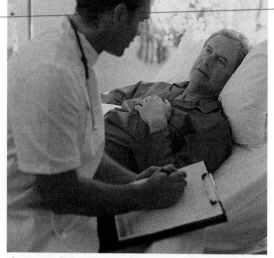

Figure 9-3 Being an active listener is an important part of communication. Identify three things in this photograph that demonstrate active listening by the nurse. (Courtesy Hamilton Medical Center, Dalton, Georgia.)

Hospitalized patients particularly may feel that their lives are out of control and that they are isolated or invisible. They may need to discuss those feelings with someone who will listen without becoming defensive (Figure 9-3).

Nurses at all levels find listening a useful and rewarding skill. Nurse managers often use listening as a tool for dealing with staff members' problems and concerns and find that no other intervention is required. Listening is a talent that can be developed; properly used, it can be an essential part of a nurse's communication repertoire.

Using Helpful Responding Techniques

There are many helpful responding techniques nurses can use to demonstrate respect and encourage patients to communicate openly. Helpful responses that have already been discussed in this chapter include being nonjudgmental, observing body language, and using active listening. Other useful responses include demonstrating empathy, asking open-ended questions, giving information, using reflection, and being silent. Each will be explained.

Empathy

Empathy consists of awareness of, sensitivity to, and identification with the feelings of another person. Nurses can empathize with patients even if they have not experienced an event in their own lives exactly like the one the patient is experiencing. If nurses have had a similar or parallel experience, empathy is possible. For example, the feeling of loss is familiar to most nurses, even though they may not personally have lost a close family member.

Empathy is different from sympathy in that the sympathetic nurse enters into the feeling with the patient, whereas the empathic nurse appreciates the patient's feelings but is not swept along with the feelings. "You seem upset about the upcoming procedure" is an example of a nursing statement that demonstrates empathy.

Open-ended questions

An open-ended question is one that causes the patient to answer fully, giving more than a yes or no answer. Open-ended questions are very useful in data gathering and in the opening stages of any nurse-patient interaction. For example, asking a patient, "Are you in pain?" may elicit only a confirming yes. Saying to him, "Tell me about your pain" is more likely to elicit information about the site, type, intensity, and duration of the pain, therefore making the nurse-patient interaction more useful.

Giving information

An essential part of nursing is providing information to patients and their significant others. Giving information includes sharing knowledge that the recipients are not expected to know. Nurses provide information when they tell patients what to expect during diagnostic procedures, inform them of their rights as patients, and teach them about their conditions, diets, or medications.

An important distinction every nurse needs to make is the difference between providing information and giving opinions. Although providing information is a helpful aspect of the nursing role, giving opinions is considered unhelpful.

Instead, nurses should encourage patients to consider their own values and opinions as primary in importance. The nurse's opinion is not relevant.

Reflection

The nurse using reflection is serving as a mirror for the patient. Reflection demonstrates understanding and acceptance. It is a method of encouraging patients to think through problems for themselves by directing patient questions back to the patient. Reflection implies respect because the nurse believes the patient has adequate resources to solve the problem without outside assistance. In response to the patient's question, "Do you think I should go through with this surgery?" the nurse can reflect the question: "Your thinking on this question is most important. Do you think you should have the surgery?" Reflection helps clarify the patient's thoughts and feelings and helps the nurse obtain additional information that may assist in developing the plan of care.

Silence

Although silent periods in social conversations may feel uncomfortable, using silence in nurse-patient relationships can be a helpful response. Using silence means allowing periods of quiet thought during an interaction without feeling pressure to "fill the gap" with conversation or activity. For example, when a patient has just been given upsetting news, sitting quietly without making any demands for conversation may be the most therapeutic response a nurse can make at that time. "Being with" patients is often just as valuable as "doing for" them and conveys respect for the patient's feelings. Professional nurses learn to use silence and find time in their busy schedules to "be with" patients.

There are many more helpful responding styles nurses can use in their interactions with patients. The five discussed here, once practiced and mastered, can be a foundation on which to build.

Culturally Sensitive Communication

Because communication is the means by which people connect, nurses must take cultural differences into consideration when planning and implementing care. No hard and fast rules can be given because communication practices are unique for each individual and vary widely, even for people from the same cultural backgrounds. Various elements to assess include dialect, style, volume, use of touch, emotional tone, gestures, stance, space needs, and eye contact (Davidhizar, Dowd, and Giger, 1998).

Culturally sensitive nurses recognize that even when individuals speak the same language, sender and receiver may perceive different meanings because of unique life experiences. Patients may be unwilling to share certain information with nurses because of cultural taboos. Nurses may inadvertently offend patients or family members by violating cultural norms concerning touch, space, and eye contact.

Later in this chapter, Box 9-6 provides strategies for communicating effectively with coworkers of different cultural backgrounds. It is easily adapted for use with patients and provides guidelines for promoting cross-cultural communication. Additional examples of cultural awareness can be found in Chapter 10, Illness, Culture and Caring.

Avoiding Common Causes of Communication Breakdown

Just as there are many factors influencing successful communication, unsuccessful communication can occur for many reasons. A sender may send an incomplete or confusing message. A message may not be received, or it may be misunderstood or distorted by the receiver. Incongruent messages may cause confusion in the receiver. In nursing situations, there are several common causes of communication breakdown. These include failing to see each individual as unique, failing to recognize levels of meaning, using value statements, using false reassurance, and failing to clarify unclear messages.

Failing to see the uniqueness of the individual

Failing to see the uniqueness of each individual is a frequent cause of communication breakdown. This failure is caused by preconceived ideas, prejudices, and stereotypes, illustrated by the

Box 9-6   Strategies to Promote Effective Communication in the Multicultural Workplace

- Pronounce names correctly; when in doubt, ask for the correct pronunciation.
- Use proper titles of respect (e.g., doctor, reverend, mister). Be sure to ask for the person's permission to use his or her first name or wait until you are given permission to do so.
- Be aware of gender sensitivities. If uncertain about the marital status of a woman or her preferred title, it is best to refer to her as "Ms." (pronounced *miz*) initially; then at the first opportunity, ask her what she prefers to be called.
- Be aware of subtle linguistic messages that may convey bias or inequality, for example, referring to a white male as "Mr." while addressing an African-American female by her first name.
- Refrain from anglicizing or shortening a person's given name without his or her permission, for example, calling a Russian American "Mike" instead of Mikhail, or shortening the name of Italian American Maria Rosaria to Rose. The same principle applies to the surname.
- Call people by their proper name. Avoid slang such as "girl," "boy," "honey," "dear," "guy," "fella," "babe," "chief," "mama," "sweetheart," or similar terms. When in doubt, ask whether a particular term is offensive.
- Refrain from using slang, pejorative, or derogatory terms when referring to persons from particular ethnic, racial, or religious groups.
- Identify people by race, color, ethnic origin, religion, or physical handicap/disability only when necessary and appropriate.
- Avoid using words and phrases that may be offensive to others. For example, "culturally deprived" or "culturally disadvantaged" implies inferiority, and "nonwhite" implies that white is the normative standard.
- Avoid clichés and platitudes, such as, "Some of my best friends are Mexicans" or "I went to school with African Americans."
- In communications, use language that includes all staff.
- Do not expect a staff member to know all the other employees of his or her background or to speak for them. They share ethnicity, not necessarily the same experiences, friendships, or beliefs.
- Refrain from telling stories or jokes demeaning to certain ethnic, racial, age, or religious groups.
  Also avoid those pertaining to gender-related issues or to persons with physical or mental disabilities.
- Avoid remarks that suggest to staff from diverse backgrounds that they should consider themselves fortunate to be in the organization. Do not compare their employment opportunities and conditions with those of people in their country of origin.
- Remember that communication problems multiply in telephone communications because important nonverbal cues are lost and accents may be difficult to interpret.

Modified with permission from Andrews MM: Transcultural perspectives in nursing administration, *J Nurs Admin* 28(11): 34, 1998.

following interchange between a 65-year-old patient and a nurse:

Patient: "My back is really hurting today. I can hardly turn over in bed."

Nurse: "I guess we have to expect these little problems when we get older."

This nurse has pigeonholed the patient in a specific group, "old people," and therefore does not react to the patient as an individual. The nurse could have promoted continued communication by responding to the patient as an individual:

Nurse: "Tell me more about your back pain, Mrs. Jameson."

Failing to recognize levels of meaning

When nurses recognize only the overt level of meaning, communication breakdown can occur. Patients often give verbal cues to meanings that lie under the surface content of their verbalizations:

Patient: "It's getting awfully warm in here."

Nurse: (Responding only to surface meaning) "I'll adjust the air conditioning for you."

This response does not help the patient express himself fully. A different type of response focuses on the symbolic level of meaning:

Nurse: "Perhaps there is something about our conversation that is making you uncomfortable."

Although it takes a lot of experience to know when and how to respond to symbolic communication, nurses should be aware of its existence.

Using value statements and clichés

Using value statements and clichés is another communication problem. **Value statements** imply that the nurse has made a judgment, either positive or negative. The use of value statements indicates that the nurse is operating out of his or her own framework without considering that the patient might feel differently. The use of **clichés**, which are trite, stereotyped expressions, is common in social conversation but should be used carefully in professional relationships. Consider the prevalence of the cliché "Have a good day." This statement has come to have little real meaning. This common error can cut off communication by showing the patient that the nurse does not understand the patient's true feelings.

Patient: "My mother is coming to see me today."

Nurse: "How nice. There's nothing as comforting as a mother's love."

This nurse has used a value statement ("how nice") and a cliché ("there's nothing as comforting as a mother's love"). She has made an assumption that the patient welcomes a visit from her mother and has failed to verify what the patient's actual wishes are. In fact, the patient and her mother may have a difficult relationship, and the patient may dread the impending visit. By assuming otherwise, the nurse has contributed to communication breakdown. This patient probably will not attempt to discuss her relationship with her mother any further with this nurse. A more helpful response would be:

Nurse: "How do you feel about her visit?"

This allows the patient to ventilate her feelings about her mother's visit, whether positive or negative. The nurse has conveyed a genuine interest in the patient's true feelings.

Giving false reassurance

Using **false reassurance** is another communication pitfall. It may help the nurse feel better but does not facilitate communication and help the patient.

Patient: "I'm so afraid the biopsy will be cancer."

Nurse: "Don't worry. You have the best doctor in town. Besides, cancer treatment is really good these days."

For a fearful patient, this type of glib reassurance does not help. This nurse has no way of knowing that the patient's concerns are not legitimate. She may indeed have cancer. A more sensitive response would be

Nurse: "Why don't we talk about your concerns?"

This kind of response keeps the lines of communication open between patient and nurse and allows the nurse to clarify any misconceptions the patient may express.

Failing to clarify

Failing to clarify the patient's unclear statements is a fifth common communication pitfall.

Patient: "I've got to get out of the hospital. They have found out I'm here and may come after me."

Nurse: "No one will harm you here."

This nurse has responded as if the patient's meaning was clear. A clarifying response might be

Nurse: *"Who are 'they,' Mrs. Johnson?"*

Confused patients or those with psychiatric illnesses often communicate in ways that are difficult to understand. It is reassuring to patients to know that nurses are trying to understand them, even if they are not always successful. Communication is facilitated by clarification responses.

Practicing Helpful Responses

Nurses can practice using helpful responses and avoiding common communication pitfalls with family members, friends, and coworkers, as well as in patient contacts. Being a good communicator takes practice and usually feels unnatural at first. Any new behavior takes time to integrate into habitual patterns. By continuing to practice, nurses soon find themselves feeling more natural. They find that these newly acquired skills are beneficial both professionally and personally. The accompanying Critical Thinking Challenge 9-1 compares the helpfulness of different types of responses in a nurse-patient interaction.

Caring Through Holistic Communication

Holistic communication is "the art of sharing emotional and factual information. It involves letting go of judgments and appreciating the patient's point of view" (Klagsbrun, 2001, p. 116). Think about those words; how reassuring would it be to you right now to have someone who, without judgment, appreciated your point of view? Virtually all nurses begin their professional lives wanting to give patients that kind of attention. But the reality of too many patients and too little time often reduces communication to its barest essentials. Proponents of holistic communication believe that it speeds the healing process, whereas using only functional or task-oriented communication, which consists of giving instructions and briefly answering questions, inhibits it.

Some nurses fear that holistic communication will take too much time when time is scarce. But when patients are listened to in this way, their anxiety decreases and they complain less, call for attention less often, feel more understood and valued, and "are more likely to comply with their treatment plan" (Klagsbrun, 2001, p. 116).

Holistic communicators actively attend to their patients through such intentional gestures as using an accepting facial expression or warm eye contact, turning toward the patient with open posture, and encouraging expression of concerns. They show a willingness to listen to whatever issues the patient needs to share by asking simple, open-ended questions such as, "How are you right now?"

Holistic communicators use the principles of active listening—that is, listening to the whole person and paying "gentle, compassionate attention to what has been said or implied" (Klagsbrun, 2001, p. 116). This kind of being present with patients means avoiding analyzing, judging, or problem solving. It means avoiding defensiveness, even when the patient is critical of you or your coworkers. In addition, it has a beneficial effect on the well-being of nurses and patients.

COMMUNICATION WITH PROFESSIONAL COLLEAGUES

This chapter has focused on nurse-patient communication as the core of the nursing process and foundation of the therapeutic use of self. In addition to patients and their families, however, nurses must also communicate effectively with an ever-increasing array of professional and unlicensed personnel including physicians; laboratory, pharmacy, and medical records personnel; other nurses; and allied health personnel, to name a few. Socialization into health care professions tends to be discipline specific. It typically does not emphasize the strengths of other disciplines and what they can offer as patient care teammates (Lindeke and Block, 2001). This tunnel vision tends to create territoriality in which each discipline defends its

CRITICAL THINKING *Challenge 9-1*

Helpful and Unhelpful Responding Techniques

Directions: Critique both interactions below, identifying each helpful and unhelpful response used by the nurse. Describe how you imagine the patient might feel at the close of each interaction. Identify what the nurse has accomplished in each instance.

Mr. Goodman has been admitted to the hospital for coronary bypass surgery. During the admission process, the following interactions might take place.

INTERACTION ONE

Nurse: Mr. Goodman, I am Mrs. Scott. Can I get some information about you now?

Patient: Okay.

Nurse: You're here for bypass surgery?

Patient: Yes, that's what they tell me.

Nurse: (Taking blood pressure) Do you have any allergies to foods or medications?

Patient: Not that I know of. I've never been in a hospital before.

Nurse: Well, your blood pressure looks good. (Silence while patient has thermometer in mouth.) This is a really nice room—just remodeled. I know you'll be comfortable here. Will your wife be coming to see you tonight? (Removes thermometer.)

Patient: My wife is sick. She hasn't been able to leave home for 2 years. I don't know what will happen to her while I am here.

Nurse: Gosh, I'm so sorry to hear that. I guess having you back home healthy is what she wants though, isn't it? And you've got a great surgeon. Well, I've got to run now. Check on you later.

INTERACTION TWO

Nurse: Good afternoon, Mr. Goodman. I'm Mrs. Scott, and I'll be your nurse this evening. If this is a good time, I'd like to ask you some questions and complete your admission process.

Patient: Okay.

Nurse: First, I'll get your temperature and blood pressure, and then we'll talk. (Silence while nurse takes vital signs.) Everything looks good. Do you have any allergies to foods or medications?

Patient: Not that I know of. I've never been in a hospital before.

Nurse: Hospitals can be a little overwhelming, especially when you've never been a patient before. Now, would you please tell me in your own words why you are here?

Patient: Well, the doc tells me I have a clogged artery, and I need a bypass. I guess they'll open up my heart.

Nurse: What exactly do you know about the surgery?

Patient: Not too much, really. He told me yesterday that I need it right away—and here I am.

Nurse: It sounds like you need some more information about what will happen. Later this evening I will come back, and we'll talk some more. Are you expecting to have visitors tonight?

Patient: No, my wife can't leave home. I don't know what she will do without me while I'm here. This came up so suddenly.

Nurse: I can see that this is a serious concern for you. We can explore some possibilities when I come back this evening. I'll plan to come around 7:15, if that suits you.

Patient: Sure, I can use all the help I can get.

---

own turf rather than promoting collegiality and collaboration. Health care delivery suffers when the members of the health care team fail to use the talents of all or experience communication breakdown.

As a general rule, nurses can use with colleagues the same communication skills that have been discussed as part of nurse-patient communication. The value of face-to-face communication cannot be overemphasized. The attitude of respect for others, regardless of position, is essential. Active listening, acceptance, and being nonjudgmental are key elements, as are the conscious use of feedback, appropriateness, efficiency, and flexibility.

Sensitivity to cultural differences and thoughtful use of electronic communication devices are both essential in today's increasingly diverse and technology-driven workplaces. Both can create communication challenges and will be discussed below.

Effective Use of Electronic Communication Devices

The past decade has brought an unprecedented proliferation of electronic communication devices such as cell phones, PDAs, e-mail, voice mail, and faxes. It is not uncommon to see nurses with "ear buds" in place talking (presumably) with other staff members even as they care for patients. This is insensitive and sends a very clear message to patients that they and their needs are secondary. The use of e-mail presents another set of problems and can lead to misunderstanding because the facial expression, tone of voice, and other contextual cues are not visible to message recipients and are therefore subject to misinterpretation. A few common-sense guidelines are useful to prevent the use of technologic communication devices from creating a barrier to nurse-patient or nurse-colleague communication:

- Give your full attention to the person you are with. Avoid checking your cell phone or PDA for messages while conversing with others.
- Adopt a courteous tone in e-mail and voice mail messages regardless of how rushed you are; remember the recipient cannot see your nonverbal communication.
- Avoid the use of jargon in verbal and written communication; use acronyms only when you are confident of their universal understanding.
- Keep messages short; include only necessary useful details without being abrupt or curt.
- When receiving a message, read, listen, and evaluate the entire message before reacting. This is particularly important when you are feeling pressed for time.

Communication in Today's Multicultural Workplace

Sensitivity to cultural differences in communication is essential in today's culturally diverse workplace. The composition of the health care workforce is being rapidly transformed by the population demographics of the nation. Diversity in age, race, gender, ethnicity, country of origin, sexual orientation, and disability is present, creating opportunities for nurses to develop skill in transcultural communication.

Culture is the lens through which all other aspects of life are viewed. Culture determines an individual's health beliefs and practices. It also affects profoundly the meaning individuals attribute to work. Different cultures view caring for the sick in widely varying ways, such as a divine calling, a religious vocation, or an occupation for the lower classes.

The meaning of work in a given culture also affects how people of that culture communicate. Andrews (1998) pointed out that verbal or nonverbal communication issues are often at the root of conflict in the multicultural health care setting. According to Andrews, the decision to speak directly with someone, send a memorandum, make a phone call or e-mail, or not to communicate at all should be made only after taking the receiving staff member's cultural preferences into consideration. Strategies for promoting effective cross-cultural communication in the workplace are found in Box 9-6.

Attention is now being paid to the cultural differences among different "generations" of nurses, all of whom can be found working side by side. Even when race and ethnicity are similar, the ages of nurses in a single setting may range from early 20s to middle 60s, a 40-year gap. This can create interpersonal challenges in the workplace. Although it is hazardous to make generalizations about groups, anecdotal evidence and research studies reveal differing opinions among age groups about what is important to them professionally and personally. Each generation experienced political events and social trends during their formative years that influence their values. These influences cut across racial and ethnic lines. The groups may differ in terms of "work ethics, communication preferences, manners, and attitudes toward authority," as well as in terms of "superficialities, such as speech habits, clothing, and hair styles," all of which can cause tensions and friction (Siela, 2006, p. 28).

The four generations include the "Veterans," also called "Traditionalists," who were born between 1922 and 1945. This group is aging out of the workforce, but some have not yet retired. Two thirds of today's workforce in all occupational groups consists of "Baby Boomers," born between 1946 and 1959. Next comes "Generation X," also known as "Twentysomethings," who were born

between 1960 and 1980. Youngest are the members of "Generation Y," also termed "Millennials," who were born between 1981 and 2000.

As you will see in Box 9-7, the characteristics and attitudes of the various groups are different. Rather than viewing these varying attitudes toward life and work as problems, professional nurses seek to understand colleagues of different generations and capitalize on the strengths each group brings to the workplace. "Knowing the characteristics and core values of each generation can help nurses of diverse ages understand colleagues who are much younger or older than they are. However,

Box 9-7   Selected Characteristics of a Multigenerational Nursing Workforce

	VETERANS (TRADITIONALISTS) B. 1922-1945	BABY BOOMERS B. 1946-1959	GENERATION X (TWENTY-SOMETHINGS) B. 1960-1980	GENERATION Y (MILLENNIALS) B. 1981-2000
Physical needs	Reaching limits of physical abilities; require rest; vulnerable to injuries	Beginning to experience physical limitations	Ample physical energy; few limitations	High levels of youthful energy
Relationship to authority	Comfortable with a directive management style; value formal lines of authority (top-down); respect for authority; rarely complain about authority	Love-hate relationship with authority; may question rules but generally follow them; comfortable bending rules	Expect authority figures to earn their respect; mistrust bureaucracy; desire frequent positive reinforcement and feedback	Not awed by authority figures; relaxed approach to the bureaucracy
Work ethic	Strong work ethic; stoic acceptance of higher work loads; belief in duty before pleasure; self-sacrificing; dedicated	Work gives meaning to life; willing to work long hours; will sacrifice for success	Little trust of work environment or loyalty to it; seek to avoid long hours and have fun on the job; desire life-work balance	High expectations of the workplace; may set unrealistic goals; need prolonged job orientation and mentoring; desire life-work balance
Decision making	Prefer to discuss process (how to do something) rather than outcomes (results)	Value consensus building	Dislike process; focused on outcomes; want to know how decisions will affect them	Highly collaborative

Continued

Box 9-7   Selected Characteristics of a Multigenerational Nursing Workforce—cont'd

Teamwork	Tend not to rock the boat	Enjoy competition; comfortable working in teams and value teamwork	Prefer to work alone; entrepreneurial	Desire to participate in decisions; team players
Psychological needs	Respect is top need; disciplined; patient	Generally optimistic; not comfortable with conflict in the workplace; feel indispensable; can be intellectually arrogant; tend to be socially conscious	Generally skeptical; tend to be pessimistic; desire accolades, whether deserved or not; motivated by money and success; seek to start at the top	Optimistic; confident; share feelings with ease; high expectations of selves; impatient to get to the top; may feel unappreciated; desire positive feedback; accept change eagerly
Formal vs. informal modes of relating	Prefer face-to-face personal discussions and handwritten notes to e-mail; unaccustomed to diversity; high expectations of younger generations can lead to frustration	Favor an informal work environment	Informal; flexible; not known for manners, etiquette, or interpersonal skills; accustomed to diversity; irreverent sense of humor; may be perceived as rude	Behave and dress casually; most tolerant of cultural diversity; desire to have fun on the job; value good manners; have best rapport with other generations
Attitude toward communication technologies	May not be technically literate; sometimes willing to learn	Many are technically literate and most are willing to learn	Technically literate	Highly proficient with technology; use the Internet for research and communication; accustomed to multitasking

Compiled from: Halfer D, Saver C: Bridging the generation gaps, *Nursing Spectrum (SE Ed.)* 4(3):28-33, 2008; Siela D: Managing the multigenerational nursing staff, *American Nurse Today* 1(3):47-49, 2006; Wieck KL: Motivating an intergenerational workforce: scenarios for success, *Orthop Nurs* 26(6): 366-371, 2007.

take care not to stereotype anyone. Each person is a unique individual with distinctive traits, which may or may not be typical of his or her generation as a whole" (Siela, 2008, p. 47).

Wise nurses do not leave their communication skills at the patient's bedside but use them throughout their personal and professional lives. Using clear, simple messages and clarifying the intent of others constitute a positive goal in all personal and professional communication. As with patients, trust must exist before communication with coworkers can be effective.

COLLABORATION SKILLS: THE KEY TO EFFECTIVE TEAMWORK

Collaboration is a complex process that builds on communication. Collaboration in health care settings is far more than simply cooperation, negotiation, or compromise. It implies working jointly with other professionals, all of whom are respected for their unique knowledge and abilities, to improve a patient's health status or to solve an organizational problem. It involves civil behavior, such as showing respect for others and sharing knowledge and authority, and is nonhierarchical (Lower, 2007). As a result, all members of the team feel their contributions are valued.

Collaboration may occur as an outgrowth of a long-standing relationship, or it can be in a fleeting encounter. It can even occur electronically. Making the most of all collaboration opportunities enhances positive patient outcomes. As mentioned earlier, schools rarely use a collaborative model of education. Once out of school, however, professionals must collaborate when a complex problem arises that is beyond one individual's ability to solve (Gerardi and Morrison, 2005).

In spite of the fact that nurses are educated as individuals, most of the time they work in teams. To work effectively on teams, collaboration skills are essential. For collaboration to occur, a variety of human and organizational factors must be in place.

Human Factors in Collaboration

Although it may seem to state the obvious, all collaborating parties must be willing to work together if the collaboration is to be successful. They must have attained a level of readiness to collaborate through education, maturity, and prior experience (Henneman, Lee, and Cohen, 1995). They must know what knowledge and expertise they bring to the table and have confidence in the worth of their contributions. They must understand their own limits and their discipline's boundaries while respecting what other professions and professionals can contribute. Above all, they must communicate effectively, trust one another, and be committed to working together (Kramer and Schmalenberg, 2003).

Box 9-8   Are You Ready to Collaborate? Key Components of Effective Collaboration

Respect for the other parties involved
Emotional maturity
Confidence in own knowledge
Willingness to learn
Cooperative spirit
Belief in a common purpose
Value unique perspectives of other disciplines
Willingness to negotiate
Know own limits
Communicate
Self-knowledge
Self-awareness (e.g., biases, values, goals)
Positive regard for opinions that differ
Not threatened by conflict

Box 9-8 contains a checklist to help you determine your readiness to collaborate.

Organizational Factors in Collaboration

Just as the people involved must have certain attributes that facilitate collaboration, the organization in which the collaboration takes place also must be supportive. According to Henneman and colleagues (1995), factors supporting collaboration include a flat, as opposed to a multitiered, organizational structure; encouragement and support of individuals to act autonomously; recognition of team accomplishments, as opposed to individual accomplishments; cooperation, as opposed to competition; and valuing of knowledge and expertise, rather than titles or roles. Collaborative organizations have values that support equality and interdependence rather than status and pecking orders. Creativity and shared vision are also valued (Kramer and Schmalenberg, 2003).

The collaborative process (Gardner, 2005) entails a number of steps if it is to be successful. They include the following:

- Identification of the stakeholders (who has a stake in the outcome?)
- Identification of the problem(s) to be solved

- Identification of barriers or roadblocks on the road to solution
- Clarification of the desired outcomes (agree on criteria for success)
- Clarification of the process (how will we approach the task?)
- Identification of who will be responsible for each step in the task
- Evaluation (have we met our criteria for success?)

Outcomes of Collaboration

Collaboration is a positive process that benefits the people involved, as individuals and as a group; the organization in which they work; and health care consumers. Increased feelings of self-worth, a sense of accomplishment, esprit de corps, enhanced collegiality and respect, and increased productivity, retention, and employee satisfaction are positive benefits of collaboration (LeTourneau, 2004). Preliminary studies show that collaboration among health care professionals holds great promise for enhancing positive patient outcomes (Kramer and Schmalenberg, 2003). Conversely, studies have shown that disruptive behavior negatively affects patient care outcomes by causing stress and resulting errors (Baggs et al, 1999; Rosenstein and O'Daniel, 2005).

Nurse-Physician Collaboration

Among the most problematic relationships that nurses encounter during practice are those with physicians. Educational, status, and gender differences must be overcome. Despite rising male enrollments in nursing schools and even more dramatic increases in female enrollments in medical schools, practicing physicians are predominantly male and practicing nurses overwhelmingly female. This leads to differences in styles of communicating and behaving that can cause challenges in collaborative relationships.

During female-dominated nursing school experiences, most nurses are encouraged to view physicians as teammates and to collaborate with them whenever possible. Male-dominated medical schools, however, tend to instill in their graduates a hierarchical model of teamwork with the physician at the top of the hierarchy. These two divergent cultures, when combined with gender differences in communication and teamwork patterns, further complicate the relationship between the two professions. Too often, gender differences are interpreted as professional differences, leading to further misunderstanding.

People realize that there are differences in communication styles and behavior among individuals of different cultures. What too few people recognize is that gender is a type of culture, because men and women grow up learning different lessons about what is appropriate adult behavior. From birth, boy babies and girl babies are dressed differently, given different toys, praised for different types of behavior, and socialized to gender-specific behavior in dozens of more subtle ways. Teachers treat boys and girls differently; authors of children's books and television scripts depict men and women differently (Heim, 1995). Is it any wonder that, as adults, men and women may have differing expectations of professional relationships?

Women tend to treat other people as equal, regardless of their position in the organizational hierarchy. They spend time chatting with others, building and maintaining relationships, and frequently make friends at work. Even when in management roles, they tend to tell people what to do indirectly. In general, they come to meetings expecting to discuss the issues and make decisions depending on the outcome of the discussion. They value the process aspects of decision making as much as the outcome and tend to seek consensus in decision making (Heim, 1995). This can cause them to seem tentative or unsure to task-oriented people.

Men tend to see other workers as above, below, or parallel to them in the organizational structure and to treat them accordingly. They tend to be task oriented and chat less, are friendly but tend not to become friends with coworkers, and are likely to tell subordinates what to do directly. In general, they come to meetings already having discussed the issues, made decisions beforehand, and lined up the votes they need to get their decisions approved. They are more goal oriented and pay less attention to process than to outcome (Heim, 1995). They tend to focus on justice issues and rule out alternatives. This can cause them to seem headstrong to more consensus-oriented people.

Beyond gender differences, medicine and nursing have differing cultures. This is sometimes termed the care-cure conflict. Differences of opinion are inevitable when the basic approach to problems is different, as they are with nursing and medicine. Conflict can be either destructive or constructive. When participants have conflict negotiation skills, conflict can lead to creative solutions and an atmosphere where diverse ideas are welcome.

In collaborative relationships, conflict can be categorized as emotionally based or task based. Emotionally based conflicts are attributable to relationships whereas task-based conflicts are a result of differences of opinion over how to approach a task or achieve a mutual goal.

Constructive conflict negotiation skills can be developed (Gerardi and Morrison, 2005). Examples of these skills include the following:

- Acknowledge the conflict.
- Recognize and affirm that positives can result from conflict.
- Facilitate debate over task issues while redirecting concerns away from the personal level.
- Promote expression of varying perspectives.
- Monitor tone of voice, eye contact, defensive nonverbal posture.
- Avoid locking into a fixed position; explore alternatives and opportunities to synthesize several ideas to create a new one.
- Share power; elicit everyone's opinions and look for win-win situations.
- Stay focused on the desired outcome.

Successful collaboration requires a focus on both relationships and the task at hand. Differences in gender culture create challenges in all aspects of personal and professional life if they are not understood. Understanding the differences in communication styles between nurses and physicians serves to increase self-awareness and minimize assumptions and erroneous interpretations. For insight into how gender culture may affect your working relationships, take the gender culture self-assessment in the Cultural Considerations Challenge on p. 218 and discuss it in a small group composed of both genders. For further study of nurse-physician collaboration, you may want to read an excellent article on the topic online: http://nursingworld.org/mods/mod775/nrsdrfull.htm (Lindeke and Sieckert, 2005).

Collaboration With Patients

Recognizing that patients often feel intimidated in health care settings and fail to say what is on their minds, The Joint Commission, a group that accredits hospitals, nursing homes, and other health care institutions, instituted the "Speak Up" initiative in 2002 (Box 9-9). This program encourages patients to question their caregivers about medicines, tests, surgeries, pain relief, and other matters of concern (Graham, 2008). Involving patients in their own care is believed to promote safety. Because patients depend on their caregivers, they are often reluctant to ask questions for fear of appearing to be unappreciative, argumentative, or seeming to challenge authority. It is therefore important for nurses to explicitly encourage patients to question anything they do not understand, to be receptive to their questions, and to avoid being defensive when patients and their families question procedures or medications. Empowering patients and families and partnering with them is the goal, and nurses can foster an atmosphere of openness and receptiveness. To learn more about the Speak Up initiative, consult The Joint Commission's fact sheet online: http://www.jointcommission.org/AboutUs/Fact_Sheets/about_speakup.htm.

Collaboration With Assistive Personnel

Relationships between registered nurses and the other members of the nursing staff, such as licensed practical nurses and patient care technicians, affect quality of care and patient outcomes (Apker et al, 2006). All too often, mutual respect and cooperation are missing in these important relationships, as the different groups feel frustrated and unappreciated. Language is often a barrier as are nonverbal and other culturally determined behaviors, such as the value placed

Cultural Considerations Challenge
Gender Culture Self-Assessment

Directions: For each of the paired statements, select the one that most accurately expresses your experiences or feelings.

COLUMN ONE

I prefer to compete to win.

I like to work where I know the hierarchy so that I know what is expected of me.

When I lead a meeting, I prefer to sit in front of the group or at the head of the table.

In arriving at a decision, I study the options, select one, and move ahead with it.

I define a "team player" as someone who follows orders, supports the leader unquestioningly, and does what is needed no matter how he or she feels.

I can disagree or even argue with my friends and not allow it to affect the friendship.

In the workplace, competent people do not worry about being nice.

I spend little time in getting to know my coworkers personally.

COLUMN TWO

I prefer to find win-win solutions.

I like to work in situations where power is equally shared.

When I lead a meeting, I prefer to sit with the group or in a circle.

In arriving at a decision, I usually ask several other people for their opinions.

I define a "team player" as someone who shares ideas, listens even when they disagree, and works collaboratively.

I expect my friends to side with me in disagreements and tend to take it personally if they do not.

In the workplace it is possible to be both competent and nice.

It is worthwhile to spend time getting to know my coworkers on a personal level.

Scoring instructions: If most of your checks were in Column One, you have a traditionally male gender style. When you work with women, you can anticipate some challenges because of differences in behavior and conversational styles. These challenges can be overcome. If most of your checks were in Column Two, you have a traditionally female gender style. When you work with men, you can anticipate some challenges because of differences in behavior and conversational styles. These challenges can be overcome. If your checks were about equally balanced between Column One and Column Two, you have a combination of male and female gender styles. You should be able to work easily with both men and women.

on schedules. Differences in beliefs, values, perceptions, and priorities create conflict, result in poor teamwork, reduce job satisfaction, and ultimately have a negative impact on patient care.

Hayes (1994) reported on team-building sessions with registered nurses and patient care technicians (PCTS) on three general hospital units. The purpose was to identify and align the needs of work-related relationships in both groups with the needs of the nursing unit. This is a key step in team building, which was the model chosen to encourage collaboration between the two groups.

Teams were defined as groups of workers with a fairly stable composition. They worked interdependently and shared a common purpose. To emphasize that the nurses and PCTs needed to

work cooperatively, researchers asked each group questions, such as the following: "What do you need from each other to make your day go better?" "What is important for you to have in the way of working relationships on this nursing unit?" "What do you need from the registered nurses?" "What do you need from the patient care technicians?" (Hayes, 1994, p. 52).

The PCTs reported needing to feel welcome, appreciated, and respected but instead reported feeling unwelcome, unrecognized, and unappreciated. They did not realize that registered nurses were expected to plan, supervise, and evaluate their work. The registered nurses expressed the need to feel competent as managers and to have PCTs comply with requests and give feedback

Box 9-9   Collaborating With Patients: The Speak Up Initiative

According to The Joint Commission, health care professionals and institutions should encourage patients to question their caregivers and recommend using the following guidelines:

Speak up if you have questions or concerns. If you still don't understand, ask again. It's your body and you have a right to know.

Pay attention to the care you get. Always make sure you're getting the right treatments and medicines by the right health care professionals. Don't assume anything.

Educate yourself about your illness. Learn about the medical tests you get, and your treatment plan.

Ask a trusted family member or friend to be your advocate (advisor or supporter).

Know what medications you take and why you take them. Medicine errors are the most common health care mistakes.

Use a hospital, clinic, surgery center, or other type of health care organization that has been carefully checked out. For example, The Joint Commission visits hospitals to see if they are meeting The Joint Commission's quality standards.

Participate in all decisions about your treatment. You are the center of the health care team.

Reprinted with permission of The Joint Commission's "Speak Up" initiative.

Box 9-10   How to Build an Effective Team

You can learn to contribute to the effective functioning of a team by adopting the following behaviors:

- Show respect for team members.
- Speak to team members clearly and concisely.
- Interact assertively and confidently.
- Work on building trust within the team.
- Help the team agree on the goal of patient well-being above all else.
- Be a collaborator by seeking, managing, and providing data to the other team members.
- Acknowledge disagreements when they arise.
- Maintain the patient focus and negotiate respectfully.
- Avoid blaming when things go wrong.
- Welcome healthy disagreement as an opportunity for additional solutions to emerge.
- Involve teammates in patient care decisions. Draw out quiet members.
- Question decisions calmly and directly when you disagree.
- Remain flexible and open-minded to others' ideas.
- Show compassion for both patients and colleagues.
- Promote a caring and supportive practice setting.

Compiled from: Apker J, Propp K, Zabava FW, Hofmeister N: Collaboration, credibility, compassion, and coordination: professional nurse communication skill sets in health care team interactions, *J Prof Nurs* 22(3):180-189, 2006; Lindeke L, Sieckert AM: Nurse-physician workplace collaboration, *Online J Issues Nurs* 10(1), 2005 (website): http://nursingworld.org/mods/mod775/nrsdrfull.htm.

about assigned activities. Some registered nurses reported that they preferred to complete work themselves rather than experience embarrassment when PCTs failed to comply with their requests.

Team-building sessions focused on identifying problematic feelings and misperceptions and correcting them. For example, in response to the PCTs' belief that their contributions to patient welfare were unappreciated, the registered nurses replied, "We could not run the unit without you" and "What you do makes the difference in how comfortable the patients feel" (Hayes, p. 53).

During team building with these groups, misperceptions were aired and discussed and expectations were clarified. Registered nurses' legitimate authority and legal responsibility for unlicensed personnel were clarified. The result was an increase in mutual respect and understanding.

Team building is an intentional process (Lindeke and Sieckert, 2005). Nurses can promote effective teamwork by modeling team-building behaviors, such as building trust and promoting a caring and supportive practice setting. Box 9-10 contains a list of team-building behaviors you can use to improve the effectiveness of your teamwork.

Summary of Key Points

- The "therapeutic use of self" means using one's personality and communication skills effectively while implementing the nursing process to help patients improve their health status.
- Phases in the traditional nurse-patient relationship include the orientation phase, the working phase, and the termination phase. Short-term patient contacts in today's streamlined care delivery system also present opportunities for connection and goal achievement.
- In long-term nurse-patient relationships, each phase has specific tasks that should be accomplished before progressing to subsequent phases.
- Acceptance of others' values, beliefs, and lifestyles is important in nursing.
- Developing awareness of biases can help nurses to prevent the intrusion of these biases into nurse-patient relationships.
- Professional nurses are aware of the boundaries of the therapeutic relationship and strive to stay within the "zone of helpfulness" at all times.
- Communication is the core of all relationships and is the primary instrument through which desired change is effected in others.
- Communication is both verbal and nonverbal and consists of a sender, a receiver, a message, feedback, and context.
- Perception, evaluation, and transmission are the three major operations in communication.
- Communication develops sequentially, beginning with somatic language and progressing to action language and then to verbal language.
- Communication may be successful or unsuccessful. Successful communication meets four major criteria: feedback, appropriateness, efficiency, and flexibility.
- Active listening is a key factor in holistic communication.
- Unsuccessful communication is caused by a variety of factors that can be identified and eliminated.
- In addition to communicating well with patients, nurses use communication skills to collaborate effectively with physicians, other nurses, unlicensed personnel, and other members of the health care delivery team.
- Professional nurses must be sensitive to sociocultural factors such as age, ethnicity, and gender that can affect communication and collaboration.

Critical Thinking Questions

1. Explain what is meant by the term "therapeutic use of self."
2. List the phases of the traditional nurse-patient relationship, and describe the tasks of each.
3. Identify ways nurses can quickly "connect" with patients and help them move toward wellness during short-term interactions.
4. Describe the negative results of boundary crossings in the nurse-patient relationship.
5. Explain why nonverbal communication may be more reliable than verbal communication.
6. List as many factors as you can that influence the communication process.
7. Identify a recent interaction you have had in which communication was incongruent. Analyze the effect of the incongruence on the communication. When are people most likely to use incongruent communication?
8. Some experts suggest that the traditional nurse-patient relationship should be reconceptualized to fit today's fast-paced health care settings. Others believe that nurses should challenge the direction of health care and advocate for a return to more traditional, patient-centered health care. Write a paragraph supporting one of these two divergent views. Share your paragraph with a small group of classmates.
9. Think of a person with whom you have experienced difficult communication. Identify which of the barriers to successful communication are functioning in that person's communication with you and analyze your responses to that person.
10. Describe a collaborative experience you have had with another health care professional.

What factors differentiated it from cooperation or compromise?

(e)volve *To enhance your understanding of this chapter, try the Student Exercises on the Evolve site at http://evolve.elsevier.com/Chitty/professional.*

REFERENCES

American Nurses Association: *Code of ethics for nurses with interpretive statements*, Washington, DC, 2001, American Nurses Association.

Andrews MM: Transcultural perspectives in nursing administration, *J Nurs Admin* 28(11):30-38, 1998.

Apker J, Propp KM, Ford WSZ, Hofmeister N: Collaboration, credibility, compassion, and coordination: professional nurse communication skills sets in health care team interactions, *J Prof Nurs* 22(3): 180-189, 2006.

Baggs JG, Schmitt MH, Mushlin AI, Mitchell PH, Eldredge DH, Oakes D, et al: Association between nurse-physician collaboration and patient outcomes in three intensive care units, *Crit Care Med* 27(9):1991-1998, 1999.

Barke J, editor: *Burns' poems and songs*, London, 1955, Collins.

Calcagno KM: Listen up…someone important is talking, *Home Healthc Nurse* 26(6):333-336, 2008.

Davidhizar R, Dowd S, Giger JN: Recognizing abuse in culturally diverse clients, *Health Care Superv* 17(2):10-20, 1998.

Gardner DB: Ten lessons in collaboration, Online J Issues Nurs 10(1):1–6, Jan 31, 2005 (website): http://www.nursingworld.org/MainMenuCategories/ANAMarketplace/ANAPeriodicals/OJIN/TableofContents/Volume102005/No1Jan05/tpc26_116008.aspx.

Gerardi DS, Morrison F: Managing conflict creatively, *Crit Care Nurs* (Suppl):(February):31-32, 2005.

Gordon RL: *Basic interviewing skills*, Prospect Heights, IL, 1992, Waveland Press, Inc.

Graham J: It's OK for patients and kin to get more involved in care, *Chicago Tribune*, (June 10):p. 4, 2008.

Hagerty BM, Patusky KL: Reconceptualizing the nurse-patient relationship, *Image J Nurs Sch* 35(2):145-150, 2003.

Halfer D, Saver C: Bridging the generation gaps, *Nursing Spectrum (SE Ed.)* 4(3):28-33, 2008.

Hayes PM: Team building: bringing RNs and NAs together, *Nurs Manag* 25(5):52-55, 1994.

Heim P: Getting beyond "she said, he said," *Nurs Adm Q* 19(2):6-18, 1995.

Henneman EA, Lee JL, Cohen JI: Collaboration: a concept analysis, *J Adv Nurs* 21(1):103-109, 1995.

Holder KV, Schenthal SJ: Watch your step: nursing and professional boundaries, *Nurs Manag* 38(2):24-29, 2007.

Johns C: *Guided reflection: advancing practice*, Oxford, 2002, Blackwell Science.

Klagsbrun J: Listening and focusing: holistic health care tools for nurses, *Nurs Clin North Am* 36(1): 115-130, 2001.

Kramer M, Schmalenberg C: Securing "good" nurse/physician relationships, *Nurs Manag* 34(7):34-38, 2003.

Leland J: In "sweetie" and "dear," a hurt for the elderly, *New York Times*, (October 7), p A-1, 2008.

LeTourneau B: Physicians and nurses: friends or foes?, *J Healthcare Manag* 49(1):12-14, 2004.

Lindeke L, Block D: Interdisciplinary collaboration in the 21st century, *Minn Med* 8(6):42-45, 2001.

Lindeke L, Sieckert AM: Nurse-physician workplace collaboration, Online J Issues Nurs 10(1), 2005 (website): http://nursingworld.org/mods/mod775/nrsdrfull.htm.

Lower J: Creating a culture of civility in the workplace, *American Nurse Today* 2(9):49-52, 2007.

National Council of State Boards of Nursing: *Professional boundaries: a nurse's guide to the importance of appropriate professional boundaries,* Chicago, 1996, National Council of State Boards of Nursing (website): https://www.ncsbn.org/Professional_Boundaries_2007_Web.pdf.

Nurse's relationship with patient results in disciplinary action, *Nurs Law Regan Rep* 43(8):4-5, 2003.

Peplau H: *Interpersonal relations in nursing*, New York, 1952, GP Putnam's Sons.

Rosenstein AH, O'Daniel M: Disruptive behavior and clinical outcomes: perceptions of nurses and physicians, *Am J Nurs* 105(1):54-65, 2005.

Ruesch J: *Disturbed communication: the clinical assessment of normal and pathological communicative behavior*, New York, 1972, WW Norton.

Siela D: Managing the multigenerational nursing staff, *American Nurse Today* 1(3):47-49, 2006.

Wieck KL: Motivating an intergenerational workforce: scenarios for success, *Orthop Nurs* 26(6):366-371, 2007.

Wright LD: When does a nurse-patient relationship cross the line?, *American Nurse Today* 2(6):52-53, 2007.

Illness, Culture, and Caring: Impact on Patients, Families, and Nurses

Kay Kittrell Chitty

10

CHAPTER

Although prevention and health maintenance activities are primary functions of nurses, many nurse-patient interactions focus on the management of illness. A unique characteristic of nursing is the emphasis on viewing patients holistically. Nurses recognize that human beings are complex organisms with physical, mental, emotional, spiritual, social, and cultural components—all of which affect how a person responds when ill. The effective nurse takes each of these dimensions into consideration when providing nursing care. This chapter explores the stages of illness, illness behaviors, cultural factors that influence how people behave during illness, and the impact of illness and culture on patients, families, and nurses. It also explores briefly the reasons why nurses need to develop balance in their lives and engage in self-care.

ILLNESS

Illnesses can be classified as either acute or chronic, and both will be discussed in this chapter. Illness is a highly personal experience.

Culture plays a powerful role in health beliefs and behaviors; it also determines how individuals and families react to illness. Nurses can be more effective in delivering care when they understand some of the factors that affect how people cope with illness.

Acute Illness

Acute illness is characterized by severe symptoms that are relatively short-lived. Symptoms tend to appear suddenly, progress steadily, and subside quickly. Depending on the illness, the patient may or may not require medical attention. The common cold is an example of an acute illness that does not usually require a health care provider's attention. Others, such as acute appendicitis, may be fatal without rapid medical intervention. Unless complications arise, people with acute illness usually return to their previous level of wellness. Some acute illnesses, such as acute myocardial infarction, may lead to chronic conditions, such as congestive heart failure.

Individuals with sudden, catastrophic injuries, such as a spinal cord injury or major stroke,

☀ EVIDENCE-BASED PRACTICE NOTE

Canadian nurse researchers Anne Dewar and Elizabeth Lee wondered how individuals with catastrophic illness and injury faced challenges that others considered unbearable and that tested the limits of human endurance. They conducted individual interviews with 28 men and women from 18 to 75 years of age. These interviewees had endured chronic conditions, such as spinal cord injuries, multiple sclerosis, or major burns, for time periods ranging from 3 to 25 years. The researchers analyzed subjects' responses using grounded theory methods, a qualitative research methodology. The theoretical framework selected by the researchers was symbolic interactionism, which seeks to determine the relationship between the individual and the social world in which he or she lives.

They found that these individuals experienced three phases in bearing their difficulties. The researchers termed these phases finding out, facing reality, and managing reality. They discovered that the individuals in their study did not progress through stages, as others have suggested, but instead the phases flowed together and were reexperienced continuously. These individuals used three enduring strategies in all phases, which the researchers termed protecting, modifying, and boosting. Protecting involved insulating oneself from further emotional pain by limiting requests for assistance and not sharing emotional distress with significant others. Modifying meant learning to manage the physical, emotional, and social aspects of a condition by learning new skills and diffusing their emotions to preserve their social support, that is, not "whining." Boosting meant efforts to enhance self-esteem, such as comparing themselves with others who were in worse condition.

Dewar and Lee concluded that "the burdens of chronic illness and injuries [are] exceedingly complex, as individuals are forced to rebuild an image of themselves, manage their daily lives, and preserve relationships with others. Social support is important but forces the sufferer to make modifications to meet the needs of others as well as his or her own" (p. 924). They recommended that nurses and other health care professionals "accept and support the individual's need to express emotions such as anger, sorrow, and despair in all phases of the illness" (p. 922).

Abstracted from Dewar AL, Lee EA: Bearing illness and injury, *West J Nurs Res* 22(8):912-926, 2000.

experience dramatic and extensive change in the blink of an eye. They face physical limitations, significant modifications in daily living, and changes in social roles for which they had no preparation. Daily, they must bear challenges that most people consider unbearable. To do so they use a variety of coping mechanisms, which differ from person to person. The Evidence-Based Practice Note describes a study of how individuals with catastrophic illnesses and injuries cope with their disabilities and describes some of the coping mechanisms they use (Dewar and Lee, 2000).

Chronic Illness

A chronic illness usually develops gradually, requires ongoing medical attention, and may continue for the duration of the person's life.

Hypertension, diabetes, and Parkinson's disease are examples of chronic illnesses; they can be treated but not cured.

It is increasingly important for nurses to understand chronic illnesses and their impact, because they are one of the fastest-growing health problems in the United States. It is estimated that one third to one half of the U.S. population has one or more chronic illnesses. Factors such as sedentary lifestyles, obesity, and the aging of the population are expected to contribute to a continued increase in the number of chronically ill Americans for the foreseeable future.

Chronic illnesses are caused by permanent changes that leave residual disability. They vary in severity and outcomes, but there is generally not an end point at which normal health is regained. Some chronic illnesses are progressively debilitating and result in premature death, whereas others are associated with a normal life span, even though functioning is impaired. Some chronic illnesses go through periods of remission, when symptoms subside, and exacerbation, when symptoms reappear or worsen.

Chronic illnesses are pervasive and life altering. They lead to altered individual functioning and disruption of family life. Long-term medical management of chronic illness can create financial hardship as well. Patients with chronic illness need to make lifestyle changes, often many changes simultaneously. They must begin doing things they are not accustomed to doing and stop doing things they normally do. Patients with diabetes, for example, must begin monitoring their blood glucose levels and change their eating habits. Box 10-1 presents the similarities and differences between acute and chronic illnesses.

Having an acute or chronic illness diagnosed can be a major life crisis. The emotional reactions of the patient and family sometimes present a greater challenge than dealing with the physical aspects of the disease. Despite the prevalence of emotional responses to illness, most medical and nursing attention is focused on physical aspects of the disease process rather than emotions. Box 10-2 describes how one patient experiences a chronic illness, systemic lupus erythematosus, and describes its impact on her feelings, family responsibilities, and relationships. As you read her thoughts and feelings, take special note of her reaction to her nurses' focus on her physical condition at a time when her emotional responses were her greatest concern.

Box 10-1   Types of Illness

ACUTE	CHRONIC
• Sudden onset of symptoms	• Gradual onset of symptoms
• Symptoms progress quickly from mild to severe	• Symptoms may be mild or vague; once illness is resolved may have remissions and exacerbations
• Patient usually returns to former level of functioning	• Illness continues through the life span
• Changes often not permanent but may progress to chronic illness	• Changes are permanent and progressive
• Does not usually require long-term behavioral change/treatment	• Requires long-term behavioral change/treatment
• May represent a life crisis	• Often represents a life crisis

Box 10-2   Comments of a Patient With a Chronic Disease: Systemic Lupus Erythematosus

If there is one thing I want to say to nurses who work with patients with chronic disease, it is "Be patient and understand our problems and feelings." When I go to the doctor's office or to the hospital, I usually leave feeling guilty because I have been impatient with everyone I saw. Guilt and anger are the two feelings I seem to have had since I was diagnosed with this disease. I alternate between being angry that I got lupus and feeling that I should be grateful for the fact that I have something I can at least live with when others are not so fortunate.

I guess the thing that bothers me most is that the nurses keep telling me what changes I need to make to take better care of myself. They never seem to understand that I am doing the best I can do. I can't possibly get the amount of rest they seem to think I need, and I can't avoid as much stress as they seem to think I should avoid. Both my husband and I work hard at our jobs, and I hate asking him and my sons to take over my responsibilities at home when I am sick, so I wind up compromising. I ask them to help some and I do more than I should. When I get the lecture from the nurses on how I should take better care of myself, I usually just nod and say that I will, even when I know that I probably won't be able to.

STAGES OF ILLNESS

Adjustment to illness is a process. Although the behaviors are different for each person, people who are ill tend to progress through certain recognizable stages. Experts from medicine, sociology, psychology, and nursing have attempted to describe the stages individuals go through when ill. The five most commonly identified stages will be discussed. The stages are disbelief and denial, irritability and anger, attempting to gain control, depression and despair, and acceptance and participation. Nurses encounter patients in each stage, so it is important to have some understanding of the types of behaviors associated with each. Remember that a person's culture affects how he or she responds to illness and that the studies by Ellis and Nowlis (1994) were done with people of individual-oriented Western cultures. Also remember that stage theories are convenient ways of conceptualizing and learning, but often human beings do not fit neatly into the identified stages.

Stage I: Disbelief and Denial

The first stage results from difficulty in believing that the signs and symptoms being experienced are caused by illness. Often, there is a belief that the symptoms will go away. Fear of illness often leads to the hope that the symptoms will subside without treatment.

Denial is a defense mechanism that people sometimes use to avoid the anxiety associated with illness. People who pride themselves on their vigor and health may downplay the significance of symptoms. If this occurs, they may avoid treatment or attempt inappropriate self-treatment. Extended denial can have serious results, because some illnesses, left untreated, may become too advanced for effective treatment.

Stage II: Irritability and Anger

As the ability to function is altered by illness, irritability results. Anger is directed toward the body because it is not performing as it should. With the current emphasis on wellness and prevention, anger may be directed inward, and guilt feelings may occur for failing to prevent the illness. Anger may also be directed toward others—spouse, family members, co-workers, or health care providers.

Stage III: Attempting to Gain Control

In this stage, people may consult their health care provider or use over-the-counter medications, folk practices, or home remedies. They are aware that they are ill and usually experience some concern or even fear about the outcome. These fears usually stimulate treatment-seeking behavior as a way of gaining control over the illness, but fears may also lead to further denial and avoidance. Family members may become involved, encouraging the person to seek treatment or follow medical advice.

Stage IV: Depression and Despair

Depression is perhaps the most common mood that occurs with illness. The ability to work is altered, daily activities must be modified, and the sense of well-being and freedom from pain are lost. Illness results in many types of loss, and depression is a normal response. The severity of the depression varies according to the severity and length of the illness, as well as the individual's personality characteristics and coping abilities. Individuals with chronic illnesses often undergo cycles of depression as remissions and exacerbations occur.

Stage V: Acceptance and Participation

By the time this stage occurs, the patient has acknowledged the reality of illness and is ready to participate in decisions about treatment. Active involvement and the hope attached to pursuing treatment usually lead to increased feelings of mastery and serve to decrease depression.

Not all individuals go through every stage, and they do not necessarily go through them at the same rate or in the same order. Those with acute illnesses may progress through stages in a different way than those with chronic illnesses. As mentioned, culture plays a major role in how people respond to illness. Box 10-3 summarizes the stages of illness.

Stage I: Disbelief and denial
Stage II: Irritability and anger
Stage III: Attempts to gain control
Stage IV: Depression and despair
Stage V: Acceptance and participation

Modified from Ellis J, Nowlis E: *Nursing: a human needs approach*, ed 5, Philadelphia, 1994, JB Lippincott.

THE SICK ROLE

Although illness is highly subjective and is experienced differently by each individual, a number of factors influence how a particular person will respond. One important factor is the cultural expectation about how people should behave when ill. Children learn the part they are expected to play as an ill person through parental modeling—that is, by observing how their parents respond to major and minor illnesses. Do their significant adult figures avoid work and other activities when ill, or do they forge ahead stoically, ignoring minor illness or pain?

Each culture generally requires that certain criteria be met before people can qualify as "sick." Talcott Parsons (1964), a renowned sociologist, identified five attributes and expectations of the sick role that guided the view of illness in Anglo-American society for decades. According to Parsons, the sick Anglo-American

1. Is exempt from social responsibilities
2. Cannot be expected to care for himself or herself
3. Should want to get well
4. Should seek medical advice
5. Should cooperate with the medical experts

In other words, Parsons' definition of the sick role includes behavior that is dependent, passive, and submissive. For decades, Parsons' sick role expectations were taught in medical and nursing schools and guided the way health care providers viewed patients' reactions to pain and illness for many years. In our multicultural society, however, this view is no longer adequate, because different cultures have differing sick role expectations.

The cultural composition of the nation and the world is changing. Nurses, regardless of their own cultural backgrounds, must strive to provide culturally competent care to patients of many diverse cultures. With more than 66 different categories of race listed in the 2000 U.S. Census, this can seem like an overwhelming task. In fact, it is probably impossible for nurses to master the subtleties of every culture they encounter. Nurses can learn about their patients' culturally determined health care and illness beliefs, values, and practices, however, by consistently performing cultural assessments. These instruments will be discussed later in this chapter.

The current Anglo-American expectation is that people should accept responsibility for their own care rather than completely submit to health care providers; this is the consumer-oriented approach to health care. There is a presumption that ill people should want to get well and should behave in a way that leads to wellness.

This expectation that ill persons should want to get well and return to their normal activities as quickly as possible means that patients should cooperate in the treatment process and, to a great extent, become submissive and compliant, placing themselves in the hands of the caretakers. Persons who refuse to take medications as ordered or who refuse to perform prescribed activities, such as adhering to an exercise program or therapeutic diet, are viewed in a negative light. Their friends and family members may become irritated at their lack of participation in getting well again. Their caregivers call them "noncompliant." Often what is missing is an understanding of the patient's perception of the illness. Shifting from a focus of caring for patients to partnering with them is helpful in overcoming negative attitudes.

In caring for patients with acute and chronic illnesses, it is important for nurses to refrain from making judgments about patients' lifestyle choices. Emphasis should be placed on encouraging and reinforcing healthy behaviors. Education and support are important role functions for the nurse, especially in the management of patients with chronic disorders.

Working with patients with chronic illnesses can be particularly challenging for nurses. The

Box 10-4   Internal and External Influences on Illness Behavior

INTERNAL INFLUENCES	EXTERNAL INFLUENCES
• Dependence/independence needs • Coping ability • Hardiness • Learned resourcefulness • Resilience • Spirituality	• Past experiences • Culture • Communication patterns • Personal space norms • Role expectations • Values • Reaction to prescribed medications • Ethnocentrism

Case Study 10-1

EXAMPLE 1: Dependence

Mrs. Johnson has been in the hospital for several days after major abdominal surgery. Even after she progressed to the point at which she could feed herself, turn over in bed, and go to the bathroom unaided, she continued to call for assistance with these activities of daily living. She now calls the nurse every few minutes, making some small request that she is quite capable of performing for herself. She is communicating to the nurse that she needs a great deal of assistance and is demonstrating overly dependent behavior.

EXAMPLE 2: Independence

One hour ago Mr. Thomas returned to his room after surgery. The nurse found him trying to get out of bed by himself. He did not call to ask for assistance, although he is still groggy from anesthesia. He says that he is used to doing things for himself and feels uncomfortable asking the nurses for help. Mr. Thomas is demonstrating behavior that is too independent for his current physical status.

inability of modern medicine to cure disease sometimes leads caregivers to feel hopeless and powerless. They may also feel overwhelmed and inadequate at times. Self-aware nurses recognize these feelings and do not allow them to interfere with the nurse-patient relationship.

Illness Behaviors

Although some behaviors are expected of sick people, there is also a wide variation in responses. Each person in whom hypertension is newly diagnosed, for example, behaves somewhat differently from other people with the same condition. Both internal and external variables affect how an individual acts when ill (see Box 10-4). An ill individual's personality has a great deal of influence on the response to illness. Past experiences with illness and cultural background also influence illness behaviors.

Internal influences on illness behaviors

Personality structure is an internal variable that determines, to a large extent, how one manages illness. Personality characteristics the nurse should consider when assessing the ill person are dependence/independence, coping ability, hardiness, learned resourcefulness, resilience, and spirituality.

Dependence and independence. Patients' needs for dependence are unrelated to the severity of their illnesses. Some patients adopt a passive attitude and rely completely on others to take care of them. Others deny they are ill or have problems with being dependent and try to continue living as independently as they did before becoming sick.

We have all encountered sick people who have expressed views such as, "I don't ask any questions—I know that my doctor and nurses know what is best for me, and I do what they tell me." Perhaps you also know someone who reacted to illness by saying, "They don't know what they are talking about. I don't need to be in bed, and I don't need to take that medicine." These two sentiments are at the opposite ends of the dependency continuum.

People who perceive themselves as helpless may be more willing to submit to health care personnel and do what they are told. Those who are used to being in charge and see themselves as independent may resent the enforced dependency of hospitalization and illness. These two different attitudes are illustrated in Case Study 10-1.

Both overly dependent and overly independent behavior can be frustrating to nurses, who sometimes become angry with patients who request help with activities they are capable of doing themselves. The patient who is too dependent requires assistance to assume gradually more responsibility. The patient who needs to be "in charge" may have problems turning control over to caregivers and is often too independent. This patient needs assistance in recognizing limitations and using available resources to meet his or her needs.

Because nurses most often focus on promoting patient independence, they may react negatively to patients who are exhibiting dependent behavior. It is important for the nurse to be aware of personal feelings about dependent behaviors and to keep in mind that these behaviors may be the patient's way of signaling an increased need for security or support. Sometimes independence may not be the desired outcome. For patients with chronic illnesses who must rely on others for assistance in meeting their needs, too much independence may actually be dysfunctional (Whiting, 1994), as well as dangerous.

Coping ability. An individual copes with disease or illness in a variety of ways. Coping is a term that describes the methods a person uses to assess and manage demands. With an acute illness, coping is generally short-term and leads to a return to the preillness state. With chronic disorders, coping behaviors must be used continuously.

Sick people use coping methods to deal with the negative consequences of the disorder, such as pain or physical limitations. Each individual has a unique coping repertoire that is called into play to achieve a sense of control. With chronic health problems, there is a continuous need for adjustments to maintain well-being and prevent the feelings of despair that can result from high-stress conditions (Bowsher and Keep, 1995).

Hardiness and learned resourcefulness. Hardiness and learned resourcefulness are two concepts that have received attention as personal characteristics related to coping. Hardiness is viewed as a function of resistance to stressful life events (Bowsher and Keep, 1995). The interrelated dimensions of hardiness include the tendency to believe that one can influence the course of events (control), to view change as a challenge, and to feel commitment to values or goals.

The person with high levels of hardiness is believed to be better able to manage the changes associated with illness and to have less physical illness resulting from stress. Hardy people are likely to perceive themselves as having some control over a situation, even when ill. This feeling can affect a person's sense of well-being and adaptation to acute and chronic health problems.

Zauszniewski (1995) described the concept of learned resourcefulness as a characteristic useful in promoting adaptive, healthy lifestyles. Throughout life, individuals acquire a number of skills that enable them to cope effectively with stressful situations. The resulting attitude of self-control can be particularly helpful in reducing the feelings of depression and helplessness that often accompany the numerous stressors of chronic illness.

The nurse can enhance both hardiness and resourcefulness by teaching new coping skills. Stress inoculation and skills in self-regulation, problem solving, conflict resolution, and emotion control are examples of the types of educational interventions the nurse may implement.

Resilience. Scholars studying human behavior have often noted that some children did well in spite of difficult circumstances that defeated others. They attributed the differing reactions as a function of the phenomenon of resilience. Resilience is an aspect of coping that can be defined as "a pattern of successful adaptation despite challenging or threatening circumstances" (Humphreys, 2001). Resilient responses are thought to be a result of three factors:

- Disposition (i.e., temperament, personality, overall health and appearance, and cognitive style)
- Family factors such as warmth, support, and organization
- Outside support factors, such as a supportive network and success in school or work

Resilience can be thought of as both a process and an outcome. It can develop over a person's lifetime and can be taught, modeled, and learned.

The study of resilience has broadened to include adolescents and adults who face difficult, traumatic, or adverse circumstances. It has also been applied to adults with critical illness, battered women, survivors of sexual abuse, and others. You can expect to see much more about resilience as this phenomenon continues to be studied and better understood. A useful website, sponsored by the American Psychological Association, can help you further your understanding of the concept of resilience. It can be found online (http://www.apahelpcenter.org/featuredtopics/feature.php?id=6&ch=1).

Spirituality. The concept of spirituality is receiving increased interest in society as a whole, as well as in nursing. **Spirituality** is defined as "inner strength related to belief in and sense of connectedness with a higher power" (Chilton, 1998). It is generally agreed that every individual has a spiritual side that affects every aspect of his or her life. The degree of spiritual awareness, however, varies from individual to individual. This awareness can be dormant or suppressed, or it may be expressed through religious worship and prayer, although it is not necessarily manifested in overt religious practices (Cavendish et al, 2000). Religion is a specific way of organizing rituals and beliefs to create meaning. Spirituality is a larger umbrella concept under which religion resides. Spirituality is less differentiated than religion and can include concepts and beliefs from many religions and philosophies.

Spiritual growth occurs over the life span and is an internal process; as such it cannot be directly observed. Spiritual growth consists of increasing awareness of meaning, connectedness, purpose, and values in life (Cavendish et al, 2000).

The role of spiritual beliefs in health and illness has only recently been formally investigated. A growing number of scholars and health professionals think that spiritual beliefs have psychological, medical, and financial benefits that can be proved scientifically. Questions about the effects of intercessory prayer (prayer by others on behalf of a sick person) have been debated. Since 2000, $2.3 million of public funds has been expended on the study of prayer's effects. A scientifically rigorous, privately funded study of more than 1800 heart surgery patients was conducted over nearly a decade. To the disappointment of many, it found that intercessory prayer had no effect on recovery (Carey, 2006). The debate will undoubtedly continue.

One of the leading proponents of the spirituality and healing movement in American medicine is Dr. Herbert Benson, a Harvard Medical School cardiologist and founder of the Mind/Body Institute. He originated the "relaxation-response" therapy to reduce stress in patients with hypertension, chronic pain, and other stress-related illnesses. According to Benson, many people use prayer as part of the relaxation response (Benson and Klipper, 2000). The Mind/Body Medical Institute of Pathway Health Network in Boston has studied the effects of the relaxation response and asserts the following benefits (Larson, 1996; Freedman et al, 2002):

- A 36% reduction in physician visits by patients with chronic pain
- Significantly fewer postoperative complications in open heart surgery patients
- Lowered blood pressure and decreased use of medications in 80% of patients with hypertension
- A 50% reduction in health maintenance organization visits by relaxation-response users

Another indication of the importance of meeting patients' spiritual needs in health care settings is the increase in chaplain presence in some inpatient and outpatient settings. More than 90% of the patients surveyed believed that having a chaplain available was helpful, and 60% were more likely to return to a hospital with a pastoral presence in an otherwise frightening and confusing environment (Larson, 1996; Freedman et al, 2002).

The Joint Commission, the International Council of Nurses, the American Association of Colleges of Nursing, and the National Council of State Boards of Nursing all acknowledge that spiritual nursing care is a responsibility that goes beyond calling the chaplain. Yet many nurses experience barriers to rendering spiritual nursing care. These barriers range from feelings of inadequacy, lack of knowledge, embarrassment, their own spiritual uncertainty, lack of preparation, lack of privacy, lack of time, or failure to see it as a nursing role (McEwen, 2005).

Nurses are encouraged to view spirituality as one aspect of the whole human person and to assess patients for spiritual distress. They should recognize the individuality and value of each patient's spiritual beliefs and encourage their use in coping with illness. Spiritual distress is a NANDA-I (2009) diagnosis meaning "impaired ability to experience and integrate meaning and purpose in life through connectedness with self, others, art, music, literature, nature, and/or a power greater than oneself" (p. 301). Patients who question the meaning of suffering and the meaning of life, who express anger at God, or who view illness as punishment from God are experiencing spiritual distress. Spiritual distress can be painful and can hinder a patient's progress. According to Eldridge (2007), nurses can help free a patient's energy for healing by providing spiritual care.

As mentioned, not all nurses feel comfortable working in the spiritual realm. Even if you are not a religious person, you can become more comfortable with providing spiritual care. If you are religious, take care not to push your own religious beliefs on the patient. This can increase spiritual distress in patients whose beliefs are not congruent with yours.

Experts (Cavendish et al, 2000; McEwen, 2005) have identified a number of ways nurses can help patients engage their spirituality:

- Assess human responses in the spiritual domain.
- Be present for patients; listen actively.
- Allow patients to discuss beliefs in a higher power or the hereafter without introducing your own religious beliefs.
- Help patients explore what is meaningful and important in their lives.
- Value patients' inner strengths and motivations.
- Encourage patients to trust messages from an inner voice or divine providence.

- Use touch to reassure and comfort if the patient gives you permission to touch.
- Pray with patients or read scripture, if the patient requests it and you are comfortable doing so.
- Understand that how nurses connect with patients affects patient outcomes.
- Go beyond caring for physical needs, and respect and facilitate religious practices.
- Obtain assistance of spiritual care experts as requested by patients.

Nurses are participating in the use of spirituality in healing. St. Francis Hospital's Congregational Nurse Program in Evanston, Illinois, for example, is reaching 15,000 local families in an interfaith health project. After training as congregational nurses, nurses spend approximately 20 hours weekly at churches and other places of worship providing classes, counseling, and referrals. They dovetail their efforts with the spiritual beliefs and customs of each congregation. As you learned in Chapter 1, the faith community nurse concept is being implemented in numerous communities around the United States. By respecting and treating the whole person, these practitioners are affirming that a key dimension of health and healing is the spiritual dimension.

External influences on illness behaviors

External factors that bear on illness behaviors include past experiences and cultural group membership. Both directly influence how an individual perceives and responds to illness. The values that guide feelings about illness and steer a person toward particular methods of treatment are acquired primarily in the family of origin and in the culture.

Past experiences. Adults who were pampered during childhood illnesses may accept being ill fairly easily. Relying on others for care may not bother them, and they may settle into the sick role easily. Adults who received childhood messages such as "It is weak to be ill" or "One must keep going even when not feeling well" may have difficulty accepting illness and the restrictions that accompany it. Still other adults who experienced traumatic hospitalizations as children or who were threatened with injections for misbehaving may see hospitals and nurses as threatening. It is easy to understand that these adults will behave differently when ill.

Nurses should determine the patient's past experiences with illness and the health care system during a careful admission assessment. They can then use these findings to individualize care.

Culture. Culture is a pattern of learned behavior and values that are reinforced through social interactions, shared by members of a particular group, and transmitted from one generation to the next. Culture exerts considerable influence over most of an individual's life experiences. Meanings attached to health, illness, and perceptions of treatment are affected to a large degree by a person's culture. Culture determines when one seeks help and the type of practitioner consulted. It also prescribes customs of responding to the sick. Culture defines whether illness is seen as a punishment for misdeeds or as the result of inadequate personal health practices. It influences whether one goes to an acupuncturist, an herbalist, a folk healer, or a traditional health care provider such as physicians and nurse practitioners.

Beginning in the early 1970s, schools of nursing began including cultural concepts in their curricula. Increasing numbers of universities and colleges offered graduate programs in transcultural nursing. The Transcultural Nursing Society was legally incorporated in 1981, and in 1988 it began certifying nurses in transcultural nursing. Through oral and written examinations and evaluation of educational background and working experiences, a qualified nurse can become a certified transcultural nurse (CTN).

The Transcultural Nursing Society began publishing the *Journal of Transcultural Nursing* in 1989. By 1993 a resolution was adopted by the American Nurses Association's House of Delegates to identify and determine strategies to promote diverse and multicultural nursing in the workforce.

In the decades since transcultural nursing was first emphasized in educational programs, the cultural makeup of the U.S. population has undergone rapid change. Census demographers, who study population trends, predict that today's ethnic and racial minorities will outnumber non-Hispanic whites by 2042. Even sooner, by 2023, they will constitute a majority of the nation's children under 18 years of age (Roberts, 2008). These cultural shifts mean that changes in the nursing workforce are needed to deal more effectively with commonalities and differences in patients. Significant disparities exist between the health status of whites and nonwhites in the United States. For example, the death rate for heart disease is more than 40% higher in African Americans than in the white population. Similarly discouraging disparities exist in death rates for cancer and HIV/AIDS, among other diseases. Although these disparities may be due in part to education, poverty, and lifestyle factors, there is a growing unease among health professionals that racism may play a role. As a result, professional associations such as the American Nurses Association, The Joint Commission, and the federal government have all endorsed standards for culturally appropriate health care services.

In 2008, The Joint Commission announced its intention to revise and develop accreditation standards for hospitals to incorporate diversity, cultural, language, and health literacy issues into patient care processes. Some states have already passed legislation requiring health care professions to include cultural competence training into their educational and continuing education programs. The profession of nursing is largely white whereas the nation is racially more diverse than ever before, which underscores the need for culturally competent nurses. Clearly, transcultural nursing is an important field of study, practice, and research and an essential one in today's increasingly diverse society.

The culturally competent nurse. Knowledge of a patient's culture guides the nurse in understanding behaviors and planning appropriate approaches to patient needs. Because culture may also guide the patient's response to health care providers, and their interventions, it is necessary for the nurse to be knowledgeable about cultural influences. This is known as cultural competence. The U.S. Office of Minority Health defines culturally competent health care as "services that are respectful of and responsive to the health beliefs and practices and cultural and linguistic needs of diverse patient populations" (U.S. Department of Health and Human Services, 2001, p. 131). Understanding a patient's cultural background can facilitate communication and support establishing an effective nurse-patient relationship. Conversely, lack of understanding can create barriers that impede nursing care.

The shared values and beliefs in a culture enable its members to predict each other's actions. They also affect how members react to each other's behavior. When nurses work with patients from cultures different from their own and about which little is known, they lack these familiar guidelines for predicting behavior. This can cause anxiety, frustration, and feelings of distrust in both patient and nurse. Some of the issues that can arise when nurses care for patients from other cultures include stereotyping, communication difficulties, misperceptions about personal space, differing values and role expectations, ethnopharmacologic considerations, and ethnocentrism.

Stereotyping. In an effort to predict behavior, nurses may stereotype or "pigeonhole" patients from different cultures. It is important that nurses refrain from stereotyping members of cultures or ethnic groups that are different from their own. When providing nursing care, one size does not fit all. Cultural conditioning is a term that means people are culture bound. They are unconscious of their own innate values and beliefs and assume that all people are basically alike, that is, that all people share their values and beliefs.

It is important to recognize that the health care professions create cultural conditioning in their practitioners during school. Nursing is no exception. Nurses tend to hold their knowledge and beliefs about health in high regard and may devalue people who do not possess similar knowledge and beliefs. Individualized planning is always the best basis for care, whatever the patient's culture or ethnic group. Failure to individualize care often results in noncompliance, dissatisfaction with care, and poor outcomes (Taylor, 2005).

Communication. The nurse should keep in mind that patterns of communication are strongly influenced by culture. The Asian patient who smiles and nods may be communicating politeness and respect, rather than agreeing or indicating understanding. Anglo-Americans tend to value a direct approach to problems, but in other cultures subtlety and indirectness may be valued. Although Western culture values direct eye contact, some cultures view this as impolite, particularly direct eye contact between men and women.

Personal space and structure. The amount of personal space needed is another factor that varies depending on cultural experience. Some cultures use touch as a major form of communication; in others, touching between persons who are not considered family is disrespectful. Culture also has a primary influence on the type of stress its members experience at various points in their lives. Every society places stress on its members at one or more stages of development. For instance, Anglo-American adolescents are typically under great stress as they struggle with independence. Amish adolescents tend to experience less stress, because their behavior during this period of development is more rigidly prescribed by their culture.

Values. Values held by the nurse may conflict with patients' cultural values. In the Navajo culture, for example, great value is placed on keeping pain and discomfort to oneself. Letting others know how you feel is seen as weak. The nurse who expects patients to ask for medication when in pain may assume that the Navajo patient is comfortable when the opposite is actually the case. On the other hand, a nurse who values suffering in silence may underrate the discomfort of a patient who comes from a culture that promotes overt expression of discomfort.

Role expectations. The role expectations of nurses also vary from culture to culture. A common Anglo-American view of nurses is that they treat people as equals, are passive, and take direction from physicians. These patients feel free to ask questions of their nurses. Asian patients, however, may expect nurses to be authoritative, to provide directives, and to be expert practitioners who take charge. Out of respect for authority, they may not speak until spoken to and may verbally agree with anything nurses propose. Case Study 10-2 illustrates a cultural difference between patient and nurse in expressing pain.

Case Study 10-2

Cultural expression of pain

Mrs. L, a 42-year-old Asian woman, became ill and required surgery while visiting her daughter in the United States. After surgery, she was given a patient-controlled analgesia pump. The nurse explained to Mrs. L how to self-administer medication when she felt pain. Mrs. L smiled and nodded her head when asked whether she understood the instructions. Much later the nurse noticed that this patient appeared to be in great pain. After talking with Mrs. L's daughter, the nurse realized that Mrs. L had not understood how to use the equipment but was unwilling to ask for additional instructions or complain of pain.

Ethnopharmacology. Research on how people of different ethnic groups respond to medications has revealed significant differences among groups. Factors such as rate of absorption, metabolism, distribution, and elimination of drugs are affected. In addition patient adherence and education vary among groups. The field of ethnopharmacology resulted from a need to understand responses to prescribed medications and genetic variations in response to drugs. "Nurses need to be knowledgeable about drugs that may elicit varied responses in people from different ethnic groups, especially the variations in therapeutic dosages and adverse effects" (Munoz and Hilgenberg, 2005, p. 46). A basic understanding of ethnopharmacology is now considered a part of being a culturally competent nurse.

Ethnocentrism. Nurses respond to sick people on the basis not only of their formal education but also of their own socialization and culture. All too often people are unaware of their own biases and tend to be ethnocentric. Ethnocentrism is the inclination to view one's own cultural group as superior to others and to view differences negatively. For example, some nurses are intolerant of patients who do not speak English and either avoid them or spend little time with them (Kulwicki, Miller, and Schim, 2000).

The nurse who identifies how personal beliefs and expectations can influence care is better able to recognize and deal with any prejudices that may impede patient care. Cultural assessment therefore begins with self-assessment. To begin a cultural self-assessment, examine your own values. What behaviors do you expect from people who are ill? Toward what groups do you have prejudices or biases? The nurse who is frustrated by the difficulty of caring for a patient from a different culture may benefit from taking a few minutes to imagine what it would be like to be hospitalized in a foreign country. Candidly answering the questions in the Cultural Consideration Challenge 10-1 will help you begin the important process of self-assessment.

Cultural assessment. An important step in meeting the challenge of providing nursing care to diverse patients is the cultural assessment. Cultural assessments are used to identify beliefs, values, and health practices that may help or hinder nursing interventions. Dr. Madeleine Leininger, nurse anthropologist, nurse theorist, and founder of transcultural nursing, advocated that nurses routinely perform cultural assessments to determine patients' culturally specific needs (Leininger, 1999). To demystify the process, it may be helpful to think of cultural assessment as "merely asking people their preferences, what they think, who we should talk to in making a decision" (Villaire, 1994, p. 138). There are numerous cultural assessment instruments available. Some of these instruments require in-depth interviews and comprehensive data gathering, which may require more time than is available in today's health care settings.

You can continue the process of becoming a culturally competent nurse by using the Cultural Assessment Checklist in the Cultural Considerations Challenge 10-2 on p. 234. It was designed for use by home health nurses but is easily adapted for use in other settings. Its concise yet comprehensive nature takes into account the limited amount of time nurses may have to get to know new patients—but also recognizes the necessity of developing a culturally congruent plan of care if desired outcomes are to be achieved.

Cultural Considerations Challenge 10-1
Sociocultural Self-Assessment

Directions: Use your answers to these questions to better understand your own social and cultural beliefs and expectations.

1. To what groups do I belong? What is my cultural heritage? My socioeconomic status? My age-group? My religious affiliation?
2. How do I describe myself? What parts of the description come from the groups to which I belong?
3. What kinds of contact have I had with persons from different groups? Do I assume that others have the same values and beliefs that I have?
4. What makes me feel proud about my group affiliations? Am I ethnocentric in my attitudes and behavior? What would I change about my group affiliations if I could? Why?

5. Have I ever experienced the feeling of being rejected by another group? Did this experience heighten my sensitivity to other cultures or cause me to denigrate others different from myself?
6. When I was growing up, what messages did I get from parents and friends about people from groups different from mine? Do these attitudes cause me any difficulty today?
7. What are the major stereotypes I hold about people from different groups? Do these biases help or hinder me in developing cultural sensitivity?
8. To work effectively with people from different cultural groups, what do I need to change about myself?

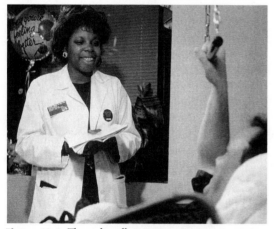

Figure 10-1 The culturally competent nurse recognizes that in today's diverse society performing a cultural assessment is an increasingly important measure that improves the effectiveness of nursing care. (Photo by Wilson Baker.)

Culturally competent nurses take cultural differences into consideration, usually interpret patient behavior accurately, and recognize problems that need to be managed. They realize that cultural norms must be included in the plan of care to prevent conflicts between nursing goals and patient/family goals. They recognize that planning culturally congruent care is the most time-effective way to achieve the desired goals (Figure 10-1).

In addition, being knowledgeable about other cultures promotes feelings of respect and enhances understanding of attitudes, behaviors, and the impact of illness. The accompanying Interview with Dr. Madeleine Leininger provides insights into her vast experience and strongly held beliefs about cultural competence in nursing. For further study in cultural competence, several websites containing valuable resources and links are http://www.transculturalcare.net, http://www.culturediversity.org, and http://www.tcns.org. Cultural competence is a process. Nurses must remember that continuous learning and sensitivity to and respect for cultural differences are qualities required of culturally competent nurses.

IMPACT OF ILLNESS ON PATIENTS AND FAMILIES

Regardless of culture, illness results in a number of changes for both patients and families. Common experiences include behavioral and

Cultural Considerations Challenge 10-2
Cultural Assessment Checklist

Patient-identified cultural/ethnic group _____

_____

Religion _____

ETIQUETTE AND SOCIAL CUSTOMS
- Typical greeting. Form of address: Handshake appropriate? Shoes worn in home?
- Social customs before "business." Social exchanges? Refreshment?
- Direct or indirect communication patterns?

NONVERBAL PATTERNS OF COMMUNICATION
- Eye contact. Is eye contact considered polite or rude?
- Tone of voice. What does a soft voice or a loud voice mean in this culture?
- Personal space. Is personal space wider or narrower than in the American culture?
- Facial expressions, gestures. What do smiles, nods, and hand gestures mean?
- Touch. When, where, and by whom can a patient be touched?

CLIENT'S EXPLANATION OF PROBLEM
- Diagnosis. What do you call this illness? How would you describe this problem?
- Cause. What caused the problem? What might other people think is wrong with you?
- Course. How does the illness work? What does it do to you? What do you fear most about this problem?

- Treatment. How have you treated the illness? What treatment should you receive? Who in your family or community can help?
- Prognosis. How long will the problem last? Is it serious?
- Expectations. What are you hoping the nurses will do for you?

NUTRITION ASSESSMENT
- Pattern of meals. What is eaten? When are meals eaten?
- Sick [comfort] foods.
- Food intolerance and taboos.

PAIN ASSESSMENT
- Cultural responses to pain.
- Patient's perception of pain response.

MEDICATION ASSESSMENT
- Patient's perception of "Western" medications.
- Possible pharmacogenetic variations.

PSYCHOSOCIAL ASSESSMENT
- Decision maker.
- Sick role.
- Language barriers, translators.
- Cultural/ethnic community resources.

Reprinted with permission of Narayan MC: Cultural assessment in home healthcare, *Home Healthc Nurse* 15(10):663-672, 1997.

emotional changes, changes in roles, and disturbed family dynamics. Illness creates stress and other emotional responses. Factors affecting responses to illness include personality before illness; suddenness, extent, and duration of required lifestyle changes; individual and family resources for dealing with the stress of illness; the life-cycle stage of the patient and family; previous experiences with illness or crisis; and social support (Lewis, 1998). Religious faith also plays a role in responses to illness.

Severe illnesses that profoundly affect physical appearance and functioning are more likely to result in high levels of anxiety and extensive behavioral changes than are short-term, non–life-threatening illnesses. The impact of a chronic

🐏 INTERVIEW   Dr. Madeleine Leininger, *FOUNDER OF TRANSCULTURAL NURSING*

Interviewer: Dr. Leininger, please tell us what you mean by the term "culturally competent."

Dr. Leininger: Culturally competent care has been defined as the culturally based knowledge with a care focus that is used in creative, meaningful, and appropriate ways to provide beneficial and satisfying care to individuals, families, groups, or communities or to help people face death or disabilities. I coined this term in 1962 as the goal of my theory of culture care diversity and universality. The term has caught hold today and is being used by many health care providers. It is now used as a requirement for The Joint Commission accreditation and with other organizations as essential to work effectively with cultures and their health care needs.

Interviewer: Please describe how a culturally competent nurse's patient care differs from that of one who is not culturally competent.

Dr. Leininger: A culturally competent nurse demonstrates the following attributes and skills: (1) Uses transcultural nursing concepts, principles, and available research findings to assess and guide care practices; (2) understands and values the cultural beliefs and practices of designated cultures so that nursing care is tailor-made or fits individuals' needs in meaningful ways; (3) knows how to prevent major kinds of cultural conflicts, clashes, or hurtful care practices; (4) demonstrates reasonable confidence to work effectively and knowingly with clients of different cultures and can also evaluate transcultural nursing care outcomes.

The nurse who is unable to demonstrate these culturally competent attributes often shows signs of being frustrated and impatient with people of different cultures. Moreover, the nurse who does not practice cultural competencies often shows signs of excessive ethnocentrism, biases, and related problems that impede client recovery and well-being.

Interviewer: How do patients respond differently when nurses take their cultural patterns into consideration when planning and implementing care?

Dr. Leininger: It is most encouraging to observe and listen to clients who have received culturally based nursing care. These clients often exhibit the following behaviors: (1) They show signs of being satisfied and very pleased with nurse's actions and decisions. (2) They make comments such as,

"This is the best care I or my family members have received from health care providers." Frequently they say, "How did you know about my values, my culture, and how to use these ideas in my care? You anticipated my needs well." (3) They appreciate the different ways the nurse incorporates their cultural needs. They express their gratitude to the nurse. (4) Clients appreciate respect for their culture shown by the nurse in care decisions and practices. (5) The clients do not experience racial biases and negative comments about their cultures or familiar lifeways.

Interviewer: With so many cultural groups in this country, knowing all one needs to know about other cultures seems overwhelming. How do you advise nurses to begin the process of becoming culturally competent?

Dr. Leininger: The nurse should first enroll in a substantive transcultural nursing course to learn the basic and important concepts, principles, and practices of transcultural nursing. This knowledge base is essential so the nurse becomes aware of common cultural needs and ways to work with a few cultures that are different. A few cultures are studied in depth, focusing on common and unique cultural features. The most frequently occurring cultures in the nurse's home or local region are studied first, and then one learns about other cultures over time, becoming sensitive and knowledgeable about these cultures. The nurse can greatly increase her or his knowledge of several cultures or subcultures by reading the literature, or by studying specific cultures when caring for people under transcultural mentors. Gradually, the nurse learns several cultures in a general way and a few in depth. As the nurse becomes increasingly knowledgeable about several cultures, comparative knowledge and competencies become evident.

There is no expectation that professional nurses can know all human cultures, as this would be impossible. An open learning attitude and mind with a sincere desire to learn as much as possible about a few cultures will help the nurse in becoming culturally knowledgeable, competent, and sensitive.

Interviewer: What signs can students look for to determine whether their nursing programs are preparing them to provide culturally competent care?

INTERVIEW   Dr. Madeleine Leininger, *FOUNDER OF TRANSCULTURAL NURSING—CONT'D*

Dr. Leininger: Nursing students will find they are able to provide culturally competent care when (or if) the following signs are evident:

- They consistently know, understand, and respect specific cultures and appreciate commonalities and differences among cultures.
- They feel a sense of confidence, creativity, and competence in their nursing care practices, see how their care fits specific cultures, and accommodate cultural differences in meaningful and creative ways.
- They go beyond common sense to actual use of culture-specific knowledge in patient care as shown in the Sunrise Model (see Chapter 13, Nursing Theory: The Basis for Professional Nursing, Figure 13-5).
- They creatively use the clients' beliefs, values, and patterns along with appropriate professional knowledge and skills that meet clients' needs.

- They prevent racial discrimination practices in nursing and in other places; they avoid cultural imposition, ethnocentrism, cultural conflicts, cultural pain, and related negative practices.
- They value and know how to use Leininger's Culture Care Theory and basic transcultural care concepts, principles, and research findings in their nursing practices to provide culturally congruent care for people's health and well-being.
- They appreciate a global perspective of nursing and value transcultural nursing to meet a growing and intense multicultural world.
- They markedly grow in their professional knowledge and sensitivities, developing a global worldview of transcultural nursing. They reach out to help cultural strangers in different living contexts.

Courtesy Dr. Madeleine Leininger.

illness is significant and continues for the lifetime of the patient. When planning holistic nursing care, the nurse must take into consideration how the family both influences and is influenced by the illness of a family member.

Impact of Illness on Patients

Illness creates a variety of emotional responses. Among the more common responses are guilt, anger, anxiety, and stress.

Guilt

Individuals may experience guilt about becoming ill, particularly if the illness is related to lifestyle choices, such as smoking. Guilt may also be associated with the inability to perform usual activities because of illness. A mother who is unable to perform child-care tasks or a father who has to take a lower-paying job because of illness may experience considerable guilt. Some cultures view certain illnesses as shameful and people who have them as guilty of cultural transgressions. Nurses who identify and encourage patients to discuss guilt feelings may help prevent the depression that can be a consequence of illness-induced alterations in lifestyle.

Anger

Anger is another common emotional response to illness, particularly in the Anglo-American culture. When patients must make sacrifices to manage their illnesses, such as giving up favorite foods or activities, they may experience anger about the changes. At times, they may feel that their bodies have betrayed them, which results in self-directed anger. Anger may also be directed toward caregivers for their inability to produce a cure, reduce pain, or prevent negative consequences of the illness. Nurses must be prepared to accept such angry feelings, to refrain from rejecting or avoiding patients who express their fears through anger, and to encourage the adaptive expression of angry feelings.

Anxiety

Anxiety is a common and universal experience. It is also a common emotional response to illness and hospitalization. Anxiety is an ill-defined, diffuse feeling of apprehension and uncertainty. Anxiety occurs as a result of some threat to an individual's selfhood, self-esteem, or identity.

A number of threats are associated with illness. Illness may alter the way people view themselves. Some illnesses result in a change in physical

Box 10-5   Levels of Anxiety

MILD ANXIETY

- Increased alertness, increased ability to focus, improved concentration, expanded capacity for learning

MODERATE ANXIETY

- Concentration limited to one thing, increased body movement, rapid speech, subjective awareness of discomfort

SEVERE ANXIETY

- Scattered thoughts, difficulty with verbal communication, considerable discomfort, purposeless movements

PANIC

- Complete disorganization, difficulty differentiating reality from unreality, constant random movements, unable to function without assistance

appearance. Often, ability to function is affected, altering relationships, work performance, and abilities to meet others' expectations. In addition, there may be concern about pain and discomfort associated with illness or treatment. Because of real and potential threats and changes arising from illness, nurses must develop skills that enable them to help patients recognize and manage anxiety.

Although the responses are similar, there is general agreement that anxiety and fear are different. Fear results from specific known causes, whereas with anxiety the cause of the feelings is unknown. For example, if you are home alone at night and you hear an unusual noise outside, most likely your heartbeat and respirations increase, your stomach tightens, and you perspire. The emotion in this situation is fear of an intruder. If you begin to have the same feelings but have heard no noises and cannot identify a source of fear, you are experiencing anxiety. Both emotions may be present at the same time. The patient who is in the hospital for an operation may experience anxiety about the unknown consequences of the surgery and fear of pain and disfigurement from the procedure itself.

Symptoms of anxiety. Nurses should be familiar with the numerous symptoms of anxiety. They are classified as physiologic, emotional, and cognitive. Signs and symptoms include increased heart rate, respirations, and blood pressure; insomnia; nausea and vomiting; fatigue; sweaty palms; and tremors. Emotional responses include restlessness, irritability, feelings of helplessness, crying, and depression. Cognitive symptoms include inability to concentrate, forgetfulness, inattention to surroundings, and preoccupation.

Responses to anxiety. Responses to anxiety occur on a continuum. The continuum is along four levels of anxiety: mild, moderate, severe, and panic. A mild level is characterized by increased alertness and ability to focus attention and concentrate. There is an expanded capacity for learning at this stage.

A person with a moderate level of anxiety is able to concentrate on only one thing at a time. Frequently, there is increased body movement (restlessness), more rapid speech, and a subjective awareness of discomfort.

At the severe level, thoughts become scattered. The severely anxious person may not be able to communicate verbally, and there is considerable discomfort accompanied by purposeless movements such as hand-wringing and pacing.

At the panic level, the person becomes completely disorganized and loses the ability to differentiate between reality and unreality. There are constant random and purposeless movements. The individual experiencing panic levels of anxiety is unable to function without assistance. Panic levels of anxiety cannot be continued indefinitely, because the body will become exhausted, and death may occur if the anxiety is not reduced. Box 10-5 lists the characteristics of each level of anxiety.

Because anxiety is such a common response to illness and hospitalization, nurses often encounter patients who are experiencing mild or moderate anxiety and, occasionally, patients who are severely anxious. When interacting with an anxious patient, the nurse should carefully assess the level of anxiety before attempting to develop the plan of care.

It is widely acknowledged that anxiety is communicated interpersonally. In other words, it is "contagious." For this reason, it is crucial that the nurse be aware of and manage personal anxiety so that it is not inadvertently transferred to patients. Likewise, self-awareness is essential to prevent absorbing patients' anxiety.

Stress

Stress is another internal variable that affects patients. Stress is both a response to illness and an important factor in the development of illness. Because illness and hospitalization involve so many alterations in lifestyle, they tend to cause a great deal of stress.

Stress is an unavoidable and essential part of life. To survive and grow, individuals must cope adaptively with constantly changing demands. The stress related to examinations, for example, motivates most students to grow by studying and learning. Although stress is unavoidable, and even sometimes desirable, some control can be exerted over the number and types of stressors (factors that create stress) encountered, and responses to the stressors can often be managed.

Hospitalized patients are removed from their usual support systems. They lose much of their control because nurses and other care providers make decisions for them. Being ill often means that they are no longer able to perform activities as they did before the illness occurred. Some patients find themselves in the role of comforting other family members rather than being comforted to avoid increasing family members' distress. Stress is a common response to all these circumstances.

Differentiating between stress and anxiety.

Stress and anxiety have some characteristics in common. The physiologic responses are similar. Anxiety is a response to a real or perceived threat to the individual, whereas stress is an interaction between the individual and the environment. Stress includes all the responses the body makes while striving to maintain equilibrium and deal with demands. Case Study 10-3 describes one example of stress and anxiety.

Case Study 10-3

Stress and anxiety

Mary S is a 32-year-old single mother and a lawyer who was recently hired by an established law firm. One morning as she prepares to take her 2-year-old daughter to the child-care center, she receives a phone call informing her that the day-care center owner was severely injured in an accident and the center will be closed indefinitely. Ms. S experiences both stress and anxiety in this situation. She has a number of demands placed on her from her workplace and from her family that lead to stress. The additional demands caused by the sudden change in her plans result in even higher levels of stress. In addition, even though none of the male lawyers has responsibility for child care, Ms. S has placed the expectation on herself that she will perform her job exactly like the men in the firm. Being late or missing work as a result of making new arrangements for child care conflicts with her self-expectations and poses a threat to her self-esteem. This threat leads to feelings of anxiety.

Internal, external, and interpersonal stressors.
Selye (1956) defined stress as the nonspecific response of the body to any demand made on it. He named this response the *general adaptation syndrome* and identified three stages through which the body progresses while responding to stress.

Stressors trigger the body's stress response. Stressors are agents, or stimuli, that an individual perceives as posing a threat to homeostasis. Stressors may come from external, interpersonal, or internal sources. External stressors include such things as noise, heat, cold, malfunctioning equipment (such as a car that will not run), or organizational rules and expectations. Interpersonal sources of stress include the demands made by others and conflicts with others. Placing unrealistic expectations on oneself is an example of an internal stressor. In the example of Mary S, an internal stressor is her expectation that her childcare responsibilities will not affect the hours she works. It is an unrealistic expectation for any single parent of a small child to expect that the child's needs will never interfere with work.

Responses to stress. Outward responses to stress are determined by the individual's perception of the stressor. Cognitive appraisal, or the way one thinks about a specific situation, determines the degree to which the situation is considered stressful. Loud music at a concert, for example, might seem less stressful to adolescents than it would to their parents.

Another factor related to the assessment of threat is whether the individual feels capable of handling the threat, that is, whether the person exhibits hardiness. The person who feels capable can be expected to feel less stress than the person who does not generally feel competent.

Stress affects the physical, emotional, and cognitive areas of functioning just as anxiety does. Physically, there is a feeling of fatigue; muscles are tight and tense. There is an increase in heart rate and respiration. The person who is under prolonged stress may be unable to sleep or eat, or there may be excessive sleeping or eating in an attempt to avoid or cope with the stress.

Emotionally, people under stress feel drained and unable to care for themselves or others. This can result in social isolation and distancing from others. They experience difficulty with enjoying life. They may have feelings of hopelessness and of being out of control. Irritability and impatience often occur.

Cognitively, stress causes decreased mental capacity and problem-solving skills. Therefore there is a tendency to have difficulty making decisions.

Stress and illness. It has been known for some time that stress plays a major role in the development of illness. More recent research has provided better understanding of the links between prolonged stress and body functioning.

The person who is under stress for long periods of time is at risk for a number of physical problems. The exhaustion that results from excessive, unmanaged stress leads to physiologic breakdowns and predisposition to a number of problems. Disorders such as hypertension, certain skin disorders, and autoimmune disorders have been termed stress-related diseases because they frequently occur in individuals who have been severely stressed.

Box 10-6   Breathing Exercises

1. Sit comfortably with feet on the floor and eyes closed.
2. Inhale slowly and deeply through the nose and fill the lungs completely. As you breathe in, imagine the oxygen flowing to all your cells. Hold your breath while slowly counting to four.
3. Slowly release all the air while thinking the word *calm*. As you breathe out, imagine the air taking all the tension out with it.
4. Repeat the cycle four times. Try to banish all thoughts except those related to your breathing, but do not fight them if other thoughts creep in.
5. When you have completed the exercise, open your eyes slowly and sit for a moment before resuming your regular activities.

Stress has been found to be related to a reduction in the immune response, which can delay healing and result in greater susceptibility to infectious disorders such as colds and flu. Long-term studies of persons with medical illnesses revealed that the more stress people experienced in a given year, the more likely they were to develop physical illness.

Coping with stress. Nurses have a role in helping patients modify their stressors. They should assess patients' abilities to recognize symptoms of stress and their usual methods of coping.

Coping with stress can be direct or indirect. In assisting patients to use direct coping, nurses help patients to identify those situations that can be changed and to take responsibility for changing them. The focus is on using problem-solving skills and planning to eliminate or avoid as many stressors as possible. It is important to realize that completely eliminating stress from one's life is neither possible nor desirable.

In helping patients use indirect coping, nurses' actions are aimed at reducing the affective (feelings) and physiologic (body) disturbances resulting from stress. Patients are taught techniques such as deep breathing, muscle relaxation, and imagery, which help them cope more effectively with stress (Boxes 10-6 and 10-7).

Box 10-7 Relaxation Exercises

Get into a comfortable position in a place where you will not be interrupted. First focus on slow, deep breathing. Close your eyes and begin to think about the muscle sensations in your body. Identify where you are feeling tense. Slowly inhale as you stretch like a cat; then exhale and allow the tension to flow out.

NECK AND SHOULDERS
- Slowly bend your head forward and backward, then side to side three times. Bring your shoulders up as if you were trying to touch them to your ears. Slowly relax and feel the difference in tension.

ARMS AND HANDS
- Make a tight fist in one hand and tighten the muscles throughout your arm. Slowly release the muscles from the shoulder to the hand. Repeat with the other arm and hand.

HEAD
- Make a wide smile and hold for a count of five. Slowly relax your face muscles and let your jaw go loose. Tightly close your eyes and feel the tension. Slowly give up the tension and allow your eyes to remain gently closed.

STOMACH
- Make your abdominal muscles tight by pushing them out as far as possible. Make your abdomen hard and feel the tension. Slowly relax your muscles and notice the difference.

LEGS AND FEET
- Holding your leg still, curl your toes down to point to the floor. Do first one leg and then the other. As you tighten your muscles, feel the tension. Then slowly relax.
- Sit quietly for a few moments and feel the relaxation in your body before you resume your activities.

To help patients to manage stress, nurses must be skilled in assessing and managing their own personal stress. Nurses who are feeling stressed themselves have difficulty assisting patients in dealing with similar problems. The questions in Box 10-8 can help you identify your own sources of stress and develop self-awareness so that you can be effective in helping patients deal with their stress. For further exploration of stress management approaches for patients and nurses, complete the University of Chicago Hospitals' self-study module online (http://www.nurse.com/ce/CE424/CoursePage).

Coping with stress through education. Patient education is a major part of nursing practice, and nurses have a professional responsibility to ensure that their patients' learning needs are met. When patients are competent in the knowledge and skills they need to manage their illnesses, they tend to feel more masterful and less stressed.

Nurses who embrace the teaching aspects of the role can assist patients in acquiring new methods of coping with stressors through learning. Historically, nurses considered patient teaching as an integral part of the nursing role. Changes in the health care system have led to a diminution of this aspect of nursing for several reasons. These reasons include lack of time; the short-term nature of many nurse-patient relationships; poor preparation in teaching-learning principles and techniques; the attitude that teaching is a low-priority nursing intervention; lack of emphasis on patient teaching as an indicator of quality care; lack of privacy; refusal of third-party insurers to pay for patient teaching; and lack of confidence that patients really want to be compliant, among others. Nevertheless, nurses have information that can make a positive impact in how patients and their families cope with the stresses of illness. Professional nurses consider patient and family teaching an important, high-priority nursing intervention.

Box 10-8   Personal Stress Inventory

	VERY OFTEN	SOMETIMES	RARELY OR NEVER
1. I feel tense and anxious and have some nervous indigestion.			
2. People at home, school, or work make me feel tense.			
3. I eat, drink, or smoke in response to tension.			
4. I have tension or pain in my neck or shoulders.			
5. I have headaches or insomnia.			
6. I have trouble turning off my thoughts long enough to feel relaxed.			
7. I find it difficult to concentrate on what I am doing because I worry about other things.			
8. I use alcohol, tranquilizers, or other medications to relax or sleep.			
9. I feel a lot of pressure at work or school.			
10. I do not feel that my work is appreciated.			
11. My family does not appreciate what I do for them.			
12. I feel I do not have enough time for myself.			
13. I have difficulty saying "no."			
14. I wish I had more friends with whom to share experiences.			
15. I do not have enough time for physical exercise.			

Scoring: Give yourself 2 points for every check in the Very Often column, 1 point for every check in the Sometimes column, and 0 points for every check in the Rarely or Never column. Total the number of points. A score of 20 to 30 represents a high level of stress. If you scored in this range, you should take steps to reduce your stress level. A score from 10 to 19 means that you are experiencing midlevel stress. You should monitor your stress and begin relaxation exercises. A score of 9 or under means that you are experiencing relatively low stress at the present time.

Box 10-9   Barriers to Patient Learning

- High anxiety
- Sensory deficits (e.g., vision, hearing)
- Pain
- Fatigue
- Hunger/thirst
- Shortness of breath
- Cultural expectations
- Language barriers
- Differing health values
- Low literacy
- Lack of motivation
- Environmental factors (e.g., noise, lack of privacy)

As a first step, nurses must identify factors that can create barriers to learning (Box 10-9). One factor is anxiety. Mild anxiety improves learning by increasing the ability to focus on the task. As anxiety increases, however, the ability to listen, focus, and concentrate decreases. Information is not retained, and the patient is unable to make the cognitive connections required for learning to take place.

Physiologic factors may also impede learning. For instance, visual or hearing deficits must be overcome. Unmet physiologic needs, such as fatigue, shortness of breath, hunger, and thirst, decrease the patient's attention to learning. Pain dramatically impairs the ability to learn, and fatigue diminishes the energy required to learn.

Nurses who assess and ensure that patients' physiologic needs are met enhance their readiness to learn.

Culture also influences learning. Understanding the meaning of illness in the patient's culture is an early step that will help the nurse determine the educational needs of the patient and family and effectively provide culturally congruent patient education. Learning can be impeded when patient and nurse have different languages and patterns of learning. When the nurse works toward an educational goal that is not seen as desirable by a patient of another culture, their cultural values may be in conflict. Self-awareness on the part of the nurse is essential to avoid allowing cross-cultural barriers to occur. In all patient teaching, and especially in a cross-cultural situation, individualizing patient teaching is essential. Learning appropriate greetings and phrases in the patient's language and obtaining the services of an interpreter also show sensitivity to cultural differences. Always show respect for folk remedies valued by the patient and family and make every effort to incorporate them into the Western health care treatment plan. Nurses must recognize that low literacy rates are a problem among patients of all cultures, including native-born Americans. This may require communicating in simple language both orally and with handouts that the patient can understand. It is also helpful when handouts are written in the patient's native language, reflect an appropriate reading level, and depict images and examples of the cultural group in a positive manner (Cutilli, 2006).

Lack of motivation and readiness are often significant barriers to education. The patient may still be reeling from an unexpected adverse diagnosis and may not be able to focus on learning. The patient may not be motivated to learn what the nurse believes is important to teach. Patients with an external locus of control, for example, believe that nothing they can do will make a difference and may not be motivated to learn about their own illnesses. Often, nurses believe that simply pointing out what patients need to know is sufficient to motivate them.

It is usually more effective to assist patients to make their own decisions about the knowledge they need. This approach may require greater effort initially, but it is ultimately more efficient to assess patient motivation and readiness first, before engaging in patient teaching.

The nurse who is preparing to teach should also assess and manage the environment. A setting that is private, comfortable, and free of distractions is beneficial to the learning process. Once barriers have been identified and removed to the extent possible, nurses must plan patient education using sound principles of learning and teaching-learning concepts. Although it goes beyond the scope of this text to review all the complexities of learning, certain basic ideas should be considered. The patient's prior experiences, gender, culture, cognitive style, and motivation are all important determinants of learning. The nurse-teacher's knowledge, flexibility, creativity, communication skills, confidence in the patient's ability to learn, and ability to motivate all facilitate or impede learning. Boxes 10-10 and 10-11 review simple principles of adult learning and teaching-learning concepts that are useful in working with patients.

Impact of Illness on Families

Families are best understood as systems, which means that change in one member changes the functioning of the total family. It is important to remember that the entire family system is affected by a member's illness. Whether the ill family member is hospitalized or cared for in the home, illness drastically increases stress in a family and disrupts usual family function.

The most important factor in how a family tolerates stress is the individual and group coping abilities. Families already experiencing difficulties may find that their problems are intensified to the point of disruption when acute or chronic illness occurs.

A sick family member has to give up responsibility to other family members. The family must continue to fulfill its usual functions while

Box 10-10 **Principles of Adult Learning**

- Prior experiences are resources for learning.
  Example: If the patient enjoys gardening, try to link health maintenance suggestions to preventive maintenance of indoor/outdoor plants.
- Readiness to learn is usually related to a social role or developmental task.
  Example: New parents are usually eager to learn how to care for their first infants.
- Motivation to learn is greater when the material is seen as immediately useful.
  Example: The same new parents are more motivated to learn care of the small infant than they are to learn about disciplining toddlers.
- The learning environment must be arranged to facilitate learning.
  Example: The room is quiet, kept at a comfortable temperature, with adequate lighting, privacy, and seating.
- Physical needs are met before the teaching session.
  Example: The patient has his or her reading glasses and/or hearing aid, has been given the opportunity to toilet, and is relatively pain free.

Box 10-11 **Basic Teaching Tips for Patients and Families**

- Identify and remove, if possible, barriers to learning.
- Evaluate what the patient and family already know and what they want to know.
- When possible, frequent, short sessions work better than long ones.
- Goals for each session must be realistic.
- Be respectful of cultural differences, for example, in diet planning.
- Avoid medical jargon, acronyms such as PRN, and slang.
- The presentation should proceed from simple to complex concepts.
- Present complex concepts only after there is mastery of simpler ones.
- Patients learn best when they are actively engaged.
- Learning is enhanced when multiple senses are used: seeing, hearing, telling, and doing make the best combination.
- Practice, or frequent repetition, reinforces skill acquisition.
- Reinforce learning with return demonstrations of skills.
- When you give feedback, be sure to include positives, as well as negatives.
- Written materials should be at a fourth-grade reading level and, if possible, in the patient's native language to make reading easier for the patient.
- Evaluate patient's understanding of the information presented; provide time to clarify misunderstandings and answer questions.
- Remember to document the teaching session and your evaluation of the outcome.

dealing with the alterations imposed by the illness or absence of a member. Family members who are able to shift and assume different roles, who can share their feelings, and who seek assistance can be expected to adjust better to changes than those who are inflexible.

Both acute and chronic illness cause changes in family functioning and create stress. Chronic illness can be particularly stressful because it is never completely cured. Families experience emotional highs and lows as the patient has remissions and exacerbations. They may experience resentment and other negative feelings. Family members who must take over the sick person's responsibilities may be angry and then feel guilty about their anger. If they cannot deal directly with feelings of anger, they may

displace them onto nurses by becoming critical and demanding. Similarly, patients may feel guilty about creating hardships for loved ones. They may become convinced that they are no longer essential because others are capably taking over their roles. Family members sometimes withdraw from each other because they fear that their negative feelings may not be understood and accepted. This mutual withdrawal leads to feelings of isolation for both patients and family members.

Families are often confused or uncertain about how to treat the sick member. They may have problems accepting and responding appropriately to the patients' dependency needs. As discussed earlier, patients may react to illness with either overly dependent or overly independent behaviors. Nurses need to monitor whether family members foster dependence, thereby keeping the patient from becoming more independent. Nurses should also be aware that some families are uncomfortable with the ill person being in a dependent role and do not allow the necessary dependency for recovery. For example, if a man who is very much in control in a family has a heart attack and is in the coronary care unit, family members may have difficulty seeing the usually strong father in a helpless position. They may continue to bring family problems to him. Other families may find it difficult to shift responsibilities back to the formerly ill member as he or she becomes able to resume role functions, thereby prolonging dependence.

The nurse needs to recognize the anxiety in the family and take steps to reduce it. Talking with family members, explaining what is happening and what to expect, and teaching them how to participate in their loved one's care can help the family considerably. During hospitalizations, it may be helpful to allow family members to be present during invasive procedures such as central line placements and chest tube insertions. Their presence can comfort and support the patient and allay family members' anxiety about such procedures (Mangurten et al, 2005).

Some families find that becoming active in seeking information, such as through the Internet, helps them manage their anxieties. Support groups and chat rooms, where family members can express their concerns and hear from others with similar issues, are also helpful. Nurses can help family members use these adaptive coping activities effectively by assisting them to find credible websites and evaluate the information

---

Box 10-12   Seven Levels of Evidence

Patients, families, and nurses must bear in mind that not all published material, including material found on the Internet, has merit. It may or may not be based on evidence. Listed below are seven levels of evidence, ranging from least reliable to most reliable.

- *Level 1:* Ideas, editorials, letters, and opinion papers
- *Level 2:* Case reports, case studies, and reports of unusual happenings, such as adverse reactions
- *Level 3:* Information based on laboratory studies
- *Level 4:* Information based on animal studies
- *Levels 5 and 6:* Studies involving human subjects with increasing levels of complexity, scope, and rigor (for example, systematic research reviews, research-based protocols, and clinical practice guidelines)
- *Level 7:* Clinical trials are the "gold standard." Bear in mind that many nursing-related problems are not amenable to clinical trials because of potential risk to research subjects.

Modified from McKibbon A: *PDQ evidence-based principles and practice,* Hamilton, Ontario, Canada, 1999, Decker, pp. 7-12.

---

they find online. Box 10-12 lists seven "levels of evidence" within health care literature, ranging from least reliable and trustworthy to most reliable and trustworthy.

Other families find that activism helps them control their anxiety. The News Note on p. 246 tells how one man's activism has become a powerful force in the search for a cure for a rare form of abdominal cancer.

The nurse should assess family functioning and the ability of the family to provide support for the patient within the family's cultural context. Observe for feelings of anger, resentment, and guilt and assist the family in identifying adaptive methods of expressing these feelings. The nurse needs to determine the level of knowledge of the family members and assist them to

news note

Norman Scherzer was compelled to look for help on the Internet following his wife Anita's diagnosis with abdominal cancer. In a patient-run chat room he discovered information about another, more aggressive type of cancer that seemed to match her symptoms more closely. This led the Scherzers to a physician who confirmed a different diagnosis: gastrointestinal stromal tumor (GIST). GIST, Mr. Scherzer learned online, is a rare but deadly cancer that seemed to show a positive response to the drug Gleevec, originally made to treat leukemia. He also learned on the Internet that a clinical trial of Gleevec with GIST patients was under way. Anita had not responded to conventional chemotherapy, and her husband succeeded in getting her into the new clinical trial in August 2000. As a result her tumors shrank by 75 percent, and the Scherzers were able to celebrate their fortieth wedding anniversary in the fall of 2001.

Mr. Scherzer went on to develop a website and newsletter and to establish a group he termed the Life Raft Group (http://www.liferaftgroup.org). The group grew from three original members to more than 125 GIST patients and their caregivers. They share information about Gleevec with each other, doctors, and the company that makes the drug, Novartis AG. The Life Raft Group studied side effects from the drug and presented their findings to Novartis. They also published the report on their website.

This is a prime example of how patient activists are using the Web in new ways to help others find reliable and comprehensive, yet understandable health information online.

Modified from Landro L: The best way to get reliable health information, *Wall Street Journal*, Nov 12, 2001, p R 10.

Box 10-13   Potential Reactions to Illness in a Family Member

- Frightened
- Resentful
- Angry
- Guilty
- Exhausted
- Feelings of uselessness
- Feelings of hopelessness
- Distrust of health care providers
- Critical and demanding behavior
- Withdrawal from the situation
- Confusion
- Deny seriousness of patient's illness
- Promote dependence by patient

identify concerns and make realistic plans. Providing information and including the family in the planning can result in increased support for the patient and in effective care.

Nurses must be prepared to accept the anger and distrust that often is directed toward care providers who are unable to cure disease or relieve the negative consequences of illness. Understanding that anger expressed by patients and families is not personally directed can enable nurses to assess patients objectively and respond to feelings expressed in a nondefensive manner. Box 10-13 summarizes common examples of family feelings and behaviors that nurses need to recognize, acknowledge, and explore in a sensitive manner with the family.

Caregiver stress is common in families of patients with prolonged, progressive illnesses, such as Alzheimer's disease. Symptoms of caregiver stress include denial, anger, social withdrawal, anxiety, depression, exhaustion, sleeplessness, irritability, lack of concentration, and health problems (Alzheimer's Association, 2008). The Alzheimer's Association website is a useful resource for learning more about the important phenomenon of caregiver stress. Information can be found online: http://www.alz.org/living_with_alzheimers_caregiver_stress_lwa.asp.

Despite the numerous stresses, role strains, and adjustments necessitated by illness of a family member, many families find that there are also positive experiences in illness. Finding new activities to share and working together to meet challenges can lead to feelings of closeness and teamwork that were not present before. Previously unrecognized individual strengths may be identified as new roles and responsibilities are assumed. New meanings for the entire family may emerge as values are reassessed, priorities are shifted, and roles become more flexible.

IMPACT OF CAREGIVING ON NURSES

Caring is the foundation of professional nursing practice. Caring meets the essential human need for love and belongingness and assists nurses to provide high-quality nursing care. A caring attitude toward patients, their families, and colleagues begins with the caregiver—the nurse. Most nurses are not accustomed to caring for themselves, tending to put the needs of others before their own. Finding a balance between caring for others and self-care can be a challenging, lifelong pursuit.

Caring for Self While Caring for Others

Nurses often report that the needs of patients and families, as well as their own spouses and children, take priority over their own needs. They are left feeling stretched, overwhelmed, frustrated, unappreciated, and resentful. This has been termed compassion fatigue (Henry and Henry, 2004). Negative feelings interfere with the ability to maintain a caring attitude and drain caring out of our interactions with others. One nurse stated it well: "As a registered nurse, I try to connect with patients the best I can. Trust develops with personal rapport. When I'm busy and overworked, I become task oriented and don't have time to work on the trust building" (Roy, Turkel, and Marino, 2002, p. 10). Another used the empty pitcher analogy: "When I have given all I can give, I can't give any more until I get my own pitcher refilled" (Wisdom, 2008).

Although the NANDA-I diagnosis "caregiver role strain" refers to family caregivers, not professional nurses, some of the defining characteristics of this diagnosis are the same for nurses: anger, stress, impatience, increased emotional lability, frustration, lack of time to meet personal needs, low work productivity, gastrointestinal upset, difficulty performing/completing required tasks, lack of support, and insufficient time (NANDA-I, 2009, pp. 201-203). These descriptors could also be applied to nurses who feel overwhelmed with competing demands in their work and professional lives.

Nursing theorist Jean Watson described caring as the essence of nursing practice. Caregivers who are filled with stress and negativity cannot provide an atmosphere conducive to healing. The inescapable conclusion is that we must learn to care for ourselves to truly care for others. Dr. Watson is founder of the Center for Human Caring in Colorado and a renowned nurse theorist, speaker, and author. She has identified the consequences of caring and noncaring for nurses (Watson, 2005). The consequences of caring for nurses include:

- Emotional: spiritual sense of accomplishment, satisfaction, purpose, and gratification
- Preserved integrity, fulfillment, wholeness, and self-esteem
- Living own philosophy
- Respect for life and death
- Reflective; increased knowledge
- Love of nursing

The consequences of noncaring for nurses include:

- Hardened attitude
- Oblivious to needs of patients and coworkers
- Robot-like manner
- Depression
- Fear
- Fatigue; worn-down feeling

Dr. Watson's work also includes the consequences of caring and noncaring for patients. She identified the consequences of caring for patients as:

- Emotional-spiritual: Well-being, dignity, self-control, personhood
- Physical: Enhanced healing, saved lives, safety, energy, fewer costs, more comfort, less loss

- Trust relationships; decrease in alienation, closer family relationships

The consequences of noncaring for patients, according to Dr. Watson, include:

- Humiliation, fear, out of control, despair
- Helplessness, alienation, vulnerability
- Lingering bad memories
- Decreased healing, lack of trust, detachment

Professional nurses must stay tuned to themselves to avoid the consequences of noncaring for themselves and their patients. This is a lofty goal and a lifelong challenge. How does one go about maintaining the ability to be caring? Diann Uustal (2009), an early proponent of work-life balance, recommended "creating a balanced life rather than merely maintaining a balancing act" (p. 7). She reminded us of the announcement heard before every airline departure, ". . . put on your own oxygen mask first, before assisting others who may need it" (p. 13). That announcement has a lot of relevance to our lives as professional caregivers. Just as airline passengers in an emergency depressurization need oxygen before they can help others, nurses need to meet their own needs so that they will have the physical and emotional energy to care for others.

Choosing to work in a milieu that supports caring and professional nursing practice is one strategy to reduce the stress nurses feel while at work. There is probably no more stressful working environment for nurses today than the hospital. Because of the nursing shortage and the expense involved in hiring and orienting new staff, nursing leaders in hospitals are focusing on retention. They realize that the atmosphere can help nurses cope with stress in the workplace thereby enhancing retention. One example can be seen in the initiatives designed to create a "Caring Practice Environment" at Hamilton Medical Center in Dalton, Georgia (Wisdom, 2008):

- Development of a caring vision, mission, and philosophy for the department of nursing, involving all the nurses through surveys, focus groups, and interviews
- Implementation of Caring Groups, monthly meetings with trained facilitators to promote

humor, stress reduction, conflict resolution, and focus on care for self and fellow nurses

- A caring/healing room, open 24 hours a day, that provides massage therapy, paraffin treatments for hands and feet, aromatherapy, and soothing music. These services are available on a rotating and as-needed basis.
- Incorporation of new graduate nurses into a mentoring program with veteran nurses to help them integrate both clinically and socially into the world of nursing and to the caring environment

Other activities you as an individual can do to reduce compassion fatigue and facilitate self-renewal include finding a coach or a mentor. Refer to Chapter 6, Becoming a Nurse, for more information about how to select and use a mentor.

The Magnet Recognition Program

Another program that supports nurses is the American Nurses Credentialing Center's (ANCC's) Magnet Recognition Program. This program formally recognizes health care organizations that have a proven level of excellence in nursing care. The Magnet program was developed by the ANCC "to recognize health care organizations that provide the very best in nursing care and uphold the tradition of professional nursing practice" (ANCC, 2006). Achieving Magnet designation demonstrates the importance of nursing and nurses to the entire organization and signals the importance of quality care and a positive practice environment for nurses. It recognizes the caliber of the nursing staff, which validates nurses for their hard work and elevates the self-esteem of the entire nursing staff. According to the physician-authors of *YOU: The Smart Patient* during an appearance on *Good Morning America,* "Nurse Magnet hospitals are where the best nurses work, the morale is highest, and the hospital has the most resources. [As a patient] You want to be where the nurses want to be" (Oz and Roizen, 2006).

As of October 2009, there were more than 350 Magnet-designated health care facilities in the United States and the District of Columbia. These facilities are "nurse friendly," have low turnover and vacancy rates, and provide opportunities for professional and personal growth. All these factors lead to better patient care and greater career satisfaction. You can learn about Magnet facilities in your state at the ANCC's website (http://www.nursecredentialing.org/MagnetOrg/getall.cfm).

Developing and Maintaining a Life-Work Balance

Nurses who feel chronically exhausted and irritable at home and at work; who worry more than usual, cannot seem to complete tasks, lack concentration, and/or are forgetful; and who have diminished self-confidence should be aware that these symptoms indicate a need for more self-care. Keeping the balance between work and personal responsibilities takes conscious and continuous effort. Often it is achieved only fleetingly. To remain energized and fully engaged in your profession, however, you can learn strategies to help you develop and maintain a life-work balance. Just as nurses use care plans to organize how they care for patients, they can also identify how to create balance in their own lives.

Diann Uustal, in her book *Caring for Yourself, Caring for Others: The Ultimate Balance* (2009), recommended taking stock periodically using the guidelines listed in Box 10-14. Read these guidelines, and think about how you can begin now to apply them in your busy life. This can be the beginning of a lifelong effort to maintain balance so that you can continue to be the caring person you want to be in all your life roles, personal and professional.

Box 10-14   Create a Balanced Life Care Plan for Yourself

Read the following ideas and reflect on their practical application in your life.

- Taking personal responsibility for your health—physically, emotionally, intellectually, socially, and spiritually—is not easy, but it is the first step. Like it or not, there is no one who can do a better job of taking care of yourself than you.
- Start today with the changes you know are healthful. Make your choices one meal at a time or one day at a time. Do not beat yourself up if you do not always stick to the care plan.
- Balance. Try to stay in balance from a holistic perspective. What this means is different to each of us and different at various stages in our own lives.
- Increase your happiness quotient. Identify the things that bring you happiness and joy and enhance your quality of life. Try to do something pleasurable or satisfying each day.
- Identify and decrease the stressors in your personal and professional life. Develop strategies for decreasing the overall level of stress in your life. Some situations and habits can be corrected easily; others will take a real commitment and time to change.
- Make sure your goals and expectations are realistic. Unrealistic goals are self-defeating. Make sure the goals are measurable, manageable, and meaningful to you, not to please somebody else.
- Give yourself permission to relax and take some time for yourself each day. Learn to take "mental health breaks," no matter how brief. Enjoy the time without thinking about what you should be doing, so you can return refreshed.
- Prioritize your commitments based on your values. Make sure you give appropriate time and attention to the relationships that have stability and meaning over time.
- Learn to say "no" if you are pressured and overcommitted. Learn to say no without feeling guilty. Practice thinking that every problem is not your sole responsibility.
- Treat yourself like you treat your best friend. Do something special and "be-friend" yourself.

(Continued)

Box 10-14   Create a Balanced Life Care Plan for Yourself—cont'd

- Be a person of encouragement—to yourself. Be affirming to yourself. Do not "dump" on yourself or put yourself down.
- Make your physical fitness a priority. Commit to a balanced fitness program that includes stretching, aerobic exercise, and strength exercises. Sneak exercise into your daily life and exercise with a friend.
- Nutrition. Eat a balanced diet low in fat and cholesterol; take a multivitamin; drink lots of water and limit refined sugar intake. Practice portion control. If necessary, consult a dietitian.
- Sleep. Know how much you need and plan to get it. A pattern of too little sleep can injure your health. Avoid trying to be more productive by sleeping less. That can be counterproductive.
- Pay attention to your spiritual growth. Is your faith a first resort or a last resort when all else fails? What does it mean to be "spiritual?" Is being a part of a faith community important to you?
- Challenge yourself intellectually and develop your intellectual curiosity. Try to learn something new every day, no matter how small or insignificant it may seem.
- Stay connected with healthy people. Set time aside and plan for fun with people who can help you lighten up and enjoy some free time. Get out and do things you enjoy doing.
- Try a little "creative neglect" with the "basement people" (we all have them) in your life, especially when you are tired or handling too much. Spend as little time as possible with people who affect you negatively.
- Make sure you get enough "alone time." How much time alone each of us needs varies, so find out what is right for you. Most caregivers spend very little time alone. Check out your balance.
- Express your creativity through music, painting, needlework, sports, decorating, acting, or whatever lets you share yourself from the inside out.
- Don't be afraid to talk with a friend or a professional counselor to help you clarify your direction and put you back in balance again.

Reproduced from Uustal DB: *Caring for yourself, caring for others: the ultimate balance,* ed 2, Jamestown, RI, 2009, Sea Spirit Press, pp. 96-98.

Summary of Key Points

- Illness is a highly personal experience.
- Reactions to illness are culturally determined.
- Sick people may progress through stages of disbelief and denial, irritability and anger, attempting to gain control, depression, and acceptance and participation.
- Although every culture has expectations about how sick people should behave, previous experience and personality characteristics also affect individuals' responses to illness.
- Culturally competent nurses perform cultural assessments to determine how best to work with patients and families.
- Because of the stress and anxiety involved with illness, it is important for the individual to have methods of coping.
- Coping ability is enhanced in people who exhibit personality characteristics of hardiness, learned resourcefulness, and resilience.
- Patients' spiritual beliefs often play a role in stress reduction and can be used in nursing interventions.
- Providing holistic care means that nurses must consider their patients' physical, mental, emotional, spiritual, social, cultural, and family strengths and challenges to personalize care.
- The family is a system in which a change in one member affects all the other members.
- Illness causes alterations in usual family functioning that can result in emotional changes, including anger and guilt.
- The nurse needs to assess both how the family is influencing the patient and how the family is being influenced by the member who is ill.

- An understanding of the cultural factors that affect behaviors associated with illness can provide a better framework for the delivery of nursing care that is both effective and satisfying to patients, families, and nurses.
- As nurses view responses to illness in a cultural context, they are better able to understand and accept the unique ways in which individuals and families react to illness, thereby providing more effective nursing care.
- Caring is the emotional cornerstone of professional nursing practice.
- Creating a work-life balance, in which caring for self has a high priority, is the key to sustaining a caring approach to others.

Critical Thinking Questions

1. If you or someone close to you has been hospitalized, how did the nurses and family members encourage or discourage dependent behaviors? Independent behaviors?
2. Would it be easy or difficult to allow yourself to be bathed and have other intimate needs met by nurses of the same gender? Of the opposite gender? Of your cultural group? Of a different cultural group? Identify the reasons for your comfort or discomfort.
3. If possible, identify your own cultural group's response to illness. What are your family's characteristic responses to illness of a member?
4. Interview someone from another cultural background to learn how he or she perceives illness. Prepare several specific questions to ask about the meaning, causes, treatment, and feelings engendered by both acute and chronic illnesses. How does his or her culture tend to view nurses?
5. In a small group, discuss aspects of spiritual nursing care that you have used, feel comfortable using, or do not feel comfortable using. Appoint a group member to monitor those interventions that primarily benefit the patient and those that primarily benefit the nurse. Discuss the appropriateness of each. Report back to the larger class and discuss with your professor.

6. Speculate about the potential changes in the family of a husband and father of four small children who has experienced a severe illness and will be unable to work for an extended period. What stressors is this family likely to encounter? How might these stressors be different if his wife (the mother of the four children) were the sick family member?
7. Identify the ways you show a caring attitude toward patients and toward yourself. If you do not often care for yourself, analyze the reasons.
8. Working in a small group, design a nurse-friendly work setting and present it to the entire class. Be prepared to give rationales for your choices.

Ⓔvolve *To enhance your understanding of this chapter, try the Student Exercises on the Evolve site at http://evolve.elsevier.com/Chitty/professional.*

REFERENCES

Alzheimer's Association: Symptoms of caregiver stress 2009 (website) http://www.alz.org/living_with_alzheimers_caregiver_stress_lwa.asp.

American Nurses Credentialing Center: *ANCC magnet program: recognizing excellence in nursing services,* 2009 (website): http://www.nursecredentialing.org/Magnet/ProgramOverview.aspx.

Benson H, Klipper MZ: *The relaxation response, Twenty fifth anniversary update,* New York, 2000, HarperCollins.

Bowsher J, Keep D: Toward an understanding of three control constructs: personal control, self-efficacy, and hardiness, *Issues Ment Health Nurs* 16(1):33-50, 1995.

Carey B: Long-awaited medical study questions the power of prayer, *New York Times,* March 31, 2006 (website): http://www.nytimes.com/2006/03/31/health/31pray.html?ex=1145937600&en=3cd622f0fc1f109b&ei=5070.

Cavendish R, Luise BK, Horne K, et al: Opportunities for enhanced spirituality relevant to well adults, *Nurs Diagn* 11(4):151-163, 2000.

Chilton B: Recognizing spirituality, *Image J Nurs Sch* 30:400-401, 1998.

Cutilli CC: Do your patients understand? Providing culturally congruent patient education, *Orthop Nurs* 25(3):218-224, 2006.

Dewar AL, Lee EA: Bearing illness and injury, *West J Nurs Res* 22(8):912-926, 2000.

Eldridge CR: Meeting your patients' spiritual needs, *American Nurse Today* 2(10):51-52, 2007.

Ellis J, Nowlis E: *Nursing: a human needs approach*, ed 5, Philadelphia, 1994, JB Lippincott.

Freedman O, Orenslein S, Boston P, Amour T, Seely J, Mount BM: Spirituality, religion, and health: a critical appraisal of the Larson reports, *Ann R Coll Physicians Surg Can* 35(2):90-93, 2002.

Henry J, Henry L: Self-care begets holistic care, *Reflect Nurs Leadersh* 30(1):26-27, 2004.

Humphreys JC: Turnings and adaptations in resilient daughters of battered women, *Image J Nurs Sch* 33(3):245-251, 2001.

Kulwicki AD, Miller J, Schim SM: Collaborative partnership for culture care: enhancing health services for the Arab community, *J Transcult Nurs* 11(1):31-39, 2000.

Landro L: The best way to get reliable health information, *Wall Street Journal*, Nov 12, 2001:p R10.

Larson L: Heaven and hospitals: the role of spirituality in healing, *AHA News* 32(1):7, 1996.

Leininger M: Personal communication, 1999.

Lewis KS: Emotional adjustment to a chronic illness, *Lippincotts Prim Care Pract* 2(1):38-51, 1998.

Mangurten JA, Scott SH, Guzzetta CE, Sperry JS, Vinson LA, Hicks BA, et al: Family presence: making room, *Am J Nurs* 105(5):40-49, 2005.

McEwen M: Spiritual nursing care: state of the art, *Holist Nurs Pract* 19(4):161-168, 2005.

McKibbon A: *PDQ evidence-based principles and practice*, Hamilton, Ontario, Canada, 1999, Decker, pp 7-12.

Munoz C, Hilgenberg C: Ethnopharmacology, *Am J Nurs* 105(8):40-49, 2005.

NANDA: *Nursing diagnoses: definitions and classification, 2009-2011*, Oxford, 2009, NANDA International.

Narayan MC: Cultural assessment in home health care, *Home Healthc Nurse* 15(10):663-672, 1997.

Oz MC, Roizen MF: Your hospital stay could kill you: 90,000 Americans die from hospital infections each year, ABC News (website) http://abcnews.go.com/GMA/OnCall/story?id=1785701&page=2, March 30, 2006.

Parsons T: *The social system*, New York, 1964, Free Press.

Roberts S: A generation away, minorities may be the US majority, *New York Times*, Aug 13, 2008:p A-1.

Roy MA, Turkel MC, Marino F: The transformative process for nursing in workforce redevelopment, *Nurs Adm Q* 26(2):1-14, 2002.

Selye H: *The stress of life*, New York, 1956, McGraw-Hill.

Taylor R: Addressing barriers to cultural competence, *J Nurs Staff Dev* 21(4):135-142, 2005.

U.S. Department of Health and Human Services: Office of Minority Health: *National standards for culturally and linguistically appropriate services in health care*, Washington, DC, March 2001, Final report.

Uustal DB: *Caring for yourself, caring for others: the ultimate balance*, ed 2, Jamestown, RI, 2009, Sea Spirit Press.

Villaire M: Toni Tripp-Reimer: crossing over the boundaries, *Crit Care Nurse* 14(3):134-141, 1994.

Watson J: *Caring science as sacred science: caritas/love and caring-healing*, King of Prussia, Pa, June 16-19, 2005, presentation at the American Holistic Nurses Association 25th Annual Conference.

Whiting SA: A Delphi study to determine defining characteristics of interdependence and dysfunctional independence as potential nursing diagnoses, *Issues Ment Health Nurs* 15(1):37-47, 1994.

Wisdom K: Personal communication, 2008.

Zauszniewski JA: Learned resourcefulness: a conceptual analysis, *Issues Ment Health Nurs* 16(1):13-31, 1995.

The Science of Nursing and Evidence-Based Practice

Beth Perry Black

LEARNING OUTCOMES

After studying this chapter, students will be able to:
- Differentiate among bench, clinical, and translational science
- Describe the historical development of the scientific method
- Give examples of inductive and deductive reasoning
- Discuss the limitations of the scientific method when applied to nursing
- Differentiate between problem solving and research
- List the steps in the research process
- Describe the phases in the design of a qualitative study

- Discuss contributions nursing research has made to nursing practice and to health care
- Describe the relationship of nursing research to nursing theory and practice
- Identify sources of support for nursing research
- Discuss the roles of nurses in research
- Define evidence-based practice
- Differentiate between research and evidence-based practice
- Discuss the pros and cons of evidence-based practice in nursing

The word "science" often conjures up images of laboratories, white lab coats, test tubes, and molecules that leave many students a little apprehensive at the thought. In fact, many of you who are studying this chapter are working toward completion of a bachelor of science in nursing (BSN) degree, and all of you are using nursing science to shape your practice. The purpose of this chapter is to help you understand the links between nursing practice, research, and nursing's scientific base—the science of nursing.

In the mid-twentieth century, the nursing profession was preparing to achieve a higher level of scientific development. Mature professions have a strong scientific base, which was lacking in nursing at the time. Scholars and researchers realized that nursing could achieve a high level of professional status only to the extent that the discipline was based on a scientific body of knowledge unique to nursing. As a result, nursing researchers began developing knowledge unique to nursing, and nursing theorists began developing theories and testing them. Theory and research are the foundations of scientifically based nursing practice.

At the same time, nurses realized that professionalization of patient care practices was also needed. Until that time, nurses relied on traditional techniques to manage common patient problems. More unusual problems were often managed by trial and error or intuition. However, these were no longer acceptable ways to care for patients. The impetus toward evidenced-based practice was developing, which required nurses to base their care and activities on research-based knowledge. This necessitates a strong link between the work of nurse researchers and nurses in practice. The development of the nursing process became a means of adapting a scientific framework to the management of patient care, so that nurses were no longer depending on hit-or-miss techniques but were shaping care in direct response to the individual needs of the patient. The nursing process is presented in depth in Chapter 8.

An understanding of the scientific method is helpful in appreciating both nursing research and the nursing process.

SCIENCE AND THE SCIENTIFIC METHOD

Science is research based on one or more past scientific achievements or accomplishments that are acknowledged by the scientific (academic) community as providing a foundation for further study or practice (Kuhn, 1970). Good science requires that research be based on the previous work of others in the same academic discipline or be related to work of others from other disciplines. This is a safeguard that ensures that knowledge development is based on sound principles and theory rather than simply the product of a creative idea that is not based on any known science. Sound science and creativity are not mutually exclusive; creativity has led to many interesting and useful research developments that in turn guide nursing practice.

The scientific community is specific to each academic discipline, meaning that nurse researchers and scholars acknowledge and judge scientific developments in nursing, just as the chemistry academic community establishes the parameters of what constitutes good research and science in chemistry. Social scientists such as sociologists and anthropologists have their own theoretical foundations and foci of research. Common to research in all disciplines, however, is the use of an orderly, systematic way of thinking about and solving problems. This systematic way of thinking is traditionally known as the scientific method, used by scientists for centuries to discover and test facts and principles.

The more traditional form of "doing science" required standardized experimental designs, measurable variables and outcomes, and statistical analyses; this form is often referred to as quantitative research. Because nursing is interested in phenomena that may not be amenable to traditional quantitative research, a significant number of noted researchers in nursing use qualitative techniques to explore human responses in health and illness. Data collection techniques

falling under the rubric of qualitative research include narrative interviews and participant observation, among others. A more recent development in nursing research is the use of mixed methods, a means of examining phenomena of interest using both qualitative and quantitative methods. Regardless of whether a researcher uses quantitative, qualitative, or mixed methods, all good research has a theoretical basis and is carried out in a systematic, disciplined way that furthers the development of a discipline's knowledge base.

Basic, Clinical, and Translational Science

Traditionally, scientists divided scientific knowledge into two categories: pure and applied. Pure science or pure research, often referred to as bench science, summarizes and explains the universe without regard for whether the information is immediately useful. When Joseph Priestley discovered oxygen in 1774, he did not have an immediate use for that information. Therefore that discovery could be classified as pure science, that is, information gathered solely for the sake of obtaining new knowledge. Applied science or applied research sought to use scientific theory and laws in some practical way. How supplemental oxygen is best used in the care of premature infants with respiratory distress syndrome is an example of applied science. Applied science is usually referred to as clinical science now—taking to the patient's bedside those findings that may be useful in curing, managing, or preventing diseases or managing symptoms.

More recently, however, scientists have recognized importance of a third type of research—translational research that serves as a conduit between the "bench and the bedside." Translational research takes the findings in the laboratories and develops them for use at the bedside. In turn, translational research takes the findings from clinical research done at the bedside to ask new questions and to direct new research at the bench level. In 2004, the National Institutes of Health (NIH), an agency of the U.S. federal government and the largest source of public funding for research, launched an ambitious new initiative known as the Roadmap for Medical Research. The purpose of the Roadmap effort is to enhance the way that American biomedical research is conducted, making it more streamlined and flexible in responding to the health needs of society, while still maintaining the high standards required of excellent scholarship and science. One of the key innovations of the Roadmap effort was to enhance translational science by funding the Clinical and Translational Science Awards (CTSA) initiative. The CTSA initiative holds great promise in advancing interdisciplinary research, shortening the time from "bench to bedside" and enhancing patient care in a multitude of ways. The NIH website (http://nihroadmap.nih.gov/) provides a comprehensive description of translational science and the Roadmap effort to enhance clinical and translational science. Over the course of your nursing career, you will see many changes in practice and medical therapies as a result of this new initiative in research.

Inductive and Deductive Reasoning

Research requires the use of one of two kinds of logic: inductive reasoning or deductive reasoning. In inductive reasoning, the process begins with a particular experience and proceeds to generalizations. Repeated observations of an experiment or event enable the observer to draw general conclusions. For example, a researcher may be interested in the responses of the families of hospice patients to ongoing bereavement support for 1 year after the death of the patient. After interviewing 10 family members and finding a generally positive response to the support, inductive reasoning may lead the researcher to infer that this is an effective intervention on the basis of this group's response. In other words, the particular experience of 10 families leads to a generalization that everyone would benefit from this sort of support. This type of inference leads to the development of probabilities but not certainties, unless every single member of all families of every hospice patient who died were studied—a study that would be impossible to conduct.

Scientists also use deductive reasoning, a process through which conclusions are drawn by logical inference from given premises. Deductive reasoning proceeds from the general case to the specific. For example, if the premises "All family members of hospice patients benefit from bereavement support for 1 year" and "Mrs. Compton is the wife of a hospice patient" are accepted, the conclusion "Mrs. Compton will benefit from hospice support for 1 year" can be drawn. It may be entirely possible, however, that Mrs. Compton, although a family member of a hospice patient, will not benefit from bereavement support at all. In deductive reasoning, the premises used must be correct or the conclusions will not be. Conclusions drawn through deductive processes are called valid rather than true. *Valid* is a term meaning "soundly founded," whereas *true* means "in accordance with the fact or reality" (Flexner, Stein, and Su, 1980). It is possible for a conclusion to be solidly founded without being true for everyone. There is a subtle but real difference between the words *valid* and *true*.

As seen by these examples, neither inductive nor deductive processes alone are adequate. If scientists used only deductive logic, experience would be ignored. If they used only inductive logic, relationships between facts and principles could be overlooked. A combination of both types of reasoning processes in science unifies the theoretical and the practical, which is the basis for the scientific method and research.

Limitations of the Strict Definition of Scientific Method in Nursing

Polit and Beck (2004, p. 16) asserted that the "traditional scientific approach used by quantitative researchers has enjoyed considerable stature as a method of inquiry and it has been used productively by nurse researchers studying a wide range of nursing problems. This is not to say, however, that this approach can solve all nursing problems." There are at least three reasons why the scientific method as implemented exclusively with quantitative techniques has limitations when applied to phenomena of interest to nursing.

The first and most obvious drawback is that health care settings are not comparable with laboratories. Certain phenomena of interest to nurses are not amenable to study in a lab setting and in fact are not amenable to study in tightly controlled circumstances. For instance, in the discussion of inductive/deductive logic regarding bereavement support, measurement of the family members' grief and distress in response to the intervention of bereavement support for a year is not possible in the laboratory setting by conventional measures. The phenomenon of grief may be of great interest to hospice nurses; the systematic examination of an intervention and the measurement of outcomes are not a particularly good fit with the laboratory setting. Grief subsequent to death of a family member is a human response that occurs in real-world settings. Research techniques generic to qualitative research may be more appropriate to the aims of this research.

Second, human beings are far more than collections of parts that can be dissected and subjected to examination or experimentation. A strength of nursing is its holistic view of patients, whereas the basis of the scientific method is to reduce a problem into manageable problem statements, each of which can be tested. Because humans are complex organisms with interrelated parts and systems, the classic scientific method loses much of its usefulness in the examination of complex human phenomena.

A third limitation of the scientific method as the only approach to solving patient problems is its claim to objectivity; it fails to consider the meaning of patients' own experiences, that is, their subjective view of reality. Nurses are keenly aware, however, that patients' perceptions of their experiences, or subjective data, are just as important as objective data and may have significant effects on their health behaviors. Again, referring to the bereavement example, let us assume that a well-designed, reliable, and valid instrument (such as a questionnaire) can measure Mrs. Compton's grief. After 1 year, her grief scores are lower, and it appears that she has benefited from bereavement support during this time. However, this approach fails to take into consideration Mrs. Compton's own experience of grief and her perception of the support intervention. If she still feels sadder than she believes she should after a year of support, the intervention may be a failure although her "grief scores" are lower. Her perception of her grief and her response are key elements of her experience that cannot be measured objectively and retain the meaning of her situation.

WHAT IS NURSING RESEARCH?

If you are a college or university student, you may have been introduced to research through your basic psychology or sociology courses, in which you may have been required to participate in some way in your professor's research project. Although some of these experiments are interesting, in some cases, the only research to which you may have been exposed was surveys or questionnaires. This kind of orientation may lead you to wonder what research has to do with your ability to care for patients.

Nursing research, however, has a different focus that you will likely find more clinically applicable and therefore more valuable than the experiments that you participated in while studying Psychology 101. The NIH's National Institute of Nursing Research (NINR) describes its mission:

"to promote and improve the health of individuals, families, communities, and populations. NINR supports and conducts clinical and basic research and research training on health and illness across the life span. NINR seeks to extend nursing science by integrating the biological and behavioral sciences, employing new technologies to research questions, improving research methods, and developing the scientists of the future. NINR supports research relevant to its mission, in order to provide a sound scientific basis for changes in clinical practice. In keeping with the importance of nursing practice in various settings, NINR's major emphasis is on clinical research" (http://www.nih.gov/about/almanac/organization/NINR.htm)

The rest of this chapter describes some basic concepts of nursing research. The purpose is to introduce nursing research, demonstrate its merit, and provide a basic vocabulary. The ultimate goal is for nurses to participate in the research process and apply research findings to clinical practice. This is a key component to what is known as evidence-based practice.

Nursing research is the systematic investigation of **phenomena** (events or circumstances) related to improving patient care. Much nursing research arises out of clinical observations. Although a research topic may be in a new area of investigation, much can be gained from choosing research problems that are connected to work already done, thereby building the body of knowledge of nursing. A problem may be amenable to research if these criteria are met:

1. A conceptual framework exists or can be constructed from research that already has been done; that is, the researcher's ideas about the problem fit logically and dovetail with what is already known about the topic.

2. The proposed research project is based on related research findings published in professional journals or is supported by similar ongoing research in other settings, thereby building nursing knowledge.

3. The proposed research is carefully designed so that the results will be applicable in similar situations or will generate hypotheses for further research and testing.

In addition to building nursing knowledge, studies that build on previous work are more likely to receive financial support. Research is expensive and often requires funding beyond what one nurse, hospital, or university can supply. Nurses who want to do research usually find it necessary to obtain outside funding or compete with other aspiring researchers for limited internal (from within the agency) funding. Therefore to receive funding, nurses must do research that interests others, has demonstrated significance, and has support from reviewers who examine the proposed research for the specific funding agency and make recommendations about whether to fund it or not.

Furthermore, research that is not based on or is not related to previous foundational work may have inadvertent violations of human participants' rights. In other words, it is hard to justify asking people to participate in research if there is no real connection to previous work or theory that supports the idea that an intervention works or a problem is significant. Researching or testing an intervention in humans just to see whether it works or that seemed like a "good idea" ignores potential shortcomings or may fail to anticipate problems if adequate foundational work is not done before instituting the research. In fact, such research will not receive approval from a federal human participants' review board if significant linkages with previous research are not demonstrated. This review board (commonly known as the institutional review board [IRB]) approval must occur before any research involving humans is undertaken.

Thus although nursing research may be broadly defined as anything that interests nurses and helps them provide better care, controversy exists over what can legitimately be included. When choosing a research question, the wise nurse researcher considers the practical issues of background and financial support. An important source of funding and support for nursing research is the NIH's NINR, created in 1992 from what had previously been known as the National Center for Nursing Research (NCNR). NINR supports basic, translational, and clinical research aimed at establishing a scientific basis for nursing practice. Although its budget has quadrupled since NCNR was first created, NINR is still able to fund only a small portion of the research proposals it receives. To establish priorities for funding, the National Nursing Research Agenda (NNRA) was launched in 1987. In 2006 NINR published its plan for the next 5 years that was built on past progress in nursing research. The priorities of current research efforts that NINR anticipates continuing to support are listed in Box 11-1.

Research is different from **problem solving**. Problem solving is specific to a given situation and is designed for immediate action, whereas research is **generalizable** (transferable)

Box 11-1   National Institute of Nursing
Research (NINR) Priorities,
2006-2011

Chronic illness
Quality and cost-effectiveness of care
Health promotion and disease prevention
Management of symptoms
Adaptation to new technologies
Health disparities
Palliative care at the end of life

National Institute of Nursing Research: *Strategic planning for the 21st century*, Bethesda, Md, National Institutes of Health, 2005 (website): http://www.ninr.nih.gov/AboutNINR/NINRMissionandStrategicPlan/

to other situations and deals with long-term solutions rather than immediate ones. For example, Mrs. Abney is an elderly patient who frequently is found wandering in the halls of the nursing home, unable to find her way back to her room. This is quite distressing to her and time-consuming for the nursing staff that help her find her way "home." A nurse notices that Mrs. Abney has no difficulty recognizing her daughter, so she tapes a photograph of the daughter to Mrs. Abney's door. Now Mrs. Abney can find her room easily. She is less agitated, and the nursing staff time can be spent elsewhere.

Mrs. Abney's case is an example of problem solving, an effective intervention in one set of circumstances that has immediate application. However, the solution that worked for Mrs. Abney may not work for all confused patients. In fact, it may not continue to work for Mrs. Abney if her cognitive abilities decline further. Remember that nursing research was developed in response to the professional and scientific mandate that nursing care be based in evidence and not simply on trial and error. On an occasional basis, creative problem solving such as that of Mrs. Abney's nurse is required on a per-case, situational basis. But this sort of trial-and-error problem-solving approach is not adequate to base one's professional practice in a substantial and sustained way. Table 11-1 contrasts problem solving and research.

EVIDENCE-BASED PRACTICE: BRIDGING THE GAP BETWEEN RESEARCH AND PRACTICE

The best efforts of nurse researchers are fruitless unless nurses make use of their research findings to improve patient care in their day-to-day practices. Patients have become more knowledgeable consumers of health care, and nurses must ensure that they provide the latest and best available care. One way to ensure positive patient outcomes is through evidence-based practice.

Evidence-based practice (EBP) means using the best available research findings "to make clinical decisions that are most effective and beneficial for patients" (Cope, 2003, p. 97). Cleary-Holdforth and Leufer (2008) include patient preference in their definition of EBP, under the assumption that nursing values the individual for whom nurses are caring, and who is a partner in care planning. They also put "significant value" on the experience, expertise, clinical judgment, and decision-making skill of the practitioner (p. 43). Archie Cochrane, a British epidemiologist, is credited with beginning the EBP movement. His work ultimately was reflected in the development of the Cochrane Library, which holds the Cochrane Database of Systematic Reviews. Systematic reviews are important means of reviewing data collectively across a number of studies. Clinicians and scholars recognized that practice was improved when critical appraisal of the best evidence is the foundation for practice (Cleary-Holdforth and Leufer, 2008). The Centre for Evidence-Based Medicine (EBM) at Oxford University in England defines EBM as "the conscientious, explicit, and judicious use of current best evidence in making decisions about the care of individual patients. The practice of evidence-based medicine means integrating individual clinical expertise with the best available external clinical evidence from systematic research" (Sackett, Rosenberg, Gray et al, 1996, p. 71). The motivation behind EBP was the belief that most of health care practice was based on intuition, experience, clinical skills, and guesswork, rather than science. The value of EBP in clinical practice,

Table 11-1   Comparison of Problem Solving and Research

Characteristic	Research	Problem Solving
Type of problems addressed	Widely experienced	Situation-specific
Conceptual basis	Theoretical framework	Often none; trial and error
Knowledge base needed	Extensive review of literature to determine latest thinking and research	Practical knowledge, common sense, and experience
Scope of application	Generalizable to similar situations	Useful in immediate situation; transferability must be determined

as well as in learning situations, was recognized, and its study and use spread rapidly to nursing.

In nursing, EBP requires that you be cognizant of research that supports the specific interventions (Alfaro-LeFevre, 2006). Basing one's practice on published work or reliable texts is an element of critical thinking and a good means of improving clinical judgment. Focusing on evidence of effective interventions is a good means of preventing one's practice from deteriorating into routine or traditional care based on what has always been done without concern for advances in care. Pursuing continuing education, attending professional conferences, reading journals, and obtaining membership in professional organizations are good means of staying current and keeping aware of new evidence of best practices.

Questions regarding best practices are raised daily by nurses in direct patient care roles. Nurses in practice commonly question procedures and routines, asking if there is a better way to achieve the outcomes of patient care. Most nurses in bedside practice are not equipped to study those questions; however, answers may already be available in the nursing literature. An important focus of professional nursing education is to learn how to seek out and critique research findings to implement best practices in one's own nursing practice. One way to streamline the process of examining research literature is a process known as PICO, an acronym for a four-step process: P—population of interest, I—intervention, C—comparison, O—outcome (Cleary-Holdforth and Leufer, 2008). By using PICO as a framework, you can eliminate looking at research that may not address

specifically enough the particular problem or intervention you are interested in.

Differences of opinion exist among nurses regarding what types of studies constitute the strongest evidence and what weight to give to each (Salazar, 2003). The use of systematic review of clinical research regarding a particular patient problem poses certain obstacles in examining published reports of research. Some nurses disagree, for example, about the relative merits of randomized controlled trials, long considered the gold standard in research, versus descriptive and qualitative studies.

Systematic reviews of the research and clinical literature—such as those that can be done on databases such as the Cumulative Index of Nursing and Allied Health Literature (CINAHL), the Educational Resources Information Center (ERIC), and PubMed—require that the reviewer have some idea of what type of research method best captures the phenomenon of interest (Macnee, 2004). Careful use of the research literature may result in the decision to forgo certain practices, even when tradition suggests "this is how it's always been done." Research is used to both support certain practices and discourage others.

Where do clinical expertise, intuition, and patient preference come into the hierarchy of importance in planning care? These issues are being debated in numerous EBP conferences and symposia. Each of these has significance in planning care for patients; however, basing practice on clinical expertise, intuition, and patient preference without having a thorough knowledge of research that supports care is unprofessional, demonstrating evidence of a lack of critical thinking about the management of one's own practice.

Sigma Theta Tau International, Honor Society of Nursing, has a long history of support of nursing research and dissemination of research findings through its publications. This association has adopted a position statement on evidence-based nursing that demonstrates the importance of EBP to its members. You can read this position statement in Box 11-2.

Box 11-2   Sigma Theta Tau International's Position Statement on Evidence-Based Nursing

As a leader in the development and dissemination of knowledge to improve nursing practice, the Honor Society of Nursing, Sigma Theta Tau International, supports the development and implementation of evidence-based nursing (EBN). The society defines EBN as an integration of the best evidence available, nursing expertise, and the values and preferences of the individuals, families and communities who are served. This assumes that optimal nursing care is provided when nurses and health care decision-makers have access to a synthesis of the latest research, a consensus of expert opinion, and are thus able to exercise their judgment as they plan and provide care that takes into account cultural and personal values and preferences. This approach to nursing care bridges the gap between the best evidence available and the most appropriate nursing care of individuals, groups, and populations with varied needs.

The society, working closely with key partners who provide information to support nursing research and EBN around the world, will be a leading source of information on EBN with an integrated cluster of resources, products and services that will foster optimal nursing care globally. The society, along with its strategic partners, will provide nurses with the most current and comprehensive resources to translate the best evidence into the best nursing research, education, administration, policy and practice.

Sigma Theta Tau International: *Position statement on evidence-based nursing,* 2005 (website): http://www.nursingsociety.org/research/main.html#ebp.

THE RESEARCH PROCESS

The nursing research process is the same as the research process in any other academic discipline; nursing research, however, focuses on a nursing-related problem. Research starts with a problem or stimulus. The stimulus for a research project may be an observation that something related to practice or patients' responses needs to be addressed. There may be insufficient data for resolving a problem, or the literature is unclear, or the data presented in the literature are conflicting. When there is a need for more information and no adequate information or conflicting information exists, research is the means to resolve, clarify, or inform.

Whether using quantitative or qualitative techniques or mixed methods, all research must be rigorously planned, carefully implemented, and scrupulously analyzed. Therefore most research follows a formal order known as the research process. Students in baccalaureate nursing programs often take a semester-long course in nursing research in which both qualitative and quantitative methods are described, so this chapter will attempt only a brief introduction to the research process. Steps in the research process include the following:

1. Identification of a research problem
2. Review of literature
3. Formulation of the research question or hypothesis
4. Design of the study
5. Implementation
6. Drawing conclusions based on findings
7. Discussion of implications
8. Dissemination of findings

Each step will be discussed briefly.

Identification of a Research Problem

Research problems generally come from three sources: clinical situations, the literature, or theories. Clinical situations are rich sources for research problems. Nurses are in a prime position for identifying problems and issues for research. For instance, a common issue among nurses in gerontological settings is the propensity for some elderly patients to wander and get lost. There are several issues related to this problem, including characteristics of patients that tend to wander, time of day this occurs, staffing issues, and medications. Is the nurse seeking to identify patients at high risk for wandering, or is the nurse more interested in preventing nighttime wandering, specifically? A nurse who has identified a clinical problem that may lead to research will have a number of questions to consider as the research is being formulated. Streamlining the problem into a researchable question is a primary goal early in the research process.

Second, sometimes researchers become interested in a problem because it has been published in the literature. They may decide to **replicate** (repeat) the study or may design a similar one to test part of the original study in a new way. For example, suppose that the nurses in the previous scenario read an article in their professional journal about an innovative means of minimizing wandering among elderly patients. In a discussion at their staff meeting about the article, one of the nurses suggests that this approach may not work on this unit for several reasons. The nurses decide to consult with a nurse researcher at the local university to discuss replicating the study on their unit to determine whether in fact this innovative intervention will work under the conditions that are in place here or to determine what prevents the intervention from working.

The third source of research problems—theory—relates to testing theoretical models. In Chapter 13, you will read about several types of nursing theory that have been developed. Theoretical models are designed to predict patients' responses to nursing actions; whether or not a model actually does predict patients' responses can be tested through research. The researcher can create certain conditions and determine whether, in fact, the events happen as the theoretical model predicted. Again, consider the nurses on the gerontology nursing unit. Suppose that one of the nurses who has a psychiatric nursing background noted that some psychiatric patients will wander, but using Peplau's theory of interpersonal relations as basis for their psychiatric

practice, the nurses on the unit found that patients who formed excellent relationships with their primary nurses were the least likely to wander. The nursing staff decided to test this theory in their elderly patients, using Peplau's theoretical model as a basis for their intervention, predicting that the formation of a trusting relationship between patient and primary nurse would result in less nighttime wandering among patients without cognitive impairment. A "real life" example of the use of Peplau's theory to guide an ongoing research project is found in Box 11-3. This study also illustrated the interrelationship between nursing theory, research, and practice.

Review of the Literature

Once a problem is identified, the research literature must be reviewed. A review of the literature (ROL) is comprehensive and covers all relevant research and supporting documents to support the research. Doing a thorough ROL requires a great deal of library time or computer search efforts and detective work. Computer-generated searches of the literature can assist tremendously with this step but cannot totally replace the efforts of a dedicated researcher. A major study with many parts requires huge review efforts, usually involving multiple investigators (researchers) in the work to make sure that the literature review is comprehensive and reflects the current state of the science.

The ROL is essential to locate similar or related studies that have already been completed and on which a new study can build. The review is helpful in creating a **conceptual framework**, or organization of supporting ideas, on which to base the study. The ROL answers the question, "What have other researchers and theorists written about this problem?" Sometimes the literature review causes the researcher to rethink or reconceptualize the initial problem, especially if the problem has been studied a variety of ways or if findings in other work are unimpressive or statistically insignificant.

Nursing is a relatively new discipline with a growing but limited knowledge base, especially in comparison with other disciplines such as

Box 11-3   A Research Study of a Nursing Intervention Guided by Theory

Hildegard Peplau has been called the "founder of psychiatric–mental health nursing" because she started the first graduate programs that prepared nurses to do advanced-practice functions such as psychiatric–mental health diagnosis, psychotherapy, and care of persons with complex mental health needs. In 1991, I was developing her Interpersonal Theory of Nursing (ITN) to guide intervention for depressive symptoms. We were exchanging letters, and she wrote, "Linda, you need to get to mothers as early as possible so that they can create the kind of relationships with their very young children that foster healthy emotional growth." Now, 15 years later, we are scientifically testing a new form of interpersonal psychotherapy done in the home of low-income, depressed mothers of infants and toddlers. The exciting part of this project is to see master's-prepared psychiatric–mental health nurses use the incredibly rich "laboratory" of the mother's interpersonal life—her interactions with her child, her exchanges with her significant others, and her relationship with the nurse—to help her change the very sources of her depression. We are trying to help these mothers take charge of themselves and their lives and, in doing so, reduce the risk of more depressive episodes for themselves and, later, for their children. The ITN gives the interventionists a framework for constructing interventions to help these mothers solve the deeply difficult issues they face and learn new strategies for reducing their depressive symptoms. We would be lost without Dr. Peplau's road map. We are so indebted to her work that we call our project "HILDA"!

• *Linda Beeber, PhD, RN, FAAN University of North Carolina at Chapel Hill*

Courtesy Linda Beeber.

medicine and some of the humanities. Because nursing has a holistic view of patients and problems, and the nursing literature may not be sufficiently broad, often the ROL has to include research outside of the discipline of nursing.

For instance, if a researcher is interested in a phenomenon such as perinatal loss, an ROL must include what has been written in nursing about the phenomenon of perinatal loss, including all aspects such as early and late miscarriage, stillbirth, and elective termination. However, because this is a subject that has many social, ethical, and psychological issues at stake, a thorough ROL would include literature from sociology, anthropology, ethics, and psychology and may include work from public health (epidemiology). In addition, literature from the medical field, such as maternal-fetal medicine and reproductive genetics, would be reviewed.

As the researcher reviews the literature, he or she will find that other researchers commonly cite some specific papers. These "classics" in research, despite being older papers, have a place in a new ROL. Otherwise, most researchers find that literature published within the past 5 years tends to be adequate. Although the review of literature is a tedious task, it is a crucial step in ensuring that the research to be undertaken will be scientifically sound and theoretically congruent with work that has already been completed.

A caveat is in order here about the use of Internet resources for scholarly work. Although there is much information available on the Internet about almost any topic you can imagine, much of this work is not peer reviewed and should be used with caution. The Internet is best used as a tool for disciplined, organized searches of established databases such as CINAHL, MEDLINE, PubMed, and PsycINFO. These online catalogs will lead you to peer-reviewed articles that have a place in scholarly work. Increasing your informational literacy (Fitzpatrick and Montgomery, 2004) strengthens your review of the literature by allowing you increased access to scientific publications that have met the challenges of peer review. Box 11-4 lists some important measures to take in establishing the credibility and usefulness of Internet resources for research. Even while you are a student, this information is important as you perform research for your assignments and prepare for clinical activities.

Box 11-4   Evaluating Information Sources on the Internet

It is often difficult to know when you are accessing credible information on a website and when you are not, particularly in health care, which has many competing commercial interests. Nursing, Midwifery and Allied Health Professions (NMAP) is part of a gateway system created in the United Kingdom to improve the quality of Internet searches for health-related information. NMAP recommends a six-step process in evaluating Internet resources. You may want to adopt some of these practices to ensure that you are retrieving the best available information from credible sources.

1. Follow any links as far as you can to find out details about a resource. The home page, help files, and frequently asked questions (FAQs) are good starting places.
2. Analyze the URL. This will give you an idea about the source of the information. For instance, .edu is a U.S.-based educational institution, .com is a U.S.-based commercial establishment, and .org is a U.S.-based organization. A country code such as .UK for the United Kingdom is added if the URL is not based in the United States.
3. Examine the information in the resource. Check for thoroughness via a site map or search facility on the website. See who the developers of the website consider to be their target audience—professional health care providers, patients, families. Check for links

to other credible websites. Then, assess the accuracy of the information. This poses a big task for a student who may not yet have the background to assess a site adequately. You should ask a professor or other expert to help you. Remember that some sites have commercial interests whose information may not be entirely accurate or it may be slanted in such a way to increase sales of a product.

4. Determine how accessible and easy the resource is to use. How available and reliable is the server? Are there restrictions on its use? Do you have to pay to use the site? Cumbersome websites with poor information are a waste of time, yielding little if any useful data.
5. Obtain additional information about the resource. Double-check the reliability of information on the Internet site you are considering using. Is the site sponsored by a credible agency? How much is this site used? A trustworthy site with reliable information should generate substantial Internet traffic.
6. Compare the resource to other similar sites and materials. The website should have basic information that is similar to that of other reliable sources. If the information is very different, look for another website. You must trust that the website's basic information is correct.

From Nursing, Midwifery and Allied Health Professions: *How to evaluate an Internet-based information source* (website): http://www.vts.intute.ac.uk/he/tutorial/nurse/ (accessed April 2009).

Formulation of the Research Question or Hypothesis

Once researchers have identified a research problem, are thoroughly knowledgeable about the relevant literature, and have chosen or created a conceptual framework that helps to focus and support the topic, they will formulate the research question. If the researcher is interested in determining and describing certain characteristics of a situation, he or she may simply pose the situation as a question. For example, "What are the characteristics of mothers who have difficulty

initiating breast-feeding with their newborns?" is a research question asking about specific characteristics of a population (mothers with breast-feeding difficulties). If comparing the relationship of two variables, a different type of question might be asked, such as "What is the relationship between maternal age, parity, and difficulty in initiating breast-feeding?" This question demonstrates that the researcher has some idea that these variables are related (and that the literature supports this idea), but the exact nature of the relationship is not known or hypothesized.

If conducting an experiment, researchers must have a hypothesis (educated or informed speculation as to what the outcome will be so that hypothesis-testing statistics may later be applied. For example, "Younger mothers with no previous children will demonstrate later initiation of breast-feeding than older and experienced mothers" is a testable hypothesis. The form and content of the research question are key to the development of the rest of the study. Larger, more complex studies will have multiple questions or hypotheses to address.

Design of the Study

Once the research questions are identified or hypotheses are generated, the study must be designed. Numerous forms of research designs exist, but experimental and nonexperimental designs are the two major categories. If the purpose of the research is to determine the effect of an intervention or to compare the responses of participants to two or more differing treatments, for example, the research will have an experimental design. If not, the research will have a nonexperimental design. The main difference between experimental and nonexperimental research is whether or not the researcher manipulates, influences, or changes the participants in any way by the testing of an intervention or medication or other substance.

True experimental designs provide evidence of a cause-and-effect relationship between actions. For example, testing the hypothesis "Patients who receive preoperative teaching need less pain medication in the first 72 hours postoperatively than those who do not" would provide evidence of a cause-and-effect relationship between teaching and perception of pain. Experimental designs require quantitative measures to determine whether there are statistically significant differences between the conditions being tested.

Sometimes it is impossible to conduct a true experimental study with human beings, because to do so might endanger them in some way. In those instances, modified experimental studies are used. In this case, a new intensive form of educational intervention before surgery might be tested

against the usual form of preoperative teaching. Because preoperative teaching of patients regarding pain management is standard care and an expected behavior of all nurses in that setting, denying that care to patients would be unethical and inappropriate. The experimental design could, however, test a new intervention against the usual care received by preoperative patients.

Nonexperimental designs are occasionally referred to as "descriptive" or "exploratory" research because the investigator is seeking to increase the knowledge base about a nursing phenomenon by doing careful, disciplined research. There are many types of nonexperimental designs: surveys, descriptive comparisons, evaluation studies, and historical-documentary research, among others. Ethnography is a qualitative methodology well suited for descriptive or exploratory research. Nonexperimental designs may be either quantitative or qualitative, or they may use a combination of both.

Whether the researcher chooses an experimental or nonexperimental design influences the data collection process. The data collection process includes selection of data collection instruments, design of the data collection protocol, the data analysis plan, participant selection, and informed consent and institutional review plans.

Data collection instruments

When designing a study, researchers must consider how the data will be collected. Data collection instruments, sometimes called data collection tools, range from simple survey forms to complex radiographic scanning devices. The selected instrument used must be reliable, or accurate. A reliable instrument is one that yields the same values dependably each time the instrument is used to measure the same thing. The tool must also be valid, which means that it must measure what it is supposed to be measuring. The ideal instrument is highly reliable and provides a valid measure of the condition, such as weight, temperature, or depression.

If body temperature is being measured, a thermometer is an obvious data collection tool. When measuring an abstract factor, such as anxiety or depression, the best data collection tool is not as clear. The selection of a data collection instrument answers the question, "What tool(s) will we use to collect the data?" To minimize measurement errors, beginning researchers should choose instruments with established reliability and validity that have been published and widely used, rather than designing their own. Inexperienced researchers will occasionally make the mistake of designing a questionnaire that they believe is a valid measure of the construct (condition) they want to study. However, this is a serious flaw in the research and must be avoided.

Data collection protocol

Another aspect of designing the study is deciding on the data collection protocol (procedure). The quality of the data depends on strict adherence to the plan. If, for example, the plan calls for administering a questionnaire to renal dialysis patients after dialysis, the data collectors must be sure to give the questionnaire to all participants—and only after their treatments. The protocol for data collection must be explicit and used by everyone who is collecting data for the study. Data collected in the wrong way or at the wrong time are unusable, introducing error into the study that can and must be avoided.

Data analysis plan

It may seem premature to decide how the data will be analyzed before they are even collected, but careful planning for the analysis is important. The research design is developed with data analysis in mind. The analysis must be part of the planning process, because the data and the protocols for collecting them depend on how the data will be analyzed. Unless the nurse researcher is an expert in statistics or there is already a statistician on the research team, consultation with a statistician well versed in human participant research is recommended in designing the data analysis plan, which answers the question, "What will we do with the data once we gather them?"

Qualitative analysis, notably, begins immediately with the collection of data, because the data themselves often drive the shape and design of the research. Qualitative analysis is a very difficult and exacting procedure that requires extensive training. Although some researchers believe that qualitative research is "easier" than quantitative research, in fact they are similar in the disciplined approach to data analysis that is required to produce usable, meaningful results.

Participant selection

Once the researcher knows what is to be done, the specifics of who will be included are decided. The individual people being studied are referred to as **participants** (formerly "subjects"). If the researchers plan to study pain control in postoperative patients, for example, they have to decide the specific type of surgery and the age, sex, ethnicity, and geographic location of the patients, as well as a variety of other factors, in planning the participant selection. Qualitative studies use different sampling strategies, that is, the participants are selected for study in a different manner than is typically used in quantitative studies. Qualitative researchers often use a strategy known as "purposeful sampling"; potential participants are selected for the study specifically rather than randomly, as is sometimes used in quantitative studies. These participants exhibit some kind of trait or have some type of experience that the researcher is studying.

Informed Consent and Institutional Review

Next, researchers who use human participants must plan to protect their rights by asking them to sign an **informed consent** form that describes the details of the study and what participation means. Any risks involved in participating must be explained. No one should be pressured in any way to participate, and the **confidentiality** (privacy) of participants must be ensured. See the Cultural Considerations Challenge.

A related step when studying humans is the submission of the proposal to the institution, such as a hospital or clinic, where the research will take place for review by a federally approved board known as the **institutional review board (IRB)**. An IRB is composed of individuals from the

Cultural Considerations Challenge
Informed Consent

If researchers who use human participants must plan to protect their rights by asking them to sign an informed consent form that describes the details of the study and what participation means, what measures would researchers need to consider when participants are recent immigrants? How might potential risks involved in participating best be explained? How might researchers ensure that these participants do not feel pressured to participate? What assurances might they desire concerning confidentiality that other participants might not need?

Additionally, consider the circumstance where potential participants do not speak English. What are the risks to these persons? How can these risks be minimized?

community and different academic disciplines and exists to ensure that research is well designed and does not violate the policies and procedures of the institution or the rights of the participants. Only after the IRB approves the proposal can the study begin. All persons conducting research or assisting with the management of data must demonstrate evidence that they have taken an online course on the protection of the rights of human participants (http://www.citiprogram.org). The protection of the rights of participants is the primary consideration of all research involving humans. Modification of any aspect of the research requires that the IRB be notified and approval procured before the change is implemented.

Implementation

Up until this point, only planning has taken place. Careful planning is, however, the key to a successful study. In the implementation phase, the actual study is conducted. The two main tasks during this phase are data collection and data analysis.

Data collection

Data (research-generated information) should be collected only by those who are thoroughly familiar with the study. All research assistants should understand the purpose of the data and the importance of accuracy and careful record keeping. No matter who is collecting the data, the integrity of the project is ultimately the responsibility of the primary researcher.

Data analysis

If all goes well, data are analyzed exactly as proposed. In analyzing the data, most researchers use the same statistical consultants who assisted in planning the study. The researcher works closely with the statistician in interpreting, as well as analyzing, the data. The nurse researcher is in charge, however, and he or she has the final word on what interpretations are made from the data.

Analyzing the findings of qualitative research presents formidable challenges for several reasons. First, the data are voluminous, often consisting of lengthy dialogues between researchers and participants. Next, dialogues must be transcribed verbatim, yielding hefty stacks of pages. The investigator then faces the task of organizing the transcripts, identifying themes, and arranging the themes into meaningful patterns. Fortunately, computer programs are available to assist in this process; however, nothing substitutes for contemplation (by humans!) in determining the nuances of meanings in narrative data such as those assimilated in qualitative designs.

Drawing Conclusions Based on Findings

In writing the research report, the findings directly related to the research question are presented first. Findings are presented factually—without value judgments. The facts must speak for themselves. Accurate presentation of the facts is the only requirement. After findings related to the research question are reported, unexpected findings can be reported. Conclusions are then drawn. Conclusions answer the question, "What do these findings mean?" Here researchers can be more reflective about the findings, discussing what was anticipated versus what was found in the study, and suggesting alternative work to clarify findings.

Discussion of Implications

Researchers are always alert to the implications of their studies. Implications are suggestions of things that should be done in the future. Every good study raises more questions than it answers. In nursing studies, there may be indications for modifications in nursing education or nursing practice. Nearly every study has implications for further research, and if the findings turn out as expected, almost all studies should be carefully replicated. Replication can answer these and other questions: "What needs to be known to develop more confidence in the findings? Will the research instrument produce similar results in a similar population in a different geographic location? Will the procedure be effective with patients having a slightly different diagnosis, condition, or type of surgery? Will age make a difference? Will cultural beliefs make a difference? What else do we need to know to improve the care of patients?"

Dissemination of Findings

Findings from a research study must be disseminated so that others can learn from the work that was done. Dissemination refers to the process of publication and presentation of findings. Most funding agencies want to know in advance how the researcher plans to disseminate findings because letting others know about the findings is very essential. The two major vehicles for dissemination of knowledge are articles published in professional journals and presentations given at conferences. Prominent nursing research journals include *Research in Nursing & Health (RINAH), Nursing Research (NR), Journal of Nursing Scholarship* (published by Sigma Theta Tau International), *Nursing Inquiry, Journal of Advanced Nursing, Advances in Nursing Science (ANS),* and the *Western Journal of Nursing Research.* These journals are not specific to any particular type of nursing but publish articles of wide interest in nursing. Professional nursing organizations may have their own research journals targeting specific nursing interests, such as *JOGNN: Journal of Obstetric, Gynecologic, & Neonatal Nursing,* published by the Association of Women's Health, Obstetric and Neonatal Nurses (AWHONN), and the

Journal of the Association of Nurses in AIDS Care (JANAC), published by the Association of Nurses in AIDS Care (ANAC).

A review process, called peer review, is the method most journals use to determine whether to publish a research report. During peer review, a manuscript is circulated anonymously to a review panel typically consisting of three experts in the area of study. They evaluate its appropriateness and accuracy and recommend that it be published, that it be revised and then resubmitted with changes, or that it be rejected. Most research that is carefully conceived, conducted, and presented can get published, although the researcher must be persistent and resilient in taking criticism and reworking manuscripts.

A somewhat easier, yet still discriminating, route to dissemination is presentation at one or more of the numerous nursing research conferences. Many research conferences also use the peer-review process. In general, however, the proportion of abstracts (summaries of research) selected for presentation at conferences is higher than the proportion of manuscripts chosen for publication. In addition to oral presentation of research papers, conferences offer the opportunity for nurses to present their findings in poster sessions, especially appropriate when work is preliminary or is still in progress. Posters allow for brief explanations of the research method and findings in written form, usually a 3- × 4-foot poster that is professionally designed.

Whether research is published or presented at conferences, it is important to disseminate research results to other nurses, who may choose to use the results either to improve patient care practices or to replicate the study.

RELATIONSHIP OF NURSING RESEARCH TO NURSING THEORY AND PRACTICE

Relationships among nursing research, practice, and theory are circular. As mentioned earlier, research ideas are generated from three sources: (1) clinical practice, (2) literature, and (3) theory.

Questions about how best to deal with patient problems regularly arise in clinical situations. As shown in the earlier example of Mrs. Abney, the elderly lady who could not find her room, problems often can be "solved" for the present. However, when the same questions recur, long-term answers may be needed. Research develops solutions that can be used with confidence in different situations.

Published articles about nursing research often generate interest in further studies. If there is published research on a particular nursing care problem, other researchers may be stimulated to investigate the subject further and refine the solutions. This is how nursing knowledge builds.

Nursing theorists also generate research ideas. They piece together postulates or premises that "explain" what has been discovered. The explanation is "tested" to determine whether it is robust or strong enough to be useful. If so, there may be more implications for applications in clinical practice.

Nursing research journals are filled with clinical studies that have made a difference in patient care. A few examples of changes in nursing practice stimulated by research include the following:

1. Improved care of patients with skin breakdown from pressure ulcers
2. Decreasing light and noise in critical care units to prevent sleep deprivation
3. Using caps on newborns to decrease heat loss and stabilize body temperature
4. Positioning patients after chest surgery to facilitate respiration
5. Scheduling pain medication more frequently after surgery
6. Preoperative teaching to facilitate postoperative recovery

Nursing research findings not only improve patient care but also affect the health care system itself. For example, research studies have demonstrated the cost-effectiveness of nurses as health care providers. This is discussed further in Chapter 14.

A final point about the influence of research on practice is a reminder about the relationship of research and professionalism. In Chapter 3, the characteristics of professions were presented. One of the criteria commonly mentioned is a scientific body of knowledge that is expanded through research. Nursing research enhances the status of nursing as a profession by expanding nursing's scientific knowledge base. Refer back to Box 11-3 for an example that may clarify the interplay between nursing research, practice, and theory; then take this chapter's Critical Thinking Challenge 11-1.

CRITICAL THINKING *Challenge 11-1*

Evidence-based practice (EBP) is a movement in nursing that is gaining widespread support. Well-informed nurses are likely to provide better care than those who are not well informed. Yet the mention of the word "research" is likely to send many novice (and experienced) nurses running for cover!

Some nursing journals are heavily research oriented, whereas others are more clinically oriented. For example, the Association of Women's Health, Obstetric and Neonatal Nurses (AWHONN), a large professional nursing association, publishes two journals: *JOGNN*, which generally publishes research-based articles; and *Nursing for Women's Health*, which is oriented toward clinical issues in women's health. Your school's library is likely to subscribe to these journals and others like them.

Sit down with back issues of each of these journals or others of interest to you, making sure that one is research based and the other is clinically based. Read the table of contents of each and assess your interest in each topic. Which ones appeal to you? Why? Do you find yourself drawn to one type of journal over another? How hard will it be to maintain EBP once you are out of school and in the work setting? What can you do to ensure that you remain current in your practice and up-to-date with research findings once you no longer have easy access to a school library?

SUPPORT FOR NURSING RESEARCH

Nursing research is expensive, and support takes many forms. It can include encouragement, consultation, computer and library resources, money, and release time from researchers' regular teaching responsibilities. Each of these forms of support is important, but none alone is adequate. Early in the development of nursing research, encouragement was often the only support available, and not all nurse researchers had that. Gradually over the years, more sources of funding have been identified, but financial support can still be difficult to obtain, particularly for new researchers. Figure 11-1 introduces you to a new nurse researcher who has been successful in obtaining funding outside of nursing to support her important work on the epigenetics of breast cancer.

In addition to the NINR discussed earlier in this chapter, many other federal agencies accept proposals that meet their funding guidelines when submitted by qualified nurse researchers. These include the 26 other centers and institutes of the NIH, such as the National Institute on Aging, the National Cancer Institute, the National Institute of Mental Health, the National Institute on Alcohol Abuse and Alcoholism, and the Eunice Kennedy Shriver National Institute of Child Health and Human Development. Competition with researchers from other disciplines is strong, however, and generally only experienced nurse researchers are successful in obtaining funding from these sources.

Nursing associations also fund nursing research. The American Nurses Foundation, Sigma Theta Tau, and many clinical specialty organizations provide research awards, even for novice researchers. State and local nursing associations sometimes have seed money for pilot projects. Universities, schools of nursing, and large hospitals also may provide small amounts of research funds. Generally, however, finding adequate funding for large-scale studies continues to be a problem faced by researchers.

ROLES OF NURSES IN RESEARCH

The *Code of Ethics for Nurses* states: "The nurse participates in the advancement of the profession through contributions to practice, education, administration, and knowledge development" (American Nurses Association, 2001). Ideally, every nurse should be involved in research, but, practically, all nurses should, as a minimum, use research results to improve their practices. Evidence-based nursing practice requires staying informed about current literature, especially studies done in one's own specific area of clinical practice.

As seen in Table 11-2, in addition to using research to improve practice, all professional nurses can contribute to one or more aspects of the research process. Baccalaureate nurses can read, interpret, and evaluate research for applicability to nursing practice. Through clinical practice they can identify nursing problems that need to be investigated. They can also participate in the implementation of scientific studies by helping principal researchers collect data in clinical

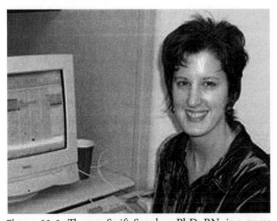

Figure 11-1 Theresa Swift-Scanlan, PhD, RN, is a nurse researcher at the University of North Carolina at Chapel Hill. In 2009, Dr. Swift-Scanlan received a 3-year Career Catalyst in Disparities Research award from the Susan G. Komen Foundation. Over the next 3 years, she will explore DNA methylation changes and environmental exposures that may contribute to the greater prevalence of aggressive breast cancer subtypes seen in African-American women. The ultimate goal of this work is to decrease breast cancer morbidity and mortality by identifying markers that can better inform screening approaches and treatment planning. The type of data that she generates is shown in the photo on the right. (Courtesy Theresa Swift-Scanlan.)

Table 11-2 Levels of Educational Preparation and Participation in Nursing Research

Level of Preparation	Level of Research Participation
Student nurse	Consumer
BSN nurse	Problem identifier
	Data collector
MSN nurse	Replicator
	Concept tester
Doctoral nurse	Theory generator
Postdoctoral nurse	Funded program director

BSN, Bachelor of science in nursing; *MSN,* master of science in nursing.

settings or elsewhere. These beginning researchers must know enough about the purpose of the research to follow the research protocols explicitly or know when it is necessary to deviate from the protocol for a patient's well-being. Baccalaureate nurses also can help disseminate research-based knowledge by sharing useful research findings with colleagues.

The master's-prepared nurse may be ready to replicate studies that have been previously conducted. Researchers cannot be sure that their findings are true until studies are repeated with similar results. Nurse researchers have learned that it is not necessary (or even desirable) always to generate a totally new and disconnected idea to do research. As mentioned earlier, to be most useful, research must be based on a conceptual framework and related to previous research.

Depending on education, clinical and research experiences, and interests, some nurses at the master's level are better prepared to conduct research than others. In addition to education and experience, a crucial factor is the support system the nurse has available. To do research, nurses need time, money, consultation, and participants. With rich resources in a research environment, master's-prepared nurses can and do make vital research contributions.

Nurses with doctor of philosophy (PhDs) or other doctoral degrees are more favorably positioned to receive research funding than are nurses without doctorates. Researchers across the United States in all professions and academic disciplines compete for a limited pool of research dollars available each year. Only those nurses with strong academic and experiential backgrounds and the best proposals succeed in obtaining federal funding.

Research in nursing provides the avenue for creative, scholarly endeavors driven by a desire to improve the care for patients. It is our hope that you will find research to be an important part of your professional practice both as a consumer of research and as an adherent to EBP and, in the future, you will conduct research of your own.

Summary of Key Points

- The scientific method is a systematic, orderly process of solving problems. It has been used for centuries and is applicable in many different situations.
- Research can occur in labs (bench research) or at the bedside (clinical research). Translational research is a means of connecting more efficiently the work that is generated in labs and directly within patient populations.
- Both inductive reasoning and deductive reasoning are necessary to combine the theoretical and the practical aspects of the scientific method.
- For safety and ethical reasons, there are limitations on research with human subjects.
- Nursing research is defined as the systematic investigation of phenomena of interest to nursing with the goal of improving care.
- The major steps in the research process are identification of a research problem, review of the literature, formulation of the research question, design of the study, implementation, drawing conclusions based on findings, discussion of implications, and dissemination of findings.
- Nurse researchers have made significant contributions to improvements in nursing care practices.
- Nursing research is related to and informed by nursing theory and nursing practice and in turn influences them.

- Nurses of all educational backgrounds have a role in research.
- Evidence-based nursing practice is the goal of nursing research.

Critical Thinking Questions

1. Why is nursing called an applied science? Explain why you agree or disagree with this description.
2. Name and describe the two types of reasoning used in the scientific method. Explain why neither alone is adequate to advance knowledge.
3. List and discuss each step of the research process.
4. Explain why a purely experimental model is an inadequate one for nursing.
5. Go to your college library or online and see which nursing research journals are in the collection. Scan through some recent issues and notice the types of studies reported. Compare them with studies done 20 years ago. What similarities and differences do you note?
6. Read a research article that interests you. See whether you can identify each of the steps in the research process. If not, what is missing? Discuss with your teacher and classmates what the significance of the missing steps might be.
7. Find out what research is being done in your school or hospital. If possible, talk with those involved, including data collectors, data analysts, research directors, participants, families of participants, and nurses who work on units where research is being conducted. What do they know about the research? What are their concerns? What do they hope will be learned from the research?
8. Obtain job descriptions for nurses at varying experience levels at different agencies. Are research functions included in the job descriptions? If not, what research functions do you think might be appropriate to include?
9. As a class, explore the evidence-based practice websites and debate the pros and cons of evidence-based practice.

ⓔvolve *To enhance your understanding of this chapter, try the Student Exercises on the Evolve site at http://evolve.elsevier.com/Chitty/professional.*

REFERENCES

Alfaro-LeFevre R: *Applying the nursing process: a tool for critical thinking*, Philadelphia, 2006, Lippincott Williams & Wilkins.

American Nurses Association: *Code of ethics for nurses with interpretive statements*, Washington, DC, 2001, American Nurses Publishing.

Cleary-Holdforth J, Leufer T: Essential elements in developing evidence-based practice, *Nurs Stand* 23(2):42-46, 2008.

Cope D: Evidence-based practice: making it happen in your clinical setting, *Clin J Oncol Nurs* 7(1):97-98, 2003.

Fitzpatrick JJ, Montgomery KS, editors: *Internet for nursing research: a guide to strategies, skills and resources*, New York, 2004, Springer.

Flexner SB, Stein J, Su PY, editors: *The Random House dictionary*, New York, 1980, Random House.

Kuhn TS: The structure of scientific revolutions, In Nurath O, editor: *International encyclopedia of unified science*, ed 2, Vol 2, Chicago, 1970, University of Chicago Press.

Macnee CL: *Understanding nursing research: reading and using research in practice*, Philadelphia, 2004, Lippincott Williams & Wilkins.

National Institute of Nursing Research: *NIH Almanac*, Bethesda, Md, 2009, National Institutes of Health (website): http://www.nih.gov/about/almanac/organization/NINR.htm

Nursing, Midwifery and Allied Health Professions: *How to evaluate an Internet-based information source* (website): http://www.vts.intute.ac.uk/he/tutorial/nurse/ (accessed April 2009).

Polit DF, Beck CT: *Nursing research: principles and methods*, ed 7, Baltimore, 2004, Lippincott Williams & Wilkins.

Sackett DL, Rosenberg WM, Gray JA, et al: Evidence-based medicine: what it is and what it isn't, *BMJ* 312:71-72, 1996.

Salazar MK: Evidence-based practice: relevance to occupational health nurses, *AAOHN J* 51(3):109-112, 2003.

Sigma Theta Tau International: *Position statement on evidence-based nursing*, 2005 (website): http://www.nursingsociety.org/research/main.html#ebp.

Conceptual and Philosophical Bases of Nursing

Kay Kittrell Chitty

After studying this chapter, students will be able to:
- Describe the components and processes of systems
- Explain Maslow's hierarchy of human needs and its relationship to motivation
- Recognize how environmental factors such as family, culture, social support, the Internet, and community influence health
- Explain the significance of a holistic approach to nursing care
- Apply Rosenstock's health beliefs model and Bandura's theory of perceived self-efficacy to personal health behaviors and health behaviors of others

- Devise a personal plan for achieving high-level wellness
- Define and give examples of beliefs
- Define and give examples of values
- Cite examples of nursing philosophies
- Discuss the impact of beliefs and values on nurses' professional behaviors
- Explain how nurses and organizations educating and employing nurses can use a philosophy of nursing
- Identify personal beliefs, values, and philosophies as they relate to nursing.

There are certain basic concepts, or ideas, that are essential to an understanding of professional nursing practice; they are the building blocks of nursing. These concepts are person, environment, and health. Everything professional nurses do is in some way related to one of these basic interrelated concepts and is guided by beliefs, values, and statements of philosophy. In this chapter we will explore how these concepts relate to each other and to nursing.

SYSTEMS

An understanding of systems will assist you in understanding the interplay among nursing's basic concepts. General systems theory was originally developed by Ludwig von Bertalanffy in 1936 (von Bertalanffy, 1968). Von Bertalanffy, a biologist, believed that a common framework for studying several similar disciplines would allow scientists and scholars to organize and communicate findings and more readily build on the work of others. He described a system as a set of interrelated parts that come together to form a whole that performs a function. Each part is a necessary or integral component required to make a complete, meaningful whole. These parts are input, throughput, output, evaluation, and feedback.

Components of Systems

The first component of a system is input, which is the raw material, such as information, energy, or matter that enters a system and is transformed by it. For a system to work well, input should contribute to achieving the purpose of the system.

A second component of a system is throughput. Throughput consists of the processes a system uses to convert raw materials into a form that can be used, either by the system itself or by the environment or suprasystem. Output is the end result or product of the system. Outputs vary widely, depending on the type and purpose of the system.

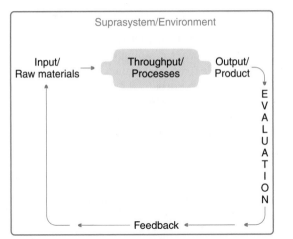

Figure 12-1 Major components of a general systems model.

Evaluation is the fourth component of a system. Evaluation means measuring the success or failure of the output and consequently the effectiveness of the system. For evaluation to be meaningful in any system, outcome criteria, against which performance or product quality is measured, must be identified.

The process of communicating what is found in evaluation of the system is called feedback, the final component of a system. Feedback is the information given back into the system to determine whether or not the purpose, or end result, of the system has been achieved. Figure 12-1 depicts the components of systems and illustrates how they relate to one another.

Examples of Systems

It may be helpful to use a simple example to clarify the components of systems. In a college system, the raw material, or input, consists of students, faculty, ideas, the desire to learn, and knowledge. For high-quality input, students need to be ready to learn, and the faculty should be knowledgeable and well prepared to teach. The processes (throughput) whereby ideas, knowledge, and skills are transmitted must be clear and understandable. In this example, throughput consists of learning experiences such as lectures, seminars, and laboratories. The output, or product, of the

system is educated graduates. For evaluation of the output, a standardized examination of reading comprehension, mathematics, and analytic skills may be used. Student scores on the comprehensive examination provide feedback to the faculty and administrators. If students score well, the system has achieved its purpose. If not, changes need to be made in the input or in the system itself—for example, admitting brighter students, hiring more talented faculty, or designing more effective courses and curricula.

Systems are usually complex and consist of several parts called subsystems. Let us examine a hospital as a system. Technically, it is a system for providing health care, but the success of the system depends on the functioning of many subsystems. The subsystems include the laboratory, radiology, housekeeping, laundry, central supply, medical records, dietetics, nursing, pharmacy, and medical staffs. Each of these subsystems is a system itself. All the subsystems function collaboratively to make the health care system—the hospital—work.

Open and Closed Systems

Continuing with the example, the hospital and all its subsystems are open systems. An open system promotes the exchange of matter, energy, and information with other systems and the environment. The larger environment outside the hospital is called the suprasystem. A closed system does not interact with other systems or with the surrounding environment. Matter, energy, and information do not flow into or out of a closed system. There are few totally closed systems. Even a completely balanced aquarium, for example, often thought of as approaching a closed system, needs light, air, and additional water and nutrients from time to time.

Two more points are essential to a beginning understanding of systems. First, the whole is different from and greater than the sum of its parts. Stated another way, the system is different from and greater than the sum of its subsystems. Anyone who has ever been in a hospital, for example, knows that what happens there is different from and more than the sum of the following equation: laundry + pharmacy +

nurses + physicians = hospital. The second point involves synergy. Synergy occurs when all the various subsystems and the people who compose them collaborate to work with patients and their families.

Dynamic Nature of Systems

The final point to be made about systems is that change in one part of the system creates change in other parts. If the hospital admissions office, for example, decides to admit patients only between the hours of 8:00 AM and 10:00 AM, that decision creates changes in the nursing units, housekeeping, the business office, surgery, the laboratory, and other hospital subsystems. If that change was implemented without prior communication to the other subsystems and coordinated planning, it could create chaos in the system.

The exchange of energy and information within open systems and between open systems and their suprasystems is continuous. The dynamic balance within and between the subsystems, the system, and the suprasystems helps create and maintain homeostasis, or internal stability.

All living systems are open systems. The internal environment is in constant interaction with a changing environment external to the organism. As change occurs in one, the other is affected. For example, walking into a cold room (change in the external environment) affects a variety of physiologic and psychological subsystems of a person's internal environment. These, in turn, affect a person's blood flow, ability to concentrate, and feeling of comfort, for example (changes in internal environment).

Application of the Systems Model to Nursing

Why is it necessary for nurses to understand systems? Nurses work within systems every day. Using the hospital example, nurses work within the nursing department's system, within a particular unit's system, and with a team system, among others. All three are open systems interacting with one another and the environment. If nurses are to work effectively in such complex systems, they need to have an understanding of how systems operate.

Box 12-1 Key Concepts About Systems

- A system is a set of interrelated parts.
- The parts form a meaningful whole.
- The whole is different from and greater than the sum of its parts.
- Systems may be open or closed.
- All living systems are open systems.
- Systems strive for homeostasis (internal stability).
- Systems are part of suprasystems.
- Systems have subsystems.
- A change in one part of a system creates change in other parts.

At the individual patient level, the openness of human systems makes nursing intervention possible. Understanding systems helps nurses assess relationships among all the factors that affect patients, including the influence of nurses themselves. Nurses who understand systems view patients holistically, including the subsystems (such as respiratory system and gastrointestinal system) and suprasystem (for example, family, culture, and community). These nurses appreciate the influence of change in any part of the system. For instance, when a patient with diabetes has pneumonia (change in subsystem), the infection increases the blood glucose level and may result in hospitalization. Hospitalization may in turn adversely affect the patient's role in the family and community (change in suprasystem). Key concepts of systems are summarized in Box 12-1. With this brief introduction to systems as a foundation, we can now examine the three basic concepts that are fundamental to the practice of professional nursing.

PERSON

The term person is used to describe each individual man, woman, or child. There are various different approaches to the study of person. This chapter briefly examines the concept of people as systems with human needs.

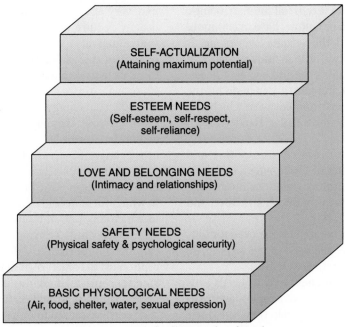

Figure 12-2 Maslow's Hierarchy of Needs.

As mentioned previously, each individual is an open system with numerous subsystems that make up the whole person. For example, there are circulatory, musculoskeletal, respiratory, gastrointestinal, genitourinary, and neurologic subsystems that compose the physiologic subsystem. There are also psychological, social, cultural, and spiritual subsystems that combine with the physiologic subsystem to make up the whole person. Each person is unique and different from all other persons. This uniqueness is determined both genetically and environmentally and is the basis for holistic nursing care—that is, nursing care that takes all the aspects of the person into consideration.

Certain personal characteristics are determined before birth by the genes received from one's parents. Genetically determined characteristics include eye, skin, and hair color; height; gender; and a variety of other features. Other characteristics about persons are determined by the environment. The availability of loving parents or parent substitutes, availability of sufficient nutritious foods, cultural beliefs, degree of educational opportunities, adequacy of housing, quality and quantity of parental supervision, and safety are all examples of environmental factors that influence how a person develops.

Human Needs

In addition to having personal characteristics, people have inborn needs. A human need is a requirement for a person's well-being. In 1954 psychologist Abraham Maslow published *Motivation and Personality*. In this classic book, Maslow rejected earlier ideas of Freud, who believed that people are motivated by unconscious instincts, and Pavlov, who believed humans were driven by conditioned reflexes. Instead, Maslow presented his human needs theory and explained that human behavior is motivated by intrinsic human needs. He identified five levels of needs and organized them into a hierarchical order, as shown in Figure 12-2.

Maslow's Hierarchy of Needs

According to Maslow, the most basic level of needs consists of those necessary for physiologic survival: food, oxygen, rest, activity, shelter, and sexual expression. These are needs all human beings, regardless of location or culture, have in common.

Maslow identified the second level of needs as safety and security. These include physical, as well as psychological, safety and security needs. Psychological safety and security include having a fairly predictable environment with which one has some familiarity and relative freedom from fear and chaos.

The third level of needs consists of love and belonging. To a greater or lesser extent, each person needs close, intimate relationships; social relationships; a place in the social structure; and group affiliations.

Next in Maslow's hierarchy is the need for self-esteem. This includes the need to feel self-worth, self-respect, and self-reliance.

Maslow called the highest level of needs self-actualization. Self-actualized people have realized their maximum potential; they use their talents, skills, and abilities to the fullest extent possible and are true to their own nature. People do not stay in a state of self-actualization but may have "peak experiences" during which they realize self-actualization for some period of time. Maslow believed that many people strive for self-actualization, but few consistently reach that level (Maslow, 1987). He also believed that people are "innately motivated toward psychological growth, self-awareness, and personal freedom. As he saw it, we never outgrow the innate need for self-expression and self-development, no matter how old we are" (Hoffman, 2008, p. 36).

Assumptions about needs

Maslow's hierarchy rests on several basic assumptions about human needs. One assumption is that basic needs must be at least partially satisfied before higher-order needs can become relevant to the individual. For example, a starving person can hardly be concerned with self-esteem until a life-sustaining level of nutrition is established.

A second assumption about human needs is that individuals meet their needs in different ways. One person may need 8 or 9 hours of sleep to feel rested, whereas another may require only 5 or 6 hours. Each individual's sleep needs

may vary at different stages of life. Older people usually require less sleep than younger people. Individuals also eat different diets in differing quantities and at differing intervals. Some prefer to eat only twice a day, whereas others may snack six or eight times a day to meet their nutritional needs. Sexual energy also varies widely from person to person. The frequency with which normal adults desire sexual activity is determined by a broad range of individual factors.

Even though sleep, food, and sex are considered examples of basic human needs, the manner in which these needs are met, as well as the extent to which any one of them is considered a need, varies according to each individual. It is therefore extremely important to determine a person's perceptions of his or her own needs to be able to provide appropriate, individualized nursing care. If a patient is uncomfortable eating three large meals, such as those served in most hospitals, nurses can help that person by saving parts of the large meals in the refrigerator on the nursing unit and serving them to the patient between regularly scheduled meals. This is a simple example of what is meant by the term individualized nursing care, which recognizes each individual's unique needs and tailors the plan of nursing care to take that uniqueness into consideration.

Adaptation and human needs

Another aspect of human needs that must be considered is the nature of people to change, grow, and develop. Carl Rogers, a well-known psychologist, built his theory of personhood based on the idea that people are constantly adapting, discovering, and rediscovering themselves. His book *On Becoming a Person* (Rogers, 1961) is considered a classic in psychological literature. Rogers' idea that a person's needs change as the person changes is important for nurses to remember. The human potential to grow and develop can be used by nurses to assist patients to change unhealthy behaviors and to reach the highest level of wellness possible.

The concept of adaptation is also helpful in understanding that people admitted to hospitals and removed from their customary, familiar environments frequently become anxious. Even the most confident person can become fearful when in an uncertain, perhaps threatening, situation. Under these circumstances, nurses have learned to expect people to regress slightly and to become more concerned with basic needs and less focused on the higher needs in Maslow's hierarchy. A "take-charge" professional person, for example, may become somewhat demanding and self-absorbed when hospitalized. As you will see in Chapter 13, several nursing theorists based their theoretical models on adaptation.

Homeostasis

When a person's needs are not met, homeostasis is threatened. Remember that homeostasis is a dynamic balance achieved by effectively functioning open systems. It is a state of equilibrium, a tendency to maintain internal stability. In humans, homeostasis is attained by coordinated responses of organ systems that automatically compensate for environmental changes. When someone goes for a brisk walk, for example, heart rate and respiratory rate automatically increase to keep vital organs supplied with oxygen. When the individual comes home and sits down to read the newspaper, heart rate and breathing slow down. No conscious decision to speed up or slow down these physiologic functions has to be made. Adjustments occur automatically to maintain homeostasis.

Individuals, as open systems, also endeavor to maintain balance between external and internal forces. When that balance is achieved, the person is healthy, or at least is resistant to disease. When environmental factors affect the homeostasis of a person, the person attempts to adapt to the change. If adaptation is unsuccessful, disequilibrium may occur, setting the stage for the development of illness or disease. How individuals respond to stress is a major factor in the development of illness. Stress and illness are discussed more fully in Chapter 10, and you may wish to review that information now.

ENVIRONMENT AND SUPRASYSTEM

The second major concept basic to professional nursing practice is environment, or the suprasystem. Environment includes all the circumstances,

influences, and conditions that surround and affect individuals, families, and groups. The environment can be as small and controlled as a premature infant's isolette or as large and uncontrollable as the universe. Included in environment are the social and cultural attitudes that profoundly shape human experience.

The environment can either promote or interfere with homeostasis and well-being of individuals. As seen in Maslow's hierarchy of needs, there is a dynamic interaction between a person's needs, which are internal, and the satisfaction of those needs, which is often environmentally determined.

Nurses have always been aware of the influence of environment on people, beginning with Florence Nightingale, who understood well the elements of a healthful environment in which restoration and preservation of health and prevention of disease and injury were possible. Concerns about the health of the public have led governmental entities at local, state, and national levels to promulgate standards and regulations that ensure the safety of food, water, air, cosmetics, medications, workplaces, and other areas in which health hazards may occur. Environmental systems to be discussed in this section are family systems, cultural systems, social systems, and community systems.

Family Systems

The most direct environmental influence on a person is the family. The quality and amount of parenting provided to infants and growing children constitute a major determinant of health. We call this the family system. Children who are nurtured when young and vulnerable, who are allowed to grow in independence and self-determination, and who are taught the skills they need for social living have the opportunity to grow into strong, productive, autonomous adults.

Nuclear and extended families

For most of the history of humankind, immediate and extended families were relatively intact units that lived together or lived within close proximity to one another. In the extended family, children were nurtured by a variety of relatives, as well as by their own parents. This closeness was profoundly affected by industrialization, which fostered urbanization. When families ceased farming, which was a family endeavor, and moved to cities where fathers worked in factories, the first dilution of family influence on children began. The nuclear family (mother and father and their children) moved away from former sources of nurturing, as older relatives such as grandparents, aunts, and uncles often stayed in rural areas.

During World War II, more women began to work, taking them out of the home and away from young children for hours each day. The increased geographic mobility of families since World War II has had a destructive effect on the role of extended family in the lives of children, as nuclear families often live half a continent or more away from grandparents and other family members. The intense attention children traditionally received from adult relatives diminished, sometimes to the detriment of the child's well-being.

Single-parent families

There are more single-parent families in the United States than ever before, most of which are headed by women. As of 2007, U.S. Census data revealed that there were more than 11.7 million single-parent families in the United States. Of these there were 9.9 million single women heading households with children under 18 years of age and no father present. In addition to single mothers, there were also 1.7 million single custodial fathers in the United States in 2007 (U.S. Census Bureau, 2007).

Life is challenging for single parents of both sexes who must perform the breadwinner role, as well as nurturing roles, in the family. The combination of bearing multiple roles alone over long periods of time can be extremely stressful, even exhausting, to single parents.

There is increasing evidence that long-term stress affects the mental and physical health of these adults, which, in turn, affects their parenting abilities. A 2000 study by nursing faculty at the University of Kentucky (Peden et al, 2004) found that low-income single mothers with children between the ages of 2 and 6 years have a high prevalence of depressive symptoms, with more than 75% scoring in the mild to high range of depressive symptoms. These symptoms included negative thinking and chronic stressors, potentially affecting the entire family's quality of life. The researchers concluded that the combination of low income and single parenting of small children increases the risk of depression and that negative thinking, instead of chronic stressors, might be more amenable to nursing intervention (Peden et al, 2004).

Although many single parents manage stress well and are able to provide excellent parenting, some children's needs are neglected. The impact of this neglect can be seen in the health, behavior and school performance of children who have not learned the skills they need to be successful. With nearly 40% of all children in the United States being born to unmarried women in 2006 (Martin et al, 2009), the trend to single-parent households is likely to continue.

The examples given here represent only a few of the ways families influence the well-being of individuals. There are many others. Understanding a patient's family and home environment is part of a complete nursing assessment. Modification of the home environment may be needed, particularly when a person is returning home with a physical disability, or where there is neglect or abuse. Nurses, social workers, and others involved in care planning must collaborate to ensure that needed changes occur.

Cultural Systems

Culture is an extremely important environmental influence affecting individuals. Culture consists of the attitudes, beliefs, and behaviors of social and ethnic groups that have been perpetuated through generations. Patterns of language, dress, eating habits, activities of daily living, attitudes toward those outside the culture, health beliefs and values, spiritual beliefs or religious orientation, and attitudes toward children, women, men, marriage, education, work, and recreation all are influenced by culture.

According to U.S. Census Bureau estimates, there were 33.5 million foreign-born Americans in 2003, representing 11.7% of the entire U.S. population (Larsen, 2004). Undoubtedly these figures have risen since the last updated information became available. The United States has become a truly multicultural society. Because basic beliefs about health and illness vary widely from culture to culture, nurses need to develop cultural competence to meet the needs of culturally diverse patients. For example, "A traditional Vietnamese folk remedy, *ventouse* . . ., involves placing a heated cup on the skin. It's believed that as the cup cools, it draws away excess energy or 'wind' causing the illness" (Grossman, 1994, p. 58). This practice can cause bruising, which can be mistaken for a sign of abuse. This is just one indication that cultural beliefs of patients have great relevance to nurses. Most cultural differences are more subtle than this and can escape the notice of nurses who have not developed cultural competence.

Effective nurses learn to be aware of and to respect cultural influences on patients. Whenever possible, they pay attention to patients' cultural preferences. They recognize that some cultural groups attribute illness to bad fortune. Individuals from cultures with these beliefs do not see themselves as active participants in their own health status. This attitude is a challenge for nurses who value the collaboration of patients in their own health care planning.

These are only two examples of the influence of cultural beliefs on the nurse-patient interaction. Wise nurses realize that integration of a patient's cultural health beliefs into the individualized care plan can make a strong impact on that patient's desire and ability to get well.

Understanding the relationship between culture and health is the basis for "transcultural nursing," a field of nursing practice initiated by nurse-anthropologist Madeleine Leininger. Additional discussion of the influence of culture on nursing practice can be found in Chapter 10.

Cultural Considerations Challenge
Working With the "Passive" Patient

Most professional nurses value engaging patients in their own care planning. These nurses encourage participation and independence in their patients. In some cultures, however, patients expect the caregivers to make decisions for them and resist efforts toward self-determination and self-care. In other cultures the head of the family (matriarch or patriarch) is the individual who makes decisions, not the patient himself or herself. How can you modify your usual nursing attitudes and practices to work effectively with patients who, for cultural reasons, resist working toward self-care? What challenges will this present to your own beliefs?

Social Systems

In addition to family and cultural systems, individuals are also influenced by the social system in which they live. Social institutions such as families, neighborhoods, schools, churches, professional associations, civic groups, and recreational groups may constitute a form of social support. Social support also includes such factors as family income; presence in the home of a spouse; proximity to neighbors, children, and other supportive individuals; access to medical care; coping abilities; and educational level.

Social change

Holmes and Rahe (1967) published a study of the relationship of social change to the subsequent development of illness. They found that people with many social changes that disrupt social support, such as death of a loved one, divorce, job changes, moving, or unemployment, were much more likely to experience illness in the following 12 months than people with few social changes. Both positive and negative changes created the need for social readjustment. In 1995 this study was updated, and the Recent Life Changes Questionnaire (Box 12-2) was devised to reflect more accurately contemporary concerns (Miller and Rahe, 1997). Numerous other researchers have

Box 12-2   Recent Life Changes Questionnaire

The following 74 potential life changes inquire about recent events in a person's life. A 6-month total equal to or greater than 300 Life Change Units (LCU), or a 1-year total equal to or greater than 500 LCU, is considered indicative of high recent life stress.

LIFE CHANGE EVENT	LIFE CHANGE UNITS
Health	
An injury or illness that:	
Kept you in bed 1 week or more or sent you to the hospital	74
Was less serious than above	44
Major dental work	26
Major change in eating habits	27
Major change in sleeping habits	26
Major change in your usual type and/or amount of recreation	28
Work	
Change to a new type of work	51
Change in your work hours or conditions	35
Change in your responsibilities at work	
More responsibilities	29
Fewer responsibilities	21
Promotion	31
Demotion	42
Transfer	32
Troubles at work	
With your boss	29
With co-workers	35
With persons under your supervision	35
Other work troubles	28
Major business adjustment	60
Retirement	52
Loss of job	
Laid off from work	68
Fired from work	79
Correspondence course to help you in your work	18
Home and Family	
Major change in living conditions	42
Change in residence	
Move within the same town or city	25
Move to a different town, city, or state	47
Change in family get-togethers	25
Major change in health or behavior of family member	55
Marriage	50
Pregnancy	67
Miscarriage or abortion	65
Gain of a new family member	
Birth of a child	66
Adoption of a child	65
A relative moving in with you	59

Box 12-2   Recent Life Changes Questionnaire—cont'd

LIFE CHANGE EVENT	LIFE CHANGE UNITS
Spouse beginning or ending work	46
Child leaving home	
To attend college	41
Because of marriage	41
For other reason	45
Change in arguments with spouse	50
In-law problems	38
Change in the marital status of your parents	
Divorce	59
Remarriage	50
Separation from spouse	
Because of work	53
Because of marital problems	76
Divorce	96
Birth of grandchild	43
Death of spouse	119
Death of a family member	
Child	123
Brother or sister	102
Parent	100
Personal and Social	
Change in personal habits	26
Beginning or ending school or college	38
Change of school or college	35
Change in political beliefs	24
Change in religious beliefs	29
Change in social activities	27
Vacation	24
New, close, personal relationship	37
Engagement to marry	45
Girlfriend or boyfriend problems	39
Sexual difficulties	44
"Falling out" of a close personal relationship	47
An accident	48
Minor violation of the law	20
Being held in jail	75
Death of a close friend	70
Major decision regarding your immediate future	51
Major personal achievement	36
Financial	
Major change in finances	
Increased income	38
Decreased income	60
Investment and/or credit difficulties	56

Continued

Box 12-2   Recent Life Changes Questionnaire—cont'd

LIFE CHANGE EVENT	LIFE CHANGE UNITS
Loss or damage of personal property	43
Moderate purchase	20
Major purchase	37
Foreclosure on a mortgage or loan	58

From Miller MA, Rahe RH: Life changes scaling for the 1990s, *J Psychosom Res* 43(3):279-292, 1997. Reprinted with permission.

found additional evidence that social support has a direct relationship to health.

Social support

Individuals vary in their need and desire for social support. When assessing patients, nurses need to remember that adequacy of social support should be determined by the patient, not by the nurse. When it is determined that strengthening social support is desirable, nurses can provide information, give positive affirmation, use empathy, be present for patients, serve as advocates, and provide validation and encouragement (Finfgeld-Connett, 2005). They can also encourage patients to use interest groups, parenting classes, marriage enrichment groups, religious groups, formal and informal educational groups, and self-help groups to develop stronger support from the social environment.

Increasingly, people receive support online—in chat rooms and through other computer-based forums. People with new insulin pumps, for example, can "talk" online with hundreds of others who have similar pumps, ask questions, and get helpful tips to assist them. There are literally dozens of online support groups, ranging from those for Alzheimer's caregivers to weight loss groups, and these can be a useful source of social support.

Poverty

Because it is the world's wealthiest country, one would expect poverty in the United States to be low. Sadly, this is not the case. The U.S. Census Bureau reported in 2008 that more than 37 million Americans were living at or below the poverty level (U.S. Census Bureau, 2008). The U.S. Department of Health and Human Services determines the poverty level annually. In 2008 "poverty level"

was considered a total income of $10,400 or less for a single person, $21,200 or less for a family of four, and $35,600 or less for a family of eight (U.S. Department of Health and Human Services, 2008).

People living in poverty have diminished access to health care for a variety of reasons. In 2007 more than 18 percent of all children under the age of 18 years were living below the poverty level (U.S. Census Bureau, 2008). The numbers are even more worrisome for different ethnic groups; for example, 34.1% of single-parent African-American families and 29.7% of Hispanic families were living below the poverty level. Lack of money often means adequate nutrition and health care are not attainable, adversely affecting the health status of all family members. Indeed, the World Health Organization (WHO) now considers poverty to be the most influential determinant of health.

A 2004 study by the U.S. Department of Health and Human Services highlighted some of the hardships experienced by poor and near-poor families. Factors such as food insecurity or hunger, inability to pay mortgage or rent, and disconnection of telephone, gas, and electricity for nonpayment featured prominently in the findings about these families (Center on Budget and Policy Priorities, 2004).

Nurses often do not understand or appreciate the complex societal forces that contribute to poverty and may even blame the poor for their situation. Misconceptions can lead to stereotyping and insensitivity to the feelings and concerns of the poor. This discourages them even further from seeking health care they need.

A study conducted by Canadian nursing professors (Reutter et al, 2004) revealed that only 13% of the 740 basic baccalaureate students surveyed had ever lived in a poor neighborhood and only 7% had ever received public assistance. One third of these students reported receiving most of their information about poverty from the news media. They felt they had limited exposure to poverty. The researchers recommended that colleges of nursing increase coursework related to poverty, provide opportunities for students to work with people living in poverty, and facilitate student involvement with groups and organizations that advocate for public policy and societal solutions to poverty (Reutter et al, 2004).

Community, National, and World Systems

The health status of people is also influenced by the larger systems in which they live. The types and availability of jobs, housing, schools, and health care, as well as the overall economic well-being, profoundly affect the citizens in a community. Although nurses may not think they have an obvious role, they can be instrumental in improving the community systems. Identifying health needs and bringing these to the attention of community planners, offering screening programs, serving on health-related committees and advisory boards, and lobbying political leaders can bring about positive change in a community. Nurses have also become politically active by running for elected offices at local, state, and national levels. They can energetically support political candidates who have sound environmental platforms. More information about political activism in nursing is provided in Chapter 15.

On a broader perspective, environment also includes the nation, the world, and the universe. A seemingly isolated incident such as an earthquake in China or an outbreak of cholera in Zimbabwe can have worldwide health repercussions. Nurses can contribute to a healthier world environment by supporting, promoting, and, when possible, participating in humanitarian responses to international disasters.

Nurses' potential impact on the environment/ suprasystem

Individual nurses, in the interest of ecological health, can choose to engage in a variety of environmentally sound practices in their personal lives and encourage others to do the same. These include turning off unused lights and computers, recycling household trash and hazardous materials such as batteries and paint, using pump rather than aerosol sprayers, avoiding insecticides and unnecessary use of gardening chemicals, staying abreast of product and toy recalls, buying energy-efficient appliances and automobiles, carpooling, walking or biking when possible instead of driving everywhere, and refusing to buy from or invest in companies that engage in environmentally unsound practices such as polluting air and water or cutting down rain forests.

As professionals, nurses can also contribute toward a healthier environment. Did you know that health care facilities are among the largest producers of waste in the nation? Even as nurses work to promote health, that very work creates all types of pollution, including biohazardous waste, which ultimately adversely affects health (Lauer, 2009). A decade ago, hospitals were a major source of mercury pollution. This highly toxic substance, once used in thermometers, blood pressure measuring devices, and other medical devices, ultimately flowed into the environment, where it contaminated water. Through the oceans' food chain, mercury in contaminated water becomes concentrated in the bodies of predator fish such as tuna and swordfish, which are eventually consumed by humans. Even in small doses, mercury poses serious health risks to pregnant women and young children. Nurses were instrumental in encouraging their employers to avoid purchasing and using mercury-containing devices and to dispose of them properly when they are discarded. Health Care Without Harm is an international coalition of 473 organizations in more than 50 countries, working to transform the health care sector so it is no longer a source of harm to people and the environment. Health Care Without Harm worked for more than a decade to reduce hazardous waste, specifically mercury, emanating from health care facilities. This organization encourages nurses to become "environmental health activists." You can learn more about Health Care Without Harm at its website: http://www.noharm.org. In other efforts to reduce environmental pollution, some health care facilities have established committees, sometimes called "green teams," dedicated to identifying and recommending environmentally sound products and procedures. Nurses can volunteer to serve on these committees or to start one. They can recommend recycling, the purchase of polyvinyl chloride (PVC)–free products, fewer disposable products, and fewer products with wasteful packaging. They can educate themselves about reducing carbon emissions and advocate for sustainable policies in their workplaces. You can join the movement of nurses to prevent environmental disease. Refer to the website http://www.luminaryproject.org to learn how others are addressing these important issues and how you can help.

HEALTH

Health is the third major concept fundamental to the practice of professional nursing. Health is best viewed as a continuum rather than as an absolute state. Each individual's health status varies from day to day, depending on a variety of factors, such as rest, nutrition, and stressors. Illness is also not an absolute state. People can have chronic illnesses such as diabetes or seizure disorders and still work, take part in recreational activities, and maintain acceptably healthy, meaningful lives. Figure 12-3 depicts the health-illness continuum.

Defining Health

Health "is as hard to define as love or happiness, and even harder to trap and keep" (Zuger, 2008). Yet many individuals and organizations have made attempts to define health. WHO defined

health as "a state of complete physical, mental, and social well-being and not merely the absence of disease or infirmity" (WHO, 1947, p. 29). This definition was the first official recognition of health as multidimensional. The WHO definition presented a holistic view of health that reflected the interplay between the psychological, social, spiritual, and physical aspects of human life.

A holistic view of health focuses on the interrelationship of all the parts that make up a whole person. Jan Christian Smuts (1926) first introduced the concept of holism in modern Western thought by emphasizing the harmony between people and nature. When viewing health holistically, individual health practices must be taken into account. Health practices are culturally determined and include nutritional habits, type and amount of exercise and rest, how one copes with stress, quality of interpersonal relationships, expression of spirituality, and numerous other lifestyle factors. As a profession, nurses value a holistic view of health.

Parsons (1959) defined health as "the state of optimum capacity of an individual for the effective performance of his roles and tasks." This definition focused on the roles individuals assume in life and the impact health or illness has on the fulfillment of those roles. A few examples of roles that are familiar may include the student role, the parent role, the breadwinner role, and the friend role. Given the activities inherent in each of these roles, it is easily seen that the state of health profoundly influences how people carry out their roles in life.

Yet another description of health is the opposite of illness (Dunn, 1959). In his classic text *High-Level Wellness*, Dunn (1961) described health as

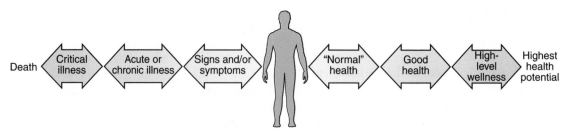

Figure 12-3 The health-illness continuum—a holistic health model.

a continuum with high-level wellness at one end and death at the other. He described high-level wellness as functioning at maximum potential in an integrated way within the environment. A prisoner of war kept in solitary confinement and given a diet of rice for many months certainly would have difficulty maintaining health. If the prisoner keeps active, both physically and mentally, and retains a positive outlook, however, he is likely to be healthier than the prisoner who does none of these things. Using Dunn's definition and taking his environment into consideration, the prisoner may even be said to have attained high-level wellness.

Pender et al (2006) described health promotion as "approach behavior," whereas prevention is "avoidance behavior" (p. 5). This may be a useful concept for nurses to keep in mind when seeking to help patients expand their positive potential for health.

A National Health Initiative: Healthy People 2000 and 2010

A remarkable national initiative to improve the health of the nation is now in its third decade. The Healthy People initiative was an unprecedented cooperative effort that grew out of the 1979 surgeon general's report on health promotion and disease prevention titled *Healthy People*. That report laid the foundation for a national prevention agenda. Federal, state, and territorial governments, as well as hundreds of private, public, and nonprofit organizations and concerned individuals, worked together for the first time ever. These partnerships resulted in Healthy People 2000, an effort designed to stimulate a national disease prevention and health promotion agenda to improve significantly the health of all Americans in the last decade of the twentieth century. On September 6, 1990, former U.S. Secretary of Health and Human Services Louis W. Sullivan released a report to the United States titled *Healthy People 2000*. He reported that progress on priority areas was mixed, but enough success was achieved to continue the project.

The second phase of the project, called Healthy People 2010, was launched in January 2000. It was developed by the Healthy People Consortium, an alliance of more than 350 national membership organizations and 250 state health, mental health, substance abuse, and environmental agencies. In addition, more than 11,000 public comments on the draft document were provided through an interactive website. Healthy People 2010 consists of a revised set of health objectives for the nation, with two overarching goals: to increase quality and years of healthy life and to eliminate health disparities. Under these two goals are 28 focus areas that provide more specific targets. To measure the health of the nation during the decade, 10 leading health indicators will be used. Each leading health indicator reflects an important health issue and has one or more of the 28 objectives linked with it. These indicators reflect the high-priority public health concerns in this country at the beginning of the twenty-first century. Box 12-3 contains the essential elements of Healthy People 2010, which is currently under revision.

Healthy People 2010 offers a simple but powerful idea: provide health objectives in a format that enables diverse groups to combine their efforts and work as a team. It is a road map to better health for all and can be used by many different people, states, communities, professional organizations, and groups to improve health. The initiative has partners from all sectors (U.S. Department of Health and Human Services, 2003).

Partners are encouraged to integrate Healthy People objectives into their programs, special events, publications, and meetings. An example is provided by the Division of Public Health Nursing of the Los Angeles County Health Department, which has shifted its focus from providing care for individuals within families to improving the health of entire communities. Nurses in this department integrated the 10 leading health indicators of Healthy People 2010 into their public health nursing practice model. This means that these nurses consider the leading health indicators as they assess and diagnose communities with which they work. This ensures consistency within the division and with national priorities (Smith and Bazini-Barakat, 2003)—a perfect

Box 12-3   Healthy People 2010 at a Glance

Healthy People 2010 is a comprehensive set of disease prevention and health promotion objectives for the nation to achieve over the first decade of the new century. Created by scientists both inside and outside of government, it identifies a wide range of public health priorities and specific, measurable objectives.

OVERARCHING GOALS
1. Increase quality and years of healthy life
2. Eliminate health disparities

FOCUS AREAS
- Access to quality health services
- Arthritis, osteoporosis, and chronic back conditions
- Cancer
- Chronic kidney disease
- Diabetes
- Disability and secondary conditions
- Educational and community-based programs
- Environmental health
- Family planning
- Food safety
- Health communication
- Heart disease and stroke

- HIV
- Immunization and infectious diseases
- Injury and violence prevention
- Maternal, infant, and child health
- Medical product safety
- Mental health and mental disorders
- Nutrition and overweight
- Occupational safety and health
- Oral health
- Physical activity and fitness
- Public health infrastructure
- Respiratory diseases
- Sexually transmitted diseases
- Substance abuse
- Tobacco use
- Vision and hearing
- Physical activity
- Overweight and obesity
- Tobacco use
- Substance abuse
- Responsible sexual behavior
- Mental health
- Injury and violence
- Environmental quality
- Immunization
- Access to health care

From U.S. Department of Health and Human Services: *Healthy People 2010: fact sheet,* 2006 (website): http://www.healthypeople.gov/About/hpfact.htm.

example of how the Healthy People initiative can be implemented at the local level.

When federal, state, and local health entities combine their efforts, improvements in the health of citizens can be made. Convincing individual Americans to change their lifestyles, however, even when to do so would result in improved health, remains a challenge. As can be seen from this review of the Healthy People project over nearly 30 years, changing health beliefs and health behaviors is a slow process. You can learn more about Healthy People 2020 and check progress toward its revision, Healthy people 2020, online (http://www.healthypeople.gov/hp2020).

Health Beliefs and Health Behaviors

Health is affected by health beliefs and health behaviors. **Health behaviors** include those choices and habitual actions that promote or diminish health, such as eating habits, frequency of exercise, use of tobacco products and alcohol, sexual practices, and adequacy of rest and sleep (Figure 12-4). Much is known about health-promoting behaviors, and this information has been available to the public for many years. Yet people do not readily change their behaviors even when they know they should. We will examine several theories about why people change their health behaviors—or why they do not.

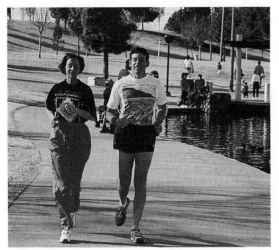

Figure 12-4 More Americans are engaging in healthy behaviors such as regular exercise, yet obesity is still on the rise.

Health beliefs model

Rosenstock (1966, 1990) was one of the first scholars interested in determining why some people change their health behaviors whereas others do not. For example, when the surgeon general's report on smoking first came out in 1960, some people immediately quit smoking. Over the years, evidence condemning smoking has accumulated and been widely communicated, yet many intelligent people still smoke. Rosenstock wondered why. He formulated a model of health beliefs that illustrates how people behave in relationship to health maintenance activities and has worked to refine it for three decades. Rosenstock's **health beliefs model** included three components:

1. An evaluation of one's vulnerability to a condition and the seriousness of that condition
2. An evaluation of how effective the health maintenance behavior might be
3. The presence of a trigger event that precipitates the health maintenance behavior

Using Rosenstock's health beliefs model, a smoker chooses to participate in a stop-smoking program depending on his perception of smoking-related heart disease and his personal susceptibility to it. If, because of family history, he believes that he is susceptible to heart disease and that it may cause his death prematurely and if he believes that not smoking will substantially reduce his risk, he is likely to participate in the program. If, however, the stop-smoking program is at an inconvenient location, scheduled at an inconvenient time, or not affordable, he is less likely to participate. If his sibling, who also smokes, has a massive heart attack, he may be motivated to attend the stop-smoking program despite the inconvenience and cost. The illness of his sibling is what Rosenstock termed "a cue to action," or a trigger event. A trigger event propels a previously unmotivated individual into changing health behaviors.

Self-efficacy and health-related behaviors

Albert Bandura (1997), a cognitive psychologist, developed an approach designed to assist people to exercise influence over their own health-related behaviors. He observed that whether or not people considered altering detrimental health habits depended on their belief in themselves as having the ability to modify their own behavior. He called this belief in their own abilities perceived **self-efficacy**. High belief in one's self-efficacy leads to efforts to change, whereas low perceived self-efficacy leads to a fatalistic lack of change.

Bandura identified four components needed for an effective program of lifestyle change: information, skill development, skill enhancement through guided practice and feedback, and creating social supports for change (Bandura, 1992). Using Bandura's model, a man wishing to stop smoking needs knowledge of the potential dangers of smoking; guidance on how to translate concern into action; extensive practice and opportunities to perfect new, nonsmoking skills; and strong involvement in a social network supportive of nonsmoking.

Locus of control and health-related behaviors

The **locus of control** concept proposed that people tend to be influenced by either an internal or external view of control. People who believe that their health is internally controlled, that is, by what they themselves do, are said to have an internal locus of control. Those who believe their health is determined by outside factors or chance are said to have an external locus of control. A number of studies have hypothesized that internally controlled people tend to see themselves as responsible for their own health status and are therefore more amenable to change. Research findings have been inconsistent, however. Although health locus of control is a concept of general relevance to health, it requires continued attention in research aimed at better understanding behavior and health (Steptoe and Wardle, 2001).

Nurses and health beliefs models

There are numerous other models of health beliefs and health behavior ranging from simple to complex. Many are being tested through empirical studies in attempts to identify the key to motivating people to improve their health choices and behaviors. No single theory of behavior has yet fully explained the complex state called health. It is important for nurses to recognize the following:

- Health is relative, ever changing, and affected by genetics, environment, personal beliefs, and cultural beliefs.
- Health affects the entire person—physically, socially, psychologically, and spiritually.
- Individuals' health beliefs are powerful and influence how they respond to efforts to change their health behaviors.
- Individuals needing or desiring change may lack knowledge, motivation, sense of self-efficacy, and support.
- Unhealthy behaviors may persist in spite of increased knowledge.
- Various models of health beliefs can be used to assess individual, family, and group readiness to change.
- Health professionals must realize that multiple interventions are necessary to bring about change and only modest changes in behavior can be expected (Dunbar-Jacob, 2007).
- The burden of action is mutually shared by patient, health care providers, and population-focused entities such as public health programs.

Influence of the Internet on Health

With more than three quarters of adult Americans having online access, the Internet has an impact on every aspect of life. People shop; make travel and restaurant reservations; check out and download the latest music, movies, plays, and books; and meet potential spouses online. Is it any wonder, then, that they also seek information about health online? The Internet, with its ready availability of information, ranging from the latest clinical trials and research studies to the most popular herbal remedies and diet fads, has changed the way we learn about health.

With the proliferation of health information sites, estimated at more than 2200 in 2008 (Tanaka, 2008), Americans are now armed with more information than has ever before been available to consumers. Patients are demanding to be equal partners in making health care decisions once decided only by the professionals they consulted. Health care practitioners encounter numerous patients each day who enter examining rooms with printouts of the latest research and advice, culled from the mountains of data available.

Support groups are available by the score. There is no need to dress, drive across town, or even leave the comforts of home to be in touch with dozens of people who share similar concerns or health problems. Cyberspace support groups have another advantage not shared by face-to-face groups: anonymity.

Some people are concerned about the validity of information available on the Internet (Chase, 1999). In fact, there is a lot of misinformation transmitted along with well-founded information from respected sources. The difficulty for the average citizen is telling the difference. Box 12-4 contains some helpful hints to improve the likelihood of obtaining valid health information from online sources. In addition to concerns about the validity of Internet information, a new type of hypochondria has emerged. Termed "cyberchondria," it refers to the tendency of some web users to jump to the worst possible conclusion after consulting websites, for example, thinking a lingering cough after a cold is due to a terminal disease (Markoff, 2008).

Increased reliance on the Internet for health information is expected to continue. This is

Box 12-4   Assessing Health-Related Sites on the Internet

- Determine who sponsors the site. This should be disclosed on the site itself.
- Be skeptical. Evaluate the source to determine whether there is self-interest on the part of the sponsor. For example, a drug company promoting one of its products.
- Make sure the author's name is clearly indicated, including credentials. Is the author qualified on this topic? Whom does the author work for?
- What is the purpose of the site—to inform or to sell something?
- Is the material dated and revised frequently to ensure it is current?
- Is there editorial review of the content by a reputable authority or professional peers?
- Does the material consist of scientific information rather than testimonials?
- Determine who runs the website. University, government, and reputable medical organization sites may prove objective and less commercial than those run by companies or individuals wishing to profit.
- Is the information unbiased, and are you referred to other sources that can validate it?

- For chat rooms, go online and "lurk" before getting involved. Monitor conversations or read postings before deciding whether you want to participate.
- Find out whether the group has a moderator who can control monopolizers, commercial pitches, and inappropriate behavior by other participants.
- For interactive sites, be sure to read and understand the privacy policy.
- Until you are confident about the quality of information, cross-check it with print and electronic sources and discuss it with your health care provider.
- Use the U.S. Department of Health and Human Services' Healthfinder site to find online support groups (http://www.healthfinder.gov).
- Be highly suspicious of reports of "miracle" cures. Rumors and unsupported claims are rampant on the Internet and cause untold harm. Use Quackwatch to check out claims that sound too good to be true (http://www.quackwatch.com).

From Chase M: Health journal: a guide for patients who turn to the Web for solace and support, *Wall Street Journal,* Sept 17, 1999, p B1; Beyea SC: Evaluating evidence found on the Internet, *AORN J* 72(5):906-910, 2000; and Ahmann E: Supporting families' savvy use of the Internet for health research, *Pediatr Nurs* 26(4):419-423, 2000.

understandable, since the Internet is readily available, day or night, whereas getting an appointment with a primary care provider can take days or weeks. Nurses have an obligation to adapt to this new influence on health by helping their patients obtain sound advice from online sources. Sharing legitimate websites and guidelines for assessing the quality of information is a way to help patients become better consumers of online health data. This means that nurses themselves must be knowledgeable and stay up-to-date on both helpful and unhelpful websites. Nurses also should be nondefensive when patients question traditional advice, citing the Internet as their source. Use these exchanges as opportunities to correct misinformation, if needed.

Perhaps you will learn something new yourself. Visit Evolve for WebLinks related to the content of this chapter: http://evolve.elsevier.com/Chitty/professional/.

Devising a Personal Plan for High-Level Wellness

Each individual nurse has a personal definition of health, certain health beliefs, and individual health behaviors. How nurses view health behaviors in their own lives affects nursing practice, both directly and indirectly. The personal health practices of nurses play a direct role in their effectiveness in counseling patients on health-related matters. Patients are more likely to adopt health-related behaviors such as not smoking and

---

Box 12-5   Self-Assessment: Developing a Personal Plan for High-Level Wellness

Nurses' personal health behaviors send a powerful message to consumers of nursing care. Are you in a position to demonstrate that you practice what you preach? By answering the following questions, you can assess how well you are meeting your responsibilities in this area of nursing.

1. I weigh no more than 10 pounds over or under my ideal weight.
   T   F

2. I eat a balanced diet, including breakfast, each day.
   T   F

3. Of the total calories in my diet, less than 30 percent come from fat.
   T   F

4. I exercise aerobically at least three times each week.
   T   F

5. I get at least 7 hours of sleep each night.
   T   F

6. I do not smoke or use any other form of tobacco.
   T   F

7. I use alcohol in moderation (or not at all) and take mood-altering medication only when prescribed by my physician.
   T   F

8. I identify and control the sources of stress in my life.
   T   F

9. I have a balanced lifestyle, with work and diversional activities both playing important roles.
   T   F

10. I have friends, neighbors, and/or family members who are sources of social support for me.
    T   F

11. I practice responsible sex.
    T   F

Directions for scoring: If you could not honestly answer "True" to all 11 questions, you need to set goals to enable you to do so.

1. On a piece of paper, begin your personal plan for high-level wellness. Write down at least two things you can do to address each "False" answer you gave to the self-assessment questions.

2. Share your health goals with one other person in your class. Make a contract with that person to serve as your "health coach."

3. Review your progress with your health coach at least once a week for the remainder of the term.

4. Begin your quest for high-level wellness today!

---

maintaining a healthy weight when the caregiver promoting these behaviors also engages in them. Yet nurses' own health behaviors are far from exemplary. Studies have shown that in spite of nurses' knowledge, no difference exists between the health behaviors of nurses and those of the general population (Pratt, Overfield, and Gill-Hilton, 1994).

Nurses have a professional responsibility to model positive health behaviors in their own lives, but nurses are individuals too. Being or becoming a healthy role model may require some effort. If you are not the positive role model for health you would like to be, Box 12-5 can help you get started.

PUTTING IT ALL TOGETHER: NURSING

Nursing integrates concepts from person, environment, and health to form a meaningful whole. Figure 12-5 depicts the relationships among nursing's major concepts and illustrates how they overlap to create nursing's sphere of interest and influence. This is termed the holistic approach to nursing.

Holistic Nursing

Holistic nursing care nourishes the whole person, that is, the body, mind, and spirit. Not surprisingly, the root word for nurse and nurture are the same Latin word, *nutrire*, which means

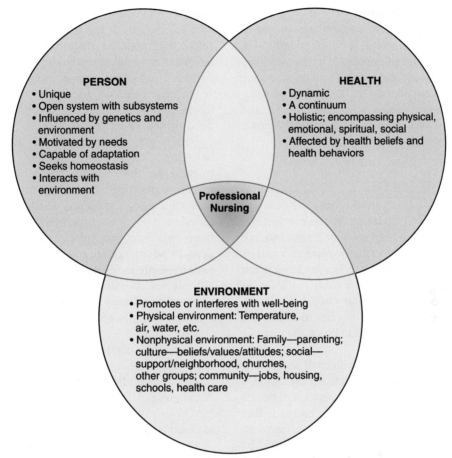

PERSON
- Unique
- Open system with subsystems
- Influenced by genetics and environment
- Motivated by needs
- Capable of adaptation
- Seeks homeostasis
- Interacts with environment

HEALTH
- Dynamic
- A continuum
- Holistic; encompassing physical, emotional, spiritual, social
- Affected by health beliefs and health behaviors

Professional Nursing

ENVIRONMENT
- Promotes or interferes with well-being
- Physical environment: Temperature, air, water, etc.
- Nonphysical environment: Family—parenting; culture—beliefs/values/attitudes; social—support/neighborhood, churches, other groups; community—jobs, housing, schools, health care

Figure 12-5 Concepts and subconcepts basic to professional nursing.

"to nourish." Let us look now at eight factors that contribute to a holistic approach to nursing.

1. Nursing is an example of an open system that freely interacts with, influences, and is influenced by external and internal forces.
2. Nursing is the provision of health care services that focus on assisting people in maintaining health, avoiding or minimizing disease and disability, restoring wellness, or achieving a peaceful death.
3. Nursing involves collaborating with patients and their families to help them cope and adapt to situations of disequilibrium in an effort to regain homeostasis.
4. Nursing is integrally involved with people at points along the health-illness continuum.
5. Nursing care is provided regardless of diagnosis, individual differences, age, beliefs, gender, sexual preference, or other factors. As a profession, nursing supports the value, dignity, and uniqueness of every person and takes their culture and belief system into consideration.
6. Nurses require advanced knowledge and skills; they also must care about their patients.
7. Nursing requires concern, compassion, respect, and warmth, as well as comprehensive, individualized planning of care, to facilitate patients' growth toward wellness.
8. Nursing links theory and research in an effort to answer difficult questions generated during nursing practice.

With an understanding of nursing's major concepts as a backdrop, we will now begin to examine the relationship of nurses' attitudes, beliefs, values, and philosophies to the way they practice; review philosophies of nursing that were developed by an individual, a division of nursing in a hospital, and a school of nursing; and assist readers in beginning to develop their own philosophies of nursing.

BELIEFS

Certain beliefs have evolved during the development of professional nursing. Specific statements of beliefs have been published for more than half a century. The most recent code was generated by the members of the American Nurses Association (ANA) and published in the *Code of Ethics for Nurses With Interpretive Statements* (ANA, 2001). Statements such as the *Code* exist to affirm the beliefs of the profession and to guide the practice of nursing.

A belief represents the intellectual acceptance of something as true or correct. Beliefs can also be described as convictions. Groupings of beliefs form codes and creeds. Beliefs are opinions that may be, in reality, true or false. They are based on attitudes that have been acquired and verified by experience. Beliefs are generally transmitted from generation to generation, are stable, and are resistant to change.

Beliefs are organized into belief systems that serve as road maps for thinking and decision making (Grube, Mayton, and Ball-Rokeach, 1994). Individuals are not necessarily aware of how their beliefs interrelate or how their beliefs affect their behavior.

Although all people have beliefs, relatively few have spent much time examining their beliefs. In nursing, it is important to know and understand one's beliefs because the practice of nursing frequently challenges a nurse's beliefs. Although this conflict may create temporary discomfort, it is ultimately good because it forces nurses to consider their beliefs carefully. They have to answer the question: "Is this something I really believe, or have I accepted it because some influential person

[such as a parent or teacher] said it?" Abortion, advance directives, the right to die, the right to refuse treatment, alternative lifestyles, and similar issues confront all members of contemporary society. Professional nurses must develop and refine their beliefs about these and many other issues. This is often difficult to do, but it pays dividends in self-awareness.

Beliefs are exhibited through attitudes and behaviors. Simply observing how nurses relate to patients, their families, and nursing peers reveals something about those nurses' beliefs. Every day nurses meet people whose beliefs are different from, or even diametrically opposed to, their own. Effective nurses recognize that they need to adopt nonjudgmental attitudes toward patients' beliefs. A nurse with a nonjudgmental attitude makes every effort to convey neither approval nor disapproval of patients' beliefs and respects each person's right to his or her beliefs (Figure 12-6).

An example of differences in beliefs that directly affect nursing is the position taken by some religious groups that all healing should be left to a divine power. For members of such groups, seeking medical treatment, even lifesaving measures such as blood transfusions, insulin for diabetes, or chemotherapy for cancer, is not condoned. From time

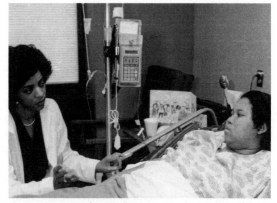

Figure 12-6 Professional nurses make every effort to maintain a nonjudgmental attitude toward patients. A nonjudgmental attitude is one of nursing's values. (Courtesy Emory University, Nell Hodgson Woodruff School of Nursing.)

to time, there have been news reports of parents who are charged with criminal acts because they did not take a sick child to a physician. According to the advocacy group Children's Healthcare Is a Legal Duty, about 300 children have died in this country over the past 25 years after parents withheld medical care on the basis of religious beliefs (Johnson, 2009). Typical of such incidents was a 2002 case reported in Georgia when the parents of a 19-year-old severely injured in an automobile accident refused to give permission for their unconscious Jehovah's Witness son to continue receiving blood transfusions. Speaking for their son, the parents asserted that he would rather die than receive a blood transfusion. Although a judge subsequently ordered the blood transfusion, it came too late, and he died less than 24 hours after the court order was issued (Eustis, 2002). More recently, an 11-year-old girl died of untreated diabetic ketoacidosis in Wisconsin (Sataline, 2008). Her parents were charged with reckless endangerment despite their claim that the charges violated their constitutional right to religious freedom. Both parents were convicted of second-degree reckless homicide and were sentenced to 30 days in jail each for the next 6 years in October 2009 (Fitzsimmons, 2009). Cases such as this have an impact on patients, families, the health care professionals involved, and the court system and often create a frenzy of media coverage.

Because you are in a health profession, you clearly have beliefs about the value of modern medicine. Think about how your health care beliefs differ from those of the families just described. What feelings might you have if assigned to work with a family with these beliefs? From this brief consideration, you may be able to appreciate how difficult it can be to maintain a nonjudgmental attitude toward the beliefs of patients. Nevertheless, it is essential.

Three Categories of Beliefs

People often use the terms *beliefs* and *values* interchangeably. Even experts disagree about whether they differ or are the same. Although they are related, beliefs and values are differentiated in this chapter and discussed separately.

Theorists studying belief systems have identified three main categories of beliefs:

1. Descriptive or existential beliefs are those that can be shown to be true or false. An example of a descriptive belief is "The sun will come up tomorrow morning."
2. Evaluative beliefs are those in which there is a judgment about good or bad. The belief "Gambling is immoral" is an example of an evaluative belief.
3. Prescriptive (encouraged) and proscriptive (prohibited) beliefs are those in which certain actions are judged to be desirable or undesirable. The belief "Every citizen of voting age should vote in every election" is a prescriptive belief, whereas the belief "People should not engage in sexual intercourse outside of marriage" is a proscriptive belief. Prescriptive and proscriptive beliefs are closely related to values (Rokeach, 1973, pp. 6, 7).

VALUES

Values are the freely chosen principles, ideals, or standards held by an individual, class, or group that give meaning and direction to life. A value is an abstract representation of what is right, worthwhile, or desirable. Values define ideal modes of conduct and reflect what the individual or group endorses and tries to emulate. Values, like beliefs, are relatively stable and resistant to change.

Although many people are unaware of it, values help them make small, day-to-day choices, as well as important life decisions. Just as beliefs influence nursing practice, values also influence how nurses practice their profession, often without their conscious awareness. Diann B. Uustal (1985), a contemporary nurse who has written and spoken extensively about values, said, "Everything we do, every decision we make and course of action we take is based on our consciously and unconsciously chosen beliefs, attitudes and values" (Uustal, 1985, p. 100). Uustal also asserts, "Nursing is a behavioral manifestation of the nurse's value system. It is not merely a career, a job, an assignment; it is a ministry" (Uustal, 1993, p. 10). She believes that nurses must give "caring attentiveness and presence" to their patients and to do otherwise "is equivalent to psychological and spiritual abandonment" (Uustal, 1993, p. 10). Do you agree or disagree with these statements?

Nature of Human Values

Values evolve as people mature. An individual's values today are undoubtedly different from those of 10, or even 5, years ago. Rokeach (1973, p. 3) made several assertions about the nature of human values:

1. Each person has a relatively small number of values.
2. All human beings, regardless of location or culture, possess basically the same values to differing degrees.
3. People organize their values into value systems.
4. People develop values in response to culture, society, and even individual personality traits.
5. Most observable human behaviors are manifestations or consequences of human values.

Authorities agree that values influence behavior and that people with unclear values lack direction, persistence, and decision-making skills (Raths, Harmin, and Simon, 1978). Because much of nursing involves having a clear sense of direction, the ability to persevere, and the ability to make sound decisions quickly and frequently, effective nurses must have a strong set of professional nursing values. A number of professional nursing values are listed in Box 12-6.

Process of Valuing

Valuing is the process by which values are determined. There are three identified steps in the process of valuing: choosing, prizing, and acting.

1. Choosing is the cognitive (intellectual) aspect of valuing. Ideally, people choose their values freely from all alternatives after considering the possible consequences of their choices.
2. Prizing is the affective (emotional) aspect of valuing. People usually feel good about their values and cherish the choices they make.
3. Acting is the kinesthetic (behavioral) aspect of valuing. When people affirm their values

publicly by acting on their choices, they make their values part of their behavior. A real value is acted on consistently in behavior.

All three steps must be taken, or the process of valuing is incomplete (Uustal, 1998). For example, a professional nurse might believe that learning is a lifelong process and that nurses have an obligation to keep up with new developments in the profession. This nurse would choose continued learning and appreciate the consequences of the choice. He or she might even publicly affirm this choice and feel good about it. If the nurse follows through consistently with behaviors such as reading journals, attending conferences, and seeking out other learning opportunities, continued learning can be seen as a true value in his or her life.

Values Clarification

Nurses, as well as people in other helping professions, need to understand their values. This is the first step in self-awareness, which is important in maintaining a nonjudgmental approach to patients.

Considering your reactions to the following statements can help in beginning to identify some nursing values you hold:

1. Patients should always be told the truth about their diagnoses.
2. Nurses, if asked, should assist terminally ill patients to die.
3. Severely impaired infants should be kept alive, regardless of their future quality of life.
4. Nurses should never accept gifts from patients.
5. A college professor should receive a heart transplant before a homeless person does.
6. Nurses should be role models of healthy behavior.

As you react both emotionally and intellectually to these statements, something about your personal and professional values is revealed. Determining where you stand on these and other nursing issues is an important step in clarifying your values. A variety of values clarification exercises have been developed to stimulate self-reflection and help people understand their values. Box 12-7 contains a values clarification exercise you may want to complete to assist you further in understanding the valuing process.

Box 12-6   Professional Nursing Values

• Accountability and responsibility for own actions	• Knowledge
• Altruism	• Listening attentively
• Balancing cure and care	• Nonjudgmental attitude
• Benevolence	• Objectivity
• Caring as a foundation for relationships	• Openness to learning
• Collaborative multidisciplinary practice	• Partnerships with patients
• Compassion	• Patient advocacy
• Competence	• Patient education
• Concern	• Presence (being fully present)
• Continuous improvement of service	• Promotion of health
• Cooperative work relationships	• Promotion of patient self-determination and patient preferences
• Courage	• Providing care regardless of patient's ability to pay
• Dependability	
• Empathy	• Quality care (physical, emotional, spiritual, social, intellectual)
• Ethical conduct	
• Flexibility	• Reliability
• Focus on patient-defined quality of life	• Respect for each person's dignity and worth
• Health promotion	• Responsibility
• Holistic, person-centered care	• Responsiveness
• Honesty and authenticity in communication	• Sensitivity
• Humaneness	• Sharing decision making
• Humility	• Sharing self through nursing interventions
• Illness prevention	• Stewardship; responsible use of resources
• Individualized patient care	• Subordination of self-interest
• Integrity—personal and professional	• Support of fellow nurses
• Involvement with families	• Teamwork
• Kindness	• Trust in self, others, and the institution

Courtesy Diann B. Uustal (2006).

Values Undergirding *Nursing's Social Policy Statement*

Professional groups, such as nursing, "have collective identities that are evidenced by their actions. These actions stem from a set of values and choices. . . . [B]y examining the actions of groups . . ., their basic values can be logically inferred" (Mohr, 1995, p. 30).

Organized nursing, through the ANA, sets forth the values that undergird the profession. This is done in a document published from time to time that is designed to serve as a resource for nurses in various practice settings, in education, and in research. It guides nursing practice and also informs others, including the public, about nursing's social responsibility. (This important document was under revision in 2009 and expected to be published in the summer of 2010. Information about how to access the latest version of *Nursing's Social Policy Statement: The Essence of the Profession* [in press] can be found on the Evolve website: http://evolve.elsevier.com/Chitty/professional/.) The social policy statement sets forth several underlying values and assumptions on which the statement is based:

• Humans manifest an essential unity of mind, body, and spirit.
• Human experience is contextually and culturally defined.

Box 12-7   Clarifying Your Values

Once you have identified a value, it is important to assess its significance to you and to clarify your willing-ness to act on the value. The following clarifying questions are organized on basis of the steps of the valuing process and can help you answer questions about what you value. First, identify a value (or values) that is (are) important to you. Write your value(s) below:

_____

_____

_____

   Next, use the questions below to assess the importance of a belief or attitude and to determine whether it is a value. Rephrase the questions to suit your own style of conversation.

CHOOSING FREELY
 1. Am I sure I've thought about this value and chosen to believe it myself?
 2. Who first taught me this value?
 3. How do I know I'm "right"?

CHOOSING AMONG ALTERNATIVES
 4. What other alternatives are possible?
 5. Which alternative has the most appeal for me and why?
 6. Have I thought much about this value/alternative?

CHOOSING AFTER CONSIDERING THE CONSEQUENCES
 7. What consequences do I think might occur as a result of my holding this value?
 8. What "price" will I pay for my position?
 9. Is this value worth the "price" I might pay?

COMPLEMENT TO OTHER VALUES
10. Does this value "fit" with my other values, and is it consistent with them?
11. Am I sure this value doesn't conflict with other values I deem important to me?

PRIZE AND CHERISH
12. Am I proud of my position and value? Is this something I feel good about?
13. How important is this value to me?
14. If this were not one of my values, how different would my life be?

PUBLIC AFFIRMATION
15. Am I willing to speak out for this value?

ACTION
16. Am I willing to put this value into action?
17. Do I act on this value? When? How consistently?
18. Is this a value that can guide me in other situations?
19. Would I want others who are important to me to follow this value?
20. Do I think I'll always believe this? How committed to this value am I?
21. Am I willing to do anything about this value?
22. How do I know this value is "right"? Are my values ethical?

From Uustal DB: *Clinical ethics and values: issues and insights in a changing healthcare environment,* East Greenwich, RI, 1993, Educational Resources in Healthcare. Reprinted with permission.

- Health and illness are human experiences. The presence of illness does not preclude health nor does optimal health preclude illness.
- The interaction between the nurse and patient occurs within the context of the values and beliefs of the patient and the nurse.
- Public policy and the health care delivery system influence the health and well-being of society and professional nursing.

Chapter 5 contains more about values and their relationship to nursing practice.

PHILOSOPHIES AND THEIR RELATIONSHIP TO NURSING CARE

Philosophy is defined as the study of the principles underlying conduct, thought, and the nature of the universe. A simple explanation of philosophy is that it entails a search for meaning in the universe. You may have learned about philosophers such as Plato, Aristotle, Bacon, Kant, Hegel, Kierkegaard, Nietzsche, Locke, Descartes, and others in nonnursing classes. These philosophers were searching for the underlying principles of reality and truth. Nursing philosophies and theories often derive from or build on the concepts identified by these and other philosophers.

Philosophy begins when someone contemplates, or wonders about, something. If a group of friends sometimes sits and discusses the relationship between men and women and ponders the differences in men's and women's natures and approaches to life, one might say that they were developing a philosophy about male and female ways of being. It is important to remember that philosophy is not the exclusive domain of a few erudite individuals; everyone has a personal philosophy of life that is unique.

People develop personal philosophies as they mature, usually without being aware of it. These philosophies serve as blueprints or guides and incorporate each individual's value and belief systems. Nurses' personal philosophies interact directly with their philosophies of nursing and influence professional behaviors.

Branches of Philosophy

Before examining professional philosophies, we briefly explore the discipline of philosophy itself. Philosophy has been divided into specific areas of study. This section reviews six branches: epistemology, logic, aesthetics, ethics, politics, and metaphysics.

1. Epistemology is the branch of philosophy dealing with the theory of knowledge itself. The epistemologist attempts to answer such questions as "What can be known?" and "What constitutes knowledge?" Epistemology attempts to determine how we can know whether our beliefs about the world are true.

2. Logic is the study of proper and improper methods of reasoning. In logic, the nature of reasoning itself is the subject. Logic attempts to answer the question, "What should our thinking methods be in order to reach true conclusions?" Chapter 8 presents a method of logical thinking that nurses use to plan and implement effective patient care, called the nursing process.

3. Aesthetics is the study of what is beautiful. It attempts to answer the question, "Why do we find things beautiful?" Painting, sculpture, music, dance, and literature are all associated with beauty. Judgments about what is beautiful, however, differ from individual to individual and culture to culture. For example, Eastern music may sound discordant to the Western ear and vice versa.

4. Ethics is the branch of philosophy that studies standards of conduct. It attempts to answer the question, "What is the nature of good and evil?" Moral principles and values make up a system of ethics. Behavior depends on moral principles and values. Ethics, therefore, underlie the standards of behavior that govern us as individuals and as nurses. Bioethics is a term describing the branch of ethics that deals with biological issues. Bioethics and nursing ethics are complex areas of study that are explored in Chapter 5.

5. Politics, in the context of a discussion of philosophy, means the area of philosophy that deals with the regulation and control of people living in society. Political philosophers study

the conditions of society and suggest recommendations for improving them. They attempt to answer the question, "What makes good governments?"

6. Metaphysics is the consideration of the ultimate nature of existence, reality, human experience, and the universe. Metaphysicians believe that through contemplation we can come to a more complete understanding of reality than science alone can provide. They ask the question, "What is the meaning of life?" and explore the fundamental nature of all reality.

This brief review of the major branches of philosophy is presented as a backdrop for the discussion of philosophies of nursing.

Philosophies of Nursing

Philosophies of nursing are statements of beliefs about nursing and expressions of values in nursing that are used as bases for thinking and acting. Most philosophies of nursing are built on a foundation of beliefs about people, environment, health, and nursing. Each of these four foundational concepts of nursing is discussed in some detail earlier in this chapter.

Individual philosophies

If asked, most nurses could list their beliefs about nursing, but it is doubtful that many have written a formal philosophy of nursing. They are influenced on a day-to-day basis, however, by their unwritten, informal philosophies. It is useful to go through the process of writing down one's own professional philosophy and revising it from time to time. Comparing recent and earlier versions can reveal professional and personal growth over time. It is also helpful to read one's philosophy of nursing from time to time to make sure daily behaviors are consistent with deeply held beliefs. Box 12-8 contains one nurse's philosophy of nursing.

Collective philosophies

Although few individuals write down their nursing philosophies, it is common for hospitals and schools of nursing to express their collective beliefs about nursing in written philosophies. In

fact, both hospitals and schools of nursing are required by their accrediting bodies to develop statements of philosophy. Philosophical statements should be relevant to the setting. They are intended to guide the practice of nurses employed in that setting. Examining some of these statements clarifies what constitutes a collective philosophy of nursing.

Box 12-8   One Nurse's Philosophy

I believe that the essence of nursing is caring about and caring for human beings who are unable to care for themselves. I believe that the central core of nursing is the nurse-patient relationship and that through that relationship I can make a difference in the lives of others at a time when they are most vulnerable.

Human beings generally do the best they can. When they are uncooperative, critical, or otherwise unpleasant, it is usually because they are frightened; therefore, I will remain pleasant and nondefensive and try to understand the patient's perception of the situation. I pledge to be trustworthy and an advocate for my patients.

I realize that my cultural background affects how I deliver nursing care and that my patients' cultural backgrounds affect how they receive my care. I try to learn as much as I can about each individual's cultural beliefs and preferences and individualize care accordingly.

My vision for myself as a nurse is that I will provide the best care I can to all patients, regardless of their financial situation, social status, lifestyle choices, or spiritual beliefs. I will collaborate with my patients, their families, and my health care colleagues and work cooperatively with them, valuing and respecting what each brings to the situation.

I am individually accountable for the care I provide, for what I fail to do and to know. Therefore, I pledge to remain a learner all my life and actively seek opportunities to learn how to be a more effective nurse.

I will strive for a balance of personal and professional responsibilities. This means I will take care of myself physically, emotionally, socially, and spiritually so I can continue to be a productive caregiver.

Philosophy of nursing in a hospital setting. First, look at the philosophy of nursing of Memorial Health Care System in Chattanooga, Tennessee, found on the Evolve website: http://evolve.elsevier.com/Chitty/professional/.

This philosophy describes a commitment to excellence in nursing service, practice, and leadership. Notice statements with which you might agree or disagree. Remember that this is the philosophy of nursing in a hospital setting. Before taking a position in a hospital or health care agency, it is a good idea to ask for a copy of the philosophy of nursing of that institution. Read it carefully and make sure you accept the beliefs and values it contains, for it will influence nursing care in that setting.

Philosophy of a school of nursing. Now examine philosophical statements of a school of nursing. The philosophy of the faculty in the Department of Nursing at the University of North Florida is found on the Evolve website: http://evolve.elsevier.com/Chitty/professional/.

After reading this philosophy, identify the similarities and differences between the philosophy of nursing in the hospital setting and the one in this school of nursing. What differences in focus can you identify?

An important point about philosophies of nursing is that they are dynamic; they change over time. When a collective philosophy is writ-

ten, it reflects the existing values and beliefs of the particular group of people who wrote it. When the group members change, the philosophy may also change. Therefore once a collective philosophy is written, it should be "revisited" regularly and modified to reflect accurately the group's current beliefs about nursing practice.

DEVELOPING A PERSONAL PHILOSOPHY OF NURSING

Your philosophy of life, whether or not you can articulate it, is the basis of your day-to-day behavior. It consists of the principles that underlie your thinking and conduct. Therefore developing a philosophy of nursing is not merely an academic exercise required by accrediting bodies. Having a written philosophy can help guide nurses in the daily decisions they must make in nursing practice.

Writing a philosophy is not a complex, time-consuming task. It simply involves writing down your beliefs and values about nursing. It answers the questions: "What is nursing?" and "Why do I practice nursing the way I do?" Whether individual or collective, a philosophy should provide direction and promote effectiveness.

Box 12-9 is designed to help you begin to develop your own personal philosophy of nursing. After you write a beginning philosophy, save it. As you progress through your educational program, take it out and revise it regularly, saving

---

Box 12-9   Philosophy of Nursing Work Sheet

Purpose: To write a beginning philosophy of nursing that reflects the beliefs and values of _____
_____[your name].

Today's date is _____.

I chose nursing as my profession because nursing is _____.

I believe that the core of nursing is _____.

I believe that the focus of nursing is _____.

My vision for myself as a nurse is that I will _____.

To live out my philosophy of nursing, every day I must remember this about:

1. My patients: _____.

2. My patients' families: _____.

3. My fellow health care professionals: _____.

4. My own health: _____.

each version. After you graduate, look back at all the different versions and see how your philosophy of nursing has changed over time.

Summary of Key Points

- Knowledge of systems and human motivation can be used to understand nursing's major concepts.
- Persons are viewed as unique open systems who are motivated by needs.
- Maslow organized human needs into a hierarchy consisting of five levels that range from basic physiologic needs, which are common to all people, to self-actualization, which is attained by few.
- Environment consists of all the circumstances, influences, and conditions that affect an individual. The physical environment and family, cultural, social, and community systems all have an impact.
- Health is dynamic and viewed as a continuum.
- Nurses view health holistically, including its effect on an individual's physical, emotional, social, and spiritual functioning, as well as its effect on the family.
- Health is affected by health beliefs and health behaviors.
- As an open system, nursing integrates person, environment, and health into a meaningful whole.
- Nursing assists people to achieve health at the highest possible level, given their environmental and genetic constraints.
- People develop beliefs and values that affect their attitudes and behaviors.
- Beliefs and values influence how nurses practice their profession.
- Nurses need to be aware of their beliefs and values to prevent the unintentional intrusion of personal values into nurse-patient relationships.
- A statement of beliefs can be called a philosophy.
- The purpose of developing a philosophy of nursing is to shape and guide nursing practice.
- Philosophies can express either individual beliefs or the collective beliefs of a group, such as a nursing faculty.

- As nurses progress professionally, they develop ideas about the practice of nursing that they agree with and support. From these, they develop their own personal philosophies of nursing.
- As nurses mature in the profession, they may find that their philosophies about nursing change, even though underlying values may not.

Critical Thinking Questions

1. Discuss systems in relation to your family. What are the family equivalents of inputs, throughputs, subsystems, suprasystems, outputs, evaluation, and feedback? Does your family tend to be an open or closed system?

2. Describe Maslow's hierarchy of needs and place yourself on the hierarchy today, 1 week ago, and when you were a senior in high school. Were you at a different level each time? Consider what factors—internal and external—may have been involved in your placement at each of these times. If possible, compare and discuss your findings with at least one other person.

3. Write your own personal definition of health and share it with one other person. Evaluate your definition in terms of holism.

4. What are factors that influence an individual's personal health behaviors? Make a list of your health behaviors, including those that promote health and those that diminish health. Analyze why you continue both the healthy and the nonhealthy behaviors. Identify factors that could influence you to make more health-generating choices.

5. Using a search engine, assess the array of support groups online. Enter the discussion group of one group that interests you, and simply observe. How would you evaluate the quality of the support and information being shared?

6. Look through your local Yellow Pages under "Social Services" and "Organizations." What types of social support do you find that might be useful to patients? Compare these with the online choices. Which type of support—face-to-face or online—is more appealing to you? Why?

7. Conduct an assessment of your community in terms of one of the following: availability of jobs, quality of public education, availability of health services, environmental hazards, and quality of air and water. What is the impact of the factor you selected on the health of the community's citizens? What can you do to strengthen the environmental health of your community?

8. Find out what your state and community are doing to link their health objectives to those of the Healthy People initiatives. Discuss these in class. Design a project to assist your school of nursing to support the national effort.

9. Name two of your health-related values. How did these become your values? Describe how you expect these values to influence your nursing practice.

10. Read "One Nurse's Philosophy" in Box 12-8. Then identify at least 10 of that nurse's professional values, using the list in Box 12-6, "Professional Nursing Values." Can you identify other values that are not listed?

11. Obtain the philosophy of the department of nursing of a facility where you work or have clinical labs. Compare it with the philosophical statements of Memorial Health Care System found on the Evolve website: http://evolve.elsevier.com/Chitty/professional/. What are three common elements and three differences? Which of the two statements is most congruent with your own beliefs about nursing?

12. Obtain the philosophy statement of the faculty of your school of nursing. What concepts are included? Which beliefs do you agree with and disagree with? Why?

13. Using the work sheet in Box 12-9, write a beginning personal philosophy of nursing. Share your philosophy with one other person.

14. Discuss how the focus on "the bottom line" affects your own and nursing's professional values.

15. Discuss how having or not having a philosophy of nursing might influence a nurse's practice.

⊖volve *To enhance your understanding of this chapter, try the Student Exercises on the Evolve site at http://evolve.elsevier.com/Chitty/professional.*

REFERENCES

Ahmann E: Supporting families' savvy use of the Internet for health research, *Pediatr Nurs* 26(4):419-423, 2000.

American Nurses Association: *Code of ethics for nurses with interpretive statements,* Silver Spring, Md, 2001 (website): http://www.nursesbooks.org.

American Nurses Association: *Nursing's social policy statement,* ed 2, Washington, DC, 2003 (website): http://www.nursesbooks.org.

Bandura A: *Self-efficacy: exercise of control,* New York, 1997, WH Freeman.

Bandura A: A social cognitive approach to the exercise of control over AIDS infection, In DiClemente RJ, editor: *Adolescents and AIDS: a generation in jeopardy,* Newbury Park, Calif, 1992, Sage Publications.

Beyea SC: Evaluating evidence found on the Internet, *AORN J* 72(5):906-910, 2000.

Center on Budget and Policy Priorities: *Census data show poverty increased, income stagnated, and the number of uninsured rose to a record level in 2003,* News release, 2004 (website): http://www.cbpp.org/cms/?fa=view&id=620.8-26-04pov.htm.

Chase M: Health journal: a guide for patients who turn to the Web for solace and support, *Wall Street Journal* B1, Sept 17, 1999.

Dunbar-Jacob J: Models for changing patient behavior, *Am J Nurs* 107(6):20-25, 2007.

Dunn HL: High-level wellness for man and society, *Am J Public Health* 49(6):786-792, 1959.

Dunn HL: *High-level wellness,* Thorofare, NJ, 1961, Slack.

Eustis R: *Parents: son would have chosen death over blood,* 2002 (website): http://www.rickross.com/reference/jw/jw90.html.

Finfgeld-Connett D: Clarification of social support, *Image J Nurs Sch* 37(1):4-9, 2005.

Fitzsimmons EG: Wisconsin couple sentenced in death of their sick child, *The New York Times,* October 7, 2009, p. A-16.

Grossman D: Enhancing your cultural competence, *Am J Nurs* 94(7):58-62, 1994.

Grube JW, Mayton DM, Ball-Rokeach SJ: Inducing change in values, attitudes, and behaviors: belief system theory, *J Soc Issues* 50(4):153-173, 1994.

Hoffman E: The Maslow effect: a humanist legacy for nursing, *Am Nurs Today* 3(8):36-37, 2008.

Holmes TH, Rahe RH: The social readjustment rating scale, *J Psychosom Res* 11(2):213-218, 1967.

Johnson D: Trials for parents who chose faith over medicine, *New York Times*, (Jan 21):p A-23, 2009.

Larsen LJ: The foreign-born population in the United States, 2003, *Curr Popul Rep*, p 20-551, 2004.

Lauer M: Reducing health care's ecological footprint: how nurses can slow the flow of health care waste, *Am J Nurs* 109(2):56-58, 2009.

Markoff J: Microsoft examines causes of "cyberchondria," *New York Times*, (Nov 25):p B-3, 2008.

Martin JA, Hamilton BE, Sutton PD, Ventura SJ, et al: *Births: final data for 2006, National Vital Statistics Reports, 57(7)*, Hyattsville, MD, 2009, National Center for Health Statistics.

Maslow AH: *Motivation and personality*, ed 3, New York, 1987, Harper & Row.

Miller MA, Rahe RH: Life changes scaling for the 1990s, *J Psychosom Res* 43(3):279-292, 1997.

Mohr WK: Values, ideologies, and dilemmas: professional and occupational contradictions, *J Psychiatr Nurs* 33(1):29-34, 1995.

Parsons T: Definitions of health and illness in light of American values and social structure, In Jaco EG, editor: *Patients, physicians and illness*, New York, 1959, Free Press, 165-187.

Peden AR, Rayens MK, Hall LA, et al: Negative thinking and the mental health of low-income single mothers, *Image J Nurs Sch* 36(4):337-344, 2004.

Pender NJ, Murdaugh C, Parsons MA: *Health promotion in nursing practice*, ed 5, Upper Saddle River, NJ, 2006, Prentice-Hall Health.

Pratt JP, Overfield T, Gill-Hilton H: Health behaviors of nurses and general population women, *Health Values* 18(3):41-46, 1994.

Raths L, Harmin M, Simon S: *Values and teaching*, ed 2, Columbus, Ohio, 1978, Charles Merrill.

Reutter L, Sword W, Meagher-Stewart D, et al: Nursing students' beliefs about the relationship between poverty and health, *J Adv Nurs* 48:299-309, 2004.

Rogers C: *On becoming a person*, Boston, 1961, Houghton Mifflin.

Rokeach M: *The nature of human values*, New York, 1973, Free Press.

Rosenstock IM: The health belief model: explaining health behavior through expectancies, In Glans K, Lewis FM, Rimer BK, editors: *Health behavior and health education: theory, research, and practice*, San Francisco, 1990, Jossey-Bass, 39-62.

Rosenstock IM: Why people use health services, part II, *Milbank Mem Fund Q* 44(3):94-124, 1966.

Sataline S: A child's death and a crisis for faith, *Wall Street Journal*, (June 12):p D-1, 2008.

Smith K, Bazini-Barakat N: A public health nursing practice model: melding public health principles with the nursing process, *Pub Health Nurs* 20(1):42-48, 2003.

Smuts JC: *Holism and evolution*, New York, 1926, Macmillan.

Steptoe A, Wardle J: Locus of control and health behaviour revisited: a multivariate analysis of young adults from 18 countries, *Br J Psychol* 92(4):659-673, 2001.

Tanaka W: *Health tips on your iPhone*, Forbes.com, Aug 25, 2008 (website): http://www.forbes.com/2008/08/25/healthy-web-sites-tech-personal-cx_wt_0825health.html/.

U.S. Census Bureau: *America's families and living arrangements*, 2007 (website): http://www.census.gov/population/www/socdemo/hh-fam/cps2007.html (Table FG5).

U.S. Census Bureau: *Current population survey: 2008 annual social and economic supplements*, 2008 (website): http://www.census.gov/hhes/www/poverty/poverty07/pov07hi.html.

U.S. Department of Health and Human Services: *Healthy People 2010: fact sheet*, 2006 (website): http://www.healthypeople.gov/About/hpfact.htm.

U.S. Department of Health and Human Services: *Healthy people 2010: implementation*, 2003 (website): http://www.healthypeople.gov/Implementation/default.htm#partners.

U.S. Department of Health and Human Services: *HHS poverty guidelines*, 2008 (website): http://aspe.hhs.gov/poverty/08computations.shtml.

Uustal DB: *Values and ethics in nursing: from theory to practice*, East Greenwich, RI, 1985, Educational Resources in Nursing and Wholistic Health.

Uustal DB: *Clinical ethics and values: issues and insights in a changing healthcare environment*, East Greenwich, RI, 1993, Educational Resources in Healthcare.

Uustal DB: *Caring for yourself, caring for others: the ultimate balance*, ed 2, East Greenwich, RI, 2009, Educational Resources in Healthcare.

von Bertalanffy L: *General systems theory: foundations, development, applications*, New York, 1968, George Braziller.

World Health Organization: *Constitution*, Geneva, 1947, World Health Organization.

Zuger A: Healthy right up to the day you're not, *New York Times*, (Sept 30):p F-3, 2008.

Nursing Theory: The Basis for Professional Nursing

Beth Perry Black

LEARNING OUTCOMES

After studying this chapter, students will be able to:
- Explore elements of selected nursing philosophies, nursing conceptual models, and theories of nursing
- Consider how selected nursing theoretical works guide the practice of nursing
- Understand how the course of study in schools of nursing is shaped by nursing philosophy or theory
- Delineate the role of nursing theory for different levels of nursing education
- Describe the function of nursing theory in research and theory-based practice

Theory is a word that is used frequently in daily language, such as "I have a theory about that" or "In theory, this should work." The word *theory* in this context means that the person has some idea about a phenomenon and the way this phenomenon works in the world. When people say, "I have a theory . . ." about a certain phenomenon or situation, they are demonstrating something about their own distinct orientation or way of seeing the world. *Theory* comes from the Latin and Greek word for "a viewing" or "contemplating."

Nursing as a profession has a distinct theoretical orientation to practice. This means that the practice of nursing is based on a specific body of knowledge that is built on theory. This body of knowledge shapes and is shaped by how nurses see the world. The word **theory** has many definitions, but generally it refers to a group of related concepts, definitions, and statements that describe a certain view of nursing **phenomena** (observable occurrences) from which to describe, explain, or predict outcomes (Chinn and Kramer, 1998). Theories represent abstract ideas rather than concrete facts. New theories are always being generated, although some theories are useful for many years. When new knowledge becomes available,

theories that are no longer useful are modified or discarded. Although nursing theory has been traced back to Florence Nightingale, most nursing theory was developed in the second half of the twentieth century (Alligood, 2002a; Tomey and Alligood, 2002).

So why is theory important? First, nursing as profession is strengthened when nursing knowledge is built on sound theory. As seen in Chapter 3, one criterion for a profession is a distinct body of knowledge as the basis for practice. Nursing has knowledge that is distinct from, although related to, other disciplines such as medicine, social work, sociology, and physiology, among others. The development of nursing knowledge is the work of nurse researchers and scholars. The evolution of the profession of nursing depends on continued recognition of nursing as a scholarly academic discipline that contributes to society. In today's research environment, where theory is developed and tested, interdisciplinary collaboration is now considered to be a critical approach to the development of knowledge. Use of nursing theory in other disciplines is not yet common, however (March and McCormack, 2009).

Box 13-1   Nursing Theory and the Professional Nurse

Theory guides the professional nurse in

- Organizing patient data
- Analyzing patient data
- Understanding connections between pieces of data
- Discriminating between important and less pertinent data
- Making sound clinical judgments based on evidence
- Planning effective nursing interventions
- Predicting outcomes of interventions
- Evaluating outcomes of interventions

Second, theory is a useful tool for reasoning, critical thinking, and decision making (Alligood, 2002c; Alligood and Tomey, 2002; Tomey and Alligood, 2002). The ultimate goal of nursing theory is to support excellence in practice. Pilson (2009) argued that subspecialties of nursing, not simply basic nursing, should be theory based, which will assist novices to become experts, therefore improving patient care. Nursing practice settings are complex, and a vast amount of information about each patient is available to nurses. Nurses must analyze this information to make sound clinical judgments and to generate effective interventions. From organization of patient data to the development and evaluation of interventions, theory provides a guide for nurses in developing effective care. Box 13-1 shows how theory guides nursing practice.

Several words are used to describe abstract thoughts and their linkages. From the most to least abstract, these include metaparadigm, philosophy, conceptual model or framework, and theory. Metaparadigm refers to the most abstract aspect of the structure of nursing knowledge (Fawcett, 2000; March and McCormack, 2009). The metaparadigm of nursing consists of the major concepts of the discipline—person, environment, health, and nursing—that were discussed in Chapter 12. Simply stated, these four concepts comprise the metaparadigm of nursing;

that is, these are the concepts (abstract notion or idea) of most importance to nursing practice and research. Nursing philosophies, models, and theories contain most or all of these concepts.

A philosophy is a set of beliefs about the nature of how things work and how the world should be viewed (Sitzman and Eichelberger, 2004). A nursing philosophy begins to put together some or all concepts of the metaparadigm. For instance, Florence Nightingale, whose work will be considered in more detail later in this chapter, wrote *Notes on Nursing: What It Is and What It Is Not,* in which her basic philosophy of nursing is described in detail. A conceptual model or framework is a more specific organization of nursing phenomena than philosophies. As the words *model* or *framework* imply, models provide an organizational structure that makes clearer connections between concepts.

Theories are more concrete descriptions of concepts that are embedded in propositions. Propositions are statements that describe linkages between concepts and are more prescriptive; that is, they propose an outcome that is testable in practice and research (Alligood, 2002c). For example, Peplau's book *Interpersonal Relations in Nursing* (Peplau, 1952) contains a theory that describes very specific elements of effective interaction between the nurse and patient. Using concepts from nursing's metaparadigm, Peplau created a theory delineating elements of excellent and effective practice in psychiatric nursing. She linked abstract concepts such as health and nursing to create a concrete, useful theory for practice. Peplau's theory will be described later in this chapter.

The primary source—the original writings of the theorist—is the best source for in-depth understanding of theoretical works. Explanatory texts written by other scholars can be very helpful in interpreting primary sources. Explanatory texts introduce students to the theoretical basis of the discipline of nursing from a nursing science perspective that is much broader than any one of the primary sources. That is, these explanatory texts trace the historical development of the philosophy, model, or theory and specify criteria (standards) by which to analyze, critique, and evaluate them. Texts such as these were first published in the early 1980s with a completely different purpose than the theorists' original writings. They are designed to contribute to the general understanding of nursing theory and theoretical developments in nursing in a unique but complementary way. Undergraduate and graduate students, faculty, and practicing nurses have found that these explanatory texts on nursing theory make a significant contribution to their knowledge and understanding of nursing science in its own right.

In this chapter, three types of nursing theoretical works will be presented: philosophies, conceptual models, and theories. Selected works from each of these three types provide a broad overview of theory within the discipline of nursing. This introduction is designed to help you develop a beginning understanding of nursing theory on which to build as you pursue your nursing education and career in the profession of nursing.

NURSING PHILOSOPHIES

Chapter 12 introduced nursing philosophy and discussed its function in nursing practice and educational institutions. A philosophy provides a broad, general view of nursing that clarifies values and answers broad disciplinary questions such as the following: "What is nursing?" "What is the profession of nursing?" "What do nurses do?" "What is the nature of human caring?" "What is the nature of nursing practice and the development of practice expertise?" Three philosophies representing different positions in the development of nursing theory are presented here. Table 13-1 contains questions that represent the different views of the same patient situation among nurses who subscribe to the philosophies of Florence Nightingale, Virginia Henderson, and Jean Watson, whose work is presented here.

Nightingale's Philosophy

Florence Nightingale was born in 1820, in Florence, Italy. She was the daughter of a wealthy English landowner and his wife, Fanny, whose

Table 13-1 Three Philosophies of Nursing: Three Different Responses to the Same Patient Situation

Florence Nightingale	What needs to be adjusted in this environment to protect the patient?
Jean Watson	How can I create an environment of trust, understanding, and openness so that the patient and I can work together in meeting his needs?
Virginia Henderson	What can I help this patient do that he would do for himself if he could?

goal in life was to find a suitable husband for her daughters. Florence was very close to her father, and he undertook the responsibility for her education, teaching her a classical curriculum of Greek, Latin, French, German, Italian, history, philosophy, and mathematics. At 25 years of age, after deciding to remain unmarried, Florence announced her decision to go to Kaiserswerth, Germany, to study nursing, over the strong objections of her parents. At that time, nursing was considered the pursuit of working-class women. Her persistence in the face of her parents' opposition proved to be a sustained characteristic over the course of her life. This trait enabled her to accomplish work that most women of the time would not have had the education or willingness to achieve.

Nightingale's work represents the beginning of professional nursing as we know it today. In *Notes on Nursing: What It Is and What It Is Not* (1969, originally published in 1859), Nightingale wrote her philosophy of health, illness, and the nurse's role in caring for patients. Importantly, she made a distinction between the work of nursing and the work of physicians by identifying health as the major concern of nursing rather than illness. Her writing about nursing reflected the sociohistorical context in which she lived, making a distinction between the work of nursing and the work of household servants, who were common in her day and often cared for the sick.

Nightingale's unique perspective on nursing practice focused on the relationship of patients to their surroundings. She set forth principles that were foundational to nursing and remain relevant to nursing practice today. For example, her description of the importance of observing the patient and accurately recording information and her principles of cleanliness still shape hospital-based nursing practice today. Nightingale focused the profession on what has become known as the metaparadigm of nursing: person (patient), health (as opposed to illness), environment (how the environment affects health and recovery from illness), and nursing (as opposed to medicine).

Using Nightingale's philosophy in practice

Nightingale believed that the health of patients was related to their environment. She recognized the importance of clean air and water and of adequate ventilation and sunlight and encouraged the arrangement of patients' beds so that they were in direct sunlight. In her writing, she described both the necessity of a balanced diet and the nurse's responsibility to observe and record what was eaten. Cleanliness of the patient, the bed linens, and the room itself were essential. Nightingale recognized the problem of noise in hospital rooms and halls, which foreshadowed the attention given to excess noise in inpatient settings in recent years. Rest is important in the restoration of health; Nightingale believed that sudden disruption of sleep was a serious problem. The relationship of health to the environment seems obvious today, but for nursing in the second half of the nineteenth century, Nightingale's work was radically different.

Nightingale recognized nursing's role in protecting patients. Nurses were newly responsible for shielding patients from possible harm by well-meaning visitors who may provide false hope, discuss upsetting news, or tire the patient with social conversation. Nightingale even suggested that the nurse's responsibility for patients did not end when the nurse was off duty. This view underpins the system of primary nursing found in some settings today. Interestingly, Nightingale

suggested that patients might benefit from visits by small pets, an idea that has been newly revisited in long-term care settings.

The nurse whose practice is guided by Nightingale's philosophy is sensitive to the effect of the environment on the patient's health or recovery from illness. This philosophy provided the foundational work for theory development that proposed changing patients' environments to effect positive changes in their health. Nightingale promoted the view that nurses' primary responsibility was to protect patients by careful management of their surroundings.

Henderson's Philosophy

Virginia Henderson was born in 1897 in Kansas City, Missouri, and was named for the state her mother longed for and to which the family returned 4 years later. Although she received an excellent education from a family friend who was a schoolmaster, and from her father who was a former teacher, Henderson did not receive a traditional education that awarded a diploma. This delayed her entry into nursing school. During World War II, she studied under Annie Goodrich at Teachers College, Columbia University, where, after numerous interruptions, she received her bachelor's and master's degrees. By the time she died in 1996, Virginia Henderson was internationally known and regarded by many as "the Florence Nightingale of the twentieth century."

One hundred years after Nightingale, Virginia Henderson's work first was published, emerging at a time when efforts to clarify nursing as a profession emphasized the need to define nursing. Henderson's philosophical approach to nursing is contained in her comprehensive definition: the "unique function of the nurse. . . is to assist the individual, sick or well, in the performance of those activities contributing to health or its recovery (or a peaceful death) that he would perform unaided if he had the necessary strength, will or knowledge" (Henderson, 1966, p. 15). Although Henderson, pictured in Figure 13-1, was recognized for many contributions to nursing throughout her long career, her early work remains particularly noteworthy and relevant, defining nursing and specifying the role of the nurse in relation to the patient. Henderson's relationship with one of her former students, who recognizes the ongoing contributions of Henderson's work to nursing, is described in Box 13-2.

Henderson's philosophy linked her definition of nursing that emphasized the functions of the nurse with a list of basic patient needs that are the focus of nursing care. She proposed an answer to questions similar to those addressed by Nightingale a century earlier: "What is the nursing profession?" and "What do nurses do?" Henderson described the nurse's role as that of a substitute

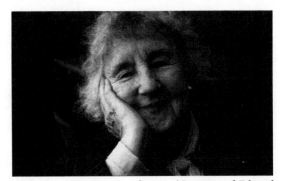

Figure 13-1 Virginia Henderson. (Courtesy of Edward J. Halloran.)

Box 13-2   Remembering Virginia Henderson

Although I had known Virginia Henderson from the time when I was a graduate student at Yale, geography later brought us more closely together. Knowing her family lived in Virginia (mine was in Connecticut), whenever I traveled by car from North Carolina to Connecticut I called and asked if she wanted a ride back home with me and I could drop her off in Virginia en route to North Carolina. Six times we made the 8-hour ride together. Our conversations were wide-ranging because we were both world travelers. We talked much about politics; most about nurses—"see a nurse before you go to a doctor" as a solution to health care cost, quality, and access problems; some about patients—"give them their records" as a most important patient education tool; and some about our large extended families. I was introduced to two of Virginia Henderson's sisters when they were all in their 90s. Four brothers and a sister had predeceased them but Frances [Fanny] had maintained the old family homestead so all who could come were welcomed to stay. Come they did for over two generations of reunions, weddings, funerals, and holidays, especially Christmas.

What was most amazing to me about our time together was that Virginia Henderson never said anything to me about our profession that she had not written down somewhere for all nurses to read. Yale's School of Nursing asked me to address the topic of her writing in their Bellos Lecture the year they celebrated her 90th birthday. I read her textbook, *Principles and Practice of Nursing*, sixth edition, and discovered any number of conversations I had experienced with her over the years. In preparing the *Virginia Henderson Reader: Excellence in Nursing*, I discovered even more. Her writings are conversational, that is, completely without the jargon of the medical and nursing professions. Her description of nursing is best used by nurses to tell patients what can be expected—to paraphrase—I'm here to help you do what you would do for yourself if you had the strength, will, or knowledge and do so for you to become free of my help as rapidly as possible. It is quite reassuring for a patient to know what the nurse is going to do.

Virginia Henderson's writings are timeless. The information in *The Nature of Nursing* and *Basic Principles of Nursing Care* is as relevant today as the day the books were written. *The Nature of Nursing* is the most important document written about nurses and nursing in the twentieth century because it provided evidence of effective and efficient nursing. If you read her work, you can have a conversation with her, too.

* *Edward J. Halloran, RN, MPH, PhD,*
  Fellow, American Academy of Nursing

Courtesy Edward J. Halloran.

Box 13-3   Henderson's 14 Basic Needs of the Patient

1. Breathe normally.
2. Eat and drink adequately.
3. Eliminate body wastes.
4. Move and maintain desirable position.
5. Sleep and rest.
6. Select suitable clothes—dress and undress.
7. Maintain body temperature within normal range by adjusting clothing and modifying the environment.
8. Keep the body clean and well groomed and protect the integument (skin).
9. Avoid dangers in the environment and avoid injuring others.
10. Communicate with others in expressing emotions, needs, fears, or opinions.
11. Worship according to one's faith.
12. Work in such a way that there is a sense of accomplishment.
13. Play or participate in various forms of recreation.
14. Learn, discover, or satisfy the curiosity that leads to normal development and health and use the available health facilities.

Reprinted with permission of Henderson V: *The nature of nursing: a definition and its implications for practice, research, and education,* New York, 1966, Macmillan.

for the patient, a helper to the patient, or a partner with the patient.

Henderson identified 14 basic needs (Box 13-3) as a general focus for patient care. She proposed that these needs shaped the fundamental elements of nursing care. The function of nurses was to assist patients if they were unable to perform any of these 14 functions themselves. Although these needs can be categorized as physical, psychological, emotional, sociological, spiritual, or developmental, thoughtful analysis reveals a holistic view of human development and health.

The first nine needs emphasize the importance of care of the physical body: breathing, eating and drinking, elimination, movement and positioning, sleep and rest, suitable clothing, maintenance of suitable environment for the body temperature, cleanliness, and avoidance of danger or harm. Next, she included psychosocial needs such as communication and spirituality, including worship and faith. She concluded with three developmental needs: the need for work and the sense of accomplishment; the need for play and recreation; and the need to learn, discover, and satisfy curiosity. Henderson saw all 14 needs as aspects of patients' lives that are amenable to nursing care. They continue to be used today in philosophical statements of schools and departments of nursing.

Using Henderson's philosophy in practice

Nurses whose practice is consistent with Henderson's philosophy adopt an orientation to care from the perspective of the 14 basic needs. Henderson's clarity about the role and function of the nurse is a strength of her work. This philosophy is easily applied to a variety of patient care settings, from brief outpatient encounters in which a limited number of needs are addressed to a complex setting such as intensive care where patients are extremely vulnerable. Henderson used her definition of nursing and the basic needs approach in her well-known case study of a young patient who had undergone a leg amputation. Using this case, Henderson demonstrated how the nurse's role changes on a day-to-day, week-to-week, and month-to-month basis in relation to the patient's changing needs and the contributions of other members of the health care delivery team (Henderson, 1966).

Watson's Philosophy

Jean Watson is a more recent contributor to the evolving philosophy of nursing. Born in West Virginia, she earned her BSN degree from the University of Colorado in 1964, her MS from the University of Colorado in 1966, and her PhD from the University of Colorado in 1973. Six years later, she published her first book, *The Philosophy and Science of Caring.* In this initial work, she called for a return to the earlier values of nursing and emphasized the caring aspects of nursing. Watson's work is recognized as human science. Caring as a theme is reflected in her other

Box 13-4   Watson's 10 Carative Factors

1. The formation of a humanistic-altruistic system of values
2. The instillation of faith-hope
3. The cultivation of sensitivity to one's self and others
4. The development of a helping-trust relationship
5. The promotion and acceptance of the expression of positive and negative feelings
6. The systematic use of the scientific problem-solving method for decision making
7. The promotion of interpersonal teaching-learning
8. The provision for a supportive, protective, and/or corrective mental, physical, sociocultural, and spiritual environment
9. Assistance with the gratification of human needs
10. The allowance for existential-phenomenological forces

Reprinted with permission of Tomey AM, Alligood MR: *Nursing theorists and their work*, ed 5, St Louis, 2002, Mosby.

professional accomplishments, such as the Center for Human Caring at the University of Colorado in Denver, where nurses can incorporate knowledge of human caring as the basis of nursing practice and scholarship. Watson proposed 10 factors (Box 13-4), which she labeled *carative* factors, a term she contrasted with *curative* to differentiate nursing from medicine.

Watson's work (1979, 1988, 1999) addressed the philosophical question of the nature of nursing as viewed as a human-to-human relationship. She focused on the relationship of the nurse and the patient, drawing on philosophical sources for a new approach that emphasized how the nurse and patient change together through transpersonal caring. She proposed that nursing be concerned with spiritual matters and the inner knowledge of nurse and patient as they participate together in the transpersonal caring process. She equated health with harmony, resulting from unity of body, mind, and soul, for which the patient is primarily responsible. Illness or disease was equated with lack of harmony within the mind, body, and soul experienced in internal or external environments (Watson, 1979). Nursing is based on human values and interest in the welfare of others and is concerned with health promotion, health restoration, and illness prevention. Watson's most recent work (1999) interprets her earlier works in light of postmodern thought for the twenty-first century. Watson recognized the scientific method as a tool for systematic solutions to problems and a guide for making decisions.

Using Watson's philosophy in practice

Watson's carative factors guide nurses who use transpersonal caring in practice. Carative factors specify the meaning of the relationship of nurse and patient as human beings. Nurses are encouraged to share their genuine selves with patients. Patients' spiritual strength is recognized, supported, and encouraged for its contribution to health. In the process of transpersonal relationships, nurses develop and encourage openness to understanding of self and others. This leads to the development of trusting, accepting relationships in which feelings are shared freely and confidence is inspired. Even a core element of practice such as patient teaching can be carried out in an interpersonal manner true to the philosophy and nature of the caring relationship.

The nurse guided by Watson's work has responsibility for creating and maintaining an environment supporting human caring while recognizing and providing for patients' primary human requirements. In the end, this human-to-human caring approach leads the nurse to respect the overall meaning of life from the perspective of the patient. Watson's (1988) work formalized the theory of human caring from this philosophy. Key aspects of nursing's metaparadigm evident in Watson's work are environment (one that supports human caring), person (both the patient and the nurse), health (in terms of health promotion and illness prevention), and nursing (what nurses contribute to the encounter with the patient).

Clinical example: Watson's philosophy of caring

Understanding how philosophy guides practice can be hard, but an example drawn from a nurse's clinical practice may help. Anna, a hospice nurse, had a patient who was very ill with lung cancer, and who had received both chemotherapy and radiation with the hope of achieving a long remission. The patient, a 60-year-old woman named Mavis, was what some people would refer to as a "character"—full of opinions that she would share with anyone who came close, still smoking, still cursing. Mavis' cancer did not respond to the various therapies, and metastases developed in her brain, causing occasional seizures. It was clear that Mavis was terminally ill. Her abrasive personality did not allow many people to get near her, but she had a particular fondness for Anna, who understood Mavis in a way that few did. They connected on a deep level, and, although they never talked in great depth about Mavis' impending death, Mavis revealed that one of her unfulfilled plans was to be baptized. She did not remember her baptism from childhood and did not want to die without having that memory.

Although nothing in the nursing texts says it is a good idea to take a weakened patient who has weeks to live out into the January cold to church for an immersion baptism, it was Anna's human-to-human caring approach that allowed her to respect the meaning of this event from Mavis' point of view. On a bitterly cold night with a howling wind, Mavis was baptized by a friend who was a minister, her family in attendance, her turban covering her bald head. Mavis told Anna that she was free to die now. Within days she took to her bed. On one of her final days, the family called Anna frantically because Mavis had called for her all day. The on-call nurse covering the weekend simply could not console her, and Mavis' cries for her hospice nurse made the family muster the courage to call Anna on her day off. Anna, knowing Mavis as she did, responded, and when she arrived at the bedside, she asked Mavis what she could do to help her. Mavis' response: "I just wanted to see if you would come." Anna said simply, "I am here." Mavis lapsed into a peaceful coma that evening. Her last words had been to Anna.

Anna practiced nursing with the philosophy that human-to-human relationships are primary in professional practice. In the confines of this deeply caring relationship, Mavis found acceptance and peace from her nurse and was guided into a calm death. Although the nurse whose guiding philosophy is based on human relationships must set clear professional boundaries, this philosophical approach to the practice of nursing raises the possibility of exquisite experiences between humans that transcend the nurse-patient relationship, just as Anna and Mavis experienced.

NURSING CONCEPTUAL MODELS

Conceptual models (or conceptual frameworks) are the second type of theoretical work that provides organizational structures for critical thinking about the processes of nursing (Alligood, 2002c; Fawcett, 2000). These are broad conceptual structures that provide comprehensive, holistic perspectives of nursing by describing the relationships of specific concepts. Models are less abstract and more formalized than the philosophies just discussed in this chapter; models are more abstract, however, than theories of nursing, which will be discussed later. Theories are built from conceptual models much as buildings are constructed from blueprints. The blueprints show the general relationships between parts of the building and are adaptable; conceptual models provide a preliminary view of the relationship between concepts of nursing that can be used to build theory.

Three conceptual models will be presented in the following section. These models represent different decades in the development of nursing theory: they are models developed by Dorothea Orem, Imogene King, and Sister Callista Roy. The focus and perspective of each model are discussed, followed by a brief overview of how that model guides nursing practice. Table 13-2 contains questions that represent how the same patient situation is viewed differently by nurses whose practices are based on the models of Orem, King, or Roy.

Table 13-2   Three Models of Nursing: Three Different Responses to the Same Patient Situation

Dorothea Orem	What deficits does this patient have in providing his own self-care?
Callista Roy	How can I modify this patient's environment to facilitate his adaptation?
Imogene King	What goals can we set together to restore him to health?

Orem's Self-Care Model

Dorothea Orem, born in 1914 in Baltimore, Maryland, first received her diploma in nursing in the 1930s, soon followed by a BS in nursing education in 1939. Six years later she earned an MS in nursing education (Sitzman and Eichelberger, 2004, p. 85). Working as a nurse in a number of roles, Orem first published her concept of self-care in 1959. She continued to develop her conceptual model over several decades, with the sixth edition of her work *Nursing: Concepts of Practice* published in 2001. Over the years Orem formalized three interrelated theories: theory of self-care, theory of self-care deficit, and theory of nursing system. Her model focuses on the patient's self-care capacities and the process of designing nursing actions to meet the patient's self-care needs. In this model, the nurse prescribes and regulates the nursing system on the basis of the patient's self-care deficit, which is the extent to which a patient is incapable of providing effective self-care. An underlying assumption of Orem's model is that "ordinary people in contemporary society want to be in control of their lives" (Pearson, Vaughan, and FitzGerald, 2005, p. 104). Nursing is needed in the presence of an actual or potential self-care deficit (Orem, 2001) when persons cannot provide their own care adequately. Orem's work is widely used in nursing education and practice, providing a comprehensive system for nursing practice in a variety of clinical settings.

Orem and nursing practice

In Orem's model, appropriate care for the patient is developed through a series of three operations: diagnostic, prescriptive, and regulatory. To determine the patient's ability to provide effective self-care, the nurse initiates a diagnostic operation that begins with the establishment of the nurse-patient relationship. This includes contracting with the patient to explore current and potential self-care demands. Factors such as age, gender, and developmental status, as well as sociocultural and environmental factors, are examined in relation to universal, developmental, and health requirements and related self-care actions of the patient. In other words, the patient's baseline ability to provide adequate self-care is assessed by the nurse to determine the extent to which the patient is limited in providing his or her own effective care. These limitations are self-care deficits.

Prescriptive operations occur when therapeutic self-care requisites (based on deficits) are determined and the nurse reviews various methods, actions, and priorities with the patient. This is a planning stage in which the nurse confirms with the patient the nurse's assessment of the patient's needs and begins to formulate a plan of care. In regulatory operations, the nurse designs, plans, and produces a system for care (Berbiglia, 2002). Systems of care range from wholly compensatory, which is the most comprehensive form of care for patients with few (if any) abilities to provide care for self, to supportive-educative, in which the patient has the ability to provide effective self-care, but needs to work with the nurse to further develop these abilities or acquire additional information to promote self-care (George, 2002).

King's Interacting Systems Framework and Theory of Goal Attainment

Imogene King was born in 1923 and received her basic nursing education from St. John's Hospital School of Nursing in St. Louis, Missouri, in 1945. Three years later she completed her bachelor of science in nursing education from St. Louis University; in 1957 she earned her master of science in nursing degree from St. Louis University. In 1961 she completed her doctor of education (EdD) degree from Teachers College, Columbia University, in New York City. Much of her career was spent in academic settings including

Ohio State University, Loyola University, and the University of South Florida (Johnson and Webber, 2005, p. 158).

Although King first published early forms of her theoretical work in 1971, *A Theory for Nursing: Systems, Concepts, Process,* published 10 years later in 1981, contained her first claim to a nursing theory (King, 1981). This complex theory focused on persons, their interpersonal relationships, and social contexts with three interacting systems: personal, interpersonal, and social. Within each of these three systems King identified concepts that provide a conceptual structure describing the processes in each system. Significantly, the focus of the nurse is on phenomena of importance to the patient; unless attention is paid to concerns of the patient, mutual goal setting is unlikely to happen (Sieloff, Frey, and Killeen, 2006, p. 254).

King's interacting systems form a framework to view whole persons in their family and social contexts: the personal system identifies concepts that provide an understanding of individuals, personally and intrapersonally (within the person); the interpersonal system deals with interactions and transactions between two or more persons; and the social system presents concepts that consider social contacts, such as those at school, at work, or in social settings. King's work is unique because it provides a view of persons from the perspective of their interactions (or communications, both verbal and nonverbal) with other people at three levels of interacting systems.

Using King's model in practice

When using King's work, nurses focus on goal attainment for and by the patient. The traditional steps of the nursing process—assessment, planning, goal setting, intervention, and evaluation—are augmented in several ways. The steps of the process describe the type of action the nurse is taking, and at each step the nurse gathers and uses information to provide care. Like the nursing process, King's model is not linear: steps occur simultaneously as the nurse and patient work to identify goals and the best means to attain those goals.

The focus of nursing care is guided by concepts at each of the system levels. For example, the personal system leads the nurse to pay close attention to the patient's perceptions, the interpersonal system guides the nurse to explore the patient's roles and the stresses in each role, and the social system cues the nurse to consider influences on the patient's decision making. In this model, for instance, the nurse providing care for a young woman who is a mother will recognize that the patient's maternal role will influence her decisions regarding her health, keeping the best interests of her children in addition to her own health in mind as she makes health-related decisions.

Interaction with the patient is an important component of King's goal attainment model. Nurses are aware of their communication with patients, identifying steps from the first encounter to the attainment of the specified goal. King describes these steps as a progression from perception, judgment, action, reaction, and interaction to transaction (King, 1981). These steps involve increasing involvement between the nurse and the patient, requiring a deep understanding of the goals of the patient within the various contexts of the patient's life to plan and provide effective nursing care. King emphasized the importance of joint goal setting by nurse and patient, reminding nurses that this relationship involves mutuality. King's process provided a structure for the nurse to monitor the relationship's progress. King clearly specified that the goal of nursing is attaining or regaining health.

Roy's Adaptation Model

Sister Callista Roy was born in Los Angeles, California, in 1939. Her first degree was a bachelor of arts in nursing from Mount St. Mary's College in Los Angeles. She then earned a master's degree in pediatric nursing and sociology, followed by a PhD in sociology from the University of California, Los Angeles. She is a member of the order of Sisters of Saint Joseph of Carondelet. Roy is currently on the faculty of the William F. Connell School of Nursing at Boston College. Although the Roy adaptation model has been in use for 35 years, Sister Roy continues to update, revise, and refine it for use in practice, research, theory, and administration (Roy and Zhan, 2006, pp. 268, 269).

Sister Callista Roy first presented her model as a conceptual framework for a nursing curriculum in 1970 (Pearson et al, 2005, p. 123). In 1976 she published *Introduction to Nursing: An Adaptation Model,* and followed with a second edition in 1984 (Roy, 1976, 1984). Roy updated all of her writing in a comprehensive text in 1999 (Roy and Andrews, 1999). Her model is widely used for education, research, and nursing practice today. She focused on the individual as a biopsychosocial adaptive system and described nursing as a humanistic discipline that emphasizes the person's adaptive or coping abilities. Roy's work is based on adaptation and adaptive behavior, which is produced by altering the environment. According to Roy, the individual and the environment are sources of stimuli that require modification to promote adaptation in the patient. Roy viewed the person as an adaptive system with physiologic, self-concept, role function, and interdependent modes.

Roy's model provides a comprehensive understanding of nursing from the perspective of adaptation. When the demands of environmental stimuli are too high or the person's adaptive mechanisms are too low, the person's behavioral responses are ineffective for coping. Effective adaptive responses promote the integrity of the individual by conserving energy and promoting the survival, growth, reproduction, and mastery of the human system. Nursing promotes the patient's adaptation and coping, with progress toward integration as the goal (Phillips, 2002).

Using Roy's model in practice

The nurse using Roy's model focuses on the adaptation of the patient and on the environment. Adaptation, specifically patients' adaptation behavior and stimuli in the internal and external environments, is assessed and facilitated. On the basis of these assessments, the nurse develops nursing diagnoses to guide goal setting and interventions aimed at promoting adaptation. Simply stated, the nurse modifies the environment to facilitate patient adaptation.

Observable behavior is recognized and understood in the context of Roy's physiologic, self-concept, role function, and interdependent modes. Descriptions of the behaviors included in each mode provide the nurse with a means of making evaluative judgments about the patient's progress toward the goal of adaptation (Phillips, 2002). Roy's model is very widely used in nursing practice and has been described comprehensively in the literature (Alligood, 2002b; Phillips, 2002; Roy and Andrews, 1999).

Clinical example: Roy's adaptation model

A clinical example of Roy's model will help you understand her work in a real world context. Mr. Elderd was referred to a home health agency for wound management. He had a very large open wound on his forehead as a result of a wide excision of several significant basal cell carcinomas. Dean, his nurse, was surprised to see that the wound extended completely to Mr. Elderd's skull. Mr. Elderd was out of work as a result of this wound, saw friends infrequently, and was some what depressed. His wife, although well-meaning, spent hours each day fixing him high-calorie "treats" because she liked to cook and found it was a good way to release her own anxiety about her husband's condition.

Dean's nursing practice was shaped by Roy's adaptation model. In his initial assessment of the home environment, he noticed the cleanliness of the home, the evidence of vigorous family and social ties, adequacy of income, availability of good nutrition, and other indicators of health. What Dean did not understand was why Mr. Elderd's wound was not healing. After Dean's assessment, he believed that there was some "missing link" in Mr. Elderd's adaptive abilities, but he was not sure whether the ineffective coping was psychological, environmental, or physiologic.

Dean visited Mr. Elderd daily for 3 weeks, and, although the wound did not become infected, it showed very little evidence of closure. Dean expressed his concern to Mr. Elderd and decided to ask Mr. Elderd again some basic questions related to his fundamental health practices, including nutrition, activity, sleep, and elimination. Mr. Elderd commented almost off-handedly that he was sleeping fine except that he had to get up to go to the bathroom several times each night. His wife chimed in from the kitchen, "But that's no different than from the day. He is always going to the bathroom. I told him to quit drinking so much water all the time!" Dean, being the experienced nurse that he is and seeking ways to assist patients with all forms of adaptation, realized the likely problem. He called Mr. Elderd's physician and asked for an order to draw a blood chemistry including glucose. Sure enough, Mr. Elderd had undiagnosed diabetes. Mrs. Elderd's stream of goodies from the kitchen aggravated the problem to the point that Mr. Elderd was experiencing polyuria and polydipsia, both signs of diabetes. With aggressive blood glucose level management with insulin, a change in diet, and increasing exercise, Mr. Elderd's wound began to heal almost immediately. He did not require a skin graft as had been feared. The use of Roy's adaptation model allowed Dean to see Mr. Elderd's situation as a function of a variety of maladaptive coping efforts. Correcting the diabetic problem became the foundation for Mr. Elderd's eventual healing and resumption of his usual life activities.

THEORIES OF NURSING

Nursing theories are the third type of theoretical work in the structure of nursing knowledge to be reviewed in this chapter. Fawcett (2000) classified theories according to their breadth and depth. For example, a **grand theory** is a very broad conceptualization of nursing phenomena, while a **middle-range theory** is narrower in focus and makes connections between grand theories and nursing practice (Parker, 2006, p. 7). Theories are less abstract than models and usually propose specific outcomes. Three theories are presented here that are well known and commonly used to shape nursing practice. Table 13-3 contains questions that represent the differing foci of care of nurses whose practices are shaped by the theories

Table 13-3   Three Theories of Nursing: Three Different Responses to the Same Patient Situation

Ida Orlando	How can I best figure out what my patient needs through my interaction with him?
Madeleine Leininger	What are the best ways to provide care to my patient that are culturally congruent?
Hildegard Peplau	Within the relationship with my patient, how can I best help him understand his health problems and develop new, healthier behaviors?

of Hildegard Peplau, Ida Orlando, and Madeleine Leininger.

Peplau's Theory of Interpersonal Relations in Nursing

Peplau, born in 1909, was one of the earliest nurse theorists who recognized the importance of the work of nursing rather than continuing to define and delineate nursing (Pearson et al, 2005, p. 179). After receiving her basic nursing training at the Pottstown, Pennsylvania, Hospital School of Nursing in 1931, Peplau studied interpersonal psychology at Bennington College in Vermont, receiving a bachelor of arts degree. Later she received a master of arts degree in teaching and supervision of psychiatric nursing, followed by an education doctorate (EdD) from Teachers College, Columbia University, in New York City. Although Peplau's first book, *Interpersonal Relations in Nursing*, was published in 1952, it was published again in 1988, reflecting both the value of her work and nursing's continuing focus on interpersonal relationships. Peplau drew from developmental, interactionist, and human needs theories in developing her work (Pearson et al, 2005, p. 179), which grew from her interest in nursing care of psychiatric patients. Peplau believed, however, that all nursing is based on the interpersonal process and the nurse-patient relationship (Forchuk, 1993).

Peplau's theory is based on the premise that the relationship between patient and nurse is the focus of attention, rather than the patient only as the unit of attention (Forchuk, 1993, p. 7). Nursing care occurs within the context of the patient-nurse relationship. The goals of therapeutic interpersonal relationship are twofold: first is the survival of the patient; second is the patient's understanding of his or her health problems and learning from these problems as he or she develops new behavior patterns. As the nurse assists the patient in developing new behavior patterns, the nurse also grows and develops a greater understanding of the effect of universal stressors on the lives and behaviors of individual patients (Pearson et al, 2005, p. 182).

Using Peplau's theory in practice

Although Peplau's theory grew from her experience as a psychiatric nurse, her work is applicable to a wide variety of practice settings. Peplau describes a four-pronged process similar to the nursing process by which the nurse assists the patient in achieving personal growth. Completion of this process involves six roles by the nurse: counselor, resource, teacher, technical expert, surrogate, and leader (Pearson et al, 2005, p. 184). Depending on the setting, the nurse will spend more or less time in each of these roles. For instance, a nurse in a critical care unit will likely spend more time as a technical expert and less time as a counselor, whereas a nurse on a postpartum unit may act as a surrogate, guiding a new mother into independent care of her newborn infant, with less time spent as a leader.

Peplau's theory is complex. Its importance lies in the focus on what happens between the nurse and patient in a therapeutic relationship. Furthermore, Peplau was visionary in her recognition of the importance of the relationship between nurse and patient, publishing early her ideas and continuing to refine and expand her work over several decades. In Chapter 11 (p. 262), you will find a description of an ongoing study at the University of North Carolina at Chapel Hill, named the "HILDA Project." It is named after Hildegard Peplau, on whose theory the intervention being tested is based.

Orlando's Nursing Process Theory

Ida Orlando was born in New York in 1926 and, like many early nurse theorists, received her basic nursing education in a diploma program. She attended nursing school at the New York Medical College School of Nursing, and in 1951 she graduated with a bachelor of science degree in public health nursing from St. John's University in Brooklyn, New York. Three years later, she completed her master's degree in nursing from Columbia University. Her early practice settings included maternity, medicine, and emergency department nursing (Gess, Dombro, Gordon et al, 2006).

Orlando first proposed her theory of effective nursing practice in 1961 in her first book, *The Dynamic Nurse-Patient Relationship: Function, Process and Principles*. She later revised it as a nursing process theory (Orlando, 1990). Her work actually proposed both: it is a theory about how nurses process their observations of patient behavior and also about how they react to patients on the basis of inferences from patients' behavior, including what they say. Orlando's early research revealed that processing observations as specified in her theory led to effective nursing practice and good outcomes.

Orlando's theory is specific to nurse-patient interactions. The goal of the nurse is to determine and meet patients' immediate needs and to improve their situation by relieving distress or discomfort. Orlando emphasized deliberate action (rather than automatic action) based on observation of the patients' verbal and nonverbal behavior, which leads to inferences. Inferences are confirmed or disconfirmed by the patient, leading the nurse to identify the patient's needs and provide effective nursing care.

Using Orlando's theory in practice

In terms of nursing practice, Orlando's theory specified how patients are involved in nurses' decision making. When used in practice, Orlando's theory guides interactions to predictable outcomes, which are different from outcomes that occur when the theory is not used. Nurses individualize care for each patient by attending to behavior, confirming with the patient ideas and inferences the nurse draws from interactions, and identifying pressing needs.

Use of Orlando's theory improves the effectiveness of the nurse by allowing the nurse to get to the "bottom line" more quickly when observing, listening to, and confirming with patients. Therefore use of this theory saves time and energy for both the patient and the nurse.

Leininger's Theory of Culture Care Diversity and Universality

Born in 1924 in Sutton, Nebraska, Madeleine Leininger received her diploma in nursing at St. Anthony's School of Nursing in Denver, Colorado, followed by a bachelor of science degree in biological science from Benedictine College in Atchison, Kansas, 2 years later. She received her MSN from Catholic University in Washington, D.C., in 1954 and her PhD in anthropology from the University of Washington in Seattle in 1965 (Reynolds and Leininger, 1993).

The work of Madeleine Leininger (1978, 1991) in cultural care grew out of her early nursing experiences. She observed that children of different cultures had widely varying behaviors and needs. After discussing the parallels between nursing and anthropology with the famed anthropologist Margaret Mead, Leininger pursued doctoral study in cultural anthropology. Through her doctoral work she became more convinced about the relationship of cultural differences and health practices. This led her to begin developing a theory of cultural care for nursing. Leininger's work is formalized as a theory rather than as a conceptual model. It has stimulated the formation of the Transcultural Nursing Society, transcultural nursing conferences, newsletters, and the *Journal of Transpersonal Caring* and the awarding of master's degrees in the specialty area known as transcultural nursing.

The goal of transcultural nursing involves more than simply being aware of different cultures. It involves planning nursing care based on knowledge that is culturally defined, classified, and tested—and then used to provide care that is culturally congruent (Leininger, 1978). Leininger described theory as a creative and systematic way of discovering new knowledge or accounting for phenomena in a more complete way (Leininger, 1991). She encouraged nurses to use creativity to discover cultural aspects of human needs and use these findings to make culturally congruent therapeutic decisions. Her theory is broad, since it considers the impact of culture on all aspects of human life, with particular attention to health and caring practices. Leininger's theory has become increasingly relevant as global migration continues and societies become more diverse.

Using Leininger's theory in practice

Leininger specified caring as the essence of nursing, and nurses who use Leininger's theory of cultural care in their practices view patients in the context of their cultures. Practice from a cultural perspective begins by respecting the culture of the patient and recognizing the importance of its relationship to nursing care. Use of the "sunrise model" (Figure 13-2) guides the assessment of cultural data for an understanding of its influence on the patient's life (Leininger, 1991). The nurse plans nursing care, recognizing the health beliefs and folk practices of the patient's culture, as well as the culture of traditional health services. To this end, nursing care is then focused on culture care preservation, accommodations, or repatterning, depending on the patient's need. The nursing outcome of culturally congruent nursing care is health and well-being for the patient. Case applications of Leininger's theory in nursing practice may be found in Morgan (2002).

Clinical example: Leininger's theory of culture care diversity and universality

No matter how expert a nurse is in clinical practice, sometimes failure to recognize and appreciate cultural differences can undermine even the best intentions. One such situation occurred when Jan, a nurse with many years of experience providing care for HIV-positive patients in a large urban hospital, decided that she would move to a less chaotic environment. Jan applied for a job

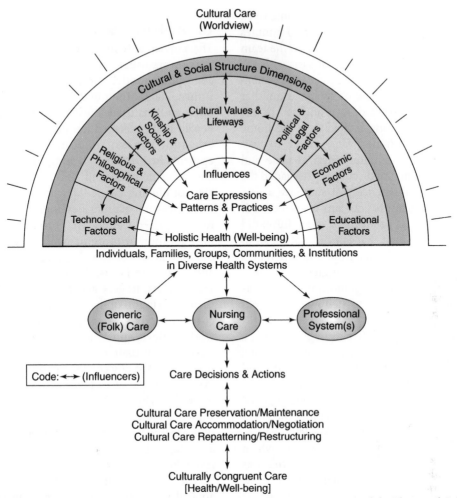

Figure 13-2 Leininger's sunrise model, created to facilitate the application in practice of the Theory of Culture Care Diversity and Universality. (Courtesy Dr. Madeleine Leininger.)

with an agency providing nursing care in the homes of low-income rural women with HIV. Jan had grown up and gone to college in a city in the northeast; her new home was in a rural county in the Deep South.

Almost immediately Jan ran into some unanticipated situations that posed problems for her. She complained at team meetings that her patients were always late for their appointments. Members of the team, each of whom had grown up nearby, explained to her that this was not unusual behavior and that she should plan "waiting time" into her daily schedule. Jan was amazed that the rest of

the team reported good visits and outcomes with their patients, and almost all seemed to be caught up with their work all the time. Jan always felt like she was running behind. She began to question her nursing skills, her knowledge base, and time management behaviors that had served her well in her previous work. Jan described herself as a "fish out of water." She decided that she would spend her "waiting time" by sitting in her car and catching up on paperwork until the patient arrived home.

One day she was invited by the patient's grandmother to wait inside but she declined, saying that she would wait in the car and "get some work done." Her patient arrived home after 20 minutes or so and Jan met with her, reporting to the team later that day that she had a great visit with the patient. Jan's pleasure was short-lived. Her patient called, demanding that she be assigned another nurse because "Jan insulted my grandma." In this community where being invited into the home was considered an honor, Jan's choice to wait instead in the car was interpreted as rude and uncaring. No amount of discussion dissuaded the patient from her insistence that she have a new nurse who "knew how to act." Jan's team met with her, but they too, as products of the culture, did not understand at first that Jan did not mean to be insulting or rude. Because the other members of the team were deeply acculturated, they knew the meaning behind the grandmother's invitation: Jan was an honored, trusted guest who was welcomed in their home.

Jan soon realized that her feelings of being a "fish out of water" in this setting were accurate; in fact she did not understand the culture and was not eager to learn about the cultural norms that so disturbed her. Importantly, she recognized that this prevented her from providing the effective patient care that she desired. She left the position and moved to a more urban area in which she knew the cultural terrain. Although this was a sad chapter in Jan's professional life, she grew from the experience in her understanding of the very deep nature of culture and its influence on the nurse-patient relationship.

THEORETICAL CHALLENGES FOR NURSING EDUCATION, PRACTICE, AND RESEARCH

These examples of nursing theoretical works illustrate the vital position of theory in nursing education, practice, and research. To continue the forward movement of nursing and to improve the quality of nursing care, nurses must engage in theory-based practice, theory-testing research, and theory-generating research. Planning educational curricula based on nursing knowledge and theory is essential to further solidifying the foundations of nursing science.

Theory-Based Education

The curricula (courses of study) of schools of nursing are usually built on one or more specific conceptual models or concepts (McEwen and Brown, 2002). The nursing profession has developed and matured since the early 1950s when Peplau first published her early work that established the modern era of nursing theory development. In 1989 and then again in 2000, Bevis and Watson published a book detailing their view of nursing curricula, with the goal "to create a new curriculum-development orientation for nursing education" (p. 1) to humanize nursing education by recognizing that there are many different modes of knowing shaped by experience and learning (Lewis, Rogers and Naef, 2006). Later, Lewis, Rogers and Naef (2006) published their description of the development of a nursing curriculum that expanded the earlier theoretical work of Bevis and Watson. Sometimes students wonder why their coursework is set up a particular way, usually couched in questions such as, "Why do we have to take this class?" or "What use will this be later?" It is important that nursing students understand that even the coursework they are undertaking is based on a philosophy or a conceptual model that shapes the way nursing is taught.

The nursing profession has evolved from an applied vocation dependent on knowledge from other disciplines to its current stage of development, with its own knowledge base. This period of growth has stimulated—and been stimulated by—the development of the nursing PhD, a research degree that generates new, discipline-specific knowledge. At the doctoral level, nurses are concerned with the philosophy of science—that is, the nature of knowledge and how it is known; the philosophy of nursing science and the generation of nursing knowledge; theory testing; and the development of new theory through research. The master's level nurse may be a primary provider in advanced practice, going beyond the generic nursing process. Master's-prepared nurses use theoretical perspectives focused on the patient for specific nursing outcomes. Many nurses conduct their first research studies as master's students, focusing on nursing practice and the testing of nursing interventions with specific patient groups.

The baccalaureate nurse is introduced to the research process and the use of theory to guide it. The research emphasis for baccalaureate-level students is on learning to critique nursing research, becoming informed consumers of research relevant to evidence-based nursing practice. (See Critical Thinking Challenge 13-1.) Baccalaureate nurses are also introduced to theory through the curriculum at their school. Many curricula of bachelor's of science in nursing programs are based on a particular nursing theoretical perspective; others introduce students to a variety of nursing theoretical perspectives. Whether the curriculum is built around one or many nursing theoretical works, the focus for the baccalaureate level is utilization and application of nursing theory as a guide for nursing practice. Associate degree nursing education programs may also use nursing theoretical works to teach the unique perspectives of nursing. Nurses with associate degrees often find middle-range theories, which are specific to patient care, useful in their practice. The importance of theory in four levels of nursing education is noted in Box 13-5.

Theory-Based Practice

How is theory translated into practice? The answer to that question lies with theory-based practice. Theory-based practice occurs when nurses intentionally structure their practice around a particular nursing theory and use it to guide them as they assess, plan, diagnose, intervene, and evaluate nursing care. Theory provides a systematic way of thinking about nursing that is consistent and guides the decision-making process as data are collected, analyzed, and used in the planning and administration of nursing

practice. Theory provides nurses with the tools to challenge the conventional views of patients, illness, the health care delivery system, and traditional nursing interventions.

We hope that these introductions to some classic nursing theoretical works will lead you to identify works that resonate with your values and that you will select one or two for in-depth study. There are many other nurse theorists whose works are more recent and complex. In addition, there are substantial numbers of nurse theorists who have developed middle-range theories that may be useful to you in specific areas of your practice as you develop your competence as a practitioner. With increased understanding and education, you can integrate the use of nursing theory in your practice.

Many benefits are gained from theory-based practice. First, you will be able to explain your

Box 13-5   Importance of Theory at Four Levels of Nursing Education

PhD in Nursing: Conducts theory testing and theory development research for nursing science development; frames practice, administration, or research in nursing works

Master of Science in Nursing: Frames advanced practice with a nursing model or theory; uses theory to guide research with practice questions

Bachelor of Science in Nursing: Learns the nursing perspective in a nursing model or theory-based curriculum or courses; uses models, theories, and middle-range theories to guide nursing practice

Associate Degree in Nursing: May have a nursing model or theory-guided curriculum or courses; may be introduced to middle-range theories for nursing practice

---

CRITICAL THINKING *Challenge 13-1*

Scan several nursing research studies that are based on nursing theory. Select one article to read carefully; note the theoretical framework on which it is based.

Describe how the authors link the study to nursing theory. Does the use of a theoretical framework strengthen the study? How or how not?

practice to other members of the health care team, sometimes as simply as "This is the way that I view this problem/situation." Your view is shaped by your theoretical orientation to practice. That is, nursing theory provides language for you to explain what you do, how you do it, and why you do it. Second, this language of practice facilitates the transmission of nursing knowledge to you as students who are new to the profession, as well as to other health professionals. Third, theory contributes to professional autonomy by providing a nursing-based guide for practice, education, and research. Finally, nursing theory develops your analytical skills, challenges your thinking, and clarifies your values and assumptions (Holder and Chitty, 1997).

Many nurses have developed their own ideas about nursing and continue to develop nursing assumptions based on education, experience, observation, and reading. Most nurses do not formally develop their own personal theories, even though their ideas influence the way they practice nursing. Wardle and Mandle (1989) studied nurses who believed that their own ideas of practice were "their theories," and they concluded that these nurses' personal theories tended to be incomplete and inconsistent as a basis for nursing practice. When you rely on your personal ideas as a basis for practice or when faculty members use their own ideas as a "framework for curricula," the outcome is ineffective. Wardle and Mandle recommended using a theory that has been tested or developed through nursing research and critiqued, analyzed, and evaluated for usefulness in nursing practice. Each of the philosophies, models, and theories presented in this chapter meets their recommendation. Application of these works in your practice with specific patient groups is an opportunity to test middle-range theories. In addition, many practice areas and patient populations may be addressed in formalized middle-range theories (Alligood, 2002d).

As you engage in theory-based practice, remember to provide feedback to nurse researchers and theorists concerning your experiences. You can do this through the Internet, where you will find groups of nurses using, discussing, and refining the theoretical works that have been discussed in this chapter. The Internet can be a powerful tool to keep you involved with nurses in practice far removed from your own location and practice setting. You can also assist these scholars and the discipline of nursing by developing manuscripts and submitting your experiences for publication, joining the many nurses who have discovered the benefits of theory-based practice.

Theory-Based Research

Great strides have been made in the last 25 years in nursing research. The expansion of graduate nursing education at the master's level and the proliferation of nursing doctoral programs played a major role, as more nurses than ever before were equipped with the knowledge and skills to conduct research. Nursing research tests and refines the knowledge base of nursing. Ultimately, research findings enable nurses to improve the quality of care and understand how evidence-based nursing actions influence patient outcomes.

Research is vital to the future of nursing, and theory is integral to research. Historically, an emphasis on method has overshadowed the subject of our research and the theory for developing nursing knowledge. In addition, many nurses have continued to use theories that address the phenomena of other disciplines—theories that do

Cultural Considerations Challenge
Using Nursing Theory to Bridge the Cultural Gap

The issue of immigration is very important in today's world. The influx of Latino immigrants into the United States has brought with it the challenges of care of persons with whom you may share no language and have little understanding of the context of their lives. Yet your professional nursing ethic demands that you provide the same level of care as you do with other patients with whom you share more in common. How can the philosophies/frameworks/theories presented in this chapter be adapted to your practice in a way that will assist you in providing excellent care under these circumstances?

not view persons holistically or provide a nursing perspective. However, more and more nurse researchers have come to understand the vital role of nursing theory in their research for knowledge development in their own discipline. These nurses are meeting the challenge of using nursing theory to structure nursing research that tests theory or that interprets the findings of qualitative research for theory development.

Summary of Key Points

- Theory development is not a mysterious activity restricted to a few nursing scholars. It is an activity that combines education, knowledge, and skill in a sustained effort.
- Nursing philosophies, models, and theories offer many perspectives on nursing, varying in their levels of abstraction and their definitions of four major concepts known as nursing's metaparadigm: person, environment, health, and nursing.
- As nurses devise theories of nursing, have them reviewed by their nursing colleagues in a peer-review process, publish them in the nursing literature, and test their efficacy in nursing practice, the discipline moves forward in the development of its unique knowledge base.
- Scholarly contributions may be made by nurses at every level of educational preparation. To the extent that nurses question, read, study, network, and write about nursing practice, they contribute to the development of nursing knowledge.
- Nurses in practice settings have invaluable insights and observations, thereby contributing to the knowledge base for nursing. Nursing theorists' early work often grew out of their clinical observations and experiences. Theorists rely on practicing nurses to test clinical interventions and explore the usefulness of their theories.
- Nurse theorists whose works were reviewed in this chapter, as well as others too numerous to include, have made significant contributions to the development of the unique body of nursing knowledge.

- Nurse scholars continue to develop and refine the works of nursing theorists. Each theoretical work has a community of scholars who use the work in their research and practice and continue to expand, clarify, and refine these original works.

Critical Thinking Questions

1. Recognizing that your understanding of the theoretical works of nursing is only beginning, which philosophy/conceptual framework/theory introduced in this chapter appeals to you the most? Which ones describe nursing in the way you think about it? What is it about these works that intrigues you?
2. In thinking about the three different examples of philosophy, conceptual frameworks, and theories, which will be the most useful to help you organize your thoughts for critical thinking and decision making in nursing practice?
3. Describe the use of nursing theory for nurses at your current level of nursing education, and how you can begin to shape your practice even during early clinical experiences.
4. Explain why theory development is important to the profession of nursing.

⊖volve *To enhance your understanding of this chapter, try the Student Exercises on the Evolve site at http://evolve.elsevier.com/Chitty/professional.*

REFERENCES

Alligood MR: The nature of knowledge needed for nursing practice. In Alligood MR, Tomey AM, editors: *Nursing theory: utilization and application,* ed 2, St Louis, 2002a, Mosby, pp 3-14.

Alligood MR: Nursing models: normal science for nursing practice. In Alligood MR, Tomey AM, editors: *Nursing theory: utilization and application,* ed 2, St Louis, 2002b, Mosby, pp 15-39.

Alligood MR: Philosophies, models and theories: critical thinking structures. In Alligood MR, Tomey AM, editors: *Nursing theory: utilization and application,* ed 2, St Louis, 2002c, Mosby, pp 41-61

Alligood MR: Areas for further development of theory-based nursing practice. In Alligood MR, Tomey AM, editors: *Nursing theory: utilization and application,* ed 2, St Louis, 2002d, Mosby, pp 453-463.

Alligood MR, Tomey AM: *Nursing theory: utilization and application*, ed 2, St Louis, 2002, Mosby.

Berbiglia V: Orem's self-care deficit theory in nursing practice, In Alligood MR, Tomey AM, editors: *Nursing theory: utilization and application*, ed 2, St Louis, 2002, Mosby, pp 239-266.

Bevis EO, Watson J: *Toward a caring curriculum: a new pedagogy for nursing*, New York, 1989, National League for Nursing.

Bevis EO, Watson J: *Toward a caring curriculum: a new pedagogy for nursing*, Boston, 2000, Jones & Bartlett.

Chinn P, Kramer M: *Theory and nursing: a systematic approach*, ed 5, St Louis, 1998, Mosby.

Fawcett J: *Analysis and evaluation of contemporary nursing knowledge: models and theories*, Philadelphia, 2000, FA Davis.

Forchuk C: *Hildegard E. Peplau: interpersonal nursing theory*, Newbury Park, Calif, 1993, Sage Publications.

George JB, editor: *Nursing theories: the base for professional nursing practice*, ed 5, Norwalk, Conn, 2002, Appleton & Lange.

Gess T, Dombro M, Gordon SC, et al: Part one: twentieth-century nursing. Wiedenbach, Henderson, and Orlando's theories and their applications, In Parker ME, editor: *Nursing theories and nursing practice*, ed 2, Philadelphia, 2006, FA Davis.

Henderson V: *The nature of nursing: a definition and its implications for practice, research, and education*, New York, 1966, Macmillan.

Holder PJ, Chitty KK: Theory as a basis for professional nursing, In Chitty KK, editor: *Professional nursing: concepts and challenges*, ed 2, Philadelphia, 1997, Saunders.

Johnson BM, Webber PB: *An introduction to theory and reasoning in nursing*, ed 2, Philadelphia, 2005, Lippincott Williams & Wilkins.

King IM: *A theory for nursing: systems, concepts, process*, New York, 1981, John Wiley & Sons.

Leininger M: *Transcultural nursing: concepts, theories, and practices*, New York, 1978, John Wiley & Sons.

Leininger M: *Culture care diversity and universality: a theory of nursing*, New York, 1991, National League for Nursing.

Lewis S, Rogers M, Naef R: Caring-human science philosophy in nursing education: beyond the curriculum revolution, *International Journal for Human Caring* 10(4):31-37, 2006.

March A, McCormack D: Nursing theory-directed healthcare, *Holist Nurs Pract* 23(2):75-80, 2009.

McEwen M, Brown SC: Conceptual frameworks in undergraduate nursing curricula: report of a national survey, *J Nurs Educ* 41(1):5-14, 2002.

Morgan MG: Leininger's theory of culture care diversity and universality in nursing practice. In Alligood MR, Tomey AM, editors: *Nursing theory: utilization and application*, ed 2, St Louis, 2002, Mosby, pp 385-402.

Nightingale F: *Notes on nursing: what it is and what it is not*, New York, 1969, Dover Publications (originally published in 1859).

Orem D: *Nursing: concepts of practice*, ed 6, St Louis, 2001, Mosby.

Orlando I: *The dynamic nurse-patient relationship: function, process and principles*, New York, 1990, National League for Nursing (originally published in 1961).

Parker M: *Nursing theories and nursing practice*, Philadelphia, 2006, FA Davis.

Pearson A, Vaughan B, FitzGerald M: *Nursing models for practice*. Edinburgh, United Kingdom, 2005, Butterworth Heinemann.

Peplau HE: *Interpersonal relations in nursing*, New York, 1952/1988, GP Putnam's Sons.

Phillips KD: Roy's adaptation model in nursing practice, In Alligood MR, Tomey AM, editors: *Nursing theory: utilization and application*, ed 2, St Louis, 2002, Mosby, pp 289-314.

Pilson EM: Using nursing theory in nursing education [letter], *AORN J* 89(2):266, 2009.

Reynolds CL, Leininger M: *Madeleine Leininger: cultural care diversity and universality theory*, Newbury Park, Calif, 1993, Sage Publications.

Roy C Sr: *Introduction to nursing: an adaptation model*, Old Tappan, NJ, 1976, Prentice Hall.

Roy C Sr: *Introduction to nursing: an adaptation model*, ed 2, Englewood Cliffs, NJ, 1984, Prentice Hall.

Roy C Sr, Andrews HA: *The Roy adaptation model*, ed 2, Norwalk, Conn, 1999, Appleton & Lange.

Roy C Sr, Zhan L: Sister Callista Roy's adaptation model and its applications, In Parker ME, editor: *Nursing theories and nursing practice*, ed 2, Philadelphia, 2006, FA Davis.

Sieloff CL, Frey M, Killeen M: Part two: applications of King's theory of goal attainment, In Parker ME, editor: *Nursing theories and nursing practice*, ed 2, Philadelphia, 2006, FA Davis, pp 244-267.

Sitzman K, Eichelberger LW: *Understanding the work of nurse theorists: a creative beginning*, Sudbury, Mass, 2004, Jones & Bartlett.

Tomey AM, Alligood MR: *Nursing theorists and their work*, ed 5, St Louis, 2002, Mosby.

Wardle MG, Mandle CL: Conceptual models used in clinical practice, *West J Nurs Res* 11(1):108-114, 1989.

Watson J: *Nursing: the philosophy and science of caring*, Boston, 1979, Little, Brown.

Watson J: *Nursing: human science and human care*, New York, 1988, National League for Nursing.

Watson J: *Postmodern nursing and beyond*, Edinburgh, United Kingdom, 1999, Churchill Livingstone/WB Saunders/Harcourt Health Sciences.

The Health Care Delivery System

Kay Kittrell Chitty

CHAPTER

14

LEARNING OUTCOMES

After studying this chapter, students will be able to:

- Describe the four basic categories of services provided by the health care delivery system
- Describe the shared governance model and explain its use in nursing
- Describe the relationship between cost-containment and quality management initiatives
- Relate two major mechanisms used to maintain quality in health care agencies
- Explain how disparities in health care disproportionately impact minority and poor populations
- Identify the key members of the interdisciplinary health care team and explain what each contributes

- Discuss seven primary roles of nurses in the health care delivery system
- Differentiate among five nursing care delivery systems in use today
- Explain the economic principles of supply and demand, free-market economies, and price sensitivity and discuss their relevance to health care costs
- Explain cost-containment efforts and their impact on nursing practice
- Describe current methods of payment for health care
- Discuss the role of nurses in managing costs
- Discuss universal health care as an outcome of health care reform

---

THE HEALTH CARE DELIVERY SYSTEM

The term *health care delivery system* as it is used in the United States is a misnomer. Far from providing health care, our system has traditionally provided care for illness, focusing on treating health problems once they have occurred rather than encouraging disease prevention through healthy living. The complexity of the system, with multiple types of financing and many different settings where patients can receive services, has resulted in a fragmented system that is difficult to understand and navigate. Although this country has the best technology, the most sophisticated procedures, and the best-educated health care providers in the world, many people do not have access to basic care, and even fewer to health promotion and maintenance services.

The U.S. government, while promising to do so for decades, has not yet devised a definitive

national health policy. A first step, however, has been taken. In 1979 the federal government initiated the Healthy People program, a science-based program that sets forth, every 10 years, national objectives focusing on health promotion and disease prevention. Every decade Healthy People sets and monitors national health objectives, building on lessons learned in the previous decade. Input is sought from both experts and the general public through a collaborative process. The two broad goals of *Healthy People 2010* were (1) to increase quality and years of healthy life and (2) to eliminate health disparities (Healthy People, 2005a). *Healthy People 2010* identified 10 leading health indicators that reflected the major health concerns of the United States at the beginning of the twenty-first century. They were physical activity, overweight and obesity, tobacco use, substance abuse, responsible sexual behavior, mental health, injury and violence, environmental quality, immunization, and access to care (*Healthy People 2010*, 2005b). These indicators were used to measure the health of the nation during the 10-year period. Healthy People is currently under revision, and new goals and objectives will be published in 2010 for the decade 2010 to 2020. You can find more information on the specific focus areas of Healthy People 2010 and the upcoming Healthy People 2020 online at http://www.healthypeople.gov.

As positive as the Healthy People initiative is, it is a voluntary program that does not mandate any real change in the health care system. Individuals, agencies, communities, and states may choose to participate in Healthy People programs or not. For real change to occur, health care reform will have to come from the national level and be mandatory. During the 2008 presidential campaign and since taking office, the Obama administration has taken steps to invigorate the reform debate. As this text goes to press in November, 2009, Congress has not yet acted on reform legislation. Time will tell if system-wide reform can be attained in the current political and economic climate.

This chapter describes the existing health care delivery system, examines nursing's role within this system, and discusses health care finance.

Major Categories of Health Care Services

Regardless of the setting in which services are provided—clinics, hospitals, homes, primary care providers' offices, or elsewhere—there are basically four major categories of health services: health promotion and maintenance, including early detection; illness prevention; diagnosis and treatment; and rehabilitation and long-term care. Each of these categories is briefly explained below.

Health promotion and maintenance

Health promotion and maintenance services assist patients to remain healthy, prevent diseases and injuries, detect diseases early, and promote healthier lifestyles. These services require patients' active participation and cannot be performed solely by health care providers. Health promotion and maintenance services are based on the assumption that patients who adopt healthy lifestyles are likely to avoid lifestyle-related diseases, such as heart attacks, lung cancers, and certain infections.

An example of health promotion and maintenance services is prenatal classes. By learning good nutritional and weight management habits, an expectant mother can take better care of herself and her baby during pregnancy and after delivery. This increases the chances of a normal pregnancy and the full-term delivery of a healthy baby. Other examples of health promotion and maintenance include education about aerobic exercise and responsible sexual activity.

Health promotion also includes the detection of warning signs indicating the presence of a disease in early stages. Early detection allows treatment to be minimal and less costly and fosters positive treatment outcomes. An example of early detection is breast self-examination and mammography, both aimed at detecting breast cancer in its early stages, thereby providing a better chance for treatment to be successful.

Illness prevention

With the increasing ability to identify risk factors, such as a family history of disease and genetic predispositions, illness prevention services are now better able to assist patients in reducing the impact of those risk factors on their health and well-being. These services require the patient's active participation.

Prevention services differ from health promotion services in that they address health problems after risk factors are identified, whereas health promotion services seek to prevent development of risk factors. For example, a health promotion program might teach the detrimental effects of alcohol and drugs on health to prevent individuals from using alcohol and drugs. Illness prevention services are used when the patient has been using alcohol or drugs and is at risk for development of health problems as a result. The boundary between health promotion and maintenance, early detection, and illness prevention is often blurred. Box 14-1 gives examples of activities in these three areas.

Box 14-1   Examples of Health Promotion and Maintenance, Early Detection, and Illness Prevention Activities

HEALTH PROMOTION/MAINTENANCE
- Health education programs (e.g., prenatal classes)
- Exercise programs
- Health fairs
- Wellness programs (worksite/school)
- Nutrition education

EARLY DETECTION
- Mammograms
- Vision and hearing screening
- Cholesterol screening
- Periodic histories and physical examinations
- Blood glucose screening
- Osteoporosis screening

ILLNESS PREVENTION
- Community health programs
- Promotion of healthy lifestyles to counteract risk factors
- Occupational safety programs (e.g., use of eye protection for work that endangers the eyes)
- Environmental safety programs (e.g., proper disposal of hazardous waste)
- Legislation that prevents injury or disease (e.g., seat belt/child restraint laws; motorcycle helmet laws)

Diagnosis and treatment

Traditionally, in the U.S. health care system, heavy emphasis has been put on diagnosis and treatment. Modern technology has enabled the medical profession to refine methods of diagnosing illnesses and disorders and to treat them more effectively than in the past. Scientific advances permit many noninvasive tests and treatments to be performed. Widely available technologies that were unheard of only a few years ago include the use of ultrafast computed tomographic (CT) scans to detect calcification in coronary arteries and live three-dimensional (3-D) ultrasonography that creates 3-D images of structures such as

the fetal face, hand, or spine. The future promises more noninvasive high technologies.

Minimally invasive surgery techniques have transformed surgical procedures, allowing incisions of an inch or less. This technology has reduced postoperative pain, reduced hospital stays from days to hours thereby reducing costs, and enabled patients to return to normal function much more rapidly.

Unfortunately, high-tech services can lead patients to feel dehumanized. This occurs when caregivers focus on machines and techniques rather than on patients. Even in high-tech settings, nurses must remember that patients benefit most when they understand their diagnoses and treatments and can be active participants in the development and implementation of their own treatment plans, in other words, when care is patient centered.

Rehabilitation and long-term care

Rehabilitation services help restore the patient to the fullest possible level of function and independence after injury or illness. Rehabilitation programs also deal with conditions that leave patients with less than full functioning, such as strokes or severe burns. Both patients and their families must be active participants in this care if it is to be successful. Rehabilitation services should begin as soon as the patient's condition has stabilized after an injury or illness. These services may be provided in institutional settings such as hospitals, in special rehabilitation facilities, in long-term care facilities such as nursing homes, or in the home and the community. The objectives of rehabilitation are to assist patients to achieve their full potential and return to a level of functioning that permits them to be contributing members of society.

Rehabilitation services also include **disease management** services. Disease management services deal with chronic diseases, such as congestive heart failure and diabetes, and ongoing conditions, such as low back pain and hypertension, that contribute to higher health care costs and a reduced quality of life, particularly for aging populations. Disease management programs focus on helping participants understand and manage their chronic conditions more effectively through phone calls or e-mails, coaching and education, symptom prevention and management, and collaboration with their providers. These steps give providers information between office visits so that they can actively manage the participant's condition before emergency or hospital services are required, thus reducing health care costs and improving the quality of life for their patients.

Long-term care is provided in residential facilities such as assisted-living homes, skilled and intermediate nursing homes, and personal care homes. Each facility is tailored to provide services that the patient or family cannot provide but at a level that maintains the individual's independence as long as possible. With the aging of the population, and with more patients surviving severe trauma and disease with impairments in physical or mental functioning or both, long-term care facilities are expected to experience continuing growth.

Classifications of Health Care Agencies

There are many agencies involved in the total health care delivery system. Organizations that deliver care can be classified in three major ways: as governmental or voluntary agencies; as not-for-profit or for-profit agencies; or by the level of health care services they provide.

Governmental (public) agencies

Many governmental (public) agencies contribute to the health and well-being of U.S. citizens. All of these public agencies are primarily supported by taxes, administered by elected or appointed officials, and tailored to the needs of the communities served.

Federal agencies. Federal agencies focus on the health of all U.S. citizens. They promote and conduct health and illness research, provide funding to train health care workers, and assist communities in planning health care services. They also develop health programs and services and provide financial and personnel support to staff them. Federal agencies establish standards of practice and safety for health care workers and conduct national health education programs on subjects such as the benefits of not smoking, prevention of acquired immunodeficiency syndrome (AIDS), and the need for prenatal care. Examples of federal agencies are the National Institutes of Health (NIH), the U.S. Department of Health and Human Services (DHHS), the Occupational Safety and Health Administration (OSHA), the Centers for Medicare & Medicaid Services (CMS), and the Centers for Disease Control and Prevention (CDC).

State agencies. State health agencies oversee programs that affect the health of citizens within an individual state. Examples of state agencies include state departments of health and environment, departments of mental health, regulatory bodies that regulate and license health professionals such as state boards of nursing, and agencies that administer Medicaid insurance programs for the poor. These agencies are not typically involved in providing direct patient care but license and support local agencies that do provide direct care.

Local agencies. Local agencies serve one community, one county, or a few adjacent counties. They provide services to both paying and nonpaying citizens. Public health departments are examples of local governmental agencies found in almost every county in the United States. All citizens, whether or not they can pay, are eligible for certain health care services through local public health departments. These services usually include immunizations, prenatal care and counseling, well-baby and well-child clinics, sexually transmitted infection clinics, tuberculosis clinics, and others. Public health nurses sometimes make home visits as well.

Voluntary (private) agencies

Citizens often voluntarily support agencies working to promote or restore health. When private volunteers support an agency providing health care, it is called a voluntary (private) agency. Support is generally through private donations, although many of these agencies apply for governmental grants to support some of their activities.

Voluntary agencies often begin when a group of individuals band together to address a health problem. Volunteers may initially perform all their services. Later, they may obtain enough donations to hire personnel, staff an office, and expand services. They may be able to secure ongoing funding through grants or organizations such as the United Way. Examples of voluntary health agencies are the American Heart Association (Figure 14-1), the American Cancer Society, the American Red Cross, and the March of Dimes.

Not-for-profit or for-profit agencies

The second major way to classify health service delivery agencies is by what is done with the income earned by the agency. A not-for-profit agency is one that uses profits to pay personnel, improve services, advertise services, provide educational programs, or otherwise contribute to the mission of the agency. A common misconception is that not-for-profit agencies do not ever make a profit. Actually, they may make profits, but the profits must be used to further the mission of the agency. Most voluntary agencies, such as the ones listed previously, are also not-for-profit agencies, as are many hospitals.

For-profit agencies distribute profits earned to partners or shareholders. The growth in for-profit health care agencies has risen over the past several decades because of the potential for health care to be very profitable.

For-profit agencies include numerous home health care companies that send nurses and other health personnel to care for patients at home. Several large national chains of for-profit health care providers also exist and have demonstrated that it is possible to provide quality patient care and make a profit while doing so. Examples include national nursing home networks, specialty outpatient centers for ambulatory surgery, heart hospitals, and rehabilitation centers. A controversial issue related to for-profit health care organizations is that they do not typically treat nonpaying patients. These people must go to publicly funded facilities that are rapidly becoming overburdened with patients who are unable to pay their bills.

Level of health care services provided

The third way in which health care services can be classified is by the level of health care services they provide. These levels have traditionally been termed primary care, secondary care, and tertiary care. A new level, subacute care, has emerged. These four levels are discussed below.

Primary care services. Care rendered at the point at which a patient first enters the health care system is considered primary care. This care may be provided in a student health clinic, community health centers, emergency departments, physicians' offices, nurse practitioners' clinics, or health clinics at worksites. The major goals of the primary health care system are providing the following:
1. Entry into the system
2. Emergency care
3. Health maintenance
4. Long-term and chronic care
5. Treatment of temporary health problems that do not require hospitalization

In addition to treating common health problems, primary care centers are, for many citizens, where

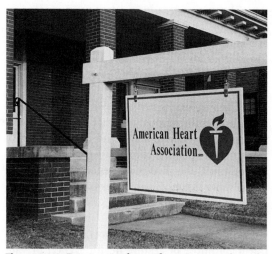

Figure 14-1 Private, not-for-profit agencies, such as the American Heart Association, provide a variety of health-related services to the citizens of their communities. (Photo by Kelly Whalen.)

much of prevention and health promotion takes place. Access to primary care in the least costly setting is now mandated by third-party payers such as insurance companies, the government, and managed care organizations.

Secondary care services. Secondary care involves the prevention of complications from disease. It includes such activities as treating temporary dysfunctions requiring medical intervention or hospitalization, evaluating long-term care, evaluating patients with chronic illness who may need treatment changes, and providing counseling or therapies that are not available in primary care settings.

Although hospitals have traditionally been associated with this level of care, other agencies increasingly provide secondary health services. They include home health agencies, ambulatory care agencies, skilled nursing agencies, and surgical centers. These settings offer skilled personnel, easy access, convenient parking, compact equipment and monitoring systems, medications and anesthesia services, and a financial reimbursement program that rewards shorter lengths of stay and home or community care.

A recent addition to secondary care is the disease management industry mentioned earlier. Health services are provided to patients with chronic diseases through outbound/inbound calls with nurses and health professionals, patients' interactive voice responses (using a touch-tone phone to respond to questions that are entered into an electronic health record), educational videos/books sent to the patient, and Internet-based tools such as e-mail and videoconferencing. To use these services, patients do not have to leave their homes; they have access to health education, coaching, and electronic tools 24 hours a day, 7 days a week. Another advantage is that patients develop a long-term relationship with their disease management nurse or health professional, which improves communication and fosters trust.

Tertiary care services. Tertiary care services are those provided to acutely ill patients, to those requiring long-term care, to those needing rehabilitation services, and to terminally ill patients. Tertiary care usually involves many health professionals working on interdisciplinary teams to design and implement treatment plans.

Examples of tertiary agencies are specialized hospitals such as trauma centers, burn centers, and pediatric hospitals; long-term care facilities offering skilled nursing, intermediate care, and supportive care; rehabilitation centers; and hospices, where care is provided to the terminally ill and their families in the hospital, in the home, or in special hospice "houses."

Subacute care services. An additional segment of health care—subacute care services—emerged in the 1990s. Subacute care is defined as inpatient care that lies between hospital care and long-term care. It is goal-oriented, comprehensive, inpatient care designed for an individual who has had an acute illness, injury, or exacerbation of a disease process. Generally, the condition of an individual receiving subacute care is less complex and does not depend heavily on high-technology monitoring or complex diagnostic procedures. The goal of subacute services is to provide lower-cost health care and create a seamless transition for patients moving through the health care system.

Subacute care is generally more intensive than skilled nursing facility care and less intensive than acute inpatient care. It requires frequent patient assessment and review of the clinical course and treatment plan for a limited time period ranging from several days to several months, until a condition is stabilized or a predetermined treatment course is completed.

Organizational Structures Within Health Care Agencies

The health care delivery system in the United States consists of a variety of agencies such as hospitals, clinics, associations, long-term care facilities, and home health services that provide any of the four major types of health services just discussed. Although the mission, category, and level of health care services provided vary, the organizational structures within them may be similar.

Organizational structure

Organizational structure refers to how an agency is organized to accomplish its mission. The organizational structure of most agencies includes a governing body or board of directors, which may also be called a board of trustees.

Board of directors. In the past, board members were often chosen from two groups: community philanthropists, who were expected to donate generously to the facility; and physicians, who practiced in the institution. Boards were large, met infrequently, and had mainly ceremonial functions.

As the health care environment became more complex, board members were chosen to represent various business and political interests of the community. They were expected to bring knowledge and expertise from the business world, as well as to have an appreciation and understanding of health care agencies and how they operate.

Boards now carry significant responsibility for the mission of the organization, the quality of services provided, and the financial stability of the organization. Boards are not involved in the day-to-day running of the agency, but they are legally responsible for establishing policies governing operations and for ensuring that the policies are executed. They delegate responsibility for running the agency to the chief executive officer (CEO). Boards of directors may or may not be paid for their services. Box 14-2 outlines a typical hospital board's primary responsibilities.

Chief executive officer. The chief executive officer (CEO) is the individual responsible for the overall operation on a daily basis. He or she usually has a minimum of a master's degree in business or hospital administration. Responsibilities include making sure that the institution runs efficiently and is cost-effective and carrying out policies established by the board. The CEO also has an important external role addressing health care issues in the community and usually sits on the

---

Box 14-2   Board of Directors' Responsibilities

- Mission development and long-range planning
- Ensuring high-quality care
- Oversight of medical staff credentialing
- Financial oversight
- Selection and evaluation of the hospital chief executive officer
- Board self-evaluation and education

Adapted from American Hospital Association: *Welcome to the board: an orientation for the new health care trustee,* Chicago, 1999, AHA Press.

---

board of directors, as well as reports to it. A chief operating officer (COO) often assists the CEO in larger organizations.

Nurses with advanced degrees and experience in administration, business, and health care policy increasingly occupy both CEO and COO positions. Boards, who are responsible for hiring CEOs, have found that the broad holistic education and clinical experience of nurses prepares them well for these positions.

Medical staff. A medical staff consists of physicians, who may be either employees of the health care organization or independent practitioners. In either case they must be granted privileges by the board of trustees to see patients at that particular institution. They cannot simply decide to admit patients to an institution. A credentials committee, composed of members of the medical staff, performs the credentialing process. This committee is charged with the responsibility of assuring the board of directors that every physician admitted to the medical staff of that facility is a qualified and competent practitioner and that, over time, each one keeps his or her skills and knowledge updated.

The medical staff, through its credentials committee, is also charged with the responsibility for credentialing nonphysician providers who admit or consult with patients. These include advanced practice nurses, psychologists, optometrists, podiatrists, and others.

Medical staff governance. In large organizations, medical staffs are usually organized by service (e.g., department of surgery, department of medicine, department of obstetrics). The entire medical staff usually elects a chief of staff. The chief of staff and the chiefs of the various services work together with the CEO and other administrative representatives through the medical executive committee to make important decisions about medical policy and physician discipline for the institution. The rules and regulations that govern these activities are called bylaws. The board of directors, to which the physicians are responsible, must officially approve the credentialing and disciplinary actions of the medical staff.

Service on committees and leadership positions of the medical staff are time-consuming activities; therefore some institutions pay members of the medical staff a fee for special services in recognition that time away from seeing patients reduces their income.

Nursing staff. The senior administrative nurse in an organization is known as the chief nurse executive (CNE) or chief nursing officer (CNO), vice president for nursing, or director of nursing. Once excluded from broad institutional decision making, nurse executives today are often members of the board of directors. Progressive organizations now recognize that the nurse executive and the chief of the medical staff are of equal importance, and this is reflected in their organizational charts.

The educational preparation of nurse executives usually includes a minimum of a master's degree in nursing, business, or health administration. Some nurse executives hold joint master's of science in nursing and business administration (MSN/MBA) or joint master's of science in health and business administration (MHA/MBA).

Nurse executives are responsible for overseeing all the nursing care provided in the institution and serve as clinical leaders and administrators. Because of the need to coordinate patient care and outcomes among all disciplines, the role may also include administrative responsibilities for departments other than nursing, such as surgery,

pharmacy, respiratory therapy, and social services, among others.

The nursing staff consists of all the registered nurses (RNs), licensed practical nurses/licensed vocational nurses, patient care technicians, and clerical assistants employed by the department of nursing. These staff members are usually organized according to the units on which they work.

Each patient care unit has its own budget and staff, for which the unit manager is responsible. The manager, who is usually a nurse, is also a communication link between the staff and the next level of management.

In large or networked organizations, there may be an additional level of management between the nurse executive and the manager of a unit. These are middle managers, known as clinical directors or supervisors. In most cases, they are also nurses, but they may come from other clinical disciplines or from a business background. These directors are responsible for multiple units or for specific projects or programs. They ensure that nursing and all other services they manage are integrated with other hospital services. They also serve as the communication link between the unit managers and the executive staff.

Other nurses combine direct patient care responsibilities with research, education, and management responsibilities, such as nurse educators, nurse researchers and clinical nurse specialists, and infection control nurses. Nurses in these roles support direct care nurses and serve as expert resources to them in their areas of specialization.

Nursing organization governance. In most health care agencies, nurses have a nursing staff organization. In some settings it serves mainly as a communication vehicle. In other more enlightened settings, nurses are expected to govern themselves through the organization, much as the medical staff is expected to govern itself through the medical staff organization.

The concept of shared governance is founded on the philosophy that employees have both a right and a responsibility to govern their own work and time within a financially secure, patient-centered system. Shared governance promotes decentralization and participation at all levels of nursing. In shared governance the role of the clinical nursing staff is to be responsible for the professional practice of their nursing unit by adhering to standards and benchmarks of quality care (Davis, 2008). The role of the nurse manager and other nurse leaders is to set expectations, facilitate, coordinate, support, and partner with the staff in achieving the identified goals. Therefore to achieve shared governance, nurse leaders must believe in the ability of their staff (Kerfoot, 2005). An example of shared governance is self-scheduling, in which staff members determine their own schedules based on established guidelines for staffing the unit set forth by the manager. The shared governance model promotes improved patient outcomes and enhanced nurse job satisfaction brought about by increased autonomy.

Health care organizations are complex entities. The way they are organized may vary, but each has an organizational chart that shows its unique structure and explains lines of authority. When considering employment in a health care organization, you can learn a great deal by examining its organizational chart to see how nursing is governed and how it relates to senior management and the board of directors. Figure 14-2 shows

an example of a basic health care organizational chart.

Maintaining Quality in Health Care Agencies

Regardless of how they are organized or the type of services they provide, maintaining high-quality services should be a goal of all health care agencies. As pressure increases to control costs, it becomes even more important to ensure that quality is not sacrificed to save dollars. This can be accomplished in a variety of ways with two chief means being accreditation processes and quality care initiatives.

Accreditation of health care agencies

Health care organizations such as hospitals, home health agencies, and long-term care facilities seek accreditation through one of two accrediting bodies approved by the CMS. They are The Joint Commission, a not-for-profit organization that serves as the nation's predominant standard-setting and accrediting body in health care (The Joint Commission, 2009), and the Healthcare Facilities Accreditation Program (HFAP), authorized by the Centers for Medicare and Medicaid Services (CMS). The goal of accreditation is to improve patient outcomes. Accreditation is important and requires that a number of standards be met

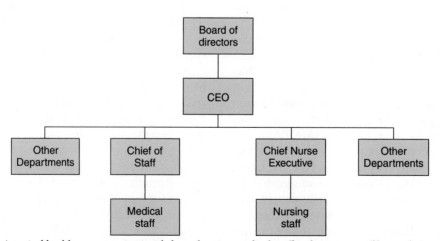

Figure 14-2 A typical health care organizational chart showing medical staff and nursing staff lines of responsibility.

in every department. Considerable resources of time and money are spent making sure accreditation criteria, set by these external accrediting bodies, are met.

Continuous quality improvement and total quality management

An additional strategy through which most organizations choose to work internally toward improvement in patient outcomes is continuous quality improvement.

The concept of continuous quality improvement (CQI) was first developed by management expert W. Edwards Deming in the 1940s when he suggested that managers in industry should rely on groups of employees, which he called quality circles, as they made decisions about how work was to be done. In today's health care systems, CQI, also called total quality management (TQM), is one of the most important concepts borrowed from industry. Rather than trying to identify mistakes after they have occurred, these systems focus on establishing procedures for ensuring high-quality patient care. Using quality improvement concepts, groups of employees from different departments decide how care will be provided. They decide what outcomes are desired and design systems and assign roles and activities to create those outcomes. Every effort is made to anticipate potential problems and prevent their occurrence. Management delegates authority to the providers of services to plan and carry out quality improvement programs. Programs in CQI/TQM reinforce the belief that quality is everyone's responsibility.

Performance improvement (PI) is another term used to describe organizational efforts to improve corporate performance. Incorporating aspects of quality management, PI focuses efforts on increasing individual and group competence and productivity. Quality can be compromised in the process of increasing productivity, however, and this must be guarded against.

Nurses are actively involved in quality and performance improvement and in accreditation processes, but these activities are not the responsibility of nursing alone. They are institution-wide initiatives, and everyone, at all levels, gets involved. Working together to improve patient care builds cooperation among departments and clinical disciplines and boosts morale.

A Continuing Challenge: Health Care Disparities

Health care disparities are defined as differences in the quality of health care provided to different populations. Most often discussed as ethnic or racial disparities, differences also have been found to exist between the treatment and treatment outcomes of men and women, as well as younger and older people. The causes of disparities may be due to race, ethnicity, gender, age, income, education, disability, sexual orientation, and place of residence (Agency for Healthcare Research and Quality, 2007). Most likely a combination of these and possibly other factors leads to disparities.

Despite decades of work by public and private groups dedicated to narrowing health care disparities attributable to race and ethnicity, there is little progress reported (Voelker, 2008). In fact, the 2007 National Healthcare Disparities Report (NHDR) noted that for minorities and poor populations, "the number of measures on which disparities have gotten significantly worse or have remained unchanged since the first NHDR [in 2003] is higher than the number of measures on which they have gotten significantly better" (Agency for Healthcare Research and Quality, 2007). Although progress has been made in some areas, reports continue to be discouraging.

Provider bias has been mentioned as a possible contributing factor to health care disparities. For example, a study examining treatment of adults with soft-tissue cancers of an arm or a leg "showed that blacks had the lowest rates of limb-preserving surgeries and the highest rates of amputations in comparison with white, Hispanic, and Asian patients" (Voelker, 2008). This study found that blacks also had the lowest rates of radiation therapy used in conjunction with surgery compared with other groups. When the changing demographics of the country, with minorities increasing, are combined with the decline in minority students entering health care fields, the possibility of provider bias is a major concern that has not been thoroughly explored as a cause of health care disparities. This chapter's Cultural Considerations Challenge contains more information about health care disparities. If this is a topic you wish to learn more about, you will find a continuing education module, "Disparities in Health Care: Focusing Efforts to Eliminate Unequal Burdens" on the continuing education website of the American Nurses Association (ANA) at http://www.nursingworld.org/mods/mod560/cebrdnvers.htm.

The Health Care Team

Within the vast array of health care settings discussed in this chapter are the people who provide care to patients—the health care team. At one time, physicians and nurses were the major members of the health care team, but as health care became complex and technology expanded, a number of other health disciplines developed. Today, there are many different health care team members who come from a variety of backgrounds. Physicians, nurses, and all the other individuals who work with patients are called the health care team, or interdisciplinary team. They are supported in their work by a number of other departments, such as nutrition services, environmental services, a pharmacy, and laboratory

---

✸ Cultural Considerations Challenge

FACTS ABOUT HEALTH DISPARITIES

The U.S. Department of Health and Human Services' Office of Minority Health and Health Disparities (OMHD) has selected six focus areas in which racial and ethnic minorities experience serious disparities in health access and outcomes:

1. Infant mortality

African-American, American Indian, and Puerto Rican infants have higher death rates than white infants. In 2000 the African-American to white ratio in infant mortality was 2.5 (up from 2.4 in 1998). This widening disparity between African-American and white infants is a trend that has persisted over the last two decades.

2. Cancer screening and management

African-American women are more than twice as likely to die of cervical cancer than are white women and are more likely to die of breast cancer than are women of any other racial or ethnic group.

3. Cardiovascular disease (CVD)

Heart disease and stroke are the leading causes of death for all racial and ethnic groups in the United States. In 2000 rates of death from diseases of the heart were 29% higher among African-American adults than among white adults, and death rates from stroke were 40% higher.

4. Diabetes

In 2000 American Indians and Alaska Natives were 2.6 times more likely to have diagnosed diabetes compared with non-Hispanic whites, African Americans were 2.0 times more likely, and Hispanics were 1.9 times more likely.

5. HIV infection/AIDS

Although African Americans and Hispanics represented only 26% of the U.S. population in 2001, they accounted for 66% of adult AIDS cases and 82% of pediatric AIDS cases reported in the first half of that year.

6. Immunizations

In 2001 Hispanics and African Americans aged 65 and older were less likely than non-Hispanic whites to report having received influenza and pneumococcal vaccines.

In addition, the following diseases and conditions disproportionately impact racial and ethnic minorities: mental health, hepatitis, syphilis, and tuberculosis.

From Office of Minority Health, Centers for Disease Control and Prevention: *Eliminating racial and ethnic health disparities,* 2009 (website): http://www.cdc.gov/omhd/About/disparities.htm.

services, among others. The decision about which of these various personnel should be involved in the care of a patient depends on the desired patient outcomes. Professional nurses must understand and appreciate the education and skills of all members of the interdisciplinary team and strive to work effectively with them. Several of the key members who are most likely to be involved in the care of patients are discussed below.

Physicians

Physicians are responsible for medical diagnosis and interventions designed to restore patient health. Although physicians have traditionally been involved mainly in restorative care, many are beginning to recognize the value of health promotion and maintenance, as well as illness and injury prevention. Some physicians are also integrating nontraditional or alternative treatment choices such as chiropractic medicine, acupuncture, herbal treatments, and massage therapy into their practices.

Physicians have completed college and 3 or 4 years of medical school and are licensed by a state board of medical examiners. Although a hospital residency is not required to practice medicine in all states, most physicians have completed one, and many do postgraduate work in a specialty area and then take examinations to become board certified in the specialty area.

Physician assistants

Physician assistants (PAs) have emerged in the last 30 years as members of the health care team. According to the American Academy of Physician Assistants (American Academy of Physician Assistants, 2009), physician assistants perform many functions of a physician under the direct supervision of a physician.

Prerequisites for entering a PA program vary, depending on the degree offered. Virtually all require that applicants have health care experience before attending a PA program, which usually lasts a little over 2 years. Beyond graduation from this program, PAs must pass a national cerifying examination and are required to be licensed by the state in which they practice. They are required to obtain continuing medical education and regularly be retested on their clinical skills. PAs may also choose to then complete a postgraduate PA program in a clinical specialty area.

Patient care technicians

Also known as certified nursing assistants, **patient care technicians** (PCTs) are unlicensed workers who are key members of the nursing staff. PCTs work under the supervision of nurses to assist with basic patient care. Their responsibilities include assisting with personal hygiene; measuring and recording vital signs, heights, weights, inputs, and outputs; collecting and testing specimens; and reporting and recording patients' condition and treatments. They also help patients meet their nutritional needs by checking and delivering food trays, assisting with feeding patients when necessary, and replenishing bedside water and ice. Additional duties include assisting patients with their mobility by turning and positioning, performing range-of-motion exercises, transferring patients to and from wheelchairs or bedside chairs, and assisting with ambulation. To become a PCT, specialized training is required in a vocational or technical school or community or junior college. Individuals who become PCTs sometimes pursue additional education to become licensed practical nurses (LPNs), also termed licensed vocational nurses (LVNs) in some states (Bureau of Labor Statistics, 2008).

Licensed practical nurses/Licensed vocational nurses

Licensed practical nurses (LPNs), or **licensed vocational nurses** (LVNs), care for patients under the direction of physicians and RNs. The supervision required varies by state and job setting. LPNs provide basic bedside care. They measure and record patients' vital signs such as height, weight, temperature, blood pressure, pulse, and respiration. They also prepare and give injections and enemas, monitor catheters, dress wounds, and give alcohol rubs and massages. They assist with bathing, dressing, and personal hygiene, moving in bed, standing, and walking. They might also feed patients who need help eating. LPNs collect samples for testing, perform routine laboratory tests, and record food and fluid intake and output. They clean and monitor medical equipment. Sometimes, they help physicians and RNs perform tests and procedures. Some LPNs help to deliver, care for, and feed infants.

LPNs monitor their patients and report adverse reactions to medications or treatments. They gather information from patients, including their health history and how they are currently feeling. They may use this information to complete insurance forms, preauthorizations, and referrals, and they share information with RNs and physicians to help determine the best course of care for a patient.

Most LPNs are generalists and work in all areas of health care. However, some work in a specialized setting, such as nursing homes or doctors' offices, or in home health care. LPNs in nursing care facilities help to evaluate residents' needs, develop care plans, and supervise the care provided by nursing aides. In doctors' offices and clinics, they may be responsible for drawing blood, measuring vital signs, making appointments, keeping records, and performing other clinical and clerical duties. LPNs who work in home health care may prepare meals and teach family members simple nursing tasks. In some states, LPNs are permitted to administer prescribed medicines, start intravenous fluids, and provide care to ventilator-dependent patients (Bureau of Labor Statistics, 2008).

Training programs for LPNs are offered in state-approved vocational or technical schools or community or junior colleges. The programs usually last 1 year. To become licensed, graduates must pass a national examination, the National Council Licensure Examination for Practical Nurses (NCLEX-PN®), developed and administered by the National Council of State Boards of Nursing.

Dietitians

Many patients require management of their nutritional intake as part of the healing process. Others need to learn how to shop for and prepare a healthy diet (Figure 14-3). Dietitians understand how the diet, whether oral or intravenous,

can affect a patient's recovery and promote and maintain health. They focus on the therapeutic value of foods and on teaching people about therapeutic diets and healthful nutrition. Dietitians have baccalaureate or higher degrees and may have completed internships in specialty areas, such as pediatrics.

Pharmacists

Pharmacists prepare and dispense medications, instruct patients and other health workers about medications, monitor the use of controlled substances such as narcotics, and work to reduce medication errors. The number and complexity of drugs available today necessitate special education and training in their preparation and dispensing and in monitoring the effects on patients. Clinical pharmacists spend time on hospital units working closely with physicians and nursing case managers to coordinate complex drug administration, such as chemotherapy. They assist in

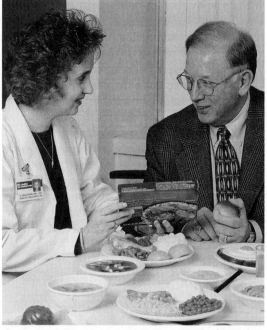

Figure 14-3 Dietitians assist patients to facilitate their own healing and health maintenance through therapeutic diets and healthful nutrition practices. (Photo courtesy Hamilton Medical Center, Dalton, Ga.)

monitoring and minimizing the drug interactions resulting from a patient taking multiple medications.

Pharmacists must obtain a doctor of pharmacy (PharmD) degree, which takes 6 years to complete, and pass a state board of pharmacy's licensure examination (U.S. Department of Labor, 2006). Depending on state licensing requirements, they may also be required to complete an internship. Certified pharmacy technicians, who are certified by state licensing boards, assist them.

Technologists

Technologists are personnel who assist in the diagnosis of patient problems.

Laboratory technologists handle patient specimens—such as blood, sputum, feces, urine, and body tissues—to be examined for abnormalities (Figure 14-4). Laboratory technologists carefully subject these body substances to various tests to determine deviations from normal ranges. Technologists have at least a bachelor's degree and are often assisted by laboratory technicians, who have 2-year degrees. They must pass a state licensing examination to practice.

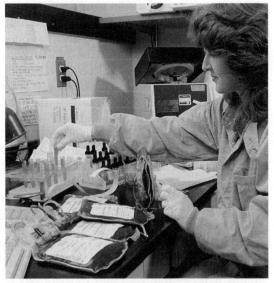

Figure 14-4 This laboratory technologist works in a critically important setting—a blood bank. Here she prepares several units of blood for administration. (Photo courtesy Hamilton Medical Center, Dalton, Ga.)

Radiology technologists perform x-ray procedures. Although patients still need routine flat-plate x-ray studies, technology in this field has become much more sophisticated. Subspecialties such as CT, magnetic resonance imaging (MRI), and positron emission tomography (PET) have developed. All of these techniques allow practitioners to see what is occurring inside the body without surgery. They also require specially educated technicians who operate multimillion-dollar equipment. Radiology technologists are educated in formal programs lasting from 1 to 4 years. In 40 states, they must be registered with the state in order to practice.

Respiratory therapists

Acutely ill or injured patients often require assistance in breathing. Respiratory therapists operate equipment such as ventilators, oxygen therapy devices, and intermittent positive-pressure breathing machines. They also perform some diagnostic procedures, such as pulmonary function tests, and blood gas analysis. With the increase in respiratory care in the home and community, these health care team members work closely with home health agencies and community health centers. Respiratory therapists must complete a 2- or 4-year educational program and obtain state licensure; in some states they must complete an internship.

Social workers

The social worker is specifically educated and trained to assist patients and their families as they face the impact of illness and injury. They serve as liaisons between hospitalized patients and the resources and services available in the community. They help patients and their families deal with financial problems caused by interruption of work or inadequate insurance benefits; they also direct them to the appropriate community support systems or facilities for home health care, long-term care, or rehabilitation. In addition to counseling patients and families, social workers are called on to assist other health care personnel to cope more effectively with the stresses associated with caring for patients in crisis. Social workers hold either a bachelor's or a master's degree and are licensed.

Therapists

Therapists help patients with special challenges. Physical therapists, or physiotherapists, assist patients to regain maximum possible physical activity and strength. They focus on assessing preillness or preinjury function, current deficits, and potential for recovery. They then develop a long-term plan for gradual return to function through exercise, rest, heat, hydrotherapy, and other measures. Physical therapists, who have a minimum of a master's degree, also supervise physical therapy assistants, who hold associate degrees.

Occupational therapists work with physical therapists to develop plans to assist patients in resuming the activities of daily living after illness or injury. They may help patients learn to cook, carry out their personal hygiene, or drive a specially equipped car. In addition, they assist patients to learn skills to return to their previous jobs or retrain patients for new employment options. Occupational therapists have bachelor's degrees. Other types of therapists include recreational therapists, art and music therapists, speech therapists, and massage therapists.

Administrative support personnel

In all organizations, administrative support staff members are needed for clerical jobs such as admitting patients, answering phones, directing visitors, scheduling patient tests, filing insurance claims, filing forms, paying bills, facilitating payroll, and other support functions. These activities require considerable time. Hiring administrative staff members frees the clinical staff to concentrate on direct patient care.

The administrative staff ensures that the operations of the facility run smoothly and that clinicians have the resources necessary to meet patient needs. These staff members also educate the clinical staff on financial constraints and work with the staff to find ways to provide quality care at the lowest possible cost.

Keeping complete and accurate medical records is an extremely important administrative function that ensures proper insurance billing, eligibility for accreditation, and legal protection of the hospital and its staff. Registered records administrators (RRAs) are vital members of the administrative staff. These professionals staff the medical records department. Many organizations today now refer to the medical records departments as "health information services."

The Nurse's Role on the Health Care Team

Whatever the setting, nurses fulfill a number of roles on the health care team. As the health care delivery system changes, the evolving role of the RN requires new competencies and skills in each of the roles described below.

Provider of care

Nurses provide direct, hands-on care to patients in all health care agencies and settings. As providers, they take an active role in illness prevention and health promotion and maintenance. They offer health screenings, home health services, and an array of health care services in schools, workplaces, churches, clinics, physicians' offices, and other settings. They are instrumental in the high survival rates in trauma centers and newborn intensive care units, among others. Nurses with advanced nursing degrees are increasingly providing care at all levels of the health care system. Their breadth and depth of knowledge, their ability to care holistically for patients, and their natural partnership with physicians make nurses some of the most sought-after and trusted care providers.

Educator

As patient and family educators, nurses provide information about illnesses and teach about medications, treatments, and rehabilitation needs. They also help patients understand how to deal with the life changes necessitated by chronic illnesses and teach how to adapt care to the home or community setting. In the current health care climate, patients are being discharged from hospitals faster than ever before. Patients and their families often must manage complex treatments, such as central lines or feeding tubes, in the home setting. A major role of the nurse as educator in today's hospital setting is to ensure continuity from inpatient to outpatient care through coordination of home care services and through discharge teaching (Bastable, 2003).

Nurses also act as educators in community settings. The major focus of the nurse in the community setting is health promotion and injury and illness prevention. Often, nurses teach classes jointly with other health care team members. For example, a nutritionist and a nurse may teach a group of expectant parents the benefits of breastfeeding their infants. Nurses also have a responsibility to understand and teach how a healthful or unhealthful environment may affect both the short-term and the long-term health of the community.

Nurses also serve as patient educators in disease management companies. By educating patients about their chronic diseases and coaching them in effective self-care behaviors, nurses work with the patient and the primary care provider to keep the patient healthier. Thus nurses as patient educators help reduce health care utilization and cost.

Nurses are often the key educators on the health care team. They teach other team members about the patient and family and why different interventions may have varying degrees of success. Nurses help other team members find cost-effective, quality interventions that are desired and needed by the patient rather than wasting resources on ineffective, inefficient, undesired, or unneeded services.

Nurses also serve as teachers of the next generation of nurses. Nursing students need educators who set high standards and ideals and who help students understand the ethical choices that all health care providers must make.

The Internet plays a significant role in health education today. It has completely transformed the access and dissemination of information for millions of Americans. Nurses functioning in the role of educator assist patients to use the Internet as an enhancement to traditional education by teaching them how to select reliable websites and evaluate the health information they find. You can find more information about assisting patients to use reliable Internet resources on the Evolve website (http://evolve.elsevier.com).

Counselor

People who experience illness or injury often have strong emotional responses. It is clear that the relationships among the emotions, the mind, and the body are critical to promotion of and restoration to health. As counselors, nurses provide basic counseling and support to patients and their families.

Using therapeutic communication techniques, nurses encourage people to discuss their feelings, to explore possible options and solutions to their unique problems, and to choose for themselves the best alternatives for action. They also serve as bereavement counselors to terminally ill patients and their families. Because nurses spend more time with patients than other professionals, they have opportunities to respond to the emotional needs of patients as they occur. Therefore the nurse's role as counselor often overlaps with the roles of social workers, psychiatrists, spiritual advisers, and mental health specialists. Nurses may, with advanced education and certification, provide psychotherapy services that extend beyond the basic counseling role.

Manager

In their daily work, all nurses are managers. The bedside staff nurse must manage the care of a group of patients, prioritize how to accomplish patient care activities during an 8- or 12-hour period, and determine staff and patient assignments. Nurses are also involved in reviewing patient cases and coordinating services so that quality care can be achieved at the lowest cost.

In addition, nurses serve in the role of managers of patient care units, outpatient clinics, or home health agencies. The effective management of nursing resources is essential. With budgets ranging from hundreds of thousands to many million dollars, nurse managers manage "businesses" larger than many small companies.

Nurse managers must have clinical and administrative expertise, including but not limited to leadership, human resources, financial, organizational behavior, system and program design, outcome research, and marketing skills.

Chief nurse executives may manage more than 1000 employees and multimillion-dollar budgets. They interact with other top executives and community leaders, often sitting on the health care organization's board of directors. Nurse executives must ensure the quality of nursing care within financial, regulatory, and legislative constraints. As noted earlier, nurses often serve as patient care executives, COOs, and CEOs. Key responsibilities of nurse managers and nurse executives are listed in Table 14-1.

Researcher

All nurses should be involved in nursing research whether or not research is a nurse's primary responsibility. According to the ANA's *Scope and Standards of Practice* (ANA, 2010), the RN integrates research findings into practice. Nurse researchers investigate whether current or potential nursing actions achieve their expected outcomes, what options for care may be available, and how best to provide care. Nursing research looks at patient outcomes, the nursing process, and the systems that support nursing services.

Outcomes research has become an integral part of the health care delivery system. Insurers and regulatory agencies require health care organizations to report outcome data related to quality of care, which requires research by nurses. Participation by all nurses in research is essential to the growth and development of the nursing profession. The increasing emphasis on evidence-based practice underscores the need for well-planned and implemented nursing research studies in all practice settings.

Collaborator

With so many health care workers involved in providing patient care, collaboration among the professions is increasingly important. The collaborator role is a vital one for nurses to ensure that everyone agrees on the same patient outcomes. Multidisciplinary teams require collaborative practice, and nurses play key roles as both team members and team leaders. Collaboration requires that nurses understand and appreciate what other health professionals have to offer. Nurses must also interpret to others the nursing needs of patients.

An often-overlooked collaborative function of nurses is collaboration with patients and families. Involving patients and their families in the plan of care from the beginning is the best way to ensure their cooperation, enthusiasm, and willingness to work toward the best patient outcomes. More in-depth information about collaboration can be found in Chapter 9.

Table 14-1 Responsibilities of Nurse Managers and Nurse Executives

Nurse Managers	Nurse Executives
Direct supervision of assigned staff and interdisciplinary collaboration	Partner with other disciplines and leaders
Manage recruitment, selection, retention, staffing, scheduling, and assigning personnel	Acquire resources for function and process and provide leadership in human resources development and management
Accept organizational accountability for services provided	Lead and direct patient care delivery
Evaluate quality and appropriateness of health care delivery for assigned areas	Accountable for continuous quality improvement for entire nursing system
Budget for assigned areas	Budget for entire nursing department and input into system-wide budget planning

Modified from American Nurses Association: *Scope and standards for nurse administrators,* ed 2, Washington, DC, 2004.

Patient advocate

Rules and regulations designed to help a complex health care system run efficiently can sometimes get in the way of a patient's treatment, and an impersonal health care system may infringe on a patient's rights. This may occur when there is an unsafe patient load, when a patient is being discharged too early, when a physician's plan of care needs revision, or when the patient's wishes are not being followed (Trossman, 2008). Therefore it is every nurse's responsibility to advocate for patients daily. Some nursing experts believe this is the most important of all the nursing roles (Sounart, 2008).

Nurses functioning as patient advocates must know how to cut through the levels of bureaucracy and red tape of health care organizations and stand up for the patient's rights, advocating his or her best interests at all times. They must value patient self-determination, that is, patient independence and decision making. In this role, nurses sometimes help patients bend the rules when it is in the patient's best interests and doing so will harm no one. Patient advocates are nurses who realize that policies are important and govern most situations well but occasionally can, and should, be broken. For example, special care units often have strict visiting hours. Family members may be allowed to see the patient for only 10 minutes each hour. If a patient's recovery will be faster if the family is present, the nurse, serving in the role of patient advocate, may allow the family members more generous visitation than the policy provides.

In conclusion, nurses must be prepared to participate both as leaders and as members of the interdisciplinary team and to assume and relinquish the leadership role to best meet the needs of patients and the team.

Types of Nursing Care Delivery Models Historically Used in Acute Care Settings

To fully understand the nurse's role on the health care team, it is important to examine the types of nursing care delivery models and how they have changed over the years.

Before World War I, nurses usually visited the sick in their homes to care for them. As hospital care improved and nursing education evolved, more sick people were treated in hospitals. Providing care to groups of patients rather than to individuals required nurses to be efficient and use their time effectively. Over the years, various types of care delivery models were designed to meet the goals of efficient and effective nursing care. Organizing patient care today often requires the professional nurse to work through other care providers, such as PCTs and LPNs, to achieve patient outcomes. It is important to remember that the delivery of high-quality patient care does not happen by chance. Each nurse manager must select a care delivery model appropriate for the unit, the acuity of the patients, and the type and number of nursing staff members available. There are a number of principles for selecting a care delivery model. Box 14-3 lists 13 principles to consider when selecting a care delivery model.

Five patient care delivery models—functional nursing, team nursing, primary nursing, case management nursing, and patient-centered care—are reviewed in this chapter.

Functional nursing

The functional approach to nursing care began in the 1950s. It grew out of a need to organize care for large numbers of patients. It focused on organizing and distributing the tasks, or functions, of care among the available staff. In functional nursing, personnel worked side by side, each performing one or two assigned tasks for all the patients on the unit. Trained nurses provided care that required high skill levels, and assistive personnel performed less-complex tasks. For example, one nurse would administer medications, another nurse performed assessments, and a nursing assistant gave baths and changed linens.

The goal of functional nursing was efficient management of time, tasks, and energy. Although this practice saved hospitals money, patient care was fragmented, because caregivers were focused on individual tasks and not the whole patient. A patient could not identify one person as "my nurse."

Box 14-3 Principles for Selecting a Care Delivery Model

The care delivery model should:
- Facilitate meeting the organization's goals
- Be cost effective
- Contribute to meeting patients' outcomes
- Provide role satisfaction for nurses
- Allow implementation of the nursing process
- Provide adequate communication among all health care providers
- Support RNs' responsibility for the overall direction of nursing care
- Be designed to give RNs the responsibility, authority, and accountability for planning, organizing, and evaluating nursing care
- Ensure that the skills and knowledge of each care provider are used for the best patient outcomes
- Ensure that communication can occur
- Ensure that the model advances professional nursing practice
- Provide for care that is perceived by the patient as a coherent whole (unity of action by a team of RNs/LPNs/others)
- Provide the work groups of RNs, LPNs, and other workers the appropriate knowledge required to meet the nursing care needs of the patient

From Rogers R: Adapting to the new workplace reality, *Info Nursing: A Publication of the Nurses Association of New Brunswick* 39(1):18-20, 2008.

Box 14-4 Advantages and Disadvantages of Functional Nursing

ADVANTAGES
- Efficient—can complete many tasks in a defined time frame
- Proficient—workers only perform tasks they are educated to do and become very efficient
- Promotes organizational skills—each worker must organize his or her own work
- Promotes worker autonomy

DISADVANTAGES
- Lacks holistic view of patient—emphasis on task, not entire person
- Lacks continuity—patients often do not know who their nurse is
- Care is fragmented
- Does not support professional practice aspects of nursing

Today, functional nursing may still be used in some settings, but its use is fading. It may still be used when there are few staff members available, such as at night, on weekends, and on holidays. Box 14-4 lists advantages and disadvantages of functional nursing.

Team nursing

In response to the frustration some nurses felt when using the functional approach to patient care, Lambertson (1953) designed **team nursing** (Figure 14-5). She envisioned nursing teams as democratic work groups with different skill levels represented by different team members. They were assigned as a team to a defined group of patients.

Team nursing has been widely used in hospitals and long-term care facilities. The team usually consists of a RN, who serves as team leader, an LPN, and one or more PCTs.

The team leader, although ultimately responsible for all the care provided, **delegates** (assigns responsibility for) certain patients to each team member. Each member of the team provides the level of care for which he or she is best prepared. The least skilled and experienced members care for the patients who require the least complex care, and the most skilled and experienced members care for the most seriously ill patients who require the most complex care.

In team nursing, the RN team leader supervises and coordinates all care for a particular shift, makes assessments, and documents responses to care. The LPN team member provides direct care by performing treatments and procedures and reporting patient responses to the team leader. The PCT provides routine direct, personal care. Today, team nursing is still used, but the model is often modified. Many of the patient-focused

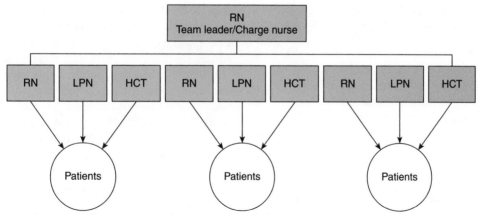

Figure 14-5 Team nursing with teams composed of RNs, LPNs, and health care technicians.

Box 14-5   Advantages and Disadvantages of Team Nursing

ADVANTAGES
- Potential for building team spirit
- Provides comprehensive care
- Each worker's abilities used to the fullest
- Promotes job satisfaction
- Decreases nonprofessional duties of registered nurses

DISADVANTAGES
- Ongoing need for communication among team members requires commitment of time
- All team members must promote teamwork, or team nursing is unsuccessful
- Team composition varies from day to day, which can be confusing and disruptive and decreases continuity of care
- May result in blurred role boundaries and resulting confusion and resentment

care models use RNs as team leaders coordinating care for a group of patients and supervising multiskilled workers who have been trained to perform a variety of comfort measures, such as positioning, and technical procedures, such as taking vital signs or drawing blood.

As with functional nursing, team nursing has both advantages and disadvantages; these are presented in Box 14-5.

Primary nursing

Developed in the 1970s as a result of the increased acuity (severity of illness) of hospitalized patients, primary nursing was designed to promote the concept of an identified nurse for every patient during the patient's stay on a particular unit. The goal of primary nursing is to deliver consistent, comprehensive care by identifying one nurse who is responsible, has authority, and is accountable for the patient's nursing care outcomes for the period during which the patient is in a unit.

In primary nursing, each newly admitted patient is assigned to a primary nurse. Primary nurses assess their patients, plan their care, and write the plan of care. While on duty, they care for their patients and delegate responsibility to associate nurses when they are off duty. Associate nurses may be other RNs or LPNs.

Patients are divided among primary nurses in such a manner that each nurse is responsible for the care of a group of patients 24 hours a day. Unless there is a compelling reason to transfer a patient, the primary nurse cares for the patient in the unit from the time of admission to the time of discharge. The primary nurse may be assisted by other care providers (such as other nurses, aides,

Box 14-6 Advantages and Disadvantages of Primary Nursing

ADVANTAGES

- High patient and family satisfaction
- Promotes registered nurse responsibility, authority, autonomy, and accountability
- Nurse can care for entire patient—physically, emotionally, socially, and spiritually
- Patient knows nurse well, and nurse knows patient well.
- Promotes patient-centered decision making
- Increases coordination and continuity of care
- Promotes professionalism
- Promotes job satisfaction and sense of accomplishment for nurses

DISADVANTAGES

- Difficult to hire all registered nurse staff
- Expensive to pay all registered nurse staff
- Nurses are not familiar with other patients making it difficult to "cover" for each other.
- May create conflicts between primary and associate nurses
- Stress of round-the-clock responsibility
- Heavy responsibility, especially for new nurses

and technicians) but retains accountability, or responsibility, for care outcomes 24 hours a day while the patient is in the unit. The primary nurse communicates effectively with associate nurses caring for the patient on other shifts and with primary nurses in other units if the patient is transferred (e.g., to the operating room or intensive care unit).

Primary nursing is used in a variety of settings and is often modified from its original form. Advantages and disadvantages of primary nursing are listed in Box 14-6.

Case management nursing

A more recent evolution in nursing care delivery is case management nursing. Begun in the late 1980s as an attempt to improve the cost-effectiveness of patient care, case management allows the nurse to oversee patient care and manage the delivery of services from all health care disciplines throughout a patient's illness. Nursing case management keeps costs down by striving to achieve predetermined daily patient outcomes within a specified time period for patients within the same diagnostic group, for example, patients having total knee replacement. The desired daily outcomes are outlined in a plan of care called a care map or critical path. You may also hear these referred to as clinical care plans or tracks.

Two models of case management nursing have evolved over time. These are characterized by either an "internal" focus, in which the case manager works within a treatment facility, or an "external" approach, in which the case manager oversees patients and the delivery of services over the continuum of an illness or chronic disease whether patients are in a treatment facility or at home. Although different in scope, these two models share the same principles of efficiency and cost-effectiveness.

In the internal model of case management, nursing case managers serve as primary nurses for patients in an identified diagnostic group, such as spinal cord injury. They not only care for these patients while on their assigned units but also manage the plans of care from admission to discharge, crossing interdepartmental lines. Although nursing case managers do not physically provide care to the patient group on units other than their own, they actively collaborate with primary nurses assigned to the patients in those units. In this nursing model, critical paths are used for all patients. A critical path is an interdisciplinary agreement showing who will provide care in a given time frame to achieve agreed-on outcomes. The use of critical paths is intended to standardize patient care and allow hospitals to plan staffing levels, lengths of stay, and other factors that heretofore could not be anticipated. Patients whose progress varies from the path are quickly identified. Once the causes for the variation are identified, team members attempt to plan solutions to reduce variances and get the patient back on track. The goal is to treat each patient by using best practices to reduce the length of stay, thereby reducing costs.

Box 14-7   Advantages and Disadvantages of Case Management Nursing

---

ADVANTAGES
- Promotes interdisciplinary collaboration
- Increases quality of care
- Is cost-effective
- Eases patient's transition from hospital to community services
- Nurse has increased responsibility

DISADVANTAGES
- Requires additional training
- Requires nurses to be off the unit for periods of time
- Is time-consuming
- Is most useful only with high-risk patients and high-cost/high-volume conditions

---

In the external model of case management, nurse case managers are part of a large network consisting of, for example, hospitals, clinics, home health agencies, and long-term care settings. They may provide services anywhere in the system, as well as when the patient is at home. They partner with patients and their families to achieve the goal of preventing hospitalizations, thereby reducing costs and minimizing disruptions to the patient's life and family.

As can be seen from the type of activities in which they engage, case managers perform complex and challenging work. Nurses generally need about 5 years of clinical experience to fill this role effectively. Social workers, psychologists, rehabilitation counselors, or other professionals may also serve as case managers. All case managers, regardless of their discipline, work to reduce the cost of providing services through coordination of providers across the continuum of care.

Advantages and disadvantages of case management nursing are shown in Box 14-7.

Patient-centered care

Patient-centered care is a contemporary care delivery model implemented by a multidisciplinary team of health professionals. It focuses on the patient's right to individualized care that takes his or her values and beliefs into consideration when planning and providing care. Nurses and other providers must be flexible, respect the patient's beliefs and wishes, and negotiate with the patient to meet patient expectations. Patient-centered care is more an attitude than a particular model of care, and traditional models, alone or in combination, may be used. The attitude of caregivers is that patients' needs have priority over the institution's needs. The model was pioneered by the Planetree Institute in 1978 after its founder experienced several "dehumanizing" hospitalizations. Patient-centered care brings together traditional and nontraditional components of care that work toward optimizing the healing environment. Such components as the architectural design of the facilities; educational programs for patients and families; emphasis on beauty, gardens, art, food, and nutrition; availability of complementary therapies such as massage and aroma therapy; emphasis on spirituality; and community interaction are the hallmarks of patient-centered care. These components are integrated with best medical practices to form a coherent continuum of care characterized by teamwork, communication, and collaboration among professionals and with patients and families. Advantages and disadvantages of patient-centered care are shown in Box 14-8.

FINANCING HEALTH CARE

The health care delivery system in the United States is under severe financial stress. Although there is renewed vigor to the public debate over health care reform, costs continue to climb, as does the number of uninsured citizens, estimated at 45.7 million in 2009. In spite of decades of effort, legislative reforms and managed-care initiatives have had little success in cutting health care costs and increasing access to health care. The nation's dilemma remains: how to provide high-quality health care services to all citizens while keeping costs down.

In 2007 the nation's health care expenditures reached $2.2 trillion and consumed 16.2% of

Box 14-8 Advantages and Disadvantages of Patient-Centered Care

ADVANTAGES
- Expedites care
- Promotes patient convenience
- Capitalizes on professional competence of team members
- Emphasizes continuum of care and reduces fragmentation of care
- Uses resources efficiently
- Fosters teamwork, collaboration, and communication

DISADVANTAGES
- Requires "right staff at right time" to meet patient needs
- Difficult to explain; uses several models of care delivery
- Requires a lot of RNs; must have both clinical and management skills

Modified from Shirey MR: Nursing practice models for acute and critical care: overview of care delivery models, *Crit Care Nurs Clin North Am* 20:365-373, 2008.

the gross domestic product (Centers for Medicare & Medicaid Services, 2008). Average annual growth of national health expenditures was expected to be 6.2% per year through 2018. If these projections are accurate, by 2018 national health spending is expected to reach $4.4 trillion and comprise just over one fifth (20.3%) of gross domestic product. Clearly these are unsustainable figures that threaten to bankrupt our national budget, even when the economy is strong.

Financial issues profoundly affect nurses and nursing practice. These issues affect nurses professionally, in their nursing practice, and personally, in the type of insurance and health services they and their families are able to afford. Therefore students of professional nursing need to understand the overall economic context in which nursing care is provided. In this section, several major concepts necessary to understanding health care

finance will be explored, including basic economic theory, the economics of nursing care, a brief historical review of the causes of health care cost escalation, cost-containment efforts, current methods of payment, and the role nurses can play in managing health care costs in their everyday work settings.

Basic Economic Theory

Nursing school curricula do not typically require undergraduates to take courses in economics, yet there is an urgent need for nurses to understand the economic context in which they practice.

Supply and demand

A basic economic theory is the law of supply and demand. According to this theory, a normal economic system consists of two parts: suppliers, who provide goods and services; and consumers, who demand and use goods and services. In a monetary environment, that is, one in which money is used as a unit of exchange, consumers exchange money for desired goods and services.

In an efficient marketplace, the market price of goods and services serves to create an equilibrium in which supply roughly equals demand, and demand roughly equals supply. When demand exceeds supply, prices rise. When supply exceeds demand, prices fall. Figure 14-6 illustrates the relationships among price, supply, and demand.

Principles of the free-market economy

In a free-market economy, consumption of any good or service is determined by an individual's ability to pay. In a pure free market, a portion of the population would be denied health care if they were unable to pay. People who support this position consider health care a privilege. Others believe that everyone should have access to basic health care and consider health care a right.

Despite the United States' leanings toward a free-market economy in general, most Americans consider health care a right, not a privilege. Rather than allowing economically disadvantaged citizens to do without health services, the federal government has taken steps to ensure

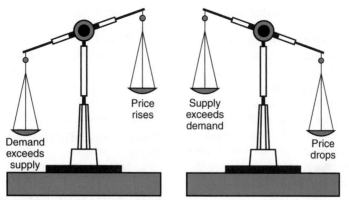

Figure 14-6 Price sensitivity in a normal economic environment.

certain groups have access to health care services through publicly funded programs such as Medicare and Medicaid. Although this is generally considered an ethical policy, it is nevertheless a policy decision that is inconsistent with free-market principles.

Price sensitivity in health care

In the days before health insurance existed, people paid their own medical bills, providers set their fees with some sensitivity to what patients could afford to pay, and many physicians used sliding-scale payment plans or accepted in-kind payments, for example, exchanging medical care for farm products or a service such as cobbler services. Health insurance created an indirect payment structure, third-party payment, that removed price sensitivity from the concern of most health care consumers because they pay only a small portion of the actual costs. A third party (the employer, insurance company, or government) pays the rest. If someone other than the consumer pays, demand can increase because the consumer is insensitive to cost. This is an important point to keep in mind when reviewing the history of health care finance. History has demonstrated that when there is little or no out-of-pocket expense to the consumer, economic equilibrium is upset because consumers use more health care services (Jacob and Rapoport, 2002).

Additional influences on the health care market

Economists have identified a number of other factors that affect the health care market in ways that violate the assumptions surrounding an effective free-market system. For example, consumers cannot always control demand for health care services. With ordinary products, a consumer can delay a purchase until there is a sale or forgo the purchase altogether. Health care is different because health care needs tend to be immediate. The consumer might suffer serious harm or even death by a delay in seeking services. Thus the health care market differs from the free market system in several key ways, as summarized in Box 14-9.

Economics of Nursing Care

Until fairly recently, few efforts were made to determine the actual cost of nursing care. The average hospital bill simply included the cost of nursing services in the general category of "room rate," just as housekeeping services, linens, and food are included in the room rate. It was assumed that the cost of nurses contributed a major portion of overall hospital expenses. During tough economic times, the first cost-reduction efforts were therefore aimed at reducing the number of nursing personnel, sometimes substituting lower-paid unlicensed personnel. Studies in the mid-1980s, however, found that nursing accounted for only

Box 14-9   Barriers to a Free Market Economy in Health Care

POOR CONSUMER INFORMATION

Individual consumers are not accustomed to "shopping" for the best available prices for medical services, supplies, and equipment. Even when the consumer is motivated to compare costs, getting that information from the suppliers of health care is difficult and time consuming. Most consumers require services quickly and cannot afford long delays to seek information, even if they have the expertise to search out the needed information.

INEFFECTIVE PRICING SYSTEM

When the price of services is based on "reasonable and customary costs of similar services" in an area, health care providers have an incentive to continue to increase their prices rather than compete by lowering prices. Eventually the new, higher price becomes the "reasonable and customary" price. Reform efforts have had some success at reducing the impact of this phenomenon by establishing prospective funding and capping reimbursement for the cost of selected services.

HEALTH CARE PROVIDERS' INTERESTS MAY CONFLICT WITH CONSUMERS' INTERESTS

Health care providers have economic interests that can be in opposition to consumer interests. Physicians, for example, act both as suppliers of health care and as demanders of patient services. When physicians are partners or stockholders in services, such as laboratories or radiographic facilities, they are more likely to order such tests, according to studies by the Department of Health and Human Services. Conversely, health maintenance organization or preferred provider organization physicians who receive incentives for not referring patients to specialists are less likely to do so.

COST EFFICIENCY IS NOT ALWAYS A MOTIVATOR FOR SUPPLIERS

Although businesses are expected to operate with cost efficiency, others, particularly some nonprofit organizations, may be influenced by other factors. By law, nonprofits cannot keep or distribute profit or surplus of funds at the end of the fiscal year, but there is no law that dictates how they spend that money. Most nonprofits operate efficiently and at the lowest cost to consumers; others have been found to use their funds to provide amenities and perks for staff and board members, such as plush exercise facilities, all-expense-paid trips, or purchases of private boxes at sports stadiums.

Modified from Maurer FA: Financing of health care: context for community health nursing. In Smith C, Maurer FA, editors: *Community health nursing: theory and practice,* ed 2, Philadelphia, 2000, WB Saunders.

20 to 28 percent of the costs of hospitalization for two thirds of the diagnosis-related groups (DRGs) examined (McKibben, 1985). Determining the cost of nursing services and developing standardized reimbursements based on costs would enhance the ability of nurse managers to control nursing resources and negotiate for a fair share of hospital financial resources, and many efforts to "cost out" nursing services were conducted.

Not knowing the exact costs of nursing services limits nursing management's ability to calculate the expense required to provide nursing care for each patient in a given DRG. Determining the best skill mix, the ratio of RNs to LPNs and PCTs in each unit, is also impaired when the cost of nursing care is unknown. It has long been recognized that different patients require different amounts of nursing time, depending in large part on how sick they are. Patient classification systems were developed to identify patients' needs for nursing care in quantitative terms to help hospitals determine the need for nursing

EVIDENCE-BASED PRACTICE NOTE

The ANA, with a coalition of other nursing associations, supported a study to improve the understanding of the economic value of the services of RNs. The objective was to quantify the economic value of professional nursing to help inform staffing decisions and policies in the nation's hospitals. A group of researchers from George Mason University in Virginia and a nearby health care policy research firm, the Lewin Group, conducted the study. They reviewed the research literature on the relationship between RN staffing levels and adverse patient outcomes for a number of nursing-sensitive **nosocomial** (hospital acquired) complications. Examples of nursing-sensitive complications include urinary tract infections, pressure ulcers, blood infections, postoperative infections, patient falls, and adverse drug events, among others. They used data from a comprehensive literature review, as well as from the 2005 Nationwide Inpatient Sample of more than 1000 hospitals sponsored by the Agency for Healthcare Research and Quality. The cost of complications—in increased length of stay, health care expenditures, and losses of national productivity—were subjected to statistical analyses to determine estimates of the economic value of nursing. The researchers reported that, as a result of increasing nurse staffing levels, patient risk of nurse-sensitive complications and hospital length of stay both decreased, "resulting in medical cost savings, improved national productivity, and lives saved." They concluded that only a portion of professional nurses' services "can be quantified in pecuniary terms, but the partial estimates of economic value presented illustrate the economic value to society of improved quality of care achieved" through higher RN staffing levels.

Modified from Dall T, Chen Y, Seifert R, Maddox P, Hogan P: The economic value of professional nursing, *Med Care* 47(1):97-104, 2009.

resources. Progress has been made (McClosky et al, 2001; Pappas, 2008; Unruh, 2008), but costing nursing services remains an inexact science. This chapter's Evidence-Based Practice Note describes a major recent study to determine the economic value of professional nursing.

When the drive to provide high-quality nursing care meets the constraints of cost containment head-on, it can create a very difficult situation. What nurses hope, as both providers and consumers of health care, is that quality will not suffer because of the emphasis on "the bottom line." The financial realities that affect the institutions in which 56.2% of nurses practice—hospitals—cannot be ignored. To stay in business, hospitals must make at least enough money to pay personnel, maintain buildings and equipment, and pay suppliers of goods and services.

The leadership of the ANA has been repeatedly outspoken in their assertion that overzealous cost-containment efforts have led to lower-quality hospital care. A strong boost to their contention that the number and mix of nurses in a hospital make a difference in patient outcomes came early in the twenty-first century with research that showed an increased patient death rate with higher nurse/patient ratios (Aiken, Clarke, Sloane et al, 2002). Other recent research focused on comparing the cost of nurse staffing in hospitals with the cost savings gained through improved patient care (Needleman, Buerhaus, Stewart et al, 2006). As research continues to demonstrate the link between nursing and quality of care, the demand for nursing services will continue to flourish.

History of Health Care Finance

Before 1945 more than 90% of Americans either paid directly from their own pockets for health care or depended on charity care. Few had private health insurance. Public insurance programs, such as Medicare and Medicaid, did not exist. After World War II, most industrialized countries began publicly financed health care systems that provided care for all citizens. The United States, however, did not adopt a public, universal access system, choosing instead to continue the private, fee-for-service system.

The entire history of health care finance in this country is a fascinating study in unintended consequences. As each initiative to improve coverage, access, and quality was implemented, it opened up unforeseen loopholes that have driven costs skyward. Providers, such as hospitals, physicians, insurers, pharmaceutical companies, and others have learned to "game the system," exploiting loopholes while protecting or enhancing their own bottom lines. All the while population growth and increases in the number of elderly and chronically ill Americans have further complicated efforts to find solutions.

If you are interested in learning more about the complex history of health care finance, including factors fueling increases in health care costs, and cost-containment initiatives through the years, refer to the Evolve website (http://evolve.elsevier.com).

Current Methods of Payment for Health Care

There are four major methods of payment for health care in use today: private insurance, Medicare, Medicaid, and personal payment. Workers' compensation is an additional mechanism for financing some health care services. Each of these is briefly explained in the following paragraphs.

Private insurance

Private insurance, also called voluntary insurance, is a system wherein insurance premiums are paid by either insured individuals or their employers or are shared between individuals and employers. Periodic payments (premiums) are paid into the insurance plan, and certain health care benefits are covered as long as the premiums are paid. Early in the development of private insurance, many treatments were covered only if they were performed in an inpatient (hospital) setting. This feature drove up the cost of services. Today most insurers stipulate that costs of hospitalization are reimbursable only if treatment cannot be performed on an outpatient basis, where costs are typically lower. Most private insurers are heavily influenced by the federal insurance program, Medicare, in determining coverage and amount of reimbursements they will pay.

Medicare

Medicare, or Title XVIII of the Social Security Act, is a nationwide federal health insurance program established in 1965. Medicare is available to people aged 65 years and older, regardless of the recipient's income. It also covers certain disabled individuals and anyone with permanent kidney failure requiring dialysis or a kidney transplant. Medicare has four basic programs.

The first program, known as Part A (Hospital Insurance), helps cover inpatient hospitalization, part-time or intermittent skilled care in nursing facilities, hospice care, and some home health care. Long-term care or custodial care is not covered. Hospice care, available to people with a terminal illness who are expected to live 6 months or less as certified by a physician, is covered under Medicare. People who paid Medicare taxes while working do not pay a Part A premium, but they do pay a deductible, and certain restrictions apply to lengths of stay and benefit periods.

Part B (Medical Insurance) is a supplementary medical insurance program that covers visits to physicians' offices and other outpatient services. It also covers some preventive services. There is a 20% co-pay for medical and other services and a $135 yearly deductible. Mental health services are covered at 50%. Part B premiums are subject to means testing, meaning that individuals with higher incomes pay more in monthly premiums than do those with lower incomes. In 2010 the premium ranged from $96.40 for individuals with a yearly income under $85,000 to $353.60 for individuals with a yearly income above $214,000 (Centers for Medicare & Medicaid Services, 2009). The Internal Revenue Service provides tax return information to Medicare to assist in verifying income.

Part C (Medicare Advantage Plans) offers a variety of managed-care options instead of the fee-for-service programs of Parts A and B. Part C plans are run by private companies approved by Medicare. Costs and services vary by plan.

Part D (Prescription Drug Coverage) is the latest addition to Medicare. Effective January 1, 2006, it is an additional supplementary insurance program that helps cover prescription drug costs. Part D has very complex regulations including a "gap" period in coverage that many find difficult to understand.

In addition to the four basic parts of Medicare, Medigap or supplemental coverage is available to Medicare-eligible individuals. It is sold by private insurance companies to help fill the "gap" between Medicare and out-of-pocket costs.

Originally intended to be a no-cost or low-cost program for the elderly, the cost of participating in Medicare has risen steadily. Although the program was originally designed to be all-inclusive, many elderly people now find they cannot afford to participate in Medicare. Ironically, some elderly are so poor that they qualify for Medicaid assistance in paying their Medicare premiums. Medicare regulations and costs change annually. For the most recent updates on Medicare, consult http://www.medicare.gov.

Medicaid

Medicaid, or Title XIX of the Social Security Act, is a group of jointly funded federal-state programs for low-income, elderly, blind, and disabled individuals. It, too, was established in 1965. There are broad federal guidelines, but states have some flexibility in how they administer the program. People must meet eligibility requirements determined by each state. Eligibility depends on income and varies from state to state. Rates of payment also vary, with some states providing far higher payments than others. The amount the federal government contributes to Medicaid varies from a minimum of 50% of total costs to a maximum of 76.8%.

The differences in eligibility and payment rates lead to wide variations in the level of care provided to the poor in different states and create disparities in care. In contrast to those on Medicare, people who receive Medicaid are not required to pay any fees to participate. Table 14-2 highlights the similarities and differences in the Medicare and Medicaid programs.

Personal (out-of-pocket) payment

Personal payment for health care services is the least common method. Few people can afford out-of-pocket payment for more than the most basic health services. At today's prices, an illness or injury severe enough to require hospitalization can quickly exhaust a family's financial reserves, forcing them into bankruptcy. A study by Harvard researchers in 2005 reported the single most commonly cited reason for declaring bankruptcy is medical bills, accounting for half of all personal bankruptcy declarations (Consumer Affairs, 2005). Generally, only those people without access to some form of private group insurance or public insurance rely on personal payment. It can take years for a family to pay a single, large medical bill.

Table 14-2   Facts About Medicare and Medicaid

	Medicare	Medicaid
Funding	Federal government	Federal and state governments
Administration	Federal government	State governments
Eligibility	People ≥65 years and certain others	Selected poor and disabled (includes some elderly)
Level of benefits	Same nationwide	Varies from state to state
Payment by recipients	Required	Usually not required; co-payments may be required in Medicaid managed care
Coverage	Inpatient care; outpatient care; prescriptions	Comprehensive inpatient and outpatient care; prescriptions

Modified from Centers for Medicare & Medicaid Services: Medicare program: general information, 2006 (website): http://www.cms. hhs.gov/MedicareGenInfo/; Centers for Medicare & Medicaid Services: *Medicaid at-a-glance 2005, a Medicaid information source,* 2005 (website): http://www.chs.hhs.gov/MedicaidGenInfo/Downloads/MedicaidAtAGlance2005.pdf.

Workers' compensation

Workers' compensation constitutes a small proportion of insurance coverage. The program varies from state to state but generally covers only workers who are injured on the job. It usually covers treatment for injuries and weekly payments during the time the worker is absent from work for injury-related causes. In the case of accidental death, the worker's family receives compensation. Companies are required by law to contribute to a compensation fund from which money is withdrawn when accidental injuries or deaths occur at work.

Figure 14-7 represents the proportion each of the major payment methods contributed to the funding of health care services in the United States in 2007.

Nurses' Role in Managing Health Care Costs

Staff nurses can play an important role in controlling health care costs. They have the most frequent and direct contact with patients and can have a positive impact by reducing unnecessary

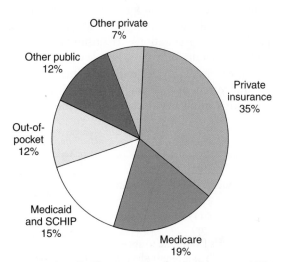

Figure 14-7 Funding sources for health care, 2007. From Centers for Medicare and Medicaid Services, Office of the Actuary, National Health Statistics Group: *The nation's health dollar, calendar year 2004: where it came from,* 2007 (website): http://www.slideshare.net/commonhealth/national-health-spending-in-2007-presentation (slide 10).

spending. Reducing spending does not have to mean sacrificing quality patient care. Many small economies can lead to large savings.

The first step is to become cost conscious. As a group, nurses tend to have poor cost awareness. When they are made aware of costs, their supply use patterns can change. Such simple methods as posting the price of supplies on shelves, cutting down on "borrowing" between units, and transferring all patients' bedside equipment, medications, and supplies carefully can make dramatic changes in per-patient expenditures. Making staff nurses aware of less-expensive alternatives is only one way they can reduce costs. Starting or expanding a revenue-generating recycling program is another measure that all hospital employees can support.

Nurses are positioned to produce even more meaningful savings by providing excellent patient care and being advocates for their patients' pocketbooks. Nurses must recognize that no matter how well-insured patients may be, they will have to pay some portion of charges personally. It may only be 20% or less, but that amount can quickly overload a family's budget.

Nurses who question unnecessary or repetitive tests, suggest generic drugs rather than name brands, and teach patients and their families how to monitor their health conditions and detect problems early to avoid repeated hospitalizations all contribute to cost management. Such nursing measures as scrupulous hand washing to prevent infections, turning patients on schedule to avoid pressure ulcers, and vigilance to reduce the risk of falls are not usually thought of as cost-containment measures, yet they are. Beginning in October 2008, Medicare no longer reimburses facilities for the treatment of eight "reasonably preventable" hospital-acquired conditions including pressure ulcers, catheter-associated urinary tract infections, falls with injury and burns, and vascular catheter-associated infections, all of which are conditions that can be prevented by nurses. Every day that a patient must be hospitalized beyond the length of stay authorized by the payer results in additional charges to the patient and costs to the hospital.

In both inpatient and outpatient settings, organizing and streamlining the flow of patients for maximum efficiency represents a huge savings for the facility and is under the control of nurses and nurse managers. Although nurses can and should look for ways to reduce costs, controlling costs must never take priority over patient care. Remembering provision 2 of the *Code of Ethics for Nurses* will assist you to maintain your ethical standards: "The nurse's primary commitment is to the patient, whether an individual, family, group, or community" (ANA, 2001).

HEALTH CARE REFORM AND UNIVERSAL ACCESS

The United States and South Africa are the two only industrialized nations that do not provide universal access to health care to all of their citizens. Despite the fact that in 2008 U.S. health care expenditures totaled more than those of any other country in the world, the U.S. infant death rate was ranked 44th of 224 of ranked nations (Central Intelligence Agency, 2009). Infant death rate is considered an indicator of a nation's health care practices.

Concerns about health care practices in the United States are not new. In the 1992 presidential campaign, candidates in both political parties, as well as nonpartisan groups, advocated some type of health care reform. These groups included nursing organizations, the American Association of Retired Persons, labor unions, the American College of Physicians, the National Leadership Coalition for Health Care Reform, and numerous members of the U.S. Congress. Most of these groups put forward specific plans for reform, including *Nursing's Agenda for Health Care Reform* by the ANA (1993), which was endorsed by more than 60 nursing organizations and associations. Early in President Bill Clinton's first term, then-First Lady Hillary Clinton led a bipartisan effort to improve access to health care. For a time, it seemed progress was being made. Despite widespread public support for reform, however, the effort ultimately failed. Lobbying against health care reform were well-funded, powerful interest groups such as the pharmaceutical, health insurance, and medical equipment industries, as well as the American Medical Association and the American Hospital Association, associations with two of the most powerful lobbies in Washington. These entities, as well as others, preferred to maintain the status quo to protect their financial interests. During the Bush administration, few steps toward reform were achieved as the terrorist attacks of September 11, 2001, and subsequent war efforts in Iraq and Afghanistan took center stage and sidelined comprehensive reform.

During the 2008 presidential campaign, concerns about access to health care, the quality of care, and disparities in care fueled renewed debate about health care in this country. To be prepared to participate in the reform efforts, the ANA revised and updated *Nursing's Agenda for Health Care Reform* and issued the report entitled *ANA's Health System Reform Agenda,* available online: http://nursingworld.org/MainMenuCate gories/HealthcareandPolicyIssues/HealthSystem Reform.aspx.

The Obama administration's campaign commitment to reform health care within his first year in office remained a priority. The economic recession, however, placed severe restrictions on what could be achieved, and partisan politics continues to create stalemates in Congress, where health care legislation must be conceived and approved. The same special interest groups that opposed change and defeated the Clinton plan again brought out their forces to oppose the administration's efforts. An encouraging early sign of President Barack Obama's commitment to change, however, was the passage of the State Children's Health Insurance Program (SCHIP), only a few weeks after he took office. This legislation expanded current SCHIP coverage to include 4 million additional children. This action, on behalf of uninsured children, was applauded by many, including nursing organizations.

Clearly, increasing the number of people covered would increase expenses unless drastic cost-management measures were put in place. As this text goes to press in November, 2009, it seems unlikely that a systematic and comprehensive reform of the entire health care system is possible. Instead, we can expect to see state-by-state efforts to address the specific current issues of concern discussed earlier. Most experts agree that reform efforts must be projected to reduce, or at least not increase, the cost of health care if they are to be supported by Congress. Despite wide-ranging differences of opinion about the specifics of health care reform proposals, some general questions should be asked in evaluating reform proposals:

1. Is there a uniform minimum set of benefits for all citizens, otherwise known as universal access?
2. Are coverage and benefits continuous and not dependent on where people live or work?
3. Are there mechanisms for controlling costs, especially administrative expenses?
4. Are provisions made for care to be provided by the most cost-effective personnel, taking quality issues and patient outcomes into consideration?
5. Are the issues of adequate facilities and personnel to ensure access for all addressed?
6. Is there an emphasis on quality care?
7. Are there incentives for healthy lifestyles and preventive care?

Further changes in nursing and health care delivery and finance are certain to be on the horizon. Most likely they will be gradual, rather than revolutionary. It remains to be seen whether these changes will improve access and quality of health care for all Americans. Health care reform legislation passed after November 2009 will be posted on the Evolve website (http://evolve.elsevier.com).

Summary of Key Points

- The health care delivery system in the United States is a complex system that provides health promotion, illness prevention, diagnosis and treatment, and rehabilitation and long-term care.
- Health care agencies may be classified as governmental or voluntary, as for-profit or not-for-profit, or according to level of care provided. A single agency may fit into all three categories.
- Health care agencies have traditionally been structured with boards of directors, chief executive officers, medical and nursing staffs, and members of a variety of other disciplines.
- Accreditation and continuous quality improvement are efforts to ensure public safety and institutional effectiveness and accountability.
- Access to comprehensive treatment and positive treatment outcomes varies among populations, creating disparities that disadvantage certain groups such as minorities and poor people. Correcting health care disparities has proved to be a complex task with only modest progress reported.
- An interdisciplinary health care team consists of an array of professionals, including physicians and physician assistants, nurses, health care technicians, licensed practical/vocational nurses, dietitians, pharmacists, technologists and technicians, social workers, various therapists, and administrative support personnel. Each member has an important part to play in ensuring the best patient outcomes.
- Historically, there have been a number of systems of nursing care delivery, each of which has advantages and disadvantages.
- Many variations and combinations of the major nursing care delivery systems are in use today.
- Nurses use a variety of roles, such as provider of care, teacher, counselor, manager, researcher, collaborator, and patient advocate, in meeting patients' needs.
- Attempts to manage costs have forced major changes in the health care delivery system.
- Health care financing in the United States is directly influenced by a basic economic disequilibrium in health care because people who do not pay directly for health care are not sensitive to the price of care.
- The entire health care system, including nurses and nursing services, has been profoundly affected by health care economic principles.
- Medicare and Medicaid programs, begun in 1965, quickly created a serious financial drain on federal and state budgets that continues today. In response, cost-containment efforts were begun by the federal government in the 1970s and persist in various old and new forms.
- Regardless of the type of cost-containment efforts used, health care costs have continued

to spiral upward. Without serious health care reform, this will continue.

- Nurses can play a role in managing health care costs by becoming more cost aware, efficient, and effective.
- System-wide health reform efforts are supported by public opinion but must pass the U.S. Congress. The Obama administration pledged to institute reform efforts within the first year of taking office, but special interest groups and opposing factors in Congress threatened to derail the process.

Critical Thinking Questions

1. Using the yellow pages of your telephone directory or a directory of social services, identify local health services in the following areas: health promotion, illness prevention, diagnosis and treatment, rehabilitation, and long-term care. Judging from the number of agencies for each service, where does the health care emphasis seem to be? What implications does this have for citizens of your community?

2. Obtain the organizational chart of a health care facility. Examine it to see how nursing fits into the overall structure. Who reports to the nurse executive, and to whom does the nurse executive report? What other administrative staff members are on the same level with the nurse executive?

3. Hold a panel discussion on reimbursement. Invite representatives from government, a managed-care organization, a hospital, a major employer, and a nonprofit charity to discuss how increases in health care costs have affected their organizations.

4. Interview nurses in the hospital, home health, disease management, and case management settings. Look for the similarities and the differences in their work and interactions with patients. How do they work together to provide seamless care for the patient?

5. Compare and contrast the five types of nursing care delivery systems from the viewpoint of the patient. If you were a consumer of nursing care, which system would you prefer? Why?

6. Look at the same question from the standpoint of the nurse. Which system would you find most satisfying in terms of your practice? Which would you like least?

7. Interview nurses in practice in an acute care setting in your community to determine what type of governance structure is used by the nursing staff. What do they see as the positive and negative aspects of the type identified?

8. In your view, is access to health care a basic right? Who should pay for it? Be prepared to defend your opinions.

9. List the basic health care services that should be provided to all citizens. Compare your list with the lists of classmates and discuss the rationale for your priorities.

10. Interview faculty members in your school to determine how they address the issue of health care disparities in their classes.

11. Should there be a limit on the percentage of national resources expended on health care? If so, how should the limit be established? Who should be responsible for determining the limit?

12. What process should be used to determine how health care resources are allocated? List criteria you would suggest to determine whether or not a person should receive a kidney transplant, a hip replacement, or a bone marrow transplant.

13. Should people with healthy lifestyles pay the same for care or insurance as those whose habits result in a greater likelihood of illness? How could such a differentiation be determined?

14. Should there be rationing of extremely expensive procedures, such as heart transplants, even if the patient is able to pay? Give a rationale for your answer.

15. List five things you as an individual nurse can do to become more cost aware and participate in managing health care costs.

⊖volve *To enhance your understanding of this chapter, try the Student Exercises on the Evolve site at http://evolve.elsevier.com/Chitty/professional.*

REFERENCES

Agency for Healthcare Research and Quality: *2007 National Healthcare Disparities Report,* Rockville, Md, February 2008, U.S. Department of Health and Human Services, Agency for Healthcare Research and Quality, AHRQ Pub. No. 08–0041 (website): http://www.ahrq.gov/qual/nhdr07/Chap1.htm.

Aiken LH, Clarke SP, Sloane DM, et al: Hospital nurse staffing and patient mortality, nurse burnout and job dissatisfaction, *JAMA* 288:1987-1993, 2002.

American Academy of Physician Assistants: *Information about PAs and the PA profession,* 2009 (website): http://www.aapa.org/about.pas.

American Hospital Association: *Welcome to the board: an orientation for the new health care trustee,* Chicago, 1999, AHA Press.

American Nurses Association: *Code of ethics for nurses with interpretive statements,* Washington, DC, 2001, American Nurses Publishing.

American Nurses Association: *Scope and standards for nurse administrators,* ed 2, Washington, DC, 2004, American Nurses Association (website): http://nursesbooks.org.

American Nurses Association: *ANA's health system reform agenda,* 2008 (website): http://nursingworld.org/MainMenuCategories/HealthcareandPolicyIssues/HealthSystemReform.aspx.

American Nurses Association: *Nursing: scope and standards of practice,* ed 2, Washington, DC, 2010, American Nurses Association.

Bastable SB: *Nurse as educator,* Sudbury, Mass, 2003, Jones & Bartlett.

Bureau of Labor Statistics, U.S. Department of Labor, *Occupational outlook handbook, 2008-09 edition, licensed practical and licensed vocational nurses* (website): http://www.bls.gov/oco/ocos102.htm.

Centers for Medicare & Medicaid Services: *Medicaid at-a-glance 2005, a Medicaid information source,* 2005 (website): http://www.cms.hhs.gov/MedicaidGenInfo/Downloads/MedicaidAtAGlance2005.pdf.

Centers for Medicare & Medicaid Services: *Medicare program: general information,* 2006 (website): http://www.cms.hhs.gov/MedicareGenInfo/.

Centers for Medicare & Medicaid Services: *National health care expenditures projections: 2008-2018,* 2008 (download available at website): http://www.cms.hhs.gov/NationalHealthExpendData/03_NationalHealthAccountsProjected.asp#TopOfPage.

Centers for Medicare & Medicaid Services: *Medicare & you 2010,* 2010 (website): http://www.medicare.gov/publications/pubs/pdf/10050.pdf.

Centers for Medicare & Medicaid Services, Office of the Actuary, National Health Statistics Group: *The nation's health dollar, calendar year 2007: where it came from,* 2007 (website): http://www.slideshare.net/commonhealth/national-health-spending-in-2007-presentation.

Central Intelligence Agency: *The world factbook: rank order—infant mortality rate,* 2009 (website): https://www.cia.gov/library/publications/the-world-factbook/geos/us.html#top.

Consumer Affairs: *Medical bills leading cause of bankruptcy, Harvard study finds,* ConsumerAffairs.com, Inc., 2005 (website): http://www.consumeraffairs.com/news04/2005/bankruptcy_study.html.

Dall T, Chen Y, Seifert R, Maddox P, Hogan P: The economic value of professional nursing, *Med Care* 47(1):97-104, 2009.

Davis DS: *Where the bedside nurse rules,* NursingSpectrum.com, Aug 5, 2008 (website): http://include.nurse.com/apps/pbcs.dll/article?AID=/20080825/PA02/108250085.

Healthy People 2010: *Healthy People 2010 fact sheet,* Rockville, Md, 2005a (website): http://www.healthypeople.gov/About/hpfact.htm.

Healthy People 2010: *What are the leading health indicators?* Rockville, Md, 2005b (website): http://www.healthypeople.gov/LHI/lhiwhat.htm.

Jacob P, Rapoport J: *The economics of health and medical care,* Sudbury, Mass, 2002, Jones & Bartlett.

The Joint Commission: *Facts about The Joint Commission,* 2009 (website): http://www.jointcommission.org/AboutUs/Fact_Sheets/joint_commission_facts.htm.

Kerfoot K: Establishing guardrails in leadership, *Nurs Econ* 23(6):334-335, 2005.

Lambertson E: *Nursing team organization and functioning,* New York, 1953, Columbia University.

Maurer FA: Financing of health care: context for community health nursing, In Smith C, Maurer FA, editors: *Community health nursing: theory and practice,* ed 2, Philadelphia, 2000, Saunders.

McClosky J, Dochterman G, Bulechek B, et al: Determining cost of nursing interventions: a beginning, *Nurs Econ* 19(4):146-155, 2001.

McKibben RC: *DRGs and nursing care,* Kansas City, Mo, 1985, American Nurses Association Center for Research.

Needleman J, Buerhaus PI, Stewart M, et al: Market watch. Nurse staffing in hospitals: is there a business case for quality? *Health Affairs* 25(1):204-211, 2006.

Office of Minority Health & Health Disparities, Centers for Disease Control and Prevention: *Eliminating racial and ethnic health disparities,* 2009 (website): http://www.cdc.gov/omhd/About/disparities.htm.

Pappas S: The cost of nurse-sensitive adverse events, *J Nurs Adm* 38(5):230-236, 2008.

Rogers R: Adapting to the new workplace reality, *Info Nursing: A Publication of the Nurses Association of New Brunswick* 39(1):18-20, 2008.

Shirey MR: Nursing practice models for acute and critical care: overview of care delivery models, *Crit Care Nurs Clin North Am* 20:365-373, 2008.

Sounart A: *Embracing the role of patient advocate,* NurseZone.com, 2008 (website): http://www.nursezone.com/nursing-news-events/more-features.aspx?ID=17938.

Trossman S: Issues up close: the personal risks of advocating for patients, *American Nurse Today* 3(8): 38-39, 2008.

Unruh L: Nurse staffing and patient, nurse, and financial outcomes, *AJN* 108(1):62-71, 2008.

U.S. Department of Labor, Bureau of Labor Statistics: *Occupational outlook handbook,* 2006 (website): http://www.bls.gov/oco/ocos079.htm.

Voelker R: Decades of work to reduce disparities in health care produce limited success, *JAMA* 299(12):1411-1413, 2008.

The Political Activism of Nursing: In Organizations and Government

Beth Perry Black

LEARNING OUTCOMES

After studying this chapter, students will be able to:
- Differentiate between politics and policy
- Explain why professions have associations
- Demonstrate an understanding of the complex role that associations play in the profession and in society
- Recognize the opportunities that associations offer to increase the leadership capacity of nursing students and registered nurses
- Explain the concept of personalizing the political process
- Cite examples of sources of both personal and professional power
- Describe how nurses can become involved in politics and policy development at the levels of citizen, activist, and politician
- Explain how organized nursing is involved in political activities designed to strengthen professional nursing and influence health policy

The 2008 presidential election of Barack Obama as the 44th president of the United States and the first African American to hold that office marked the end of a long, arduous, and sometimes rancorous national campaign. From the early days of the primary season until the final results were announced on election night, the presidential campaign was filled with debates and forums on many topics that are of interest to American citizens. Health care reform was one of the key areas of discussion during the campaign. President Obama campaigned on the issue, citing the high costs of health care and the high percentage of uninsured Americans as central concerns in his plans for reform (Figure 15-1).

Never before has the national policy-making stage seemed so close at hand to the American public. National media networks and 24-hour cable news coverage have brought life "inside the Beltway" into American living rooms and into scrutiny. Interest and involvement of American citizens in governmental processes and accountability are good for democracy. It is sometimes hard to determine, however, what is newsworthy versus what is simply interesting! A heavily covered event in the media was the First Family's new puppy, a promise from the President-elect during his acceptance speech in Grant Park, Chicago, on election night. At the same time, serious economic troubles threatened to shut down one of the country's largest automakers, and piracy off the coast of Africa threatened the lives of the American crew. The news coverage of the foundering economy and an act of piracy competed for airtime with the arrival of the First Dog at the White House. These events on the national and world stage seemed very close at hand.

National politics and policy are of great interest; however, much of the politics and policy that affect our daily lives occurs at the state and local levels. The workings of government in your state legislature and local municipalities are likely to be much less familiar to you than what is occurring nationally. Even less conspicuous are the policy-making and policy-influencing activities

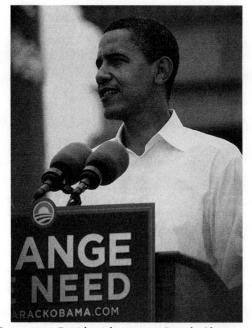

Figure 15-1 Presidential nominee Barack Obama and vice-presidential nominee Joe Biden campaign for "Change We Need" at a rally in Greensboro, NC in September 2008. (Courtesy of Beth Black.)

that occur within the professional organizations that support and shape nursing practice. Yet our day-to-day lives, both professionally and personally, are shaped to a large degree by what happens at the local and organizational levels. This chapter will focus on politics and policy making in several arenas of importance to nursing. This discussion will start with professional organizations and their roles in setting practice and policy, then will address politics and policy in government from both national and local perspectives.

Several chapters of this book cover material that is heavily influenced by government. The content of Chapter 1, the current status of nursing, will be the content of a future edition's Chapter 2, the history and social contexts of nursing. The content of both of these chapters reflects policy and politics that affect who nurses are and what we do. Chapter 4 is directly concerned with policy that affects practice. Governmental

regulation through licensure is an issue, but the influence of professional organizations to set standards and affect nurse practice acts demonstrates the two-way process that is required to keep nursing relevant and up-to-date within the health care arena. The focus on ethics in Chapter 5 describes issues of justice and autonomy, foundational principles in American jurisprudence, which shape how we understand and resolve ethical dilemmas.

Issues of nursing education (Chapter 7) are directly shaped by governmental regulation to ensure that schools of nursing produce graduates that can be entrusted to provide safe care. In Chapter 11, nursing research is shown to be heavily dependent on the financing of the National Institutes of Health's National Institute for Nursing Research and other centers and institutes funded with federal dollars. Research is key to the development of the knowledge base of nursing, which in turn protects its status as a profession and an academic discipline, and its influence in both academic and policy arenas. The previous chapter, Chapter 14, addressed the complex issues surrounding how health care is delivered and financed. This is a heavily regulated endeavor with incredibly intricate implications affecting how and where nurses practice. This completes the circle, in a sense, drawing you back to Chapter 1, the current status of nursing, and where we are going.

Furthermore, you are on the edge of a significant movement for health care reform, through which nurses do not have to be passive recipients of decisions made on their behalf about practice. Nurses are poised to participate in decisions about health care reform in which nurses, the largest single group of health care providers in the country, can have significant influence.

POLICY AND POLITICS

Policy and politics are more than what is happening in Washington, D.C. They encompass what happens to us in our daily lives, in the workplace, and in our organizations, as well as in government. Politics has two meanings. Concise definitions are as follows (http://dictionary.reference.com/browse/politics, 2009):

1. "The science of government; that part of ethics which has to do with the regulation and government of a nation or state, the preservation of its safety, peace, and prosperity, the defense of its existence and rights against foreign control or conquest, the augmentation of its strength and resources, and the protection of its citizens in their rights, with the preservation and improvement of their morals."

2. "The management of a political party; the conduct and contests of parties with reference to political measures or the administration of public affairs; the advancement of candidates to office; in a bad sense, artful or dishonest management to secure the success of political candidates or parties; political trickery."

We tend to think of politics in terms of the second definition, the one associated with political parties, campaigns, promises, and wrangling for votes, support, and position. However, the first definition is the one that has the more lasting impact on society. The government is the political body that has to do with the regulation and preservation of the nation. The politics of the second definition is the process by which we determine who will occupy the government in our representative democracy.

Policy, on the other hand refers to the following:

a plan or course of action, as of a government, political party, or business, intended to influence and determine decisions, actions, and other matters: American foreign policy or American health care policy (http://dictionary.reference.com/browse/policy, 2009).

Policy is shaped to a great degree by those who are successful in the political arena (the second definition). These are the elected officials who describe their agenda before the election to receive support, endorsements, and, ultimately, the majority of votes to be elected into office. For

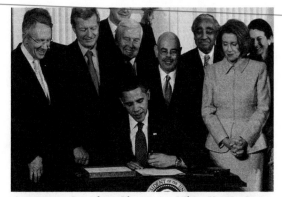

Figure 15-2 President Obama at a White House signing ceremony of the SCHIP legislation 2 weeks after taking office. He said, "I refuse to accept that millions of our children fail to reach their full potential because we fail to meet their basic needs." (Used with permission from UPI.)

instance, President Obama's agenda on health care reform was discussed and debated at length during the campaign season. That he is embarking on a complex and wide-ranging effort to make health care more affordable should be of no surprise to anyone who was paying attention to the 24-hour cable news outlets that both reported and argued the various merits of his health care campaign agenda throughout the 2008 campaign. In other words, President Obama used the politics as a process (the second definition) to achieve a goal of managing the government (first definition) so that he may influence change in health care policy with the expectation and hope of improving affordability. One of the first pieces of legislation signed by President Obama was the State Children's Health Insurance Program (SCHIP) that extended health insurance coverage to 8 million children whose parents cannot afford health insurance coverage (Figure 15-2).

Power, Authority, and Influence

A review of the concepts *power, authority,* and *influence* will help focus the discussion of policy and the remainder of this chapter. Power is strength or force that is exerted or capable of being exerted. Power in and of itself is latent.

A person who has authority has legitimacy to exert power, that is, to enforce laws, demand obedience, make commands and determinations, or judge the acts of others. Persons who have been vested with this power, for instance, through a fair and democratic process, are known as authorities, especially a government or body of government officials. Influence is a form of power that is not legitimated through official channels, that is, elections or appointments by one in authority, but influence is the action or process of producing effects on the actions, behavior, and opinions of others. For example, the issue of lobbyists got much attention in the 2008 presidential election. Lobbyists are people who try to influence government officials to act in a certain way that will benefit the constituency that hired the lobbyist to work on its behalf, that is, to exert influence.

A simple clinical example will clarify the difference among these three concepts.

Jake Wilson, RN, is an experienced labor and delivery nurse, and his patient is Ms. McLean. Ms. McLean has been in labor for several hours but is not making very much progress. Jake believes that augmenting her labor with oxytocin would be a good idea. Jake cannot begin this infusion because he does not have the authority to do so without Dr. Martin's order. Dr. Martin has both the power and the authority to write orders. Jake, because he is very experienced, understands that he can influence Dr. Martin's decision by giving Dr. Martin his expert opinion on the situation. Jake calls Dr. Martin, influences Dr. Martin to order the oxytocin, and begins the infusion in a few minutes. Ms. McLean delivers a healthy baby girl 3 hours later. Note that Jake exerted power through influencing Dr. Martin's behavior; Dr. Martin had latent power, that is, power that had not yet been used to write an order for the oxytocin; and Dr. Martin had the authority as a licensed physician to write the order and to make sure that it was enforced.

This is a common scenario between nurses who need something for their patients and physicians who hold the authority to write orders. As the patient's advocate, skilled nurses know how to influence physicians to get what their patient needs. This is not to be confused with manipulation, which is not a good personal or professional behavior. But being able to state your case on behalf of your patient clearly, without manipulation, is an excellent way of influencing the outcome in a way that you and your patient would like.

Policy

Policy involves principles that govern actions directed toward given ends; policy statements set forth a plan, direction, or goal for action. Policies may result in laws, regulations, or guidelines that govern behavior in the public arena or in the private arena. Health policy refers to public or private rules, regulations, laws, or guidelines that relate to the pursuit of health and the delivery of health services. Policy reflects the choices that an entity (government or organization) makes regarding its goals and priorities and how it will allocate its resources.

Policy decisions (e.g., laws or regulations) reflect the values and beliefs of those making the decisions. As values and beliefs change, so do policy decisions. For instance, laws limiting smoking in public buildings or private restaurants were nonexistent 40 years ago because the harmful effects of smoking and secondhand smoke were not well known. As the public became more aware of the dangers of smoking, values about smoking changed. Changes in laws followed the change in values. Laws limiting smoking and the sale and use of tobacco products have now become commonplace. Elected officials responded to the changing values of the public and recognized that the public supported the passage of laws limiting smoking. In a representative democracy, this is how policy gets changed. Officials are elected to represent and then act on the interests of their constituents, that is, the people of their state, district, or municipality.

In professional organizations, policy focuses on the rules and guidelines established by the governing body of the organization, usually a board of directors. Those guidelines or policies also reflect the values of the organization. For instance, one would expect a nursing organization such as the American Nurses Association (ANA) to focus on issues of health promotion, illness prevention, and nursing practice issues. That would be quite different from an organization such as the National Collegiate Athletic Association (NCAA), where the values of its members would be reflected in policies and recommendations that support and regulate athletics at the college level across the country.

Politics

Politics is a process that requires influencing the allocation of scarce resources. Allocation assumes that there are not enough resources for all who may want them. Those resources might be money, people, time, supplies, or equipment. Who gets what, or how those resources are allocated, is determined through the political process. Policies are the decisions; politics is influencing those decisions. There are always stakeholders, individuals with a vested interest, who try to influence those with the power to make the final decisions.

In organizations, stakeholders are the members, the larger community served by the work of the organization, and other groups or individuals affected by those decisions. For example, Patients Out of Time, an organization started by a nurse, has worked for years to educate the public and health care professionals about the therapeutic use of cannabis and to advocate for the medicinal use of marijuana (http://www.medicalcannabis.com). Stakeholders for this organization would be affected patients and families, health care providers, and those who make decisions about the laws and regulations about cannabis use. These include state and federal legislators, as well as the Food and Drug Administration (FDA), the Secretary of Health and Human Services (who oversees the policies of the FDA), and organizations such as the ANA and the American Public Health Association, both of which have been supportive of the issue (Mather, 2007).

Politics works similarly in the public arena. For example, to garner support from state legislators to increase funding for nursing scholarships, an organization or coalition of organizations must have a plan to mobilize stakeholders (those who have a particular interest tied to an issue) to lobby legislators. Such stakeholders would include administrators of nursing organizations, colleges of nursing, hospitals, nursing homes, and other health care organizations, as well as physician groups and others who know the necessity of having a competent and adequate nursing workforce. The more stakeholder support that can be mustered, the more likely it is that policymakers will appreciate the broad constituent support for the issue and the more likely they will be to vote for increased funding for nursing education and scholarships.

Linking Practice, Policy, and Politics

Leaders in nursing, from Florence Nightingale to Lavinia Dock, saw and understood the connection between their work and the larger world in which policy decisions affected what they were able to do. Nightingale could not have been successful in the Crimea without the support of Sir Sidney Herbert, Secretary of War. Lavinia Dock joined with other nurses to found the ANA, pressure hospital administrators to improve working conditions for nurses, and galvanize support for nursing registration (Lewenson, 2007, p. 23). A recent example is Karen Daley, a modern nurse who went public with her needlestick injury that resulted in human immunodeficiency virus (HIV) and hepatitis C infections. She went public to influence legislation requiring protective devices. In each instance these leaders knew that nursing practice could be improved only through legislation, regulation, or unification to create a formidable national organization. She recognized the power in her story and the extent to which her experience could influence those with authority to make nursing practice safer. Her testimony before the House Committee on Education and the Workforce's Subcommittee on Workforce Protection can be found at http://republicans. edlabor.house.gov/archive/hearings/106th/wp/ needlestick62200/daley.htm. The larger world of public policy and the work of organizations become the arena in which someone with a vision for improved health or working conditions can change the way health is delivered and improve the health of populations. With these examples in mind, we now turn our attention to professional organizations as a means of activism.

PROFESSIONAL ORGANIZATIONS

Professionals create organizations to work collectively on issues that enhance their work and their involvement in communities, ensure continued learning and competence, and use political action to influence policy makers to support the mission of the organization. Professional organizations offer a supportive way to learn leadership skills, to test ideas, and to follow these ideas to completion. Nursing has a national organization open to all graduate nurses, the ANA (http://www.nursingworld.org); a national student nurses organization, the National Student Nurses' Association (NSNA, http://www.nsna.org); and many other specialty organizations developed around particular practice areas. Nursing organizations influence public policy in a variety of ways. We will begin this section by looking at the role and function of organizations, examining why nurses do or do not join organizations, and discussing examples of collective action. Because organizations are often the catalyst for involvement in political action, we will also explore the broader area of political action in the public arena.

Joining a Professional Organization

Nurses join organizations to network with colleagues, to pursue continuing education and certification opportunities, to stay informed on professional issues, to develop leadership skills, to influence health policy, and to work collectively for job security. Yet fewer than 10 percent of the nation's registered nurses are members of the ANA (Kany, 2007) and only about 20 percent of nurses belong to one of the 100 or more specialty nursing organizations. Nurses cite issues of high cost of dues, lack of time, and lack of interest as reasons that they do not join. In some states,

complex relationships between the state nurses association, the ANA and collective bargaining units restrict ANA membership. There are also different expectations and interests among generations of nurses. Although baby boomers and older members may accept traditional organizational structures and volunteer tasks, younger colleagues prefer short-term projects, using technology such as blogs and chat rooms rather than face-to-face meetings. Sometimes young members overestimate their influence in these organizations, expecting to assume leadership positions quickly without having to work up through the ranks (Holland, 2005). As older members retire, organizations are becoming more responsive to incorporating processes and products that appeal to younger members.

Types of Associations

There are more than 100 national nursing organizations and many more state and local groups. Nurses often express confusion about which group to join. In general, associations can be classified as one of three main types:
1. Broad-purpose professional associations
2. Specialty practice associations
3. Special interest associations

The ANA is an example of a broad-purpose association. Individual nurses who belong to the ANA typically become members of their state's constituent member association.

As the nursing profession's body of knowledge and research grows and diversifies, many nurses limit their practices to specialty practice areas such as maternal/infant care, school or community health, critical care, or perioperative or emergency/trauma nursing. They often join the specialty organization for their area of clinical interest. Members of specialty practice nursing associations also may choose to belong to the ANA or one of its constituent member associations (at the state level) to support the entire profession because specialty associations focus only on standards of practice or professional needs of the particular specialty. Sixty-six specialty organizations are represented in the Nursing Organizations Alliance.

Examples of special interest organizations include Sigma Theta Tau International (the Honor Society of Nursing), which one must be invited to join, and the American Association for the History of Nursing, which focuses on a particular area of study in nursing. Comprehensive and frequently updated lists of nursing organizations are available online (http://www.nurse.org/orgs.shtml).

Nurses are connected internationally through the International Council of Nurses (ICN). The ICN is a federation of national nurse associations (NNAs) representing nurses in 118 countries. The ANA represents U.S. registered nurses in the ICN, and the NSNA represents U.S. nursing students in the ICN.

Founded in 1899, the ICN is the world's first and widest-reaching international organization for health professionals. Operated by nurses for nurses, the ICN works to ensure quality nursing care for all, sound health policies globally, the advancement of nursing knowledge, the presence worldwide of a respected nursing profession, and a competent and satisfied nursing workforce. For additional details about the ICN's activities in professional nursing practice, nursing regulation, and the socioeconomic welfare of nurses, visit the ICN home page (http://www.icn.ch).

PURPOSE AND ACTIVITIES OF ORGANIZATIONS

Organizational activities reflect their mission statements. The mission statement is generated by the membership and defines the purpose and who is served by the organization. For instance, the mission of the ANA is "to work for the improvement of health standards and availability of health care services for all people, foster high standards for nursing, stimulate and promote the professional development of nurses, and advance their economic and general welfare." This defines the association's areas of focus as practice standards, a code of ethical conduct, continuing education and conferences, and collective action around workplace issues. In 1999 the ANA House of Delegates, the elected representatives from the constituent member associations (CMAs), approved the creation of two divisions for economic and employment issues: the Center for American Nurses (CAN) (http://centerforamericannurses.org) and a collective bargaining unit, the United American Nurses (UAN) (http://www.uannurse.org/). CAN's mission is to promote safe workplace environments and to advocate for issues of appropriate staffing, generational workplace issues, and patient and provider safety. The UAN focuses on collective bargaining and is the only national union of nurses. It provides guidance, information, and support for state nursing association affiliates. The UAN is an affiliate of the AFL-CIO, the largest labor organization in the country.

Nurses and Unions

Unionization of nurses is a controversial topic. Nurses may choose to join unions to work collectively, to have control over their practice and workplace, and to work to equalize power between management and staff. This can be an effective approach if the health care organization is willing to work collaboratively with unions. Union affiliation is a highly complex process, one that is defined by rules and regulations under the National Labor Act and overseen by the National Labor Relations Board. There are limits on what issues unions can bargain; for instance, hours, pay, and benefits are included in all contracts for all unionized workers.

For nurses there are additional issues that are increasingly part of contract negotiations. These include issues such as staffing, work assignments, and shared governance responsibilities. The national nursing shortage is creating an environment in which both management and nurses themselves have a desire to create work environments that decrease turnover and ensure a competent workforce.

The UAN represents only nurses, but there are many nursing units affiliated with nonnursing unions. The Service Employees International Union (SEIU); the American Federation of Teachers (AFT); the Association of Federal, State,

County, and Municipal Employees (AFSCME); and the United Mine Workers (UMW) are all examples of organizations that have nursing units but also represent larger, nonnursing constituencies.

Nurses wonder if they should join unions. Much of that depends on where they work. If seeking a staff job in an institution in which a nursing union already exists, a nurse may be required to join the union as a condition of employment. This is called a "closed shop," meaning that management is required to bargain with the union and union membership is required as a condition of employment. An "open shop" is one in which employees are not required to join but in which an individual's contract will be dependent on what union and management have negotiated. Most nurses work in nonunion facilities. Some states are more "union friendly" than others. States in which labor unions flourish, such as in the Northeast, Northwest, and Midwest, have the vast majority of nursing unions. Smaller states, particularly in the Southeast (other than Florida) and Southwest, have few or no nurse unions. These are known as "right to work states." Though unions have made numerous attempts to organize nurses in these states, the value system of the work culture is less supportive of union affiliation by professionals.

BENEFITS OF BELONGING TO PROFESSIONAL ASSOCIATIONS

A variety of benefits result from membership in professional associations. These range from certification and discounts on travel, products, and services, to opportunities to engage in research projects and learn political action strategies.

Developing Leadership Skills

Students who join the NSNA have opportunities to learn from and socialize with their peers in school and at the state and national levels (Figure 15-3). As NSNA members, they benefit from developing leadership and organizational skills that can be vital in their professional careers and personal lives. Through the NSNA Leadership

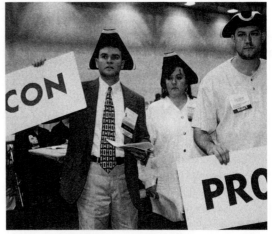

Figure 15-3 Students serving as delegates to the NSNA House of Delegates learn leadership and political skills, in addition to meeting persons with similar interests. In this photo, students voice their views—pro and con—about resolutions being considered by the delegates. (Courtesy of the NSNA.)

University, the NSNA recognizes students for their leadership and management competencies with a certificate presented at the annual NSNA convention. The NSNA Leadership University provides an opportunity for nursing students to earn academic credit for their participation in NSNA's many leadership activities. From the school chapter level to the state and national levels, nursing students learn how to work in shared governance and cooperative relationships with peers, faculty, students in other disciplines, community service organizations, and the public. In addition to preparing students to participate in professional organizations, practicing shared governance also prepares students to work in health care delivery settings that incorporate unit-based decision making, such as magnet hospitals. By participating in the NSNA Leadership University, students learn and practice the skills needed for future leadership. A list of those skills and competencies is provided in Box 15-1. For complete details about the NSNA Leadership University and all of the NSNA's programs, visit their websites (http://www.nsna.org and http://www.nsnal eadershipu.org).

Box 15-1   Attributes and Competencies Needed by Future Nurse Leaders and Managers*

- Demonstrates intellectual and analytical capacity
- Develops critical thinking ability
- Develops systems thinking
- Comprehends interdisciplinary models
- Communicates effectively
- Demonstrates effective interpersonal skills
- Listens empathetically and actively
- Adapts quickly to new situations
- Identifies global, national, and local trends
- Accepts high moral and ethical standards
- Manages conflict and masters conflict resolution skills
- Facilitates collaboration and group process
- Motivates others to participate in decision making
- Demonstrates capacity to interchange leadership/followership roles
- Mentors future leaders
- Empowers others
- Functions as a team player
- Understands strategic/tactical planning, implementation, and outcome evaluation
- Treats all human beings with respect and acceptance
- Strives for an inclusive society
- Balances professional responsibilities and personal life
- Accepts responsibility and accountability for decisions
- Demonstrates a commitment to lifelong learning
- Practices the spirit of cooperation
- Balances "high tech" with "high touch"
- Solves problems creatively
- Demonstrates the capacity for introspection and reflection
- Demonstrates the capacity to connect with the spiritual nature of human beings

Compiled by Dr. Diane J. Mancino, Executive Director, NSNA.
*These competencies and attributes are developed during participation in NSNA's leadership activities at the school, state, and national levels of the association. Visit http://www.nsnaleadershipu.org for more details.

Leadership skills are foundation blocks for nursing professional practice. Nurses have multiple opportunities to exercise leadership at the bedside, in clinical teams, and in management teams. The Nursing Alliance Leadership Academy (Nursing Organizations Alliance, 2005) was created to help nurses enhance leadership skills and focus on patients and care issues. The academy also focuses on developing political skills and policy awareness (http://www.nursing-alliance.org/content.cfm/id/nala).

Professional associations offer a supportive environment in which members can practice the acquisition of important leadership skills. Speaking publicly, planning projects, managing resources, and developing resolutions and position papers are opportunities to practice skills essential to formal leadership roles. It is no accident that nurses who are active in associations also tend to be recognized leaders in their work settings.

Certification and Continuing Education

Practicing nurses want to be recognized, through both compensation and position, for their level of professional expertise. Toward those ends, they may pursue certification in a specialty area. Certification is granted through professional associations. As discussed in Chapter 7, certification is a formal but voluntary process of demonstrating expertise in a particular area of nursing. Certified nurses may receive salary supplements and special opportunities. For information about credentials in nursing, visit the website of the ANA's subsidiary, the American Nurses Credentialing Center (ANCC), which offers a range of certification credentials (http://www.nursingworld.org/ancc).

Political Activism

As their careers develop, nurses may obtain master's-level and doctoral-level preparation or become nurse practitioners and practice independently outside an institution. These nurses desire and deserve direct reimbursement for their work, and they need state laws that mandate direct reimbursement of nurses. Others work in settings in which there are not enough registered nurses available to provide the quality of care the residents need. These nurses need laws that ensure appropriate registered nurse staffing and control educational requirements for unlicensed assistive personnel.

In each of these instances, the ANA, labor unions, and specialty organizations are involved in political action with legislators and regulators in the government arena. There are those within these organizations who develop the positions that nursing organizations believe are in nursing's best interests. There are a number of people within these organizations whose responsibilities are to advocate for legislation to support nursing's position. The process of political action and policy recommendations involves both paid staff, usually in the government affairs department, and volunteer members of the organizations, usually practicing nurses. The legislative agenda, that is, the public policy issues the organization supports, is developed by members appointed by the board of directors, as well as by staff who are experts in political and policy issues. The board of directors approves the legislative agenda. Organizations with legislative agendas depend on members to lobby legislators. They provide members with background information and also create "talking points" to use when lobbying for the selected issue. You can read about the ANA's particular legislative interests online (http://www.nursingworld.org/gova). As part of the process of encouraging nurses to lobby, information is given on the website about specific bills along with talking points for writing or speaking with congressional representatives. Association members can be very influential in lobbying legislators, particularly when the constituency is nationwide and representative of different stakeholders. Learning how to be politically active increases the power of both the individual and the organization represented.

Nursing organizations also work collaboratively through coalitions with other health professional and consumer groups. Such coalitions are focused on specific issues. For example, Health Care Without Harm (http://www.noharm.org)

is a group of 443 organizations in 52 countries whose mission is to protect health by reducing pollution in the health care industry. A nurse, Hollie Shaner McRae of Vermont, founded this organization when she became concerned about the waste created by disposable instruments in an operating room (Shaner McRae, 2002). The organization is now a significant national and international force advocating for the recycling and safe disposal of dangerous materials, such as mercury. This example demonstrates how one individual, working through organizations and coalitions of organizations, can have worldwide positive impact.

Practice Guidelines and Position Statements

Organizations serve an important function by defining practice standards, taking positions on practice issues, and developing ethical guidelines. For example, the ANA has positions on blood-borne and airborne diseases that include statements about HIV infection and nursing students. It defines ANA's recommendation of requiring educational content about such infections by qualified faculty, mandating universal precautions, and providing postexposure support for students who may sustain a needlestick injury. These statements serve to guide the organization's work in both the practice and the policy arenas and help individual nurses within workplaces to implement the policy. Guidelines and position statements are based on evidence from research, as well as opinions of nurse experts in the field. For example, ANA was involved in national coalitions and with the Occupational Safety and Health Administration (OSHA) when developing the brochure, *Blood-Borne Diseases*.

Another example is the recent revision of the *Code of Ethics for Nurses*, found inside the back cover of this book. A task force was appointed by the board of directors to review the previous Code and create revisions and recommendations. The revisions went through a process of approval by many entities within the ANA: the Congress of Nursing Practice, the Board of

Directors, and the House of Delegates, which speaks on behalf of all the members. Approval from so many groups within an organization assures "buy-in" by the membership. Buy-in is important because the Code serves as an ethical standard for all practicing nurses, whether they are ANA members or not, and is therefore of critical importance.

The NSNA also has a Code of Conduct (Box 15-2), which provides guidance for nursing students. This Code serves as the ethical foundation of student practice.

Box 15-2   National Student Nurses Association's Code of Academic and Clinical Conduct

PREAMBLE

Students of nursing have a responsibility to society in learning the academic theory and clinical skills needed to provide nursing care. The clinical setting presents unique challenges and responsibilities while caring for human beings in a variety of health care environments.

The Code of Academic and Clinical Conduct is based on an understanding that to practice nursing as a student is an agreement to uphold the trust that society has placed in us. The statements of the Code provide guidance for the nursing student in the personal development of an ethical foundation and need not be limited strictly to the academic or clinical environment but can assist in the holistic development of the person.

A CODE FOR NURSING STUDENTS

As students are involved in the clinical and academic environments, we believe that ethical principles are a necessary guide to professional development. Therefore within these environments we:

1. Advocate for the rights of all clients.
2. Maintain client confidentiality.
3. Take appropriate action to ensure the safety of clients, self, and others.
4. Provide care for the client in a timely, compassionate, and professional manner.
5. Communicate client care in a truthful, timely, and accurate manner.
6. Actively promote the highest level of moral and ethical principles and accept responsibility for our actions.
7. Promote excellence in nursing by encouraging lifelong learning and professional development.
8. Treat others with respect and promote an environment that respects human rights, values, and choice of cultural and spiritual beliefs.
9. Collaborate in every reasonable manner with the academic faculty and clinical staff to ensure the highest quality of client care.
10. Use every opportunity to improve faculty and clinical staff understanding of the learning needs of nursing students.
11. Encourage faculty, clinical staff, and peers to mentor nursing students.
12. Refrain from performing any technique or procedure for which the student has not been adequately trained.
13. Refrain from any deliberate action or omission of care in the academic or clinical setting that creates unnecessary risk for injury to the client, self, or others.
14. Assist the staff nurse or preceptor in ensuring that there is full disclosure and that proper authorizations are obtained from clients regarding any form of treatment or research.
15. Abstain from the use of alcoholic beverages or any substances that impair judgment in the academic and clinical setting.
16. Strive to achieve and maintain an optimal level of personal health.
17. Support access to treatment and rehabilitation for students who are experiencing impairments related to substance abuse and mental or physical health issues.
18. Uphold school policies and regulations related to academic and clinical performance, reserving the right to challenge and critique rules and regulations according to school grievance policy.

Other Benefits

There are many other benefits of membership, such as access to journals, newsletters, and action alerts about particular topics that need immediate response; eligibility for group health and life insurance; networking with peers; continuing education opportunities; and discounts on products and services, such as car rentals, computers, or books.

Deciding Which Associations to Join

As you decide whether to belong to an association, visit the group's website to find out more about its activities. Then ask yourself the following questions:

1. What is the mission and what are the purposes of this association?
2. Are the association's purposes compatible with my own?
3. How many members are there nationally, statewide, and locally?
4. What activities does the association undertake?
5. How active is the local chapter?
6. What opportunities does the association offer for involvement and leadership development?
7. What are the benefits of membership?
8. Does the association offer continuing education programs?
9. Does this organization lobby for improved health care legislation? How successful is it?
10. Is membership in this association cost-effective?
11. Even if I am not active, what benefit will I derive from the legislative agenda and other activities that the association undertakes to advocate for nurses and patients?

Answering these questions and speaking with current association members should provide nurses with adequate information to make reasoned decisions.

POLITICAL ACTIVISM IN THE GOVERNMENT ARENA

Now that you understand how professional organizations use collective power to influence policy decisions, let us examine how policy influences the practice of nursing. The ability of the individual nurse to provide care is significantly affected by public policy decisions. Yet too few nurses are aware of the importance of their role in influencing such policy outcomes, because they miss the connection between their own practice and the world of public policy.

As discussed in Chapter 4, state licensure of a registered nurse derives from legislation that defines the scope of nursing practice. The defined scope determines what a nurse legally can and cannot do. For example, giving intravenous medication and performing physical assessments are now accepted as actions within the scope of nursing practice. Forty years ago such activities were within the scope of the medical practice act rather than the nursing practice act. As a result of changes in education and clinical practice, nursing organizations influenced legislators to change state nurse practice acts to reflect what nurses were qualified to do.

Regulations are developed to guide the implementation of legislation. They affect practicing nurses and their work environments. For example, the rules for administering and documenting the administration of narcotic drugs are promulgated by a regulatory agency of the federal government, the FDA, a division of the Department of Health and Human Services. The way in which such regulations are written can greatly affect nurses' ability to practice.

The regulations in each state governing nursing practice flow from the state's nurse practice act. When the regulations change, for example, adding a requirement for continuing education for license renewal, it affects all nurses in the state. For advanced practice nurses, there are a variety of regulations related to prescription writing and autonomy issues. These change from time to time, and if nurses do not actively participate in changes, new regulations can restrict rather than enhance nursing authority for regulated activities.

A specific example of the impact regulatory changes can have involves advanced practice nurses, such as nurse practitioners and certified registered nurse anesthetists (CRNAs).

A November 2001 federal ruling from the Centers for Medicare & Medicaid Services (CMS) required that CRNAs must practice under the supervision of a surgeon or anesthesiologist to receive Medicare reimbursement. This change limits what many states had previously allowed nurses to do—practice "collaboratively" rather than "under the supervision of." CRNAs are working with governors in each state to get an exception (known as an "opt-out") and enable previous state laws to take precedence (http://www.aana.com/).

Broader issues affecting the nursing profession are also political in nature. Issues of pay equity, or equal pay for work of comparable value, are of concern to nurses, because they have historically been underpaid for their services. One of the earliest cases demonstrating the inequality of nursing salaries involved public health nurses in Colorado. These nurses brought a case against the city of Denver, stating that they were paid considerably less than city tree trimmers and garbage collectors. The nurses demanded just compensation for their work by demonstrating that nursing requires more complex knowledge and is of greater value to society than the other occupations.

As a result of this suit, recognition of nursing's low pay was brought to public attention; this in turn mobilized public support for increasing nursing salaries. This is an example of political action by nurses that resulted in both policy outcomes (regulations that expanded comparable pay issues to other jobs) and professional outcomes (salary increases for the individual nurse). More recently, the nursing shortage has caused concern among the public that the number of nurses available to provide care in hospitals and other agencies is inadequate. Nurses in California mobilized the public and other constituency groups to get the first legislation requiring specific nurse-to-patient ratios passed in 1999. However, the regulations were not implemented until 2004. As of June, 2009, 13 states plus the District of Columbia had implemented legislation or adopted regulations related to safe nurse-patient ratios (http://www.nursingworld.org/MainMenuCategories/ANAPoliticalPower/State/StateLegislativeAgenda/StaffingPlansandRatios_1.aspx).

Becoming Active in Politics: "The Personal is Political"

Women involved in the feminist movement in the 1960s coined the phrase "The personal is political." This statement recognized that each individual—woman or man—could use personal experience to understand and become involved in broader social and political issues. This concept enabled individuals who did not consider themselves political to gain insight into what needed to be changed in society and how they could help bring about the change. It gave power to each individual and resulted in people becoming involved in the political process—usually for the first time.

This premise of personalizing the political process has become a fundamental activity for organized nursing. Nurses at the grassroots level become involved in advocating for legislation and supporting candidates for elective office because they understand the relationship between public policy and their professional and personal lives. Most associations, such as the ANA, American Association of Colleges of Nursing, the American Hospital Association, and numerous specialty nursing organizations, actively engage in lobbying to advocate for the professional concerns of their members. Contemporary nursing leaders recognize that "being political," both through professional associations and as individuals, is a professional responsibility essential to the practice and promotion of the nursing profession.

This chapter started with a discussion about national politics, as this has been the source of a great deal of media coverage and public interest since the 2008 presidential election. But an importance premise in the earlier discussion was that much of what affects our day-to-day lives occurs at the state and local levels.

When you go to work in a practice setting, what you can and cannot do—the scope of your practice—is set by state law in the nurse practice act and is enacted by your state board of nursing. The board of nursing is also the governmental agency that licenses you and certifies your ongoing safety for practice. You may be late for work today because of work being done on an old bridge, from funding through the American Recovery and Reinvestment Act of 2009, the "stimulus package" that infused billions of dollars into repair of America's infrastructure. Because you were then in a hurry to get to work, you may be pulled over by your local police officer for speeding, and although she took pity on your work situation, she could not overlook the fact that you were both speeding and driving with an expired license, which you had been meaning to renew but had not gotten around to it. You have been very busy working extra shifts because your unit is short staffed, and the local economic conditions have required a hiring freeze, meaning that you are going to continue to be busy for a while. Each of these situations affecting your day-to-day life reflects the notion that you are always, one way or another, in some situation that involves legislation, regulation, or other form of government intervention. The personal is political, and the political is personal.

During the last 50 years of changing national and state health policies, nurses have increased their political astuteness. Through the well-orchestrated efforts of the ANA, other professional organizations, constituent member associations, and political action committees (PACs), nurses are now participating more effectively in both governmental and electoral politics than in the past. Nursing PACs raise and distribute money to candidates who support the profession's stand on certain issues. Nurses' endorsements of candidates have become a valued political asset for many local, state, and national candidates.

Nurses can make a difference in health policy outcomes. Through the political process, nurses influence policy in a variety of ways: by identifying health problems as policy problems; by formulating policy through drafting legislation in collaboration with legislators; by providing formal testimony; by lobbying governmental officials in the executive and legislative branches to make certain health policies a priority for action; and by filing suit as a party or as a friend of the court to implement health policy strategies on behalf of consumers. All major nursing professional associations engage in these activities. Because the ANA is the major organization that speaks for all nurses, specific examples of influencing public policy will be drawn largely from ANA's activities.

Capitol Update, an online newsletter published by the ANA, reports on the progress of nursing influence with the president, members of Congress and their staffs, and the regulatory agencies that set policy for health programs (http://www.capitolupdate.org/newsletter/). Such activity reflects the work of both ANA members and ANA staff. The ANA's political activity in Washington, D.C., is mirrored throughout the United States by other nursing organizations and by ANA constituent member associations conducting similar work with their state governments.

Nurses Strategic Action Teams (N-STAT) are ANA's grassroots network of nurses across the country who keep elected representatives in Congress informed about issues of concern to patients and nurses. By notifying network members, ANA can rapidly mobilize nurses to lobby their federal representatives to support or oppose particular legislation and/or rules and regulations. Through the use of telephones, fax, e-mail, and regular mail, N-STAT members can respond by sending well-timed, well-targeted messages to members of Congress.

Organized activity in identifying, financially supporting, and working for candidates who are committed to nursing and "nurse-friendly" issues has dramatically increased since the early 1990s. The electoral process is an essential function of the professional association.

Individual nurses can make a difference in policy development and elections. Either by election or by appointment, nurses need to be making health policy decisions, not just influencing them. Getting elected or appointed requires visibility, expertise, energy, risk taking, and a belief that policy and politics are critically important in achieving nursing's goals. Box 15-3 contains the story of Gale Adcock, MSN, RN, FNP (Figure 15-4), who has found that being a nurse has equipped her well for understanding issues and problems surrounding her town and in having the skills to enter the political arena locally.

Box 15-3   A Nurse's Voice in Local Politics

If it's true that all politics is local, then it doesn't get more "local" than serving as an elected official at the municipal government level.

In October 2007, I was elected to a 4-year term on the seven-member Cary Town Council, winning my nonpartisan (and first) campaign with 55 percent of the vote against two male opponents. Cary, North Carolina is a town of 134,000 residents, geographically located near the Research Triangle Park and part of the fastest-growing area in the United States. Because of explosive growth in Cary since the late 1990s, the biggest issue during the election and since taking office has been how to manage development in a smart and sustainable way that maintains a high quality of life for citizens. Smart greenfield and infill development and adequate public facilities are key concerns for Cary citizens, landowners, developers, and public officials. It is an ongoing challenge to craft policy that reflects core values, adequately meets current and future needs, and strikes a balance among the numerous stakeholders. Since taking office in December 2007, I have been committed to establishing, and then following, policies to ensure adequate roads, school capacity, and water and wastewater facilities; lessening the impact of traffic congestion; protecting air and water quality; and increasing the number of parks and greenways. Each of these issues has a defined and substantial impact on the health and well-being of Cary citizens.

And that's where being a nurse and nurse practitioner has been extremely helpful.

I began my nursing career in 1975 with a diploma in nursing, 1 year later returned to school to receive a BSN, and in 1987 completed my MSN and certificate as a family nurse practitioner. My political education started early in my nursing career. In 1980 North Carolina's nursing practice act was slated for review and sunset. I joined the North Carolina Nurses Association and worked with dozens of nurses to lobby for the 1981 passage of a stronger version of this important legislation. This was followed by successfully lobbying for third-party reimbursement for nurse practitioners (NPs) and other advanced practice registered nurses (APRNs) in 1993 (an insurance mandate); amendment to the Professional Corporations Act in 1995 (allowing nurses to incorporate across professional lines); and the Managed Care Patients' Bill of Rights in 2001 (adding antidiscrimination language). It was pretty obvious that I was hooked.

Realizing the equal importance of the regulatory side of policy making, in 2000 I began a 7-year stretch on the N.C. Board of Nursing and served as the NP representative on the Joint Subcommittee of Nursing and Medicine that is statutorily charged with promulgating rules for NP practice. (This is where I really learned to play political hardball.) Amid the many years spent lobbying others for action it hit me that I was also preparing myself for a role change—from advocate to policy maker. In 2006 I threw myself into high gear and completed a 5-month fellowship in the Institute of Political Leadership. I also joined the county Democratic women's club and began attending Chamber of Commerce events among other high-profile, nonnursing activities. I had my sights set on a N.C. House or Senate seat when the Town Council seat in my district came open, and local party officials approached me to run.

It's not a mystery why they choose a nurse to run for this office or why nurses in general are naturals for politics and policy making. We are adept at problem identification. We think critically and craft viable solutions. We are excellent listeners. We are content experts and quick studies. We are consensus builders. We understand human nature and group dynamics. We understand health in its broadest terms and advocate for it that way. Nurses have relevant skills and are capable of playing important advocacy and policy-making roles at all levels of government. Whether it's federal Medicare reimbursement policy, state funding for school nurses, or municipal ordinances forbidding smoking in public buildings, nurses can contribute and belong at all of these tables.

• *Gale Adcock, MSN, RN, FNP*

(Courtesy of Gale Adcock.)

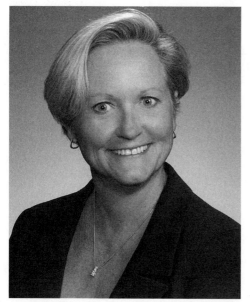

Figure 15-4 Gale Adcock, MSN, RN, FNP. (Courtesy Gale Adcock.)

GETTING INVOLVED

To get involved, a nurse must begin to understand the connections between individual practice and public policy. Once that happens, it is easy to get started. Three levels of political involvement in which nurses can participate are as nurse citizens, nurse activists, and nurse politicians.

Nurse Citizens

A nurse citizen brings the perspective of health care to the voting booth, to public forums that advocate for health and human services, and to involvement in community activities. For example, budget cuts to a school district might involve elimination of school nurses. At a school board meeting, nurses can effectively speak about the vital services that school nurses provide to children and the cost-effectiveness of maintaining the position.

Nurses tend to vote for candidates who advocate for improved health care. Here are some examples of how the nurse citizen can be politically active:

Box 15-4   Communication Is the Key to Influence

Cultivate a relationship with policy makers from your home district or state. Communicate by visits, telephone, e-mail, and letters. Letters and other messages need these elements:

- If writing a letter, use personal stationery.
- State who you are (a nursing student or registered nurse and a voter in a specific district).
- Identify the issue by a file number, if possible.
- Be clear on where you stand and why.
- Be positive when possible.
- Be concise.
- Ask for a commitment. State precisely what action you want the policy maker to take.
- Give your return address, e-mail address, and phone number to urge dialogue.
- Be persistent. Follow up with calls or letters.
- If you plan to visit your policy maker on a specific issue, be sure to make your appointment in advance in writing and indicate what issue you are interested in discussing.
- Be quick to thank and praise policy makers when they do something you like.

- Register to vote.
- Vote in every election.
- Keep informed about health care issues.
- Speak out when services or working conditions are inadequate.
- Participate in public forums.
- Know your local, state, and federal elected officials.
- Join politically active nursing organizations.
- Participate in community organizations that need health experts.
- Join a political party.

Once nurses make a decision to become involved politically, they need to learn how to get started. One of the best ways is to form a relationship with one or more policymakers. Box 15-4 contains several pointers for influencing policymakers.

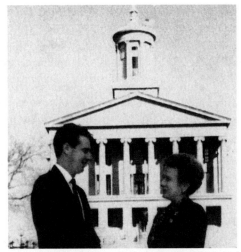

Figure 15-5 The nurse activist has a high level of involvement in selected political issues. Here she visits with one of her state legislators at the state capitol. *(Courtesy Tennessee Nurses Association. Photograph by Chip Powell.)*

Nurse Activists

The nurse activist takes a more active role than the nurse citizen and often does so because an issue arises that directly affects the nurse's professional life (Figure 15-5). The need to respond moves the nurse to a higher level of participation. For example, a nurse in private practice who has difficulty getting insurance companies to honor patients' claims for reimbursement of nursing services may become active in lobbying state legislators for changes in insurance regulations.

Nurse activists can make changes by:
- Joining politically active nursing organizations
- Contacting a public official through letters, e-mails, or phone calls
- Registering people to vote
- Contributing money to a political campaign
- Working in a campaign
- Lobbying decision makers by providing pertinent statistical and anecdotal information
- Forming or joining coalitions that support an issue of concern
- Writing letters to the editor of local newspapers
- Inviting legislators to visit the workplace

Box 15-5   Key Questions for Nurses Who Want to Make a Difference in Health Policy

1. Know the system. Is it a federal, state, or local issue? Is it in the hands of the executive, legislative, or judicial branch of government?
2. Know the issue. What is wrong? What should happen? Why is it not happening? What is needed: leadership, a plan, pressure, or data?
3. Know the players. Who is on your side, and who is not? Who will make the decision? Who knows whom? Will a coalition be effective? Are you a member of the professional nursing organization?
4. Know the process. Is this a vote? Is this an appropriation? Is this a legislative procedure? Is this a committee or subcommittee report?
5. Know what to do. Should you write, call, arrange a lunch meeting, organize a petition, show up at the hearing, give testimony, demonstrate, or file a suit?

- Holding a media event to publicize an issue
- Providing or giving testimony to legislators and regulatory bodies

Box 15-5 includes pointers on how to make a difference in health policy development.

Nurse Politicians

Once a nurse realizes and experiences the empowerment that can come from political activism, he or she may choose to run for office. No longer satisfied to help others get elected, the nurse politician desires to develop the legislation, not just influence it. Gale Adcock (Box 15-3) mentioned that she "got hooked" when she began to deal with local political issues as a nurse and as a citizen.

As of 2011 there were three nurses serving in Congress. In 1992 Congresswoman Eddie Bernice Johnson (D-TX) (Figure 15-6) was the first nurse elected to the U.S. House of Representatives. She has been consistently reelected since. The second nurse, Carolyn McCarthy (D-NY) (Figure 15-7), an LPN, was elected in 1996 as a

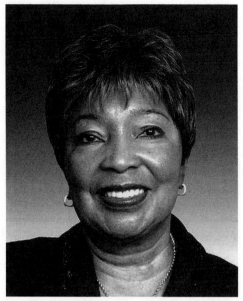

Figure 15-6 Rep. Eddie Bernice Johnson (D-TX), nurse in Congress.

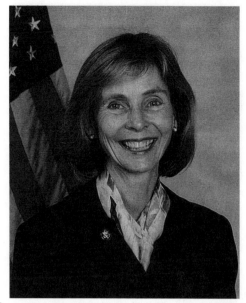

Figure 15-8 Rep. Lois Capps (D-CA), nurse in Congress.

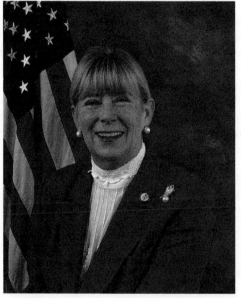

Figure 15-7 Rep. Carolyn McCarthy (D-NY), nurse in Congress.

result of her stance on gun control. Her husband was killed and her son critically injured after a lone gunman with a 9-mm semiautomatic pistol walked through a train on the Long Island Railroad and killed 25 people and wounded 19 others.

Congresswoman McCarthy was suddenly thrown into the national spotlight when she challenged the incumbent congressman running for office on his stand supporting a repeal on a ban for assault rifles. Her ability to speak passionately about the issue led to her campaign against the incumbent and her election to his seat. She has been a leader in the House of Representatives on gun control, as well as on nursing issues (McCarthy, 2007). In 1998 Congresswoman Lois Capps (D-CA) (Figure 15-8) became the third nurse to be elected to the House of Representatives. Congresswoman Capps was a long-time leader in health care and a school nurse. After her election to Congress, she drew on her extensive health care background to cochair the House Democratic Task Force on Medicare Reform, and in 2003 she founded the Bipartisan Congressional Caucus on Nursing and the Bipartisan School Health and Safety Caucus.

Two other members of Congress are high-profile "friends of nursing." Senator Richard Durbin (D-IL) (Figure 15-9) introduced legislation (S. 497) in March 2009 backed by the American Organization of Nurse Executives and other nursing groups that would provide grants to nursing schools for faculty and other resources to increase enrollment.

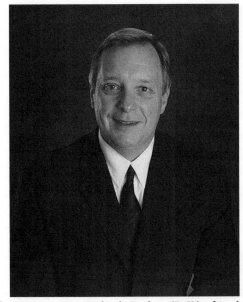

Figure 15-9 Sen. Richard Durbin (D-IL), friend of nursing.

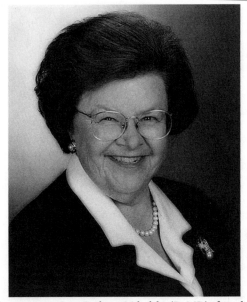

Figure 15-10 Sen. Barbara Mikulski (D-MD), friend of nursing.

Senator Barbara Mikulski (D-MD) (Figure 15-10), a senior member of the Senate Appropriations Committee, announced the 2009 Omnibus Appropriations Act in March 2009 that contained several important health care–related measures. This bill provided $171 million for nursing programs for the Advanced Nursing Education Program, the Nurse Loan Repayment and Scholarship Program, and the Nurse Faculty Loan Program, all of which are dedicated to addressing the nationwide nursing and nursing faculty shortage.

The American Recovery and Reinvestment Act of 2009 (the Stimulus Bill) has significant funding for nursing education and health-related research, with particularly generous dollars going to the National Institutes of Health. At the time of writing this chapter, the Recovery and Reinvestment Act's exact distribution of health-related dollars was yet unknown.

In March 2010, the passage of the Affordable Helath Care Act signaled the beginning of significant changes in US health care. Known as "health care reform," this legislation requires most Americans to have health insurance coverage, and will provide Medicaid coverage to an additional 16 million people. Private insurers are prohibited from denying care to persons with preexisting conditions and persons up to age 26 can be continued on their parents' insurance under certain conditions. The role of nurses will expand as a result of the increased need for affordable care. Nurses stand to gain a tremendous amount in this reform, which, ultimately, is for the improvement of care for our patients.

Nurses have shown that they can take on important and public roles in speaking for health care and for the profession of nursing. To be effective agents of change, nurses can

- Run for an elected office
- Seek appointment to a regulatory agency
- Be appointed to a governing board in the public or private sector
- Use nursing expertise as a front-line policy maker who can enhance health care and the profession

We Were All Once Novices

In general, nurses who have achieved success as leaders started with no knowledge of the political process and no expectations of the greatness they would achieve. Instead, they became involved because some issue, injustice, or abuse of power affected their lives. Instead of complaining or feeling helpless, they responded by taking an active role in bringing about change.

The mark of a leader is the ability to identify a problem, have a goal, and know how to join others in reaching that goal. A leader must ask the right questions, analyze the positive and restraining forces toward meeting the goal, and know how to obtain and use power. A leader must know how to ask for help and how to give support to those who join the effort. These are the marks of nursing leaders who have become political experts.

NURSING AWAITS YOUR CONTRIBUTION

You can apply the skills discussed in this chapter. Look to teachers, family, friends, and community leaders whom you admire. What are the leadership qualities they possess that you wish to have? These individuals can offer inspiration and serve as role models for you to imitate.

You may also choose to form a relationship with a political mentor. A mentor serves as a role model but also actively teaches, encourages, and critiques the process of growth and change in the learner. All nurses who have become political leaders have found mentors along the way to guide and support their growth. Your mentor could be a faculty member, such as the adviser to the nursing student organization or honor society, who can teach you leadership skills. Ask for help in running for a class office or student council president. If elected office does not appeal to you, use your political skills to develop a school or community project with other nursing students.

You may have a relative or friend involved in a political campaign who could help you learn about the political process. You might find a problem during a clinical experience that inhibits your ability to provide the level of care that you wish to provide. Seek a faculty member or nurse in a clinical facility who can guide you through the process of policy change within the agency or institution.

Watch the communication skills of your role models or mentors. How does your own behavior compare with theirs? What enhances or impedes your progress? Get your friends and peers to join your activity. Seek their help and support. Always thank them and be ready to offer your help and support when they need it. The importance of grassroots organization in the past election cycle demonstrated the effectiveness of getting-out-the-vote activities and becoming involved in politics at local, state, and national levels. And no matter what your political leanings or positions, it is important that, as a nurse and as a citizen of the democracy, you exercise your right to vote.

Summary of Key Points

- Professional associations are the vehicle through which nursing takes collective action to improve both the nursing profession and health care delivery.
- There are many nursing associations from which to choose, and they offer a variety of benefits to the public, to the nursing profession as a whole, and to individual members.
- Membership in professional associations is essential for professionals, but selecting which associations to join can be a challenge. Prospective members should ask key questions to help them select wisely.
- Professional organizations and professional nurses have much to offer in formulating policy decisions at federal, state, and local levels and in each branch of government.
- Today, organized nursing is involved in politics at many levels in promoting comprehensive health reform and creating a safer workplace.
- Becoming politically active is as easy as signing your name in support of an issue, registering to vote, organizing a project, or speaking out on an issue.
- Political involvement is empowering; one person can make a difference.
- The involvement of nurses in the political process benefits nurses, the nursing profession, and the recipients of health care.

Critical Thinking Questions

1. Look in a local newspaper for articles about federal legislation that support nursing's concerns, such as the Safe Staffing Act, or other

nursing-related or patient-related legislation pending in your state. Write a letter to the editor of your local paper about these bills, taking a stand on the issues.

2. Find out whether there is a student nurses association on your campus. If there is, learn all you can about it and consider joining. Get your friends to join with you. If there is not a student nurses association, consider establishing one. (Resources: Go to http://www. nsna.org; click on "Program Activities.")

3. As a student, attend a local or state nurses association meeting to gain a better sense of the issues in the profession, so that you can be prepared for what lies ahead when you graduate. How is the association addressing these issues? Do they interest you? How can you get involved?

Consider the following hypothetical situations:

4. You read in a local newspaper that students at your university have a high rate of drug and alcohol use. The following week, a story appears about a senior university student who died following a car crash. The student was driving under the influence of alcohol. How can nursing students address the need for education about drug and alcohol use? What collective action can you initiate to address this or another issue of importance to your college or university community? (Resources: Go to http://www.nsna.org; click on "Publications" to download Guidelines for Planning Community Health Projects.)

5. The demand for nursing services is increasing, but the availability of registered nurses will not meet this demand. The student nurses association chapter has formed a recruitment committee to address this issue and answer the following questions: Why are students not considering nursing as a career? Why are students considering nursing as a career? How many registered nurses will be needed in the future? Why do many nursing programs have waiting lists to enter the program? Plan a collective action project that can be implemented by the student nurses association to increase interest in

the nursing profession. (Resources: Go to http://www.nsna.org; click on "Publications" to download Guidelines for Planning Breakthrough to Nursing Projects.)

6. Students at your school must struggle to pay tuition. Many students work part-time while attending school full-time. They have taken out student loans and have applied for scholarships to help pay for tuition, books, and other school-related expenses. A faculty member announces in class that the Nurse Reinvestment Act is going before Congress for funding authorization. What collective actions can the student nurses association take to ask Congress to increase funding for undergraduate nursing education and for student loan repayment programs? (Resources: Go to http://www.nsna.org; click on "Publications" to download Guidelines for Planning Legislative Activities.)

7. A classmate asks you to share a paper you prepared for a leadership course she is now taking so that she can see how you handled the assignment. You willingly give her a copy of your "A" paper. At the end of the semester, the faculty member who teaches the leadership course calls you into her office. She shows you the paper you wrote for her course last semester, but it now has your classmate's name on it instead of yours! What collective action can the student nurses association take to prevent plagiarism and cheating? (Resources: Go to http://www.nsna.org; click on "Publications" to download the NSNA Bill of Rights and Responsibilities for Students of Nursing and the NSNA Code of Academic and Clinical Professional Conduct.)

8. Conduct a class poll. Of those in the class who are eligible to vote, how many are registered? How many voted in the last local, state, or national election? Challenge those not yet registered to become registered before the end of the current school term.

9. Because nurses have differing personal and political values, it has been a challenge to get them all united behind a single issue or candidate. If you were the president of the ANA,

what techniques would you use to convince the 2.9 million American nurses to use the power of their numbers, their knowledge, and their commitment on behalf of their profession?

10. Find out whether the members of your state board of nursing are elected or appointed. What is the composition of the board (that is, how many registered nurses, licensed practical nurses, and consumers are there, for example)? Do nurses hold most of the seats on the state board? Are there any other health professionals, such as physicians, on the board of nursing? If so, are there any nurses on the state board of medicine?

The author wishes to acknowledge the prior contributions of Judith Leavitt in the preparation of this chapter.

⊖volve *To enhance your understanding of this chapter, try the Student Exercises on the Evolve site at http://evolve.elsevier.com/Chitty/professional.*

REFERENCES

Daley K: Needlestick injuries in the workplace: implications for public policy, In Mason D, Leavitt J, Chaffee M, editors: *Policy and politics in nursing and health care*, ed 5, St Louis, 2007, Saunders.

Dictionary.com, "policy," *The American Heritage Dictionary of the English Language*, 4th ed, Boston, 2004, Houghton Mifflin Company (website): http://dictionary.reference.com/browse/policy (accessed April 10, 2009).

Dictionary.com, "politics," *Webster's Revised Unabridged Dictionary*, MICRA, Inc. (website): http://dictionary.reference.com/browse/politics (accessed April 10, 2009).

Holland K: *Dealing with generational differences: we have always done it that way*, 2005 (website): http://www.alwaysdoneitthatway.com/2005/11/20/dealing-with-generational-differences/.

Kany K: Contemporary issues in nursing organizations, In Mason D, Leavitt J, Chaffee M, editors: *Policy and politics in nursing and health care*, ed 5, St Louis, 2007, Saunders.

Lewenson S: An historical perspective on policy, politics and nursing, In Mason D, Leavitt J, Chaffee M, editors: *Policy and politics in nursing and health care*, ed 5, St Louis, 2007, Saunders.

Mather M: Reefer madness: the illogical politics of medical marijuana, In Mason D, Leavitt J, Chaffee M, editors: *Policy and politics in nursing and health care*, ed 5, St Louis, 2007, Saunders.

McCarthy C: A nurse in congress, In Mason D, Leavitt J, Chaffee M, editors: *Policy and politics in nursing and health care*, ed 5, St Louis, 2007, Saunders.

Nursing Organizations Alliance: *Nursing alliance leadership academy*, 2005 (website): http://www.nursing-alliance.org/events.cfm.

Shaner McRae H: Environmental advocacy: a nurse's journey, In Mason D, Leavitt J, Chaffee M, editors: *Policy and politics in nursing and health care*, ed 4, St Louis, 2002, Saunders.

Nursing's Future Challenges

Kay Kittrell Chitty

LEARNING OUTCOMES

After studying this chapter, students will be able to:
- Review societal influences on the nursing profession anticipated during the next decade
- Recognize the impact that changes in the health care system will have on the practice of nursing
- Discuss the role of the nurse in disaster preparedness and disaster response

- Explain trends in nursing education needed to meet society's future nursing needs
- Describe major challenges that the nursing profession must resolve to ensure it remains in control of its destiny
- Describe four major components of the American Nurses Association's Health System Reform Agenda

As you have seen throughout this textbook, the nursing profession is profoundly affected by a rapidly changing world. The challenges nurses face today relate to a variety of factors: changes in demographics, unhealthy lifestyles of many Americans, the continued deterioration of the environment, rapid change in the health care system, cost-containment pressures, advances in technology, bioterrorism, natural and man-made disasters, cultural diversity within both nursing and the wider population, blurring of professional boundaries, increasing interdisciplinary collaboration, and issues within nursing itself.

It is painfully clear that even in the United States, the wealthiest of the industrialized nations, we fall far short of the goal of having a healthy nation in spite of spending nearly $2 trillion annually on health care in recent years. An estimated 46 million Americans have no health insurance, and many others have less than enough (Leavitt, 2009). Infant mortality, the number of infant deaths per 1000 live births, is widely accepted as one of the most important indicators of the health of a nation. It is therefore distressing that in spite of upwardly spiraling health care costs, the United States ranks twenty-ninth among the developed countries in

infant mortality, behind Japan, Sweden, Spain, France, Germany, Australia, England, Wales, Canada, and others (MacDorman and Mathews, 2008). The actual rate in 2006, the last year for which data are available, was 6.71 infant deaths per 1000 live births. The Healthy People goal is 4.5, indicating that as a nation we have a long way to go (MacDorman and Mathews, 2008).

The fitness level of citizens, including young people, continues to decline as obesity increases at an alarming rate. Smoking in youth continues to increase. In addition, the threat of bioterrorism is a new challenge we must face as a profession and as a nation. All these negative trends continue even though the United States spends more of its gross domestic product (16% in 2006 compared with 8% to 10% for most major industrialized nations) on health than any other nation in the world (Davis et al, 2007). Complete overhaul of the health care system, believed by many Americans to be essential if these problems are to be addressed, has been stalled in Congress since 1994 despite efforts at reform by several recent presidential administrations.

Nursing enjoys high levels of respect and public confidence. It is a profession in heavy demand, and its practitioners enjoy more autonomy than ever.

As the health care profession with the highest number of practitioners, numbering nearly 3 million, nursing has enormous but largely untapped political power that would allow nurses to influence societal changes—rather than simply be influenced by them—if they were unified in their efforts. Yet apathy, turf issues, lack of focus, and inaction continue to divide nurses, diminishing their influence at every level of public discourse.

You might wonder what purpose is served by thinking about the future. The purpose of "futures work" is "to study potential developments, using tools and certain attitudinal alignments, to effect change in a desired direction. A deliberated future may be personal, professional or organizational, but the process is the same: creating an image of a desired result to serve as a blueprint for action. It allows us to avert, encourage, or direct the course of events" (Dickenson-Hazard, 2003), rather than simply reacting to them.

For too long, members of the nursing profession have allowed other professions to lead the way in promoting or, more often, opposing health care reforms that will benefit all our citizens. This chapter explores some of the challenges and opportunities for the nursing profession to become proactive rather than reactive in shaping both itself and health care in our nation in the future.

SOCIETAL CHALLENGES

At least six societal influences are expected to have major impact on the future of the nursing profession: demographic changes, environmental deterioration, the need to prepare for large-scale public health disasters, unhealthy lifestyles and the resulting rise in chronic illnesses, continuing need for cost containment, and governmental regulation of health care. Each of these influences is examined briefly.

Demographics

Demography is the science that studies vital statistics and social trends. Demographers examine vital statistics such as birthrates (births per 1000 people in 1 year), morbidity rates (illness), mortality rates (deaths), marriages, the ages of various populations, and migration patterns. From this wealth of information, futurists, people who try to project what will occur, draw conclusions about what these trends mean for the future.

Four demographic trends are particularly important to the future of nursing: the aging population, poverty, the cultural diversity of the population, and urbanization, including increasing levels of violence. Each has implications for nursing.

Aging population

Estimates vary, but demographers have predicted that the number of people older than 75 years of age in the United States by the year 2020 will exceed 21.8 million. The number of aging baby boomers will create an additional strain on the U.S. health care system. These "boomers" will be different from patients in the past because they will "expect more and tolerate less" (Wolf, 2003, p. 32). They will be the most knowledgeable and demanding health care consumers ever and will keep their caregivers on their toes.

Centenarians, people more than 100 years of age, represent one of the fastest-growing groups in the United States. The World Future Society predicted that by the end of the twenty-first century, the average life span will approach 100 years (Hendrick, 1995). Many elderly people are healthy, but the likelihood of illness becomes greater as people age. For example, indications are that by the age of 90 years, Alzheimer's disease will develop in one of two people (Herbert, Scherr, Beckett et al, 1995). In general, the elderly are greater users of health care than any other population segment (Valentino, 2002). Clearly, nurses of the future must be prepared to work effectively with the rising numbers of elderly patients.

Ethical issues such as euthanasia and assisted suicide will become increasingly important as technology enables people to sustain life far beyond the point of useful, meaningful existence. Society's views of assisted suicide and euthanasia are changing, as evidenced by the fact that juries twice acquitted Dr. Jack Kevorkian of charges of murder in the assisted deaths of several terminally ill people before he was ultimately convicted and sentenced to prison. Additionally, the citizens of Oregon decided by referendum to explicitly allow assisted suicide, and several other states do not consider assisted suicide a crime. Two countries, the Netherlands and Belgium, have legalized assisted suicide, and other nations are considering it. The future will gradually bring further changes in laws and attitudes toward giving individuals control over the timing and manner of their own death. As our population ages, end-of-life care, particularly pain control and other forms of palliative care, will increasingly be a focus of formal and continuing education nursing programs.

Poverty

Even though the United States is considered the world's wealthiest nation, the number of Americans living below the poverty line is increasing. This is particularly true of women, children, and the elderly. Another large group of Americans are employed yet cannot make enough money to provide adequately for their families' needs. They are known as the working poor. This group has grown since the start of the economic slump that began in late 2007. The gap between the "haves" and the "have-nots" in the United States continues to widen, creating discontent and disillusionment. Never was this more clearly seen than after Hurricane Katrina, when the poor residents of New Orleans, who were unable to evacuate, lived in inhumane conditions for days on end.

When basic needs for food, clothing, and shelter are unmet or uncertain, health care becomes an out-of-reach luxury. Children's immunizations, prenatal care for pregnant women, nutritious meals, dental care, and a variety of other health-maintaining factors are neglected. Medically indigent people, those who do not qualify for Medicaid but nevertheless cannot pay for health care, tend to put off seeking care until illness is advanced and thus harder and more expensive to treat. Conditions that can be prevented often are not because of lack of education, poor sanitation, crowded living conditions, improper shelter, homelessness, and a host of other poverty-related factors.

It is a sad reality that poverty will continue to rise in the future, creating increasing numbers of disenfranchised people, that is, people who have no power in the political system, with limited access to health care. As their numbers grow, both federal and state governments will be forced by limited resources to implement more strategies that limit health care expenditures for these vulnerable populations.

Nursing, as a profession, values providing care to all people, regardless of social and economic factors. The increasing numbers of medically disenfranchised people and pressure to limit health care expenditures will collide to create an intense values conflict for nurses of the future.

Cultural diversity

Cultural diversity refers to the array of people from different racial, ethnic, religious, social, and geographic backgrounds who make up a particular entity. Some countries, such as Japan, are homogeneous in culture. This means that most citizens have similar cultural beliefs and practices. Others, such as the United States, have a heterogeneous cultural mix. The cultural beliefs and practices of our citizens are quite different and becoming more so with every passing year.

Immigration to the United States from Southeast Asia, Central America, the Middle East, Mexico, and the islands of the Caribbean has increased in recent years as a result of civil unrest, wars, and poor economic conditions (Figure 16-1). People from these countries are the latest wave of newcomers to the United States and join the European Americans, African Americans, and others whose ancestors came to this country in the twentieth century and earlier. Each group has its own language, nutritional practices, health beliefs, folk remedies, childcare practices, and conventional wisdom about health and illness.

Nurses need to take cultural beliefs, values, and practices into consideration when planning and implementing nursing care for individuals of diverse cultural backgrounds. Culturally competent care will be more important in the future than ever before (see Cultural Considerations Challenge, below). Speaking a second language, particularly Spanish, will be an important skill that will both enhance nurses' ability to communicate with patients and increase nurses' value to health care organizations.

The nursing profession itself will become increasingly diverse as its membership reflects a heterogeneous society. In addition, global nurse migration has intensified, with the outflow of nurses from English-speaking nations to the United States being the most common route (Brush, 2008). As long as nurse migration is unchecked and uncoordinated, this trend will continue, creating further diversity within the profession. These factors emphasize the need for nurses to understand, respect, and value the contributions of both patients and coworkers of all cultural backgrounds.

Urbanization

Urbanization, that is, people moving from rural, farming areas to cities, has increased since the time of the Industrial Revolution. That trend continues today around the entire globe. *The Futurist* magazine predicted that world urbanization will reach 60% by 2030, worsening existing environmental and socioeconomic problems found in many urban areas, such as lack of sanitation and resulting epidemics (Cetron and Davies, 2008).

In this country, as cities grow, suburbs flourish, and many people who can afford to do so move away from the centers of cities. Decaying inner cities with large populations of poor people create major social problems such as homelessness, drugs, gangs, single-parent households, mental illness, violence, and crime. Despite the increase in public-private partnerships designed to revitalize inner cities and programs formulated to deal effectively with urban issues, social problems continue to grow and spill over into the suburbs and rural areas, creating further social changes. Nurses of the future will be increasingly confronted with health problems resulting from these social phenomena.

Violence is of particular concern to members of the nursing profession. Violence is present in our homes, workplaces, schools, and communities, causing untold chaos and loss. Violence is becoming a major public health problem in the United States and elsewhere, and we see the results in offices, clinics, and trauma units. Because the nursing profession cannot turn a blind eye to this

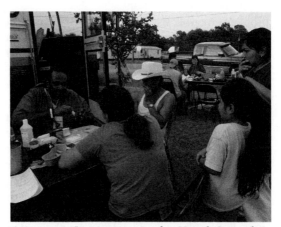

Figure 16-1 Immigration to the United States from Southeast Asia, Central America, Mexico, and the Caribbean islands is expected to continue in the next decade, contributing to sweeping demographic changes. Here nursing students and their faculty participate in a farm worker family health program for migrant workers in rural Georgia. (Courtesy Emory University, Nell Hodgson Woodruff School of Nursing.)

Cultural Considerations Challenge

THE IMPACT OF IMMIGRATION ON YOUR NURSING PRACTICE

Immigration, especially from Mexico, is a phenomenon expected to continue. In a group setting with classmates, respond to these questions:

- What effects do you anticipate that immigration may have on your own practice?
- What preparations have you made to incorporate immigrants into your practice?
- What do you believe is your professional responsibility in the care of immigrants?
- How does your personal belief system about immigration affect the way that you may react to immigrants in your work as a nurse?
- How is the immigration status (documented or undocumented) of a patient relevant to the care you provide to that patient?
- What adjustments might you need to make to accommodate persons who have migrated to the United States?

problem, we will see nurses as individuals and as a professional group increasingly take action against the rising tide of violence to protect the basic societal principles of safety and security.

Environment

Every newspaper, newsmagazine, and television news program brings disturbing reports of the deterioration of our environment. There are major environmental tragedies, such as a nuclear power plant incident in Japan and floodwaters spreading effluent from hundreds of hog farms in eastern North Carolina. These overshadow the less dramatic but insidious gradual decline in the quality of the world's air, water, and plant and animal life.

Acute and chronic respiratory diseases are increasing, as are debilitating allergic reactions to chemicals in the environment and cancers of all types (Figure 16-2). Reports of deterioration of the ozone layer, accidental lead and mercury poisonings, toxic shellfish beds, truckloads of pesticides spilling into streams and rivers, and accidental release of radioactive steam from nuclear power plants all occur with unsettling regularity.

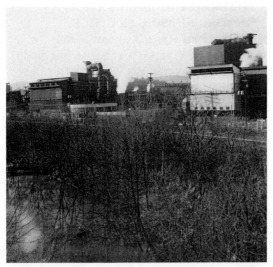

Figure 16-2 This manufacturing plant, while providing jobs to scores of workers, has polluted the air and the ground around it, as well as a nearby stream. Although the plant is slated for closure, it will take years to clean up the ground and water contaminated during its decades of operation. (Photo by Kelly Whalin.)

Meanwhile, clear-cutting of forests, destruction of wetlands by development, and relaxing of standards for polluting industries have become "business as usual." Scientists now agree that global warming is accelerating and is attributable to human activity. Still, our government and others do little to control emissions effectively.

Epidemiologists, who study the origins and spread of diseases, believe that there is a relationship between environmental decline and increases in certain diseases, including H1N1 (swine) flu and mad cow disease. Emerging diseases and multidrug-resistant strains (MDRS) of organisms currently under control, such as tuberculosis and staphylococcus, will increasingly challenge health care resources. Humans are responsible for destroying the environment, and the more human beings there are, the faster the environment will inevitably decline. Overpopulation contributes to the deterioration of the world's environment, yet too few countries are dealing effectively with issues of overpopulation, including the United States, and powerful religious groups oppose birth control.

In December 2009 the world population reached the record number of 6.8 billion people. The U.S. Census Bureau has projected that the world's population will increase to 8.8 billion by the end of 2025 (U.S. Census Bureau, 2009). Feeding, immunizing, providing potable water, and caring for this many human beings threaten to overwhelm the environmental, economic, social, and medical systems of the world. In the United States alone there is one birth every 7 seconds, one international migrant every 36 seconds, and one death every 13 seconds—for a net gain of one person every 11 seconds (U.S. Census Bureau, 2009).

At the most recent Climate Change Conference held in Copenhagen, Denmark in December, 2009, the analogy of the overloaded lifeboat was frequently used. World overpopulation, overdevelopment, and overconsumption by wealthy nations threaten to deplete the resources and destroy the environment of the entire world, not just overpopulated countries. The closely linked problems of climate change, environmental deterioration, and overpopulation are health care issues that future nurses will face, and there are no easy answers.

Disasters and Bioterrorism

Since September 11, 2001, and Hurricane Katrina in August and September 2005, many professions have reevaluated their disaster preparedness. Nurses are often at the forefront in emergency and disaster situations, but too few U.S. schools of nursing include disaster training in their curricula. As we have all so sadly witnessed, this needs to change in the future.

A disaster is defined as "an event or situation that is of greater magnitude than an emergency; disrupts essential services such as housing, transportation, communications, sanitation, water, and health care; and requires the response of people outside the community affected" (Gebbie and Qureshi, 2002). Disasters can be natural or man-made and range from earthquakes, hurricanes, and major fires to wars and major environmental contamination. The Southeast Asia tsunami of December 26, 2004, serves as a sad example of a natural disaster on a scale heretofore unseen.

Regardless of the cause of a disaster situation, no two of which are alike, the basic competencies nurses need in disaster preparedness are essentially the same. The Centers for Disease Control and Prevention (CDC) collaborated with a nurse, Dr. Kristine M. Gebbie, to develop a set of core emergency preparedness competencies for public health workers. This served as a basis on which Dr. Gebbie and another nurse, Kristin Qureshi, developed core competencies for nurses (Gebbie and Qureshi, 2002). The core disaster preparedness competencies for nurses are found in Box 16-1.

Box 16-1   Core Nursing Competencies for Disaster Preparedness

To consider themselves prepared for a major emergency or a disaster, nurses should be able to perform the following:
- Describe the agency's (your place of employment's) role in responding to a range of emergencies that might arise.
- Describe the chain of command in emergency response (to whom you would report).
- Identify and locate the agency's emergency response plan (or the pertinent portion of it).
- Describe emergency response functions or roles and demonstrate them in regularly performed drills.
- Demonstrate the use of equipment (including personal protective equipment) and the skills required in emergency response during regular drills.
- Demonstrate the correct operation of all equipment used for emergency communication.
- Describe communication roles in emergency response within your agency, with news media, with the general public (including patients and families), and with personal contacts (one's own family, friends, and neighbors).

- Identify the limits of your own knowledge, skills, and authority, and identify key system resources for referring matters that exceed these limits.
- Apply creative problem-solving skills and flexible thinking to the situation, within the confines of your role, and evaluate the effectiveness of all actions taken.
- Recognize deviations from the norm that might indicate an emergency and describe appropriate action. Participate in continuing education to maintain up-to-date knowledge in relevant areas.
- Participate in evaluating every drill or response and identify necessary changes to the plan.

In addition, nurses with managerial or leadership responsibilities should be able to perform the following:
- Ensure that there is a written plan for major categories of emergencies.
- Ensure that all parts of the emergency plan are practiced regularly.
- Ensure that identified gaps in knowledge or skills are filled.

From Gebbie KM, Qureshi K: Emergency and disaster preparedness: core competencies for nurses, *Am J Nurs* 102(1):46-51, 2002.

Until recently, nurses were not expected to know much about the types of disasters caused by bioterrorism. **Bioterrorism** refers to the use of a biologic or chemical agent as a weapon. Some futurists have predicted that bioviolence, such as genetically altering bacteria and viruses to increase their lethality and resistance to antibiotics and foster their use as weapons, could be used as a new form of warfare (Kellman, 2008; Gatti and Montanari, 2008). Nurses of the future must be able to recognize the signs and symptoms of biologic agents such as anthrax and smallpox or chemical agents such as ricin. They must know how to notify the proper authorities; assist with diagnosis, postexposure prophylaxis, and treatment; and participate in infection control.

Nurses are encouraged to keep up with emerging information to improve their readiness for possible bioterrorism by referring to the CDC's bioterrorism website (http://www.bt.cdc.gov). You can register for the CDC's free e-mail updates and training opportunities via the CDC's Clinician Registry (http://emergency.cdc.gov/coca/registry.asp).

The American Nurses Association (ANA) encourages registered nurses who are interested in helping during disasters to sign up with the appropriate group and prepare themselves for disaster work before they are needed. You will find links to various disaster-related volunteer databases on the ANA website: http://nursingworld.org/MainMenuCategories/HealthcareandPolicyIssues/DPR/VolunteerNow.aspx.

Unhealthy Lifestyles

Despite the focus on wellness and fitness in contemporary American society, unhealthy lifestyles still predominate; this trend shows no signs of changing; in fact, the number of people with bad habits is increasing.

Obesity

Every year public health officials report that there are more obese Americans than ever, even though **obesity**, defined as a body mass index (BMI) of 30 or more, has long been known to predispose people to a number of illnesses, including asthma,

cancer, cardiac disorders, type 2 diabetes, hyperlipidemia, high blood pressure, and arthritis. The accompanying News Note tells of a disturbingly rapid increase in the number of Americans who are more than 100 pounds overweight. You may want to compute your own BMI, using the formula found in Box 16-2.

Futurists predict that Americans will eat more meals in restaurants in the future, but ordering a nutritious, well-balanced meal in a restaurant is a major challenge, even to people with a working knowledge of nutritional science. In a troublesome sign that indicates acquiescence to the fast-food mentality of many families, nutritional

---

Box 16-2   Compute Your Body Mass Index

Body mass index (BMI) is a mathematical calculation used to determine whether a patient is overweight. BMI is calculated by dividing body weight in kilograms by height in meters squared (weight [kg] ÷ height [m²]) or by using the conversion with pounds (lbs) and inches squared (in.²) as shown below. This number can be misleading for very muscular people, or for pregnant or lactating women.

CALCULATE YOUR BMI

$$[Weight(lbs) \div Height(in.^2)] \times 704.5 = BMI$$

For example, if you are 5 feet 5 inches tall and weigh 134 pounds, your formula will look like this:

$$[134 \div (65 inches \times 65 inches)] \times 704.5 = 22.34$$

Being obese and being overweight are not the same condition. A BMI of 30 or more is considered obese, and a BMI between 25 and 29.9 is considered overweight. There are many factors that impact a person's health risk relative to his or her BMI, such as waist size, smoking, the types of foods regularly eaten, exercise, and medical conditions associated with obesity including diabetes, high blood pressure, high cholesterol level, and coronary artery disease.

Modified from National Heart, Lung, and Blood Institute's Obesity Education Initiative: *Calculate your body mass index,* 2009 (website): http://www.obesity.org/information/what_is_obesity.asp.

news note

EXTREME OBESITY BALLOONING: 1 IN 50 ADULTS IN U.S. AT LEAST 100 POUNDS TOO HEAVY

Americans are not just getting fatter; they are ballooning to extremely obese proportions at an alarming rate. The number of extremely obese American adults, those who are at least 100 pounds overweight, has quadrupled since the 1980s to about 4 million. That equates to about 1 in every 50 adults.

Extreme obesity once was thought to be a rare, distinct condition whose prevalence remained relatively steady over time. The new study contradicts that thinking and suggests that it is at least partly attributable to the same kinds of behaviors, overeating and underactivity, that have contributed to the epidemic number of Americans with less severe weight problems.

In fact, the findings by a RAND Corporation researcher show that the number of extremely obese adults has surged twice as fast as the number of less severely obese adults.

On the scale of obesity, "as the whole population shifts to the right, the extreme categories grow the fastest," said RAND economist Roland Sturm. He added, "These people have the highest health costs."

Sturm said health problems associated with obesity—including diabetes, heart disease, high blood pressure, and arthritis—probably affect the extremely obese disproportionately and at young ages. "There is no evidence that it (the obesity rate) is flattening out," Sturm said. "It's full speed ahead." Sturm has completed projections showing that if this problem is not addressed, the number of obese Americans will jump from about 20% of adults today to 80% by 2040, and the proportion of normal-weight people will drop from 42% today to 5% in 2040.

Sturm's study, which appeared in the *Archives of Internal Medicine,* is based on nationwide telephone surveys conducted by the U.S. Centers for Disease Control and Prevention, in which people were asked their height and weight. His report covers surveys from 1986 through 2000.

In 1986, 1 in 200 adults reported height and weight measurements reflecting extreme obesity, or a body-mass index of at least 40. By 2000 that number had increased to 1 in 50, Sturm found. Body mass index is a ratio of height to weight.

The prevalence of the most extreme obesity, people with a BMI of at least 50, grew fivefold—from 1 in 2000 to 1 in 400—Sturm said. By contrast, ordinary obesity, a BMI of 30 to 35, doubled—from about 1 in 10 to 1 in 5—based on the same surveys.

Americans tend to understate their weights, and a recent study based on actual measurements found an obesity rate of nearly 1 in 3, or almost 59 million people. Sturm said his findings probably understate the problem for the same reason.

The average man with a BMI of 40 in the study was 5 feet 10 inches and 300 pounds, while the average woman was 5 feet 4 inches and 250 pounds. Sturm said the trend largely is the result of the increasing affordability of calorie-dense food. "We've reached Nirvana," he said. "Food is cheap and plentiful. You can stuff yourself on less than a half-hour of minimum wage."

The trend is also fueled by a substantial reduction in the amount of physical activity that Americans engage in, said Linda Baumann, a nursing professor at the University of Wisconsin, Madison. School physical education budgets have been cut, suburban neighborhoods have been built without sidewalks, and "children are driven instead of walking to school," said Baumann, who is also is president of the Society of Behavioral Medicine.

Obesity researchers say the trend has to be reversed, or the health consequences will be devastating. "How can we put up with having this many people that large?" said James Hill, an obesity expert at the University of Colorado. "We have to do something quick."

Reprinted from Extreme obesity ballooning, *The Post and Courier* [Charleston, SC], 103(287): 1A, 8A, Oct 14, 2003.

consultants are now being hired by public school districts to teach cafeteria workers how to make nutritious school lunches look and taste more like fast foods. Apparently, many modern children refuse to eat anything else.

Childhood obesity has recently come to the forefront of concern as the number of overweight American children has grown. For example, the National Health and Nutrition Examination Survey (NHANES), conducted regularly by the CDC, found in its 2003-2004 survey that 13.9% of preschool-aged children, 18.8% of school-aged children, and 17.4% of adolescents were overweight. Overweight children are at risk of becoming obese, and obese children become obese adults. As obese adults, they will have children who themselves are more likely to become obese, thereby perpetuating the cycle (Jordan-Welch and Harbaugh, 2008).

As a result of pressure from health-conscious consumers, many of whom are now aging baby boomers, some fast-food restaurant chains have introduced grilled foods and other "low-fat" items. On examination, however, the fat content of some of these foods remains unacceptably high. Restaurant owners report that even when they include low-fat meals on the menu, few people order them. The majority of regular menu items are still loaded with animal fats, long known to cause cardiovascular disease, and sodium, known to aggravate a variety of health conditions. A taco salad, for example, can contain as many as 30 grams of fat, which represents about half of the recommended fat intake for an entire day.

Tobacco use

Yet another lifestyle issue is tobacco use. Smoking continues to increase among the young, especially females and minorities, both of whom are targeted for higher levels of marketing by tobacco companies. For decades, smoking has been known to cause lung cancer, emphysema and other chronic lung diseases, low–birth-weight babies, and a host of other health problems.

Lung cancer is a leading cancer killer in both men and women. There were an estimated 173,700 new cases of lung cancer and an estimated 160,440 deaths of lung cancer in the United States in 2004. The rate of lung cancer cases appears to be dropping among white and African-American men in the United States, while it continues to rise among both white and African-American women (American Lung Association, 2006).

The use of smokeless tobacco is rising, creating unhealthy oral mucous membranes and predisposing users to oral cancer. All these trends ensure that tobacco-related illnesses and deaths will rise in the future.

Lack of exercise

Lack of exercise is a troubling lifestyle issue for Americans of the future, particularly the young. The ready availability of entertainment on television is at least partly to blame. Studies show that the more television people of all ages watch, the more likely they are to be overweight. Snacking and television watching usually go hand in hand. Entire generations of Americans, raised watching several hours of television each day, are unlikely to give up the habit in the future, especially because more viewing options are added yearly. Others spend hours in front of computer screens, playing video games, or in other sedentary pursuits. These habits are expected to continue in the future.

Lack of exercise is not limited to the young, however. For every jogger seen pounding the roadways, legions of sedentary adults remain unseen at home, gradually becoming less fit and more susceptible to disease. Browsing through mail-order catalogs aimed at the affluent middle-aged population reveals a plethora of labor-saving devices being developed and marketed to make Americans even less active in the future.

Stress

Another lifestyle issue is stress. The rapid pace of modern life creates stress, yet Americans continue to step up the pace with cellular telephones, fax machines, satellite communications, personal computers, paging devices, call-waiting options, texting, and all the other fruits of modern technology. Although many Americans mourn the loss of leisure time, indications are that when given more leisure time, many people spend it working.

The instant availability of news of the latest natural and man-made disasters only serves to increase the stress the average person feels about events totally beyond his or her control. Yet few people seem willing to turn off the devices and give themselves a break from the pressure of being "always available." Given these conditions, it is little wonder that stress-related diseases are on the increase and are likely to continue in the future.

HIV/AIDS and drug abuse

The epidemics of acquired immunodeficiency syndrome (AIDS) and drug abuse are two issues that will affect the future of nursing.

HIV/AIDS. When the AIDS epidemic began in the United States early in the 1980s, the first individuals infected were homosexual men. A few years later, infection rates among intravenous drug users began to rise. By the mid-1980s, AIDS began to move into the general population of heterosexual adults, a trend already seen in other countries and now well established in the United States. As early sexual activity and IV drug abuse increased in young people, the rate of AIDS among adolescents and young adults mushroomed. Although HIV/AIDS no longer commands the headlines as it did in the early years of the epidemic, it continues to take a heavy toll on the population at home and abroad. In some African countries, for example, more than half of all adults are infected, and the number of orphaned children is increasing rapidly.

Even optimists in the medical community no longer predict a vaccine against human immunodeficiency virus (HIV), believing that it will be many years before a vaccine is discovered, if ever. Meanwhile, millions of Americans are already infected, and no cure is on the horizon. Long-term survival has become commonplace, however, because of the increasing availability of effective chemotherapy "cocktails" that stave off the devastating effects of the virus, sometimes for decades.

Because of the widespread incidence of blood-borne pathogens, nurses of the future must continue to be vigilant about protecting themselves and their patients from transmission of these diseases by scrupulously following protocols.

This epidemic, although not attracting the media attention it once did, shows no signs of ending.

Drug abuse. Drug abuse is a self-destructive lifestyle choice that continues to plague American life, particularly the youth of the nation. The impact of a drug-abusing public on nursing is multidimensional and brings up issues such as addiction, withdrawal, harm reduction, noncompliance with health care regimens, and appropriate pain management for drug abusers. Because of their lifestyle choices, drug abusers are at increased risk for many diseases such as HIV/AIDS, hepatitis, various resistant bacterial infections, liver disorders, and kidney failure.

Substance-abusing people suffer more accidents and illnesses than their nonabusing counterparts, thus requiring more medical and nursing care. They are also more likely to have unprotected sex, putting them at risk for acquiring HIV and other sexually transmitted diseases. If current trends continue, nurses of the future will be called on to provide intensive nursing care to increasing numbers of substance abusers. Nurses will be involved in the development of public policies concerning drug abuse treatment and prevention.

Given the predominance of unhealthy lifestyle choices, it is clear that nurses will play an increasingly important role in educating people about wellness and self-care in the years ahead. Nurses will also be instrumental in educating the public about how to be informed consumers of health care services. As nurses continue to provide care in acute care settings, hospitals, and clinics, their personal opinions and judgments must be put aside to be effective patient advocates and provide equal opportunities for health care to all populations.

Health Care Reform

Governmental budget deficits have reached all-time highs. For the past 30 or more years, at federal, state, and local levels, governments routinely spend more money than is generated through taxes. With the economic recession of 2008-2009 came the heavy expenditures of various economic stimulus packages, which, when combined with subsidies to major companies, quickly tripled the national debt. Even during these times of economic crisis, pressure to provide health care for the uninsured, the elderly, and the poor continues, increasing the pressure on our national and state budgets.

As mentioned earlier, our infant death rate is a national embarrassment, and our prescription drug costs are the highest in the world. Society's poor, homeless, elderly, substance abusers, patients with AIDS, and mentally ill are increasing in number and will continue to increase. Given the global economic recession, the question to be answered is, "How can we pay for health care for these vulnerable populations now and in the future when their numbers become even greater and our national resources are committed to debt repayment?"

Federal and state governments are seeking to answer that question. In most states, Medicaid is the largest and fastest-growing single state expense. Although welfare reform efforts of the 1990s removed thousands from welfare rolls, the aging of America will continue to create huge numbers of social security–eligible and Medicare-eligible citizens. The corresponding decrease in the number of those working and paying social security and income taxes will place an additional burden on the federal government's budget.

The future may bring hospital closings, continued pressures from the business community to force changes in health care financing, and significant health care reform, piece by piece if not by sweeping legislative mandate. The nursing profession stands to benefit because nursing has been shown to be a cost-effective yet high-quality alternative to traditional medical care. In addition, nurses are well equipped to provide managed care. As a profession, nursing is expected to benefit from health care reform efforts in the United States by expanding roles in prevention, community-based nursing, and advanced practice, among others.

One cost-effective method of providing basic health care to children is through school nurses. As the burden of providing care continues to shift from federal agencies to state and local agencies, local school boards will recognize the economies to be realized through school nursing. Health care reform will likely provoke a dramatic rise in state-mandated

health "safety net" services for children. Many of these services will be delivered by nurses.

Even if the cost of health care can be slowed or contained by congressional mandate, health care expenses in the United States will continue to rise. This increase will be caused by the large number of aging Americans and the growing number of impoverished ones. As the economy worsens and more citizens are covered by government-sponsored medical programs such as Medicare and Medicaid, even greater governmental regulation of health care costs and quality will be required.

Nurses will become increasingly active in developing health policies that improve access, quality, and value in the delivery of health services. Legislation mandating the direct reimbursement of nurses for their services will be a feature of most government-funded programs, despite the opposition of organized medicine and hospitals. Private insurers and managed-care companies will also authorize advanced practice registered nurses to receive reimbursement for primary health care.

Nursing, through its professional associations, will continue to be a player in health care politics in the United States. Nurses will form coalitions with consumer groups to influence consumer-friendly legislation at state and national levels. Individual nurses will become more politically active as voters, campaign workers, community health activists, and political candidates. As nursing's public profile becomes higher, public scrutiny of the profession will increase. Consumers of nursing services will exercise their political power to ensure that nurses and other primary care providers consistently offer first-class health care.

Editor's Note: As this book goes to press, health care reform is being debated in congress. Any significant reforms passed will be posted on the Evolve website: http://evolve.elsevier.com/Chitty/professional.

CHALLENGES IN NURSING PRACTICE

The societal changes just reviewed will necessarily create changes in nursing practice. Nurses in the next decade will face an ever-widening array of practice opportunities in hospital and community-based health care settings, each of which will bring its own set of challenges.

Differentiating Practice Levels

There has been considerable resistance to differentiating levels of nursing practice, even though nursing leaders have pointed out the need to do so for years. Differentiated practice means that nurses prepared in associate degree, baccalaureate degree, and higher degree programs should have different, well-defined roles and possibly even different levels of licensure. The competencies of nurses at each level could be clearly demonstrated, and nurses at each level could be held accountable for practice standards at that level. If differentiated practice became a reality, educational programs could be streamlined, employers and consumers could understand the differences, and patient care delivery systems could be reorganized to capitalize on the strengths of each level.

In the past, nurses prepared in diploma and associate degree programs opposed efforts to differentiate educational and practice levels in nursing, believing that they would be disenfranchised. Nursing leaders have been unwilling to take the risk of tackling such a potentially divisive issue. The result is that nursing is the only health care profession for which entry into practice is less than a baccalaureate degree. Many professions currently require a master's degree as the credential for entry into a profession, and educational standards are rising in all fields but nursing. This has hampered nursing in its quest for professionalism and equal status among the health care professions.

In addition to improving educational standards, differentiated practice could help nurses be more cost-effective by determining who is best suited to perform certain nursing actions. Differentiated practice can be realized in the future only if practicing nurses are willing to give up the notion that "a nurse is a nurse is a nurse" and acknowledge that different educational programs do and should prepare different types of nursing practitioners. Nurses must be willing to see the larger picture and recognize that advances in the profession benefit all nurses. They are being encouraged in these efforts by the American Association of Colleges of Nursing (AACN), which refers to differentiated practice as one of the "hallmarks of the professional nursing practice environment" in its white paper by the same title. You can read the entire document at AACN's website (http://www.aacn.nche.edu/Publications/positions/hallmarks.htm).

Health Care Reform

During the 1990s, cost-containment initiatives in hospitals eliminated layers of middle-management nurses. This represented a crisis for individual nurse managers but created an opportunity for a stronger voice for nurses involved in direct patient care. Future cost-containment measures will require nurses to demonstrate the cost-effectiveness of the care they provide. The "bottom line" will be an increasing focus of concern in all health care settings, and nurses will need resource management skills more than ever before. Nurses will find that they need business expertise as much as they need clinical expertise.

Increasingly, nurses will work with unlicensed assistive personnel, such as patient care technicians, and will delegate tasks to deliver patient care. They will need communication, collaboration, delegation, and management skills to make the new partnerships work. In addition, a variety of new health care job opportunities in quality care, case management, advanced practice, and primary care will present themselves as a result of economic pressures of managed care and health reforms (Marrilli, 2006).

Autonomy and Accountability

Shared governance, that is, participation by nurses on strong policy-making hospital committees, is a trend already seen and mandated by accreditation bodies such as The Joint Commission. Along with the empowerment of nurses, however, will come increased demand for accountability. Effective nursing care will be measured by patient outcomes. Continuous quality improvement of nursing care will be emphasized more than ever. Nurses must be able to show evidence that the care they provide makes a demonstrable difference in patient outcomes.

As more and more nursing care is provided in community settings, autonomy and accountability will become increasingly important. Nurses who function independently in homes and other community-based practice settings need additional education and experience. When the supervisory guidance of better-prepared colleagues is not readily available, novice or inexperienced nurses must assume responsibility for knowing the limits of their expertise and for seeking consultation to ensure patient safety. Professional nurses of the future will increasingly pursue baccalaureate and advanced degrees to prepare them for autonomous practice. More than ever, lifelong learning will be a requirement for professional nurses.

Technology and Nursing Informatics

All types of technology will continue to advance at a dizzying pace, as they have in the first years of the twenty-first century. Areas expected to affect nursing are nursing informatics, telecommunications, genetic engineering, alternative treatments, and the Internet.

Nursing informatics

Nursing informatics, the organization and use of nursing data, continues to change nursing practice dramatically. Computerized health information networks (CHINs) will allow immediate access to all patient data needed in refining the plan of care. The increased access to patient data will reinforce the need for patient confidentiality. Voice-activated bedside computers already allow nurses to record patient information literally "at the bedside," rather than making written notes and transferring them to the patient's chart at a later time. This practice will become even more widespread as the push for electronic health records, a campaign promise made by the Obama administration, continues. Some have even suggested that with handheld devices receiving such widespread acceptance, individuals could keep their own health records, uploading them to health care providers as needed (Eisenberg, 2008). Shifting the responsibility for keeping health records from providers to patients themselves could represent a cost savings but would require that providers be much more forthcoming in sharing information with patients than they have traditionally been willing to do.

Telecommunications

Advances in telecommunications will improve access to medical services for rural and elderly Americans. Nurses and physicians will examine and treat patients who are hundreds of miles away using two-way television systems. They will evaluate and prescribe treatments via telephone. Telemedicine will become routine for those who live in remote areas or are homebound. Nurses will be increasingly involved in telehealth, and there will be explosive growth in home telemonitoring of patients.

Genetic engineering and the genomic revolution

Genetic engineering has become more common since scientists participating in the Human Genome Project completed the initial mapping and sequencing of a composite set of human genes in 2003. This made it potentially possible to treat and prevent many more genetically transmitted and genetically predisposed diseases. It will also create ethical dilemmas of dramatic proportions as the ability to clone individuals and predetermine characteristics of human infants becomes a reality. Genetic research will also make possible individualized medications, or designer medicines. Designer medicines are drugs tailor-made to treat patients on the basis of their individual genetic makeup. A new role for nurses, the Genomics Nurse Case Coordinator, has been proposed (Lea and Monsen, 2003). Programs preparing nurses for basic practice have been encouraged to include knowledge and skills to prepare graduates for "family history assessments, screening, and case coordination for clients receiving genetic testing and gene-based therapies" (Lea and Monsen, 2003, p. 75). Genetic literacy will be a must for nurses of the future. For ideas about how you can prepare yourself to include genetic and genomic nursing competencies into your clinical practice, refer to *The Online Journal of Issues in Nursing* (Junglen et al, 2008): http://www.nursingworld.org/MainMe nuCategories/ANAMarketplace/ANAPeriodical s/OJIN/TableofContents/vol132008/No3Sept08/ ArticlePreviousTopic/IncorporatingGeneticsand GenomicsintoPractice.aspx.

The Internet

The Internet will create major changes in the way Americans view health care and their role as partners in their own care. The proliferation of websites designed to provide reliable medical and health information to the lay public will continue. Nurses will be called on to educate patients about how to evaluate and appropriately use the information they obtain from these sites.

As a result of these and other unforeseen technologic advances, nurses of the future will continue to fight the dehumanizing tendency of technologic advances such as patient monitoring devices while valuing and providing a holistic, "high-touch" environment for patients. Nurses will realize that advanced technology and traditional nursing values are not mutually exclusive. Patients can have both if nurses stay focused on the patient rather than on the machine or monitor. Advances in technology will bring new ethical dilemmas. Nurses will be more active in exploring ethical aspects of patient care, and their unique ethical perspective will be valued by other professionals. As a result, nurses will sit on ethics committees and serve as ethics consultants in greater numbers.

Practice in Community Settings

Community-based primary health care will continue to expand as cost-effectiveness remains a high priority. Nurse-managed clinics will increasingly serve underserved populations in inner city and rural areas. School nurses will be needed in large numbers, as will hospice nurses and those specializing in gerontology and chronic diseases. For nurses who are willing to work outside traditional settings and their own "comfort zones," there will be no end to the available opportunities.

Flexible scheduling and job sharing will increase in all professions and will become commonplace in nursing. Nurse entrepreneurship will flourish in the future as a result of changes in restrictive legislation, the resourcefulness and self-confidence of better-educated nurses, and the trust the public places in the nursing profession. Increasing numbers of nurses will own clinics and other health-related businesses, such as independent practice associations, free-standing wellness programs, adult day care centers, dialysis care services, and worksite health programs.

Cultural Competence

Providing culturally competent nursing care will become even more important in the future as the nation's demographics change even more dramatically than they have in the past. Nurses of the future must recognize that cultural sensitivity begins with one's fellow health care providers. If relationships within the team are strained by insensitivity and prejudice, patient care cannot be culturally sensitive. Meaningful dialogue must become a vehicle for building relationships within the work group. A united team will be capable of providing respectful, understanding, and dignified care to patients.

Effective nursing leaders of the future will provide cultural support groups and mentoring to ensure that "faculty, providers, students, patients, and others can become less inhibited about individuals who are culturally different. They can foster the courage to engage in conversations, to get to know each other, to share our worldviews, to speak out, and to trust that interactions about our specific and particular culture, on a personal level, will make a difference" (Gary, Sigsby, and Campbell, 1998, p. 277). Nurses who are unable or unwilling to become culturally aware, culturally sensitive, and culturally competent will unnecessarily limit their career potential.

Complementary and alternative therapies

As disenchantment with the cost, depersonalization, and fragmentation of traditional medicine grows, more Americans will turn away from mainstream medical care and seek other treatments

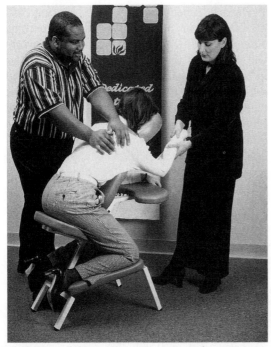

Figure 16-3 Alternative treatments, such as massage therapy, are appealing to more Americans as they take responsibility for their own health. This trend to natural healing and the use of alternative and complementary therapies is expected to increase in the future. (Courtesy Memorial Health Care System, Chattanooga, Tenn.)

Box 16-3 Complementary and Alternative Therapies

- Nearly 50% of Americans use some form of complementary and alternative therapies (CAT).
- About 80% of the world's population use herbal medicine.
- Approximately 72% people who use CAT do not tell their health care providers.
- CAT can interact with other forms of treatment to create potential risks.
- In a study, more than half of critical care nurses surveyed reported that patients and families requested common therapies (e.g., diet, exercise, relaxation, prayer), as well as massage and counseling.
- Therapies considered legitimate by more than 75% of critical care nurses surveyed included diet, exercise, massage, counseling, prayer, relaxation techniques, music therapy, meditation, pet therapy, and behavioral medicine. Those viewed as not legitimate by 25% or more of respondents included megavitamin therapy and electromagnetic/magnet therapies.

Modified from Goley A: APNs need to learn more about complementary and alternative medicine, *Top Adv Pract Nurs eJournal* 4(2), 2004 (website): http://www.search.medscape.com/medscape=search?queryText=Goley; Tracy MF, Lindquist R, Savik K, et al: Use of complementary and alternative therapies: a national survey of critical care nurses, *Am J Crit Care* 14(5):404-415, 2005.

as they take responsibility for their own health (Figure 16-3, Box 16-3). It is estimated that one half of Americans use some form of alternative medicine, such as yoga, meditation, chiropractic, homeopathy, acupuncture, aromatherapy, massage, therapeutic touch, megavitamins, and herbal remedies, among others. **Complementary therapies** include techniques that are used along with standard medical care and are a combination of Eastern and Western healing methods.

Alternative therapies are used in place of standard care. The National Center for Complementary and Alternative Medicine, a division of the National Institutes of Health, is charged with raising the standards of evidence of effectiveness of complementary and alternative therapies (CAT). Scientific evidence has too often been obscured by the lack of reliable clinical trials on the effectiveness

of various therapies (Broad, 2008). Nurses, with their holistic approach to patient care, are well positioned to assist in establishing **integrative care**, combining the best of both standard and nontraditional treatments. These therapies will increasingly become a focus of interest, study, research, practice, and publication in nursing.

Maintaining a Healthy Work Environment

No profession is free from hazards, and no workplace can ever ensure absolute security. Nursing is no exception to this sad fact of contemporary life. Occupational health hazards in nursing include needlestick injuries and possible infection with blood-borne pathogens; exposure to chemicals such as disinfectants and chemotherapeutic agents; and violence in the workplace, among others.

Additional hazards include latex allergy, a continuing concern for nurses, with a prevalence rate of approximately 8% to 12% in frequent glove users (ANA, 2006). Injuries from accidents and back strain also occur too frequently, with pain, disability, lost income, absenteeism, and decreased productivity only a few of the results.

Shift work itself is a hazard to nurses, causing a variety of physical and psychological problems, including exhaustion, depression, interpersonal problems, and accidents. Stress from work overload, inadequate staffing, and the intense feelings generated by caring for acutely ill and dying patients add to the mix of workplace hazards faced by nurses.

In addition, nurses increasingly find themselves at risk for violence in the workplace. This is not a new phenomenon, as evidenced by the fall 1999 issue of Sigma Theta Tau International's membership publication *Reflections* (now titled *Reflections on Nursing Leadership*), being devoted entirely to the issue of workplace violence.

Among the articles in that issue of *Reflections* was a report of a survey by the Colorado Nurses Association's Task Force on Violence, which conducted a seven-state study examining nurse safety. There were 586 respondents, one third of whom disclosed "that they were victims of workplace violence" in the prior year. Most nurses indicated patients were the assailants, "yet half of the nurses acknowledged that violence went unreported at work" (Carroll and Goldsmith, 1999, p. 26).

Assuring nurses of a healthy work environment is a major challenge. It is not, however, a problem that nurses can expect to be solved by others. Clearly, nurses of the future must themselves take positive, effective, united action to ensure the basic dignity and safety of practicing nurses everywhere. They must demand and use safer needlestick devices and disposal containers; high-efficiency ventilation systems; alternatives to latex gloves and products; adequate housekeeping support; adequate lifting assistance with devices or additional personnel; reduction or elimination of shift rotation and double shifts; and appropriate occupational safety and health training. Nurses themselves must use impeccable hand-washing techniques and personal protective equipment such as gloves, gowns, and masks when needed. In addition, they must demand that adequate screening security be provided to protect them against violent patients and family members.

CHALLENGES IN NURSING EDUCATION

As the profession of nursing matures, more nurses will recognize the value of bachelor's degrees for beginning professional practice and master's degrees for advanced practice. More nurses will pursue doctoral degrees to prepare for leadership roles in research, theory development, and teaching. In response, colleges of nursing will expand flexible and online educational programs to improve access. They will also develop differentiated levels of nursing education that correspond to differentiated levels of practice.

Outcome-Based Education

The quality of educational programs will continue to be judged by student competencies—that is, what students can actually do as a result of education. Nursing educational programs will monitor their graduates' activities and achievements as professional nurses. They will be required to report on graduates' accomplishments as part of the accreditation process. The emphasis on accountability of nursing education programs will increase as measures of competence in graduates are refined.

Just as nursing practice is being challenged to measure patient outcomes and adopt evidence-based practice, nursing education will be challenged to develop student outcomes and adopt evidence-based education. Faculty will modify age-old teaching/learning strategies and adopt new pedagogies (teaching methods) proved effective through research (i.e., evidence-based teaching). Passive learning, such as lectures, will be deemphasized. Critical thinking, independent decision making, and creative problem solving will assume even greater importance, fostered by role playing, simulations, and group problem solving (Davidhizar and Shearer, 2005). Faculty will be required to document evidence-based teaching as part of accreditation processes.

Accreditation of nursing education programs will become more difficult to achieve as national accrediting bodies come under increasing pressure to raise standards and to apply standards consistently. Substandard programs will be closed. This will strengthen nursing but will not help the nursing shortage.

Diversity

Students in nursing education programs will reflect the demographics of the United States and become more diverse than ever before. More men, older students, and students with baccalaureate degrees in other fields will come into nursing because of the emotional rewards, economic stability, and professional image it offers. Student bodies will become more culturally diverse, reflecting the diversity of the nation's population. Educational needs of students from different cultures will be unique and will not be adequately met with traditional teaching strategies applied to all students (Davidhizar and Shearer, 2005). Schools of nursing must strive to offer individualized, culturally competent education.

Access to education for nontraditional and traditional students will be an even greater issue. Schools will expand nontraditional curricula that enable adults to work and go to school simultaneously. Nursing courses delivered online and by distance learning technologies, such as telecommunications and satellite linkages, will increase access for students living in remote areas. Cost-minded legislators will require that state-supported schools offer fully articulated programs to qualify for state funding. Schools that fall behind in distance learning offerings will have difficulty filling their classes as more and more students seek nonresidential education.

Changes in demographics will affect the content of curricula, as well as the methods by which content is delivered. As the population

ages, the need for nurses prepared in gerontology, chronic disease management, and hospice care will give emphasis to educational programs at both undergraduate and graduate levels. Curricula will emphasize community-based care instead of traditional hospital-based care. Educational programs will develop and expand multicultural courses. Foreign languages will again become a graduation requirement in baccalaureate programs. International educational opportunities will increase as the global village concept becomes a reality. Every nursing program will have the provision of culturally competent care as an outcome criterion for its graduates.

Impact of Technology and Nursing Informatics

Technologic advances and the growth of nursing knowledge will create the need for informatics expertise in nursing education, as well as in nursing practice. Computer competence will not suffice for nurses of the future. Students will need to master sophisticated information systems to use the wealth of available knowledge to improve and document patient care and to assist in the transition to electronic health records. Faculty will be challenged to keep pace with students' acquisition of knowledge from the World Wide Web. Students of the future will become increasingly active in obtaining information from a vast array of sources available to them at the touch of a computer key. This will enable students to be more engaged in their own learning process and foster active learning.

Nursing faculty will be required to practice the profession actively to keep up with rapidly changing technologies. Maintaining faculty currency will become a greater focus in higher education. Active practice in addition to teaching will become an expected part of the faculty role. Students will be incorporated into faculty practices to obtain clinical experience. In this regard, nursing education will resemble medical education.

It will be impossible for nursing education programs to include in their curricula everything nurses of the future need to know. If, for example, genomics and disaster nursing are to be added to curricula, what will be removed? Nursing students already are overwhelmed with the amount of material they must master.

The solution to this problem is that all nurses must be educated to become lifelong learners. They must be taught to expect change and be prepared to adapt or retool their skills quickly to respond to health care marketplace demands (Jenkins, 2005). They must invest in themselves, pursuing knowledge and refreshing their knowledge base through vigorous, self-motivated continuing education efforts.

Licensing examinations will change to reflect the expansion of nursing knowledge and the increase in community-based practice and resulting autonomy. Licensure at multiple levels will become a reality. Employers of new graduates will expect to provide internships designed to enable novices to make the transition from student to practicing nurse effectively.

Collaboration

As nurses acquire more education, the resulting knowledge and self-confidence will enable them to develop collaborative relationships on an equal footing with physicians and other highly educated health care professionals. This will enable nurses to be more assertive in patient advocacy and will improve patient care and strengthen the profession.

Nursing faculty, nurse managers, and practicing nurses will join forces to strengthen educational experiences and provide mentorships for tomorrow's nurses. They will collaborate on clinical research that demonstrates the effectiveness of nursing care in terms of patient outcomes. They will collaborate with other nurses and consumer groups to remove regulatory restrictions that impede advanced clinical practice. They will work together to close the gap between education and practice.

Nurse educators will recognize the need to treat students as professionals in training and will transform nursing education attitudes from controlling students to collaborating with them. This will create a new generation of empowered nursing professionals.

Disciplinary boundaries are becoming blurred as knowledge from all disciplines is brought to bear on problems of mutual concern, such as breast cancer, domestic violence, and AIDS. Nursing must become more interdisciplinary in its focus. Only nurses with a strong sense of personal and professional identity will be able to enter fully into multidisciplinary collaboration. Those nurses who understand the value of collaboration will become the managers of care using a case-management model, and they will thrive.

Reforms in Health Care and Higher Education

As a result of health care reforms and cost-containment initiatives, nurses of the future will need to be well versed in the costs, budgeting, and financing of health care. Business education will be increasingly emphasized, particularly at the graduate level, as nurses pursue entrepreneurial roles. Nursing faculty either will return to school to prepare themselves to teach business courses or will create interdisciplinary alliances with business schools to provide nursing students with the necessary business courses.

Higher education will undergo public scrutiny and reform. It already suffers from serious underfunding, which is worsening as the economy weakens. As governmental grants are reduced or eliminated to help balance the national budget and state tax revenues decline because of constraints on consumer spending, educational programs will experience dramatic budgetary constraints. During budget shortfalls in the past, several nursing education programs, including some well-regarded ones, were closed. In many universities, autonomous schools and colleges of nursing were combined with health and human service programs into one administrative unit to save money. This often weakened the nursing program's voice on the campus. Budgets for operating expenses, equipment, and faculty salaries are under par in many locations, even though the demand for nursing education remains high and employment opportunities for graduates are strong and will remain strong for many years.

For a time, it appeared that hospitals could be a source of support for nursing education programs, but with their own significant budgetary constraints, it is unlikely that this will be a long-term solution. Hospitals, however, will support nursing education for as long as possible with financial aid to students, subsidies of faculty salaries, joint appointments of faculty, and other forms of assistance.

Graduate education programs will change to produce practitioners who can meet consumer demands. Changes in hospital-based nursing practice will force a reexamination of the clinical nurse specialist and nurse practitioner roles. The need for efficiency and cost-effectiveness will lead to a revision of advanced practice models, and educational programs will combine the two roles and emphasize community-based practice.

Curricula at all levels will be standardized and streamlined to reduce cost and confusion and improve student mobility. Fast-track curricula will proliferate. The trend toward use of multiskilled workers will force nursing faculty to identify unique aspects of nursing and to educate students for broader roles in the delivery of patient care.

Faculty Shortage/Student Shortage

In the next decade, many long-time nursing faculty members, educated at the master's level during the nurse-traineeship funding heyday of the 1960s, will retire. There will be no one to replace many of them because relatively few younger nurses are entering teaching; this shortage of teachers is attributable to the fact that nursing education salaries lag behind those in practice settings. There is already a serious shortage of nursing faculty, which will worsen as more retirements occur. This will force a major restructuring of nursing education programs and negatively affect the already problematic shortage of nurses.

Colleges of nursing routinely report turning away qualified applicants, often because of a lack of faculty to teach them. These two problems—too few faculty members and fewer students in the pipeline—combine to create a negative synergy and downward spiral in the number of

practicing nurses. The nursing profession, working in collaboration with public and private funding sources and policymakers, and employers of nurses must find a solution to these twin problems in the near future if nursing is to thrive as a profession. Creating a more desirable work environment for practicing nurses, thereby retaining nurses who might otherwise leave the profession, will attain a greater and much needed focus (Valentino, 2002).

As the faculty shortage in nursing is translated into a student shortage—and therefore to a worsening of the nursing shortage—medical schools are increasing their output of physicians. Of particular concern is the trend toward physician role expansion in the area of inpatient care by hospitalists. These are physicians who are hospital based and care for patients only while they are hospitalized. They "are predicted to care for many nonsurgical patients by 2005, thus decreasing demand for advanced practice nurses" (Wolf, 2003, p. 32). Because advanced practice nursing is the goal of many of today's undergraduate nursing students, this is a trend that bears monitoring. Outside the hospital walls, the declining number of primary care physicians entering practice will open opportunities for family nurse practitioners to fill the gap (American College of Physicians, 2006).

A CHALLENGE TO THE ENTIRE NURSING PROFESSION: FOCUS, UNITE, ACT!

Most of the important issues the nursing profession will face in the next decade cannot be resolved by any one group of nurses. These concerns will require the attention of the entire profession, working in a focused, united, active manner through nursing's professional associations. Although collective power is the only way nursing will effectively resolve these issues, fewer than 10% of all nurses belong to their professional association, a sad commentary on the priorities most nurses place on this vital aspect of professionalism.

As the largest health care profession in the United States, with more than 2.9 million registered nurses, nursing can and should have a powerful voice and presence at every table where substantive health care issues are discussed. However, nurses have historically been unwilling to throw their support behind their professional organizations. They have allowed issues of educational background, political philosophies, right-to-life, and other concerns to divide them.

If you think for a moment about other groups to which you belong—for example, a political party, church, or parent-teacher association—you do not expect to agree with every position taken by the organization or its leaders. Nurses seem to have such an expectation of their professional association, however, and use that as a reason for lack of unity. This is naïve and unrealistic. With nursing and society becoming increasingly diverse, nurses of the future must become more tolerant of differences and work hard to find common ground with their colleagues in the profession. If we fail to do so, nursing will not prosper, nor will its practitioners.

Nursing's Agenda for the Future

An encouraging development was the coming together in 2001 of 19 major nursing organizations at the Nursing Profession Summit. A $100,000 grant from the American Nurses Foundation, a branch of the ANA, enabled the ANA to convene this group, which formed a steering committee. The steering committee took leadership in identifying 10 domains (areas) that describe the work needed to accomplish the vision they set forth in a document titled *Nursing's Agenda for the Future*. This document identified what the steering committee envisioned: how nursing should look and where it should be by the year 2010. In other words, this committee developed a desired future vision for nursing and set forth areas that were to be addressed to achieve the desired vision.

The steering committee called on all nurses to review *Nursing's Agenda for the Future* and to find those objectives that match with the mission, priorities, and resources of their own entities. The intent was to involve as many nurses as possible in charting their own future (Nursing's Agenda

for the Future Steering Committee, 2002, pp. 6, 7). A more recent report prepared by the members of the ANA is entitled, *ANA's Health System Reform Agenda* (2008). This represents an update of *Nursing's Agenda for the Future.* It promotes and expands on four basic ANA beliefs (ANA, 2008):

- That health care is a basic human right and that universal access to a standard package of essential health care services should be provided to all citizens and residents;
- That the development and implementation of health policies should aim for safe, effective, patient-centered, timely, efficient, and equitable care based on outcomes research;
- That the health care system must turn away from the overuse of expensive, technology-driven, acute, hospital-based services to a more balanced one with emphasis on community-based and preventive services; and
- That a single-payer system is the most desirable option for financing a reformed health care system.

As efforts at reforming health care progress, you can monitor progress toward these goals.

You, the readers of this book, are the future of the nursing profession. You represent our best hope for building nursing into an even more powerful force for good. Look around at the other members of your class. Whether you have 25 fellow students or 125, you can accomplish far more working together than you can working in isolation. So it is with nursing's future: we can accomplish far more by working collectively. All nurses, individually and as a profession, will benefit from the results. As Mohandas Gandhi said, "Be the change you wish to see in the world."

Summary of Key Points

- Future societal changes will occur in the following areas: demographics, the environment, potential for disasters such as bioterrorism, lifestyles, economics, and governmental regulation of health care.
- Both nursing practice and nursing education will be affected by these changes.

- Nursing roles will be differentiated.
- Nursing practice will become more community based with new roles continually emerging.
- Today's nurses should be prepared to serve effectively as members of an emergency and disaster response team.
- Nurses will be able to demonstrate that the care they provide makes a positive difference in patient outcomes and is cost-effective.
- Nurses will continue to provide a warm, humanizing influence on patient care in potentially dehumanizing high-tech environments.
- Effective nurses will be culturally competent.
- The major challenges for nursing education will be to respond to societal changes rapidly with appropriate curricular modifications; to produce a steady supply of well-prepared graduates in the face of an aging faculty; to adapt to rapidly changing technology; to acquire competency needed to respond to increasing cultural diversity of students and patients; and to address the lack of human and budgetary resources in higher education.
- Active membership in professional associations is the best way for nurses to focus, unite, and act to solve the challenges facing the profession.

Critical Thinking Questions

1. As the number of elderly and obese Americans rises, the rate of chronic illness also rises. What challenges does this present for nurses of the future?
2. Take a position on the statement "Nurses of the future will have an impact on the environment that exceeds that of the ordinary citizen." Be prepared to defend your position.
3. Describe economic issues that will affect nurses of the future. How can you begin now to prepare yourself to deal with these issues?
4. Initiate a classroom debate on the issue "To assure patient safety, HIV-positive nurses should be limited in how they practice nursing."
5. As a class, brainstorm ways a school health nurse could improve pupils' health status.

Then design an educational program to prepare school nurses. Compare your curriculum with that of an existing school health nurse program.
6. Interview faculty members to identify components of your educational program that will prepare you for the culturally competent nursing needed in the twenty-first century. Report your findings to the class.
7. Using the core competencies listed in Box 16-1, evaluate your own disaster preparedness and devise a plan to become better prepared.
8. Using the GeneTests website as a resource (http://www.ncbi.nlm.nih.gov/sites/GeneTests?db=GeneTests), learn all you can about testing, counseling, and treatment for a genetic condition. These might include albinism, sickle cell disease, hereditary breast or ovarian cancer, hemophilia, hemochromatosis, Marfan syndrome, cystic fibrosis, or others of interest to you or your family. Report your findings to the class or to your family.

⊖volve *To enhance your understanding of this chapter, try the Student Exercises on the Evolve site at http://evolve.elsevier.com/Chitty/professional.*

REFERENCES

American College of Physicians: *The impending collapse of primary care medicine and its implications for the state of the nation's health care,* 2006 (website): http://www.acponline.org/fcgi/search?q=the+impending+collapse&site=ACP_Online&x=0&y=0.

American Lung Association: *Facts about lung cancer,* 2006 (website): http://www.lungusa.org/site/apps/nlnet/content3.aspx?c=dvLUK9O0E&b=2058829&content_id={62C3D98B-887D-4C19-B7AA-C558C240D450}&notoc=1#whatis.

American Nurses Association: *Workplace issues: occupational safety and health,* 2006 (website): http://www.nursingworld.org/MainMenuCategories/ANAPoliticalPower/Federal/AGENCIES/OSHA/SHLATEX11704.aspx.

American Nurses Association: *ANA's health system reform agenda,* 2008 (website): http://nursingworld.org/MainMenuCategories/HealthcareandPolicyIssues/HealthSystemReform/Agenda.aspx.

Broad WJ: Applying science to alternative medicine, *New York Times*, (Sept 30):p F-7, 2008.

Brush BL: Global nurse migration today, *J Nurs Sch* 40(1):20-25, 2008.

Carroll V, Goldsmith J: One-third of nurses are abused in the workplace, *Reflections* 25(3):24-27, 1999.

Cetron MJ, Davies O: Trends shaping tomorrow's world, part one, *The Futurist*, (March-April): p 52, 2008.

Davidhizar R, Shearer R: When your nursing student is culturally diverse, *Health Care Manag* 24(4): 356-363, 2005.

Davis K, Schoen C, Guterman S, Shih T, Schoenbaum MD, Weinbaum I: Slowing the growth of U.S. health care expenditures: what are the options? *The Commonwealth Fund* 47(1), 2007 (website): http://www.commonwealthfund.org/Content/ Publications/Fund-Reports/2007/Jan/Slowing-the-Growth-of-U-S-Health-Care-Expenditures–What-Are-the-Options.aspx.

Dickenson-Hazard N: Future study or the Magic 8 Ball? *Reflect Nurs Leadersh* 29(4):4, 2003.

Eisenberg A: Keeping your own health chart, online, *New York Times*, (Oct 12):p BU-4, 2008.

Extreme obesity ballooning: *The Post and Courier*, [Charleston, SC], 103(287):1A,8A, Oct 14, 2003.

Gary FA, Sigsby LM, Campbell D: Preparing for the 21st century: diversity in nursing education, research, and practice, *J Prof Nurs* 14(5):272-279, 1998.

Gatti AM, Montanari S: Nanopollution: the invisible fog of future wars, *The Futurist*, (May-June):p 32, 2008.

Gebbie KM, Qureshi K: Emergency and disaster preparedness: core competencies for nurses, *Am J Nurs* 102(1):46-51, 2002.

Goley A: APNs need to learn more about complementary and alternative medicine, *Top Adv Pract Nurs eJournal* 4(2), 2004 (website): http://www.medscape.com/medscape-search?queryText=Goley.

Hendrick B: The coming millennium, *Atlanta Journal/ Atlanta Constitution*, (July 16):p A12, 1995.

Herbert LE, Scherr PA, Beckett LA, et al: Alzheimer's disease, *JAMA* 273(17):1354-1359, 1995.

Jenkins A: Invest in yourself, *Nurs Stand* 20(10):69, 2005.

Jordan-Welch M, Harbaugh BL: End the epidemic of childhood obesity one family at a time: teaching big kids and their families to stop living large, *Am Nurs Today* 3(6):26-31, 2008.

Junglen L, Pestka E, Clawson M, Fisher S: Incorporating genetics and genomics into nursing practice: a demonstration, *Online J Issues Nurs* 13(3), 2008 (website): http://www.nursingworld.org/MainMenu Categories/ANAMarketplace/ANAPeriodicals/OJIN/ TableofContents/vol132008/No3Sept08/ArticlePrev iousTopic/IncorporatingGeneticsandGenomicsinto Practice.aspx.

Kellman B: Bioviolence: a growing threat, *The Futurist*, (May-June):p 25, 2008.

Lea DH, Monsen RB: Preparing nurses for a 21st century role in genomics-based health care, *Nurs Educ Perspect* 24(2):75-80, 2003.

Leavitt J: The new administration and health care reform, *Am J Nurs* 109(1):86-87, 2009.

MacDorman MF, Mathews TJ: *Recent trends in infant mortality in the United States.* NCHS data brief, No. 9, Hyattsville, Md, 2008, National Center for Health Statistics.

Marrilli T: Nursing in flux: are you ready to meet the challenge of the future? *Am J Nurs* 106(1 suppl):19-25, 2006.

National Heart, Lung, and Blood Institute, Obesity Education Initiative: *Calculate your body mass index,* 2009 (website): http://www.obesity.org/information/ what_is_obesity.asp.

Nursing's Agenda for the Future Steering Committee: *Nursing's agenda for the future: the future vision for nursing*, Washington, DC, 2002, American Nurses Publishing.

Tracy MF, Lindquist R, Savik K, et al: Use of complementary and alternative therapies: a national survey of critical care nurses, *Am J Crit Care* 14(5):404-415, 2005.

U.S. Census Bureau: *Population clock, U.S. and international,* 2009 (website): http://www.census.gov/main/ www/popclock.html.

Valentino LM: *Future employment trends in nursing, AJN 2002 career guide*, New York, 2002, Lippincott Williams & Wilkins.

Wolf G: Coming of age in health care: changes, challenges, choices, *Reflect Nurs Leadersh* 29(4):32-34, 2003.

Epilogue

You, our readers, are inheriting a rich legacy of achievement and progress in the nursing profession. While appreciating the accomplishments of those who paved the way for us, we cannot lose sight of the fact that much remains to be done. As health care professionals, you will be challenged to lead your communities in addressing the complex issues of containing health care costs, improving access to health care for the disenfranchised, decreasing health disparities, and other not-yet-imagined concerns. You will be part of the solution.

It is our hope that through using this textbook you have been inspired to develop values, beliefs, knowledge, professionalism, and desire to become a nursing leader of the future and a positive force for change in the nursing profession.

You can begin to exert your influence to improve the profession by evaluating this book. If you are willing to help in this way, please e-mail us any observations you would like to share about the helpful and not-so-helpful aspects of the current edition. With your assistance we will continue to improve this book to better meet the needs of future students.

KayKChitty1@comcast.net
beth_black@unc.edu

Glossary

A

Abstract Summary of a research report or article.

Acceptance See Nonjudgmental acceptance.

Accountability Responsibility for one's behavior.

Accreditation A voluntary review process of educational programs or service agencies by professional organizations.

Action language A developmental phase in language development of older infants. Examples include reaching for or crawling toward a desired object or closing the lips and turning the head when an undesired food is offered.

Active collaborator One who is engaged as a participant with another person.

Active listening A method of communicating interest and attention using such signals as maintaining good eye contact, nodding, and encouraging the speaker.

Acuity Degree of illness.

Acute illness Sudden, steadily progressing symptoms that subside quickly with or without treatment, such as influenza.

Adaptation A change or coping response to stress of any kind.

Adaptation model A conceptual model that focuses on the patient as an adaptive system; that is, one that strives to cope with both internal demands and external demands of the environment.

Adjudicate To decide or sit in judgment, as in a legal case.

Administrative law Law created by a governmental agency to meet the intent of statutory law.

Advance directives Written instructions recognized by state law that describe individuals' preferences in regard to medical intervention should they become incapacitated.

Advanced degrees Degrees beyond the bachelor's degree; master's and doctoral degrees.

Advanced practice Nursing roles that require either a master's degree or specialized education in a specific area.

Advanced practice nurse A registered nurse who has met advanced educational and practice requirements beyond basic nursing education.

Aesthetics Branch of philosophy that studies the nature of beauty.

Affective domain Field of activity dealing with a person's mood, feelings, values, or belief system.

Alternative educational programs Programs other than basic nursing programs, such as baccalaureate programs for registered nurses and the Excelsior Program, formerly known as the New York Regents' External Degree Program.

Alternative therapies Treatments other than traditional Western medical treatments, such as acupuncture and therapeutic touch.

Altruism Unselfish concern for the welfare of others.

Ambulatory care Health services provided to those who visit a clinic or hospital as outpatients and depart after treatment on the same day.

American Assembly for Men in Nursing (AAMN) Professional organization that seeks to encourage, support, and advocate for men in nursing.

American Association of Colleges of Nursing (AACN) A national organization devoted to advancing nursing education at the baccalaureate and graduate levels.

American Nurses Association (ANA) A professional organization that addresses ethics, clinical standards, public policy, and the economic and general welfare of nurses. Membership is limited to nurses.

American Nurses Credentialing Center (ANCC) The credentialing arm of the American Nurses Association that deals with certification of individual nurses, and approval of organizations as continuing education providers.

American Organization of Nurse Executives (AONE) An organization for high-level nursing managers, such as chief nurses. Leaders in nursing education can be associate members.

ANA Position Paper A 1965 paper published by the American Nurses Association concluding that baccalaureate education should become the basic foundation for professional practice.

Analysis The second step in the nursing process during which various pieces of patient data are analyzed. The outcome is one or more nursing diagnoses.

Ancillary workers Nonprofessional auxiliary health care workers, such as nursing assistants.

Androcentric Male-centered cultural bias.

Anxiety A diffuse, vague feeling of apprehension and uncertainty.

Applied science Use of scientific theory and laws in a practical way that has immediate application.

Appropriateness A criterion for successful communication in which the reply fits the circumstances and matches the message, and the amount is neither too great nor too little.

Articulation An educational mobility system providing for direct movement from a program at one level of nursing education to another without significant loss of credit.

Assault A threat or an attempt to make bodily contact with another person without the person's consent.

Assessment The first step in the nursing process involving the collection of information about the patient.

Assisted suicide Suicide by a person with help from another person, such as a health care provider.

Associate degree in nursing program The newest form of basic nursing education program, leading to the associate degree in nursing (ADN), consisting of 3 or fewer years, and usually offered in technical or community colleges.

Association An organization of members with common interests.

Authority Possessing both the responsibility for making decisions and the accountability for the outcome of those decisions.

Autonomy Self-determination. Control over one's own professional practice.

B

Baccalaureate degree in nursing (BSN) Degree offered by programs that combine nursing courses with general education courses in a 4- or 5-year curriculum in a senior college or university.

Balance of power A distribution of forces among the branches of government so that no one branch is strong enough to dominate the others.

Basic program Any nursing education program preparing beginning practitioners.

Battery The impermissible, unprivileged touching of one person by another.

Belief The intellectual acceptance of something as true or correct.

Belief system Organization of an individual's beliefs into a rational whole.

Beneficence The ethical principle of doing good.

Biases Prejudices, often outside the individual's awareness.

Biculturalism A term used to describe a nurse's ability to balance the ideal nursing culture learned about in school and the real one experienced in practice, using the best of both.

Bioethics An area of ethical inquiry focusing on the dilemmas inherent in modern health care.

Biomedical technology Complex machines or implantable devices used in patient care settings.

Bioterrorism The use of a biological or chemical agent as a weapon.

Birthrate The number of births in a particular place during a specific time period, usually expressed as a quantity per 1000 people in 1 year.

BRN Baccalaureate registered nurse, a term sometimes used to describe a registered nurse who has returned to school to earn a bachelor's degree.

Brown Report A 1948 report recommending that basic schools of nursing be placed in universities and colleges and that efforts be made to recruit large numbers of men and minorities into nursing education programs.

Burnout A state of emotional exhaustion attributable to cumulative stress.

C

Cadet Corps A government-created entity designed during World War II to rapidly increase the number of registered nurses being educated so they could assist in the war effort.

Capitation A cost management system in which a certain amount of money is paid to a provider annually to take care of all of an individual's or group's health care needs.

"Captain of the ship" doctrine A legal principle that implies that the physician is in charge of all patient care and thus should be financially responsible if damages are sought.

Caregiver stress A condition affecting individuals responsible for meeting the needs of others, often a family member, with a chronic condition such as Alzheimer's disease. Consists of feeling overwhelmed and a variety of other emotional and physical symptoms of stress.

Caring Watching over, attending to, and providing for the needs of others.

Case management Systematic collaboration with patients, their significant others, and their health care providers to coordinate high-quality health care services in a cost-effective manner with positive patient outcomes.

Case management nursing A field within nursing in which nurses are responsible for coordinating services provided to patients in a cost-effective manner.

Case manager An individual responsible for coordinating services provided to a group of patients. May or may not be a nurse.

CCNE Commission on Collegiate Nursing Education, the accrediting arm of the American Association of Colleges of Nursing.

Centenarian A person who has reached the age of 100 or more years.

Centers for Medicare and Medicaid Services (CMS) Federal cost-containment program that establishes standards and monitors care in the Medicare and Medicaid programs. Formerly known as Health Care Financing Administration (HCFA).

Certificate of need (CON) A cost-containment measure requiring health care agencies to apply to a state agency for permission to construct or substantially expand an existing facility.

Certification Validation of specific competencies demonstrated by a registered nurse in a defined area of practice.

Certified nurse-midwife (CNM) A nationally certified nurse with advanced specialized education who assists women and couples during uncomplicated pregnancies, deliveries, and postdelivery periods.

Certified registered nurse anesthetist (CRNA) A nationally certified nurse with advanced education who specializes in the administration of anesthesia.

Change agent An individual who recognizes the need for organizational change and facilitates that process.

Chief executive officer (CEO) The senior administrator of an organization.

Chief nurse executive (CNE) The senior nursing administrator of an organization. Also, chief nurse officer (CNO).

Chief nurse officer (CNO) The senior nursing administrator of an organization. Also chief nurse executive (CNE).

Chief of staff A physician in a health care facility, generally elected by the medical staff for a specified term, who is responsible for overseeing the activities of the medical staff organization.

Chronic illness Ongoing health problems of a generally incurable nature, such as diabetes.

Civil law Law involving disputes between individuals.

Clarification A therapeutic communication technique in which the nurse seeks to understand a patient's message more clearly.

Cliché An often-repeated expression that conveys little real meaning, such as "Have a nice day."

Clinical coordinator See Clinical director.

Clinical director Middle management nurse who has responsibility for multiple units in a health care agency.

Clinical judgment The ability to make consistently effective clinical decisions based on theoretical knowledge, research findings, informed opinions, and prior experience.

Clinical ladder Programs allowing nurses to progress in the organizational hierarchy while staying in direct patient care roles.

Clinical nurse specialist A nurse with an advanced degree who serves as a resource person to other nurses and often provides direct care to patients or families with particularly difficult or complex problems.

Closed system A system that does not interact with other systems or with the surrounding environment.

Coalition A temporary alliance of distinct factions.

Code of Academic and Clinical Conduct Code of ethics of the National Student Nurses Association.

Code of ethics A statement of professional standards used to guide behavior and as a framework for decision making.

Code of Ethics for Nurses A formal statement of the nursing profession's code of ethics.

Cognitive Pertaining to intellectual activities requiring knowledge.

Cognitive domain Area of activity that affects an individual's knowledge level.

Cognitive rebellion A stage in the educational process wherein students begin to free themselves from external controls and to rely on their own judgment.

Collaboration Working closely with another person in the spirit of cooperation.

Collective action Activities undertaken by or on behalf of a group of people who have common interests.

Collective bargaining Negotiating as a group for improved salary and work conditions.

Collective identity The connection and feeling of similarity individuals in a particular group feel with one another; group identification.

Collegiality The promotion of collaboration, cooperation, and recognition of interdependence among members of a profession.

Commission on Collegiate Nursing Education (CCNE) The accrediting arm of the American Association of Colleges of Nursing.

Common law Law that develops as a result of decisions made by judges in legal cases.

Communication The exchange of thoughts, ideas, or information; a dynamic process that is a primary instrument through which change occurs in nursing situations.

Community health nursing Formerly known as public health nursing; a nursing specialty that systematically uses a process of delivering nursing care to improve the health of an entire community.

Community-based nursing Nursing care provided for individuals, families, and groups in a variety of settings, including homes, workplaces, and schools.

Compassion fatigue A state experienced by those helping people in distress; an extreme state of tension and preoccupation with the suffering of those being helped to the degree that it is traumatizing for the helper.

Competency Refers to the capability of a particular patient to understand the information given and to make an informed choice about treatment options.

Complementary therapies Those treatments intended to augment traditional Western medical treatments such as massage therapy or acupuncture.

Completeness An element of informed consent that refers to the comprehensiveness of the information provided.

Concept An abstract classification of data; for example, "cooperation" is a concept.

Conceptual model or framework A group of concepts that are broadly defined and systematically organized to provide a focus, a rationale, and a tool for the integration and interpretation of information.

Confidentiality Ensuring the privacy of individuals participating in research studies or being treated in health care settings.

Congruent A characteristic of communication that occurs when the verbal and nonverbal elements of a message match.

Constituent Member Association (CMA) Organizational members of the American Nurses Association, such as state nurses associations or specialty nursing organizations.

Consultation The process of conferring with patients, families, or other health professionals.

Consumerism A movement to protect consumers from unsafe or inferior products and services.

Contact hour A measurement used to recognize participation in continuing education offerings, usually equivalent to 50 minutes.

Context An essential element of communication consisting of the setting in which an interaction occurs, the mood, the relationship between sender and receiver, and other factors.

Continuing education (CE) Workshops, conferences, and short courses, in which nurses maintain competence during their professional careers.

Continuous quality improvement (CQI) A management concept focusing on excellence and employee involvement at all levels of an organization.

Contracts Written agreements between workers and management that include provisions about staffing levels, salary, work conditions, and other issues of concern to either party. May also refer to an agreement between nurse and patient regarding the terms of their relationship.

Copayment The portion of a provider's charges that an insured patient is responsible for paying.

Coping The methods a person uses to assess and manage demands.

Coping mechanisms Psychological devices used by individuals when a threat is perceived.

Cost containment An attempt to keep health care costs stable or increasing only slowly.

Criminal law Law involving public concerns against unlawful behavior that threatens society.

Criteria Standards by which something is judged or measured.

Critical paths Multidisciplinary care plans outlining a patient's treatments and expected outcomes, day by day.

Cross-functional team People from all parts of an organization who contribute to a particular activity and outcome.

Cross-training Preparing a single worker for multiple tasks that formerly were performed by multiple specialized workers.

Cultural assessment The process of determining a patient's cultural practices and preferences in order to render culturally competent care.

Cultural care, theory of A nursing theory focusing on the importance of incorporating a patient's culturally determined health beliefs and practices into care.

Cultural competence The integration of knowledge, attitudes, and skills that enhance cross-cultural communication and appropriate interactions with others.

Cultural conditioning The process by which a person becomes entrenched in his or her own culture's ways; culture bound.

Cultural diversity Social, ethnic, racial, and religious differences.

Culturally competent education Nursing education that incorporates knowledge, attitudes, and skills that enhance cross-cultural communication and appropriate interactions with others.

Culturally congruent nursing care Care that incorporates knowledge, attitudes, and skills that enhance cross-cultural communication and appropriate interactions with others.

Culture The attitudes, beliefs, and behaviors of social and ethnic groups that have been perpetuated through generations.

Culture of nursing The rites, rituals, and valued behaviors of the nursing profession.

D

Data Information or facts collected for analysis.

Deaconess Institute A large hospital and planned training program for deaconesses established in 1836 by Pastor Theodor Fliedner at Kaiserswerth, Germany.

Decentralization An organizational structure in which decision-making authority is shared with employees most affected by the decisions rather than being retained by top executives.

Deductible The out-of-pocket amount individuals must pay before their health insurance begins to pay for health care.

Deductive reasoning A process through which conclusions are drawn by logical inference from given premises; proceeds from the general case to the specific.

Defining characteristics Signs and symptoms of a specific disease.

Delegate To refer a task to another.

Delegation The practice of assigning tasks or responsibilities to other persons.

Demographics The study of vital statistics and social trends.

Demography The science that studies vital statistics and social trends.

Deontology The ethical theory that the rightness or wrongness of an action depends on the inherent moral significance of the action.

Dependency The degree to which individuals adopt passive attitudes and rely on others to take care of them.

Dependent intervention Nursing actions on behalf of patients that require knowledge and skill on the part of the nurse but may not be done without explicit directions from another health professional, usually a physician, dentist, or nurse practitioner.

Designer medicines Pharmacologic agents developed for an individual, based on his or her genetic makeup.

Developmental theory A theory in which growth is defined as an increase in physical size and shape toward a point of optimal maturity.

Diagnosis Identification of a disease or condition.

Diagnosis-related groups (DRGs) A method of classifying and grouping illnesses according to similarities of diagnosis for reimbursement purposes.

Dietitian Bachelor's or master's degree–prepared nutrition expert who specializes in therapeutic diet preparation and nutrition education.

Differentiated practice Nursing practice at two levels, professional and technical, with differences in both educational preparation and clinical responsibilities.

Diploma program The earliest form of formal nursing education in the United States; usually based in hospitals, requires 3 years of study, and leads to a diploma in nursing.

Disaster An event or situation that is of greater magnitude than an emergency; disrupts essential services such as housing, transportation, communications, sanitation, water, and health care; and requires the response of people outside the community affected.

Disease A pathologic alteration at the tissue or organ level.

Disease management A process of helping patients understand and manage their chronic conditions more effectively through phone calls, coaching and education, symptom prevention and management, and collaboration with the patient's health care provider.

Disenfranchised The state of having no power or voice in a political system.

Disseminate Publish or widely distribute scientific information, such as the findings of a research study.

Dissonance Lack of harmony.

Distance learning The process of taking classes and earning academic credit through technologic means such as televised or online classes. The teacher and student may be many miles apart.

Distributed campaign A political campaign that makes extensive use of the Internet to distribute information about the candidate and to raise funds.

Documentation Written communication about a patient's condition, care, and reactions to treatments; found in the patient record/chart.

Dominant culture Mainstream culture that contains one or more subcultures.

Double effect Ethical concept encompassing the belief that there are some situations in which it is necessary to inflict potential harm in an effort to achieve a greater good.

Duty of care The responsibility of a nurse or other health professional for the care of a patient.

Duty to report The requirement, according to state law, for health professionals to report certain illnesses, injuries, and actions of patients.

E

Economic and general welfare Employment issues relating to salaries, benefits, and working conditions.

Educative instrument A tool for increasing the knowledge and power of another person.

Efficiency A criterion for successful communication that consists of using simple, clear words timed at a pace suitable to participants.

Electoral process The procedures that must be followed to select someone to fill an elected position.

Emotional intelligence Awareness of and sensitivity to the feelings of others.

Empathy Awareness of, sensitivity to, and identification with the feelings of another person.

End-of-life care Care aimed at comfort and dignity for patients who are nearing death and for their significant others.

Entrepreneur A person who envisions, organizes, manages, and assumes responsibility for a new enterprise or business.

Environment All of the many external and internal factors, such as physical and psychological, that influence life and survival.

Epidemiologist A scientist who studies the origins and transmission of diseases.

Epistemology The branch of philosophy dealing with the theory of knowledge.

Ethical decision making The process of choosing between actions based on a system of beliefs and values.

Ethics The branch of philosophy that studies the propriety of certain courses of action.

Ethnocentrism The belief that one's own culture is the most desirable.

Ethnographic research A type of qualitative research.

Ethnopharmacology The systematic study of the use of medicinal plants by specific cultural groups. Also, the study of how medicines affect people of differing racial and ethnic groups.

Euthanasia The act of painlessly putting to death a person suffering from an incurable disease; also called mercy killing.

Evaluation Measuring the success or failure of the results or "outputs," and consequently the effectiveness, of a system. It is the final step in the nursing process wherein the nurse examines the patient's progress to determine whether a problem is solved, is in the process of being solved, or is unsolved. In communication theory, it is the analysis of information received.

Evidence-based practice The use of research findings as a basis for practice rather than trial and error, intuition, or traditional methods, such as problem solving.

Exacerbation Reemergence or worsening of the symptoms of a chronic illness.

Executive branch The branch of government responsible for administering the laws of the land.

Experimental design Research design that provides evidence of a cause-and-effect relationship between actions.

Expert power Strength derived from knowledge that can influence an outcome.

Expert witness An individual called on to testify in court because of special skill or knowledge in a certain field, such as nursing.

Extended care Medical, nursing, or custodial care provided to an individual over a prolonged period of time.

Extended family A term used to describe nonnuclear family members such as grandparents, aunts, and uncles.

External degree program An alternative educational program in which learning is independent and is assessed through highly standardized and validated examinations.

External factors Values, beliefs, and behaviors of significant others that have an impact on an individual.

F

Faith community The members of a church, synagogue, mosque, or other entity who worship together and share common beliefs about religion.

Faith community nurse A specialized nurse who focuses on the promotion of health within the context of the values, beliefs, and practices of a church, synagogue, mosque, or other faith community.

False reassurance A nontherapeutic form of communication that seeks to reassure that "all will be well."

Family system The group of individuals who comprise the basic unit of family living and their interactions with one another and the larger society.

Famous trio Three famous schools of nursing founded in 1873: the Bellevue Training School, the Connecticut Training School, and the Boston Training School.

Feedback The information given back into a system to determine whether or not the purpose of the system has been achieved. A major element in the communication process.

Feminism Belief in the value and equality of women.

Fidelity An ethical principle that values faithfulness to one's responsibilities.

Flexibility A criterion for successful communication that occurs when messages are based on the immediate situation rather than preconceived expectations.

Flexible staffing A mechanism whereby nurses may work at times other than the traditional hospital shifts.

Flexner Report A 1910 study of medical education that provided the impetus for much-needed reform.

Formal socialization The process by which individuals learn a new role from the direct instruction of others.

For-profit agency A health care agency established to make a profit for the owners or shareholders.

Frontier Nursing Service Founded in Kentucky in 1925, it provided the first organized midwifery service in the United States.

Functional nursing A system of nursing care delivery in which each worker has a task, or function, to perform for all patients.

Futurist An individual who studies trends and makes predictions about the future.

G

Gatekeeper An individual, generally a primary care physician, who controls patients' access to diagnostic procedures, medical specialists, and hospitalization.

Gender-role stereotyping The practice of automatically and routinely linking specific characteristics to either males or females; also called sex-role stereotyping.

General election An election in which all registered voters may vote and may choose a candidate from any party on the ballot.

General systems theory A theory promulgated by Ludwig von Bertalanffy in the late 1930s to explain the relationship of a whole to its parts.

Generalizable Research findings that are transferable to other situations.

Generic master's degree An accelerated master's degree in nursing for people with nonnursing bachelor's degrees.

Generic nursing doctorate A doctoral degree program designed for individuals who are not already registered nurses and who possess baccalaureate degrees in other fields.

Genetic counseling Health and reproductive advice given to individuals based on their genetic makeup.

Goldmark Report A major study of nursing education published in 1923 and named *The Study of Nursing and Nursing Education in the United States*.

Governmental (public) agency An agency primarily supported by taxes, administered by elected or appointed officials, and tailored to the needs of the communities served.

Grand theory A very broad conceptualization of nursing phenomena.

Grassroots activism The involvement of a large number of people, generally widely dispersed, who are concerned about a particular issue.

Growth An increase in physical size and shape toward a point of optimal maturity.

H

Hardiness A personality characteristic that enables people to manage the changes associated with illness and to have fewer physical illnesses resulting from stress.

Health An individual's physical, mental, spiritual, and social well-being; a continuum, not a constant state.

Health behaviors Choices and habitual actions that promote or diminish health.

Health beliefs Culturally determined beliefs about the nature of health and illness.

Health care network A corporation with a consolidated set of facilities and services for comprehensive health care.

Health Insurance Portability and Accountability Act (HIPAA) Federal law, passed in 1996, designed to protect health insurance coverage for workers and their families when they change or lose their jobs.

Health maintenance Preventing illness and maintaining maximal function.

Health maintenance organization (HMO) A network or group of providers who agree to provide certain basic health care services for a single predetermined yearly fee.

Health promotion Encouraging a condition of maximum physical, mental, and social well-being.

Health promotion model A theoretical nursing model that uses illness prevention and health promotion as a basic framework.

Helping professions Professions such as social work, teaching, and nursing that emphasize meeting the needs of clients.

Henry Street Settlement A clinic for the poor founded by Lillian Wald and her colleague Mary Brewster on New York's Lower East Side.

Heterogeneous Composed of parts of differing kinds.

High-level wellness Functioning at maximum potential in an integrated way within the environment.

High-tech nursing Nursing care that involves the use of technologies such as monitors, pumps, and ventilators.

High-touch nursing Nursing care that involves the use of interpersonal skills such as communication, listening, and empathy.

Hill-Burton Act A 1946 federal law that called for and funded surveys of states' needs for hospitals, paid for planning hospitals and public health centers, and provided partial funding for constructing and equipping hospitals and health centers.

Holism A school of health care thought that espouses treating the whole patient: body, mind, and spirit.

Holistic communication Sharing both emotional and factual information and appreciating another individual's point of view.

Holistic nursing care Nursing care that nourishes the whole person—that is, the body, mind, and spirit.

Holistic nursing research Nursing research that considers the whole person—that is, the body, mind, and spirit.

Holistic values The approach to nursing practice that takes the physical, emotional, social, economic, and spiritual needs of the person into consideration.

Home health agency An organization that delivers various health services to patients in their homes.

Home health nursing Field of nursing in which nursing care is provided to patients in their own homes.

Homeostasis A relative constancy in the internal environment of the body.

Homogeneous Composed of parts of the same or similar kinds.

Hospice An agency that provides services to terminally ill patients and their families.

Hospice and palliative care nursing Specialized nursing care provided at the end of life to patients and their families in homes and residential facilities. Aimed at a comfortable and dignified death that honors the wishes of patients and loved ones.

Hospitalist Hospital-based physicians who care for patients only while they are hospitalized.

Human caring, theory of Nursing theory emphasizing the nurturing aspects of professional nursing through which curative strategies are implemented.

Human Genome Project A scientific project designed to map the genetic structure of composite human DNA, completed in 2003.

Human motivation Abraham Maslow's conceptualization of human needs and their relationship to the stimulation of purposeful behavior.

Human needs theory Theory proposed by Abraham Maslow that human motivation is determined by the drive to meet intrinsic human needs.

Human responses The problems an individual experiences as a result of a disease process.

Humanistic nursing care Care that includes viewing professional relationships as human to human rather than nurse to patient.

Humanistic nursing values The approach to professional relationships as human-to-human experiences rather than nurse-to-patient experiences.

Hypothesis A statement predicting the relationship among various concepts or variables.

I

Illness An abnormal process in which an individual's physical, emotional, social, or intellectual functioning is impaired.

Illness prevention All activities aimed at diminishing the likelihood that an individual's physical, emotional, social, and intellectual functions become impaired.

Implementation A stage of the nursing process during which the plan of care is carried out.

Incongruent Describes a confusing form of communication that occurs when the verbal and nonverbal elements of a message do not match.

Independent intervention Actions on behalf of patients for which the nurse requires no supervision or direction.

Individualized care plan A plan of care designed to meet the needs of a specific person.

Inductive reasoning The process of reasoning from the specific to the general. Repeated observations of an experiment or event enable the observer to draw general conclusions.

Inertia Disinclination to change.

Infant mortality rate The number of deaths of infants (1 year of age or younger) per 1000 live births.

Informal socialization The process through which individuals learn a new role by observing how others behave.

Informatics nurse A nurse who combines nursing science with information management science and computer science to manage and make accessible the information that nurses need.

Information technology (IT) Development of hardware and software to manage and process information.

Informed consent The process of asking individuals who are scheduled to undergo diagnostic procedures or surgery or who are potential research subjects to sign a consent form once the procedures and risks have been explained and their privacy rights have been assured.

Infrastructure Basic support mechanisms needed to ensure that an activity can be conducted.

Input The information, energy, or matter that enters a system.

Institutional review board A committee that ensures that research is well designed and protects the rights of human participants in the research.

Institutional structure The way in which the workers within an agency are organized to carry out the functions of the agency.

Integrative care Care that combines the best of both standard and nontraditional treatments, for example, pain control through both prescription medication and acupuncture.

Interdependent intervention Actions on behalf of patients in which the nurse must collaborate or consult with another health professional before or while carrying out the action.

Interdisciplinary team Group composed of individuals representing various disciplines who work together toward a common end.

Internal factors Personal feelings and beliefs that influence an individual.

Internalize The process of taking in knowledge, skills, attitudes, beliefs, norms, values, and ethical standards and making them a part of one's own self-image and behavior.

International Council of Nurses (ICN) The federation of national nurses associations, currently representing nurses in more than 120 countries.

Internship An apprenticeship under supervision.

Irrational belief A false fixed idea that is not affected by information to the contrary.

Issues management Assisting a group to resolve a particular question about which there are significant differences of opinion.

J

Jargon Specialized vocabulary used by those in the same line of work to communicate about work-related matters.

Job hopping Moving rapidly from job to job.

Judicial branch The branch of government that decides cases or conflicts of a civil or criminal nature.

Justice An ethical principle stating that equals should be treated the same.

K

Knowledge technology The use of computer systems to transform information into knowledge and to generate new knowledge; expert systems.

Knowledge-based power Authority or control based on the way information is used to effect an outcome.

L

Latent power Untapped strength.

Law All the rules of conduct established by a government and applicable to the people, whether in the form of legislation or custom.

Learned resourcefulness An acquired ability to use available resources on one's behalf.

Legal authority A group of people in whom power is vested by law, such as the powers vested in state boards of nursing by nurse practice acts.

Legislative branch The branch of government consisting of elected officials who are responsible for enacting the laws of the land.

Length of stay (LOS) The number of days a patient stays in an inpatient setting, such as a hospital.

Licensure The process by which an agency of government grants permission to qualified persons to engage in a given profession or occupation.

Licensure by endorsement A system whereby registered nurses or licensed practical/vocational nurses can, by submitting proof of licensure in another state and paying a licensure fee, receive licensure from the new state without sitting for a licensing examination.

Lifelong learner An individual who seeks continuing education and opportunities to increase knowledge throughout his or her professional life.

Lifelong learning Continuing education and increasing knowledge throughout an individual's professional life.

Lobby An attempt to influence the vote of legislators.

Locus of control The place an individual believes the power in his/her life resides, either within or outside of himself/herself.

Logic The field of philosophy that studies correct and incorrect reasoning.

Long-term care Care provided to individuals, such as people with Alzheimer's disease, who require ongoing assistance in the maintenance of activities of daily living.

Long-term goals Major changes that may take months or even years to accomplish.

Lysaught Report A 1970 report entitled *An Abstract for Action* that made recommendations concerning the supply and demand for nurses, nursing roles and functions, and nursing education.

M

Magnet hospital A designation granted by the American Nurses Credentialing Center (ANCC), a magnet hospital provides excellent patient outcomes, a high level of job satisfaction among nurses, low staff nurse turnover rate, and appropriate grievance resolution, among other factors.

Malpractice An act resulting in injury that occurs when a professional fails to act as a reasonably prudent professional would under specific circumstances.

Managed care A process in which an individual, often a nurse, is assigned to review patients' cases and coordinate services so that quality care can be achieved at the lowest cost.

Managed care organization (MCO) Any of a number of organizations that attempt to coordinate subscriber services to ensure quality care at the lowest cost.

Mandatory continuing education The requirement that nurses complete a certain number of hours of continuing education as a prerequisite for relicensure.

Maximum health potential The highest level of well-being that an individual is capable of attaining.

Medicaid A jointly funded federal and state public health insurance that covers citizens below the poverty level and those with certain disabling conditions; established in 1965.

Medical paternalism The attitude that health care providers know best and that "good" patients simply follow directions without asking questions.

Medically indigent Individuals and families who do not qualify for Medicaid or Medicare but cannot afford health insurance or medical care.

Medicare A federally funded form of public health insurance for citizens 65 years of age and older; established in 1965.

Members In professional associations, members may be individuals, agencies such as schools of nursing, or other associations. For example, in the ANA, the members are the state associations, whereas in the NLN, members may be either individuals or organizations.

Mentor An experienced nurse who shares knowledge with less experienced nurses to help them advance their careers.

Message An essential element of communication consisting of the spoken word and/or nonverbal communication.

Metaparadigm The most abstract aspect of the structure of knowledge; the global concepts that identify the phenomena of interest for a discipline.

Metaphysics The branch of philosophy that considers the ultimate nature of existence, reality, and experience.

Middle-range theory Theory that makes connections between grand theories and nursing practice.

Milieu Surroundings or environment.

Mission The special task(s) to which an organization devotes itself.

Model A symbolic representation of a concept or reality.

Modeling An informal type of socialization that occurs when an individual chooses an admired person to emulate.

Moonlighting The practice of working a second job in addition to the regular one.

Moral development The ways in which a person learns to deal with moral dilemmas from childhood through adulthood.

Moral distress Pain or anguish of a person who unwillingly participates in perceived moral wrongdoing.

Morals Established rules or standards that guide behavior in situations in which a decision about right and wrong must be made.

Morbidity rate The incidence or occurrence of a certain illness in a particular population during a specific period of time; usually expressed as a quantity per 1000 people in a specific year.

Mortality rate The number of deaths in a particular population during a specific period of time; usually expressed as a quantity per 1000 people in a specific year.

Multidrug-resistant strains Microorganisms, such as the tubercle bacillus, that have become immune to the effects of drugs that formerly were effective against them.

Multiskilled worker Individual who has been cross-trained to perform a number of tasks formerly performed by multiple specialized workers.

Mutual recognition model A system whereby a registered nurse may be licensed in the state of residency yet practice in other states, after being recognized by them, without additional licenses.

Mutuality Sharing jointly with others.

N

NANDA International (formerly North American Nursing Diagnosis Association) Group working since 1970 to establish a comprehensive list of nursing diagnoses.

National Council Licensure Examination for Practical Nurses (NCLEX-PN) The examination that graduates of practical nursing programs must take to become licensed to practice as licensed practical nurses (LPNs) or licensed vocational nurses (LVNs).

National Council Licensure Examination for Registered Nurses (NCLEX-RN) The examination that graduates of basic nursing programs must take to become licensed to practice as registered nurses (RNs).

National League for Nursing (NLN) National organization that seeks to advance the profession of nursing through advocacy and improving educational standards for nurses. Nonnurses may be members.

National League for Nursing Accrediting Commission (NLNAC) The arm of the National League for Nursing that accredits associate degree, diploma, baccalaureate, and master's programs in nursing.

National Practitioner Data Bank (NPDB) A national clearinghouse containing reports of adverse incidents involving physicians, nurses, and other health care providers that may be useful to potential employers or patients.

National Student Nurses Association (NSNA) National organization devoted to developing leadership skills in nursing students.

NCLEX-PN® See National Council Licensure Examination for Practical Nurses.

NCLEX-RN® See National Council Licensure Examination for Registered Nurses.

Negligence The failure to act as a reasonably prudent person would have acted in specific circumstances.

Network A system of interconnected individuals; useful to develop contacts or exchange information to further a career.

NLN See National League for Nursing.

NLNAC See National League for Nursing Accrediting Commission.

Nonexperimental design Research with the intent to describe or clarify a phenomenon. Not intended to test an intervention.

Nonjudgmental Describes an attitude that conveys neither approval nor disapproval of patients' beliefs and respects each person's right to his or her beliefs.

Nonjudgmental acceptance An accepting attitude that conveys neither approval nor disapproval of patients or their personal beliefs, habits, expressions of feelings, or chosen lifestyles.

Nonmaleficence The duty to inflict no harm or evil.

Nonverbal communication Communication without words; consists of gestures, posture, facial expressions, tone and loudness of voice, actions, grooming, and clothing, among other things.

Nosocomial Hospital-acquired, as a nosocomial infection.

Not-for-profit agency An organization that does not attempt to make a profit for distribution to owners or stockholders. Any profit made by such organizations is used to operate and improve the organization itself or to extend its services.

Nuclear family Term used to describe a mother and father and their children.

Nurse activist A nurse who works actively on behalf of a political candidate or certain legislation.

Nurse anesthetist A nurse with specialized advanced education who administers anesthetic agents to patients undergoing operative procedures.

Nurse citizen A nurse who exercises all the political rights accorded citizens, such as registering to vote and voting in all elections.

Nurse entrepreneur A nurse who engages in a business undertaking related to health care or nursing, such as owning a traveling nurse agency.

Nurse executive The top nurse in the administrative structure of a health care organization.

Nurse Licensure Compact An agreement among certain states, authorized by legislation, that they will honor licenses issued to registered nurses by other states in the compact.

Nurse manager A nurse who is in charge of all activities in a unit, including patient care, continuous quality improvement, personnel selection and evaluation, and resource (supplies and money) management. Formerly known as a head nurse.

Nurse politician A nurse who runs for political office.

Nurse practice act Law defining the scope of nursing practice in a given state.

Nurse practitioner A nurse with advanced education who specializes in the health care of a particular group, such as children, pregnant women, or the elderly.

Nurse-based practice A clinic, office, or home practice in which nurses carry their own caseloads of patients with physical and/or psychiatric needs.

Nurse-midwife A nurse with advanced specialized education who assists women and couples during uncomplicated pregnancies, deliveries, and postdelivery periods.

Nurse-patient relationship The interpersonal connection between a nurse and patient.

Nursing The provision of health care services, focusing on the maintenance, promotion, and restoration of health.

Nursing diagnosis A process of describing a patient's response to health problems that either already exist or may occur in the future.

Nursing goal A statement of the desired long-term or short-term outcome as a result of one or more nursing interventions.

Nursing informatics The branch of nursing that manages knowledge and data through technology with the goal of improving patient care.

Nursing information system A software system that automates the nursing process.

Nursing orders Actions designed to assist the patient in achieving a stated patient goal.

Nursing process A cognitive activity that requires both critical and creative thinking and serves as the basis for providing nursing care. A method used by nurses in dealing with patient problems in professional practice.

Nursing research The systematic investigation of events or circumstances related to improving nursing knowledge or practice.

Nursing theory A formal statement of related concepts used to explain, predict, control, and understand commonly occurring phenomena of interest to nurses.

O

Obesity A body mass index (BMI) of 30 or more.

Objective data Factual information obtained through observation and examination of the patient or through consultation with other health care providers.

Occupation A person's principal work or business.

Occupational and environmental health nurse A nurse specializing in the care of a specific group of workers in a given occupational setting.

Open posture Body position, such as squarely facing another person with arms in a relaxed position.

Open system A system that promotes the exchange of matter, energy, and information with other systems and the environment.

Open-ended question An inquiry that causes the patient to answer fully, giving more than a "yes" or "no" answer.

Organizational structure How an agency is organized to accomplish its mission.

Orientation phase The beginning phase of a nurse-patient relationship in which the parties are getting acquainted with one another.

Outcome criteria Expected results of nursing intervention.

Out-of-pocket payment Direct payment for health services from individuals' personal funds.

Output The end result or product of a system.

P

Palliative care nursing A specialty in nursing dedicated to improving the experience of seriously ill and dying patients and their families.

Paramedical Having to do with the field of medicine; generally used to describe ancillary workers such as emergency medical technicians.

Parental modeling A type of socialization that occurs when parents' behavior and responses to various stimuli influence a child's future behaviors and responses.

Participants The individuals who are studied in a research project.

Patient acuity The degree of illness of a particular patient or group of patients; used to determine staffing needs.

Patient advocate One who promotes the interests of patients. Also a nursing role.

Patient care technician (PCT) A health technician working under the supervision of a registered nurse, physician, or other health professional to provide basic patient care.

Patient classification system (PCS) Identification of patients' needs for nursing care in quantitative terms.

Patient interview A face-to-face interaction with the patient in which an interviewer elicits pertinent information.

Patient Self-Determination Act Effective December 1, 1991, this law encourages patients to consider which life-prolonging treatment options they desire and to document their preferences in case they should later become incapable of participating in the decision-making process.

Patient-centered care, also known as patient-focused care A system that emphasizes coordinating patient care to maximize patient comfort, convenience, and security.

Patients' rights Responsibilities that a hospital and its staff have toward patients and their families during hospitalization.

Pay equity Equal pay for work of comparable value.

Peer review The process of submitting one's work for examination and comment by colleagues in the same profession.

Perception The selection, organization, and interpretation of incoming signals into meaningful messages.

Performance improvement (PI) Organizational efforts to improve corporate performance, incorporating aspects of quality management.

Person An individual—man, woman, or child.

Personal payment Direct payment for health services from individuals' personal funds.

Personal space The amount of space surrounding individuals in which they feel comfortable interacting with others; usually culturally determined.

Personal value system The social principles, ideals, or standards held by an individual that form the basis for meaning, direction, and decision making in life.

Pew Health Professions Commission One of three major national groups that in 1993 issued reports or studies of nursing education in the United States.

Phenomena Occurrences or circumstances that are observable. The singular form is phenomenon.

Phenomenological inquiry/research A qualitative research approach focusing on what people experience in regard to a particular phenomenon, such as grief, and how they interpret those experiences.

Philosophy The study of the truths and principles of being, knowledge, conduct, or nature of the universe.

Physician hospital organization (PHO) A separate corporation formed by a hospital and a group of its medical staff for the purpose of joint-contracting with managed care organizations and businesses.

Planning The third step in the nursing process, which begins with the identification of patient goals.

Point-of-care technology Information system used for entering patient data directly from the bedside.

Point-of-service organization (POS) A hybrid preferred provider organization in which the consumer selects service providers within the defined network or may go outside the network and pay a higher deductible or copayment.

Policy The principles and values that govern actions directed toward given ends. Policy sets forth a plan, direction, or goal for action.

Policy development The generation of principles and procedures that guide governmental or organizational action.

Policy outcome The result of decisions made by governmental or organizational leaders who choose a certain course of action.

Political action committees (PACs) Groups that raise and distribute money to candidates who support their organization's stand on certain issues.

Politics The area of philosophy that deals with the regulation and control of people living in society; in government, it includes the allocation of scarce resources such as health care resources.

Population The entire group of people possessing a given characteristic; for example, all brown-eyed people older than age 65.

Position paper Statement pertaining to the stance a group or organization takes on an issue; for example, the American Nurses Association's 1965 *Position Paper* advocated the baccalaureate degree as the entry level into the practice of registered nursing.

Position power Authority and control accorded to an individual who holds an important role in an organization, profession, or government.

Posttraumatic stress disorder (PTSD) An anxiety disorder characterized by an acute emotional response to a traumatic event or situation.

Power grabbing Hoarding control, taking it from others, or wielding it over others.

Power in numbers The ability of a group of people to accomplish a goal that an individual acting alone is unlikely to achieve.

Power sharing A process of equalizing resources, knowledge, or control.

Powers of appointment The authority to select the people who serve in positions such as judges, ambassadors, and cabinet officials.

Practical nurse (LPN/LVN) program A 1-year educational program preparing individuals for direct patient care roles under the supervision of a physician or registered nurse.

Preceptor A teacher; in nursing, usually an experienced nurse who assumes responsibility for teaching a novice.

Preferred provider organization (PPO) A form of HMO that contracts with independent providers such as physicians and hospitals for a negotiated discount for services provided to its members.

Premium The amount paid for an insurance policy, usually in installments.

Primary care Basic health care, including promotion of health, early diagnosis of disease, and prevention of disease.

Primary election An election in which voters who are declared members of a political party choose among several candidates of that same party for a particular office.

Primary nursing A system of nursing care delivery in which one nurse has responsibility for the planning, implementation, and evaluation of the care of one or more clients 24 hours a day for the duration of the hospital stay.

Primary source The patient is considered the primary source of data about himself or herself; in a literature review, a primary source is the original writing of a theorist or author.

Principalism Use of multiple ethical principles, such as beneficence, autonomy, nonmaleficence, veracity, justice, and fidelity, in the resolution of ethical conflicts rather than a single principle.

Private insurance Insurance obtained from a privately owned company, as opposed to public or governmental insurance.

Private practice Nursing practice engaged in by some nurses with advanced education; usually provided on a fee-for-service basis, as in most medical practices.

Privileged communications The principle that information given to certain professionals is protected and is not to be disclosed even in court.

Problem solving A method of finding solutions to difficulties specific to a given situation and designed for immediate action.

Profession Work requiring advanced training and usually involving mental rather than manual effort. Usually has a code of ethics and a professional organization.

Professional A person who engages in one of the professions, such as law, medicine, or nursing.

Professional accountabilities In the shared governance model, a basic set of responsibilities of all professional nurses regardless of practice setting.

Professional association An organization consisting of people belonging to the same profession and thereby having many common interests.

Professional boundary The dividing line between the activities of two professions. The area in which a professional person functions to avoid both underinvolvement and overinvolvement, maintaining the patient's needs as the focus of the relationship.

Professional governance The concept that health care professionals have a right and a responsibility to govern their own work and time within a financially secure, patient-centered system.

Professional outcomes The impact on a profession from political action by its practitioners.

Professional practice advocacy Includes activities such as education, lobbying, and advocating individually and collectively to advance a profession's agenda.

Professional review organization (PRO) Organizations that review Medicare hospital admissions and Medicare patients' lengths of stay.

Professional socialization The process of developing an occupational identity.

Professionalism Professional behavior, appearance, and conduct.

Professionalization A process through which an occupation evolves to professional status.

Proposition A statement about how two or more concepts are related.

Prospective payment system (PPS) A cost-containment mechanism wherein providers, such as physicians and hospitals, receive payment on a per-case basis, regardless of the cost of delivering the services.

Protocol A written plan specifying the procedure to be followed.

Provider A deliverer of health care services—hospital, clinic, nurse, or physician.

Proximate cause Action occurring immediately before an injury, thereby assumed to be the reason for the injury.

Psychomotor domain Area of activity referring to motor skills or actions by an individual; for example, learning to dance is in the psychomotor domain.

Pure science Information that summarizes and explains the universe without regard for whether the information is immediately useful; also known as "basic science."

Q

Qualitative research Research that seeks to answer questions that cannot be answered by quantitative designs and that must be addressed by more subjective methods.

Quality management See Total quality management.

Quantitative research Research that uses data-gathering techniques that can be repeated by others and verified. Data collected are quantifiable—that is, they can be counted, measured with standardized instruments, or observed with a high degree of agreement among observers.

R

Reality shock Feelings of powerlessness and ineffectiveness often experienced by new nursing graduates; usually occurs as a result of the transition from the educational setting to the "real world" of nursing in an actual health care setting.

Receiver An essential element of communication; the person receiving the message.

Reengineering Radical redesign of business processes and thinking to improve performance.

Referendum An election resulting from registered voters being asked by a legislative body to express a preference on a policy issue.

Reflection A communication technique that consists of directing questions back to patients, thereby encouraging patients to think through problems for themselves.

Reflective practice A method of focusing on one's practice, both in the moment and after an event, with an open and curious mind, drawing on all the senses to know oneself more fully.

Reflective thinking The process of evaluating one's thinking processes during a situation that has already occurred, as opposed to evaluating one's thinking during the situation as it occurs.

Registered nurse (RN) An individual who has completed a basic program for registered nurses and successfully completed the licensing examination.

Rehabilitation services Those activities designed to restore an individual or a body part to normal or maximum possible function following a disease or an accident.

Reliable Yielding the same values dependably each time an instrument is used to measure the same thing.

Remission A period of chronic illness during which symptoms subside.

Replication The process of repeating a research study as closely as possible to the original.

Research process Prescribed steps that must be taken to plan and conduct meaningful research properly.

Research question A statement, question, or hypothesis that a research study is designed to answer.

Resilience A pattern of successful adaptation despite challenging or threatening circumstances.

Resocialized The outcome of a transitional process of giving up part or all of one set of professional values and learning new ones.

Resolution A written position on an issue presented to the voting members of an association for their consideration, discussion, and vote.

Respondeat superior Legal theory that attributes the acts of employees to their employer (Latin term).

Retrospective reimbursement Insurance payment made after services are delivered.

Risk management A program that seeks to identify and eliminate potential safety hazards, thereby reducing risk for patient injuries.

RN-to-baccalaureate in nursing Programs enabling registered nurses who hold associate degrees or diplomas in nursing to acquire baccalaureate degrees in nursing.

Role A goal-directed pattern of behavior learned within a cultural setting.

Role model An individual who serves as an example of desirable behavior for another person.

Role strain Stress created by difficulty experienced in adjusting to a life or occupational role.

S

Salary compression A phenomenon in which pay increases are limited during an individual's career, so that the salary of a veteran nurse may be little higher than that of a recently hired novice nurse.

Sample A subset of an entire population that reflects the characteristics of the population.

School nurse Nurse specializing in the care of school-age children or adolescents and practicing in school settings.

Scientific discipline A branch of instruction or field of learning based on the study of a body of facts about the physical or material world.

Scientific method A systematic, orderly approach to the gathering of data and the solving of problems.

Scope of practice The boundaries of a practice profession's activities as defined by law.

Secondary care An intermediate level of health care performed in a hospital having specialized equipment and laboratory facilities.

Secondary source Sources of data such as the nurse's own observations or perceptions of family and friends of the patient.

Self-actualization A process of realizing one's maximum potential and using one's capabilities to the fullest extent possible.

Self-awareness Understanding of one's own needs, biases, and impact on others.

Self-care The ability to care for oneself, that is, engage in activities of daily living without assistance.

Self-care model Nursing theoretical model based on the concept of ability to care for self.

Self-directed work team A method of decentralizing decision making using cross-functional groups united around common goals.

Self-efficacy A belief in oneself as possessing the ability to exercise control over one's own health-related behaviors.

Self-insurance Coverage in which an individual or business pays for care directly rather than purchasing insurance.

Sender An essential element of communication; the person sending a message.

Separation of powers Under the U.S. Constitution, each branch of the federal government has separate and distinct functions and powers.

Set A group of circumstances or situations joined and treated as a whole.

Sex-role stereotyping The practice of automatically and routinely linking specific characteristics to either males or females; also called gender-role stereotyping.

Sexual assault nurse examiner (SANE) Nurse trained to collect forensic evidence and provide initial counseling following rape or other sexual assault.

Shared governance Incorporation of unit-based decision making in nursing practice models. Generic term used to describe any organization in which decision making is shared.

Short-term goals Specific, small steps leading to the achievement of broader, long-term goals.

Sick role Cultural expectation about how people should behave when ill; varies from one culture to another.

Sigma Theta Tau International (STTI) The international honor society for nursing.

Sign Outward evidence of illness visible to others, for example, a rash.

Skill mix The ratio of registered nurses to licensed practical nurses and nursing assistants in a hospital unit.

Social services Services designed to assist individuals and families in obtaining basic needs, such as housing, food, and medical care.

Socialization The process whereby values and expectations are transmitted from generation to generation.

Somatic language Language used by infants to signal their needs to caretakers—for example, crying; reddening of the skin; fast, shallow breathing; facial expressions; and jerking of the limbs.

Spelman Seminary Site of the first nursing program for African Americans; founded in Atlanta, Georgia, in 1886.

Spiritual nursing care Care that recognizes, respects, and, if appropriate, facilitates the practice of a patient's spiritual beliefs.

Spirituality Belief in and sense of connectedness with a higher power.

Staff nurse The bedside nurse who cares for a group of patients but has no management responsibilities for the nursing unit.

Stage theory A theory that views human development as a series of identifiable stages through which individuals and families pass.

Stakeholders Individuals with an interest in an outcome or process.

Standard of care A guideline stating what the reasonably prudent nurse, under similar circumstances, would have done.

Standards of practice Formal statements by a profession of the accountability of its practitioners.

State board of nursing The regulatory body in each state that regulates and enforces the scope of practice and discipline of the members of the nursing profession.

Statutory law Law established through formal legislative processes.

Stereotypes Simplistic and preconceived image about a person or group.

Stereotyping Erroneous belief that all people of a certain group are alike.

Stress Any emotional, physical, social, economic, or other type of factor that requires a response or change.

Stressors Stimuli that tend to disturb equilibrium.

Subacute care A level of care between hospital-based acute care and long-term residential care.

Subjective data Information obtained from patients as they describe their needs, feelings, and strengths, as well as their perceptions of the problem.

Subsystems The parts that make up a system.

Supervision The initial direction and periodic inspection of the actual accomplishment of a task.

Suprasystem The larger environment outside a system.

Symptom An indication of illness felt by the individual but not observable to others, such as pain.

Synergy Combined action that is greater than that of the individual parts.

System A set of interrelated parts that come together to form a whole.

Systems theory See General systems theory.

T

Taxonomy A framework for classifying and organizing information.

Team nursing A system of nursing care delivery in which a group of nurses and ancillary workers are responsible for the care of a group of patients during a specified time period, usually 8 to 12 hours.

Technologists Personnel, such as laboratory technologists or radiological technologists, who assist in the diagnosis of patient problems.

Telehealth The practice of providing health care by means of telecommunication devices, such as telephones, computers, and other devices; the removal of time and distance barriers for the delivery of health care services and related health care activities through telecommunication technologies.

Telehealth nursing The delivery of nursing care services and related health care activities through telecommunication technology, such as telephones, video conferencing, and others.

Termination phase The final phase of the nurse-patient relationship wherein a mutual evaluation of progress is conducted.

Tertiary care Specialized, highly technical level of health care provided in sophisticated research and teaching hospitals.

Tertiary source Sources of patient data including the medical records and health care providers, such as physical therapists, physicians, or dietitians.

Theory A general explanation scholars use to explain, predict, control, and understand commonly occurring events.

Therapeutic milieu An environment created to foster healing.

Therapist Any of several health care workers with differing educational backgrounds who work with patients with specific deficits; examples include physical therapists and occupational therapists.

Third-party payment Payment for health services by an entity other than the patient or the provider of services, such as the government or insurance companies.

Throughput The processes a system uses to convert raw materials into a form that can be used, either by the system itself or by the environment.

Tort A civil wrong against a person; may be intentional or unintentional.

Total quality management (TQM) Management philosophy and activities directed toward achieving excellence and employee participation in all aspects of that goal.

Transcultural nursing Nursing care that is based on the patient's culturally determined health values, beliefs, and practices.

Transmission In communication theory, the expression of information verbally or nonverbally.

U

Universal care Provision of health care to all people.

Unlicensed assistive personnel (UAP) Health care personnel, such as nursing assistants and home care aides, who are not themselves licensed but are supervised by licensed individuals, such as nurses or physicians.

Urbanization The process of population migration to cities.

Utilitarianism An ethical theory asserting that it is right to maximize the greatest good for the greatest number of people.

V

Valid Measuring what it is intended to measure, as in a valid test question or research instrument.

Value ethics Ethical beliefs and behaviors that arise from the character of the decision maker.

Value statement A statement regarding the desirability of something.

Values The social principles, ideals, or standards held by an individual, class, or group that give meaning and direction to behavior.

Venting The verbal "letting off steam" that occurs when people talk about concerns or frustrations.

Veracity Truthfulness.

Verbal communication All language, whether written or spoken.

Virtue ethics The system of ethics based on a person's natural tendency to act, feel, and judge but developed through training; ethics based on the inborn moral virtue of the decision maker.

Voluntariness The degree to which an action is brought about by an individual's own free choice.

Voluntary (private) agency An agency supported entirely through voluntary contributions of time and/or money.

Vulnerable populations Groups who are at risk and unable to advocate for themselves, such as small children, developmentally challenged individuals, the frail elderly, or the socially marginalized.

W

Whistle-blower A person who speaks out against unfair, dishonest, or dangerous practices by a company or agency. Usually an employee of that company or agency.

Whole system shared governance System in which people at all levels within the organization are included in decision making.

Woodhull Study on Nurses and the Media A comprehensive 1997 study of nursing in newspapers, journals, and other print media.

Work ethic A belief on the part of an employee or group in the importance of work; an appreciation for the characteristics employers desire in employees and a commitment to exhibiting them.

Workers' compensation A federally mandated insurance system covering workers injured on the job.

Working phase The middle phase of the nurse-patient relationship, wherein goals are achieved.

Working poor Those who, although employed, are unable to earn enough to live at more than a very modest level.

Work-life balance The equilibrium between the amount of time and effort a person devotes to work and that given to other aspects of life.

Workplace advocacy Action ensuring that workers have a voice in the issues that concern them, either through collective action or through other effective means.

Y

Yale School of Nursing The first school of nursing in the world to be established as a separate university department with an independent budget and its own dean, Annie W. Goodrich.

Index

Page numbers followed by f indicate figures; t, tables; b, boxes.